CW01021112

PRACTICAL SMALL ANIMAL MRI

SOUTHERN COUNTIES
VETERINARY SPECIALISTS
FOREST CORNER FARM
HANGERSLEY RINGWOOD
BH24 3JW
TEL: 01425 485615

PRACTICAL SMALL ANIMAL MRI

Patrick R. Gavin
DVM, PhD, Diplomate ACVR

Rodney S. Bagley
DVM, Diplomate ACVIM (Internal Medicine and Neurology)

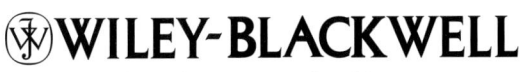
A John Wiley & Sons, Ltd., Publication

Edition first published 2009
© 2009 Wiley-Blackwell

Blackwell Publishing was acquired by John Wiley & Sons in February 2007. Blackwell's
publishing program has been merged with Wiley's global Scientific, Technical, and Medical
business to form Wiley-Blackwell.

Editorial Office
2121 State Avenue, Ames, Iowa 50014-8300, USA

For details of our global editorial offices, for customer services, and for information about how
to apply for permission to reuse the copyright material in this book, please see our website at
www.wiley.com/wiley-blackwell.

Authorization to photocopy items for internal or personal use, or the internal or personal use
of specific clients, is granted by Blackwell Publishing, provided that the base fee is paid
directly to the Copyright Clearance Center, 222 Rosewood Drive, Danvers, MA 01923. For
those organizations that have been granted a photocopy license by CCC, a separate system of
payments has been arranged. The fee codes for users of the Transactional Reporting Service
are ISBN-13: 978-0-8138-0607-5/2009.

Designations used by companies to distinguish their products are often claimed as
trademarks. All brand names and product names used in this book are trade names, service
marks, trademarks or registered trademarks of their respective owners. The publisher is not
associated with any product or vendor mentioned in this book. This publication is designed to
provide accurate and authoritative information in regard to the subject matter covered. It is
sold on the understanding that the publisher is not engaged in rendering professional services.
If professional advice or other expert assistance is required, the services of a competent
professional should be sought.

Library of Congress Cataloging-in-Publication Data

Gavin, Patrick R.
    Practical small animal MRI / Patrick R. Gavin, Rodney S. Bagley.
        p. ; cm.
    Includes bibliographical references and index.
    ISBN-13: 978-0-8138-0607-5 (alk. paper)
    ISBN-10: 0-8138-0607-0 (alk. paper)
    1. Veterinary radiography.   2. Magnetic resonance imaging.   I. Bagley, Rodney S.   II. Title.
    [DNLM: 1. Magnetic Resonance Imaging–veterinary. SF 757.8 G283p 2009]
    SF757.8G38 2009
    636.089'607548–dc22

                        2008040608

A catalogue record for this book is available from the U.S. Library of Congress.

Set in 10/12.5 pt Palatino by Aptara® Inc., New Delhi, India
Printed in Singapore by Markono Print Media Pte Ltd

1   2009

Disclaimer
The contents of this work are intended to further general scientific research, understanding,
and discussion only and are not intended and should not be relied upon as recommending or
promoting a specific method, diagnosis, or treatment by practitioners for any particular
patient. The publisher and the author make no representations or warranties with respect to
the accuracy or completeness of the contents of this work and specifically disclaim all
warranties, including without limitation any implied warranties of fitness for a particular
purpose. In view of ongoing research, equipment modifications, changes in governmental
regulations, and the constant flow of information relating to the use of medicines, equipment,
and devices, the reader is urged to review and evaluate the information provided in the
package insert or instructions for each medicine, equipment, or device for, among other
things, any changes in the instructions or indication of usage and for added warnings and
precautions. Readers should consult with a specialist where appropriate. The fact that an
organization or Website is referred to in this work as a citation and/or a potential source of
further information does not mean that the author or the publisher endorses the information
the organization or Website may provide or recommendations it may make. Further, readers
should be aware that Internet Websites listed in this work may have changed or disappeared
between when this work was written and when it is read. No warranty may be created or
extended by any promotional statements for this work. Neither the publisher nor the author
shall be liable for any damages arising herefrom.

DEDICATION

This work is dedicated to our former and current radiology and neurology residents, the animal patients, and their owners.

Rod Bagley
Pat Gavin

CONTENTS

PREFACE

Dr. Rod Bagley and I discussed writing a textbook on Veterinary MRI for several years. Rod had already published a textbook, and knew the tremendous amount of work involved. We tackled this text with enthusiasm, but also with a degree of trepidation due to the daunting task.

Our goal in writing this textbook was not to have an exhaustive referenced rehash of material that is already present in text. Our goal was to provide a useful, clinical Veterinary MRI text. We were fortunate in starting magnetic resonance imaging of the brain in 1986. Magnetic resonance imaging for spontaneous brain tumors in dogs was a foundation for our research project. MRI continued to be a cornerstone of our research project to monitor the response of the brain tumor treatment and to evaluate normal tissue toxicities.

Washington State University had the oldest teaching hospital in North America in the 1990s. In 1996, we moved into a new facility that included a 1.0 Tesla superconducting magnetic resonance unit. We were the first veterinary medical college in an U.S. university with a state-of-the-art in-house superconducting MR unit. We were enthusiastic to expand beyond the imaging of brain tumors, and our initial efforts were in spinal disease. Our initial studies were not very good, and we had to methodically evaluate numerous pulse sequences and image planes to arrive at a clinically useful study. Magnetic resonance imaging was evolving rapidly in all fields, and some of the anatomical differences with our small patients necessitated a change from previous human protocols. We became comfortable in the spine, and then advanced into imaging for other conditions of the head, orthopedic disease, thorax, and abdomen. We also embarked on the imaging of the limbs of live adult horses. Our equine studies will not be covered in this textbook and will need to be treated in a separate volume.

The superior visualization of soft tissues of the body has allowed for the imaging of virtually all disease processes. The improved conspicuity allows clinicians of multiple disciplines to have clear visualization of the disease process. This text is to provide examples of our experiences that have been gained over the past 21 years. In addition to our experiences, some of the examples come from my active collaboration with other sites. These include the IAMS Pet Imaging Centers in Vienna, Virginia, Raleigh, North Carolina, and Redwood City, California. Examples have also been used from Dr. Michael Broome's Advanced Veterinary Medical Imaging Center in Tustin, California. These centers, coupled with the Washington State University cases make up the bulk of the material for the figures in the text, but other images come from Dr. Kelley Collins, Veterinary Imaging Center in Ambler, Pennsylvania, Oakridge Veterinary Imaging in Edmond, Oklahoma, Tacoma Veterinary MRI in Tacoma, Washington, and Veterinary Neurological Centers in Phoenix, Arizona.

The images chosen are realistic examples of common abnormalities. We have endeavored to provide good quality images, but not ones that cannot be readily obtained virtually all superconducting magnets. There are no permanent magnet images due to lack of availability of such images in our files. The images are shown with the patients right on the viewers left, unless otherwise indicated. The images are generally shown with the dorsal anatomic area to the top of the image, even when acquired differently. If the dependence of the image is important, that will be given in the figure legend.

There is intentional overlap of some diseases in the various chapters. For example, neoplasia of a peripheral nerve may be covered in Chapter 2 (Section 3) on the peripheral nervous system, Chapter 3 on orthopedic disease, and Chapter 7 on MR imaging for cancer. The studies may have been requested for different reasons, that is loss of function, lameness, or for radiation therapy planning, and this redundancy should help the reader find the material for the clinical problem as presented.

We considered an exhaustive library of normal images, but discarded that notion. All studies have variability due to species, individual variation, technique, and volume averaging. Therefore, it is impossible to show an example that would fit all needs. We have given limited normal information, and have endeavored to illustrate common misunderstandings.

The text has limited information on physics, sequence selection, and artifacts. There are many superb texts that delve into these topics in great detail. We have only provided a skeleton of that material to facilitate the discussion of the case material presented in the various chapters. Magnetic resonance imaging is just now becoming an accepted modality throughout the veterinary profession. We have been fortunate to be among the early adaptors of this exciting technology. We hope this text will aid you in the continued exploration and discovery of new information.

We would like to thank Dr. Susan Kraft, DVM, PhD DACVR and Dr. Shannon Holmes for their superb contributions. Finally, we would like to thank the many students, interns, residents, and colleagues that helped us learn from our mistakes.

CHAPTER ONE

Physics

SECTION 1

Comparative Imaging

Patrick R. Gavin

Diagnostic imaging has always been a mainstay of the armamentarium for the veterinarian. Veterinarians have limited resources available as regards history and routine screening procedures. Therefore, diagnostic imaging has a major role in the workup of numerous veterinary patients. An overreliance on diagnostic imaging has been observed by numerous clinicians; however, the move toward less invasive diagnostic procedures with a high precision of diagnosis has continued to drive this phenomenon. This chapter deals with the advances in diagnostic imaging through the last 60 years.

DIAGNOSTIC RADIOLOGY

Diagnostic radiology was invented in the late 1800s. The use of diagnostic radiology was rewarding primarily in the study of skeletal structures. However, due to the cost of the equipment, lack of education, and potential risks, the modality did not penetrate veterinary medicine until approximately the 1950s. Initially, these were the colleges of veterinary medicine in North America that possessed the equipment to perform diagnostic radiographic examinations. There were no trained radiologists at that time and in some places the studies were often performed and interpreted by non-veterinarians. Clinicians did not know what to expect as they had no prior knowledge of the diagnostic modality. Clinicians were often asked if they wanted a V/D or lateral and would merely say "yes" at the answer and accept the outcome. Much was to be learned.

Diagnostic radiology advanced rapidly in veterinary medicine, and the first examinations for veterinary radiologists were performed by charter diplomates for the American College of Veterinary Radiology in

1965. Following this beginning veterinary radiology advanced rapidly. Diagnostic radiology was utilized in multiple species throughout colleges of veterinary medicine and in selected practices. By the early to mid-1970s, advanced radiographic procedures including fluoroscopy and angiography were available, though primarily at colleges of veterinary medicine. The use of diagnostic radiology expanded with improved knowledge, especially with better understanding of its diagnosis of various pathologic conditions. The use of diagnostic radiology abated somewhat with the advance of diagnostic ultrasonography; however, it has remained the stalwart of diagnostic imaging in the veterinary profession. At the current time, there is a major push to move from conventional analog film screen technology to computed and/or digital radiography. It is presumed that veterinary radiology will continue to follow the progression realized in human radiology.

NUCLEAR MEDICINE OR GAMMA SCINTIGRAPHY

The previously used term, nuclear medicine, fell out of favor with the antinuclear movement of the 1970s. Medical personnel were quick to adopt the softer terminology of gamma scintigraphy that facilitated its continued development as an imaging modality. While gamma scintigraphy has the advantage of visualizing physiologic and temporal pathologic changes, for the most part its greatest use in veterinary medicine has been static studies for the diagnosis of skeletal disease. The use of the modality for the diagnosis of skeletal disease is well documented. The challenges of using nuclear isotopes, radiation safety concerns, and time delays are well documented. Some studies have become rather routine in veterinary medicine. These include studies of the thyroid gland that have been published and have led to a better understanding of thyroid disease.

While this modality has been present since the turn of the century, it became rather commonplace in veterinary medicine in the 1980s. Its involvement as a diagnostic modality has undergone little evolution in the last two decades.

COMPUTED TOMOGRAPHY

Computed tomography (CT) was first utilized in the mid-1970s in veterinary medicine, primarily for the diagnosis of intracranial disease. The modality was modified for the study of large animal species shortly thereafter. CT has had a large expansion in the veterinary medical field. Virtually all colleges of veterinary medicine provide this diagnostic modality. In the last 10 years, extension into private veterinary practices has significantly expanded its availability. There are now numerous large specialties, and even general practices, with CT on site. Many units were purchased as used equipment, but many include state-of-the-art helical units.

CT uses the same basic physical principles as diagnostic x-ray, except it depicts the shades of gray in cross-section. It is also possible to better visualize different tissues and the pathologic change within them, if present. Therefore while the modality is similar to diagnostic x-ray, CT is superior in diagnosis because the axial images are far superior to the two-dimensional radiographic projections. CT has led a renaissance in the understanding of three-dimensional anatomy and physiologic principles.

ULTRASONOGRAPHY

Ultrasonography became a clinical imaging modality in veterinary medicine in the late 1970s. It languished in veterinary colleges through much of the 1980s as the technology advanced. The initial technology of static B-mode machines was replaced by real-time machines that allowed an approximate 80% reduction in scanning time. The resolution and utility of the studies improved at the same time. However, diagnostic ultrasonography did not hit its stride and become mainstream in the United States until approximately the 1990s. Now, most large veterinary practices (and certainly referral practices) have diagnostic ultrasonography. This modality is also available in many smaller private practices. There

have been numerous technologic advancements that have improved the quality of this modality. Increased availability of traveling diagnostic radiologists and/or interpretation via teleradiology have improved diagnostic outcomes.

Other specialists utilizing diagnostic ultrasonography, including cardiologists and internists, have further fueled the expansion of this modality in veterinary medical practice. Currently, most ultrasonographic examinations are performed by licensed veterinarians. It is this author's opinion that in the future, many of these procedures will be performed by trained ultrasonographers and interpreted by radiologists, just as occurs in the human field. In the human field, there is a greater medical liability issue, and if physician radiologists can make it work, certainly veterinary radiologists can work in this format to further advance this modality's utility in the diagnosis of our veterinary patients.

MAGNETIC RESONANCE IMAGING

Magnetic resonance imaging (MRI) came into clinical utility in the mid-1980s. It was utilized in veterinary medicine primarily as a research tool in the 1980s and early 1990s. In the mid-1990s, some areas began to use MR as a routine clinical modality. The procedure was applied to large animal imaging a few years later. However, the attitude of "not invented here" plagued the inclusion of MRI for the diagnosis of veterinary patients at many sites in the early years. Many veterinary sites had antiquated equipment or equipment with poor reliability, which gave it the aura of an unreliable diagnostic modality. However, as more sites gained modern diagnostic equipment, the utility of the modality became apparent.

Following the change of the millennium, MR became the modality of choice for the veterinary neurologist for the examination of disease processes involving the brain and spinal cord. Efforts to expand the use of the modality included corporate sponsorship of diagnostic facilities. At the time of this writing, this author is aware of more than 40 sites dedicated to MR imaging of animals using what would be considered modern state-of-the-art equipment. One limitation has been the nonavailability of appropriately trained veterinary radiologists with expertise in this modality capable of providing accurate diagnoses of clinical conditions. Currently, the American College of Veterinary Radiology does not require training time minimums in MRI for their core curriculum, as not all training sites have this modality available. Therefore many veterinary radiologists, and others, must essentially undergo "on the job training" in the use of this modality.

There is a broad spectrum of equipment options. These options span from the currently available best, including machines capable of functional MRI, commonly utilized super conducting magnets, cost-effective mid-field units, to even less expensive but less capable low field permanent magnets. It is this author's opinion that equipment generally costs what it is worth. Therefore, equipment that is more expensive is of more diagnostic worth, and conversely, equipment that costs less has less diagnostic capability. The equipment purchase balance will be finding equipment that provides the utility required for the financial reality of the practice. There has been a rapid development of equipment in the last few years.

Basic Physics

Patrick R. Gavin

It is beyond the scope of this text to do an extensive treatise of the physics of MRI. There are several excellent texts, as well as numerous study guides, and even impressive volumes of free information on the Internet that can be consulted for more in-depth information on patient MR physics. This chapter outlines the salient features of the physics of MRI to allow a better understanding of image, and artifact, production, and visualization.

Current clinical applications for MRI rely on visualization of the hydrogen atom's nucleus. This physical property was previously known as nuclear magnetic resonance, that is, the hydrogen atom nuclei resonate. The word nuclear does not refer to radioactivity, but merely refers to the nucleus of the atom. For more politically correct names it has become known as MRI. The basic physical principle is that a moving electrical charge produces a magnetic field. The size of the magnetic field is dependent on the speed of movement (magnetic movement) and the size of charge. While the hydrogen nucleus has a small electric charge it spins very fast. These physical attributes in concert with the abundance of the hydrogen nucleus within the body produce a detectable magnetic field.

Magnetic field strengths are measured in units of gauss (G) and tesla (T). One tesla is equal to 10,000 gauss. The earth's magnetic field is approximately 0.5 G. The strength of MRI is similar in strength to the electromagnets used to pick up large heavy scrap metal. Materials can be ferromagnetic, paramagnetic, supraparamagnetic, or diamagnetic. Ferromagnetic materials generally contain iron, nickel, or cobalt. These materials can become magnetized when subjected to an external magnetic field. In MR images, these materials cause large artifacts characterized by the properties of signal and distortion of the image. These artifacts can be seen in MR images even when the ferromagnetic substances are too small to be seen on conventional radiography. Commonly seen sources of these artifacts are microchips, ameroid constrictors, certain bone plates, gold-plated beads, and colonic contents.

Paramagnetic materials include ions of various metals such as iron (Fe), manganese (Mg), and gadolinium (Gd). These substances can also have magnetic susceptibility, but only about 1/1,000 that of ferromagnetic materials. These substances increase the T1 and T2 relaxation rates. Because of this property, chelates of these elements make ideal components of MR contrast agents. Gadolinium chelates are the most common agents and generally cause an increase in T1-weighted signal. This is seen as increased hyperintensity (brightness) in T1-weighted images. At very high gadolinium concentrations, as seen in the urinary bladder, loss of signal can be seen as a result of T2 relaxation effects dominating.

Supraparamagnetic elements are materials that have ferromagnetic properties. The most commonly used is super paramagnetic iron oxide (SPIO), which is an iron (Fe)based contrast agent for liver imaging. These have been used minimally in veterinary MR. Diamagnetic materials have no intrinsic magnetic moment, but can weakly repel the field. These materials include water, copper, nitrogen, and barium sulfate. They will cause a loss of signal and have been seen as a loss of MR signal in images made after the administration of barium sulfate suspensions.

Since hydrogen is the common element used to make an MR clinical image, we will discuss the process of image formation. When hydrogen is placed within a large external magnetic field, the randomly spinning protons (hydrogen nucleus) will come into alignment with the external field. Some of the protons align with the field and some align against the field, largely canceling each other out. A few more align with the field than against it. The net number aligning with the magnetic field is very small. Approximately, three protons align with the field for every one million protons as 1.0 T. This number is proportional to the external magnetic field strength. While this number appears very small, the abundance of hydrogen allows for high-quality images. For example, in a typical volume imaging element termed a voxel, the number of protons aligned with the field would be roughly 6×10^{15}.

Basic physics dictate that the energy is proportional to the nuclei's unique resonant frequency in MR; this is called the Larmor frequency. The frequency of the spinning of the hydrogen nuclei is relatively low. The resonance frequency is proportional to the external magnetic field, which for hydrogen is equal to $42.56\,MHz/T$. MRI is able to make high-quality images, not because of the energy of the spinning protons, but due to the abundance of hydrogen protons present in the body. The spinning or "resonating" of nuclei occurs because of unpaired electrons in the orbital shell. Each nucleus with this characteristic will resonate at a unique frequency. The spinning protons act like toy tops that wobble as they spin. The rate of wobbling is termed precession. These precess at the resonance or Larmor frequency for hydrogen.

If a radiofrequency (RF) pulse is applied at the resonance frequency, the protons can absorb that energy. The absorption of energy causes the protons to jump into a higher energy state. This causes the net magnetization to spiral away from the main magnetic field, designated B_0. The net magnetization vector, therefore, moves from its initial longitudinal position a distance proportional to pulse, which is determined by its temporal length and strength. After a certain length of time, the net magnetization vector would rotate 90° and lie in a transverse plane. It is at this position that no net magnetization can be detected. When the RF pulse is turned off, three things start to happen simultaneously:

1. The absorbed energy is retransmitted at the resonance frequency.
2. The spins begin to return to their original longitudinal orientation, termed the T1 relaxation.
3. While the precessions were initially in-phase, they begin to de-phase, termed T2 relaxation.

The return of the excited nuclei from the high energy state to their ground state is termed T1 relaxation (or spin–lattice relaxation). The T1 relaxation time is the time required for the magnetization to return to 63% of its original longitudinal length. The T1 relaxation rate is the reciprocal of the T1 time (1/T1). T1 relaxation is dependent on the magnetic field strength that dictates the Larmor frequency. Higher magnetic fields are associated with longer T1 times.

T2 relaxation occurs when spins in high and low energy states exchange energy but do not lose energy to the surrounding lattice as occurs in T1 relation. It is, therefore, sometimes referred to as spin–spin relaxation. This results in loss of transverse magnetization. In biological materials, T2 time is longer than T1 time. T2 relaxation occurs exponentially like T1 and is described as the time required for 63% of the transverse magnetization to be lost. In general, T2 values are unrelated to field strength. In patients, the magnetic signal decays faster than T2 would predict. There are many factors creating imperfections in the homogeneity of the magnetic field, including the magnet and patient inhomogeneities including surface contours, air–tissue interfaces, and any metal the patients may have within them, including dental work, staples, and orthopedic appliances. The sum effect of all of these inhomogeneities pronounces an effect called T2*. The T2 relaxation comes from random interactions, while T2* comes from a combination of random and fixed causes including magnet and patient inhomogeneity.

To attempt to negate the fixed causes, a 180° refocusing pulse is used. Consider the following analogy, three cars in a race going at different speeds. At the start, all the cars are obviously together, and can be thought of as being in-phase. At some time after the start of the race, there is a noticeable difference between them due to different speeds; they are in essence out-of-phase. At that time, everybody will turn around and go back toward the starting line. If it is assumed that everyone is still going at the same rate as before, then they will all arrive at the starting line together and in-phase. The time required for the atoms to come back in-phase is equal to the time it took for them to lose phase. This total time is called the "TE" or echo time. The 180° pulse is used to reverse the T2* de-phasing process. As soon as the spins come back into phase, they will immediately start to go out-of-phase again. The two variables of interest in spin echo (SE) sequences are (1) the repetition time (TR) and (2) the echo time (TE). All SE sequences include a slice-selective 90° pulse followed by one or more 180° refocusing pulses. This refocusing pulse can be applied multiple times. The use of multiple refocusing pulses is the basis for fast or turbo spin–echo imaging, FSE, or TSE respectively.

Images of T1 and T2 relaxation are produced by sampling the signal at various times. Both effects are always present; however, we will often accentuate one effect over the other such that the sequences are often properly termed T1-weighted or T2-weighted images. To produce the cross-sectional images, gradient coils are needed, which produce deliberate variation in the main magnetic field. There is one gradient coil in each Cartesian plane direction (X, Y, and Z planes). These slight variations in the magnetic field will allow for slice selection and phase and frequency encoding. The slice selection gradient will be the Z, X, and Y gradients for a patient in supine position for the transverse, sagittal, and dorsal plane sequences, respectively.

A term commonly used in discussing image formation is the signal-to-noise ratio (SNR). SNR determines the appearance of the image. This ratio is measured by calculating the difference in signal intensity between the area of interest (the patient) and the background. The difference between the signal and background noise is divided by the standard deviation of the signal from the background, which provides an indication of the variability of the background noise. SNR is proportional to the volume imaged, called a voxel, and the square root of the number of signal averages and the number of phase encoding steps. Since signal averages and phase steps are temporal parameters, SNR is closely related to image acquisition time. Decreasing the voxel size (by decreasing the field of view), increasing the phase encoding, and decreasing the slice thickness will all decrease the SNR. Increasing the voxel size (by increasing the field of view, increasing the slice thickness, or decreasing the matrix size), or decreasing the phase encoding steps will all improve the SNR. The slice selection gradient will set the slice thickness. The two dimensions of the image are then mapped depending on emitted frequency in the phase and frequency encoded directions.

All of the frequencies in the frequency encoded direction can be encoded at one time; whereas, the number of phase encodings increases the time of acquisition in a directly proportional manner. Therefore, it is common to map the signal with fewer phase encodings compared to frequency encodings (e.g., 192 × 256) to reducing scan time. Dividing the field of view by the matrix size gives the voxel area, which represents the displayed element called a pixel. The depth of the voxel is determined by slice thickness. Slice thickness is almost always the largest dimension of this imaging voxel. Therefore, the resolution perpendicular to the image plane is generally the poorest. The signal obtained for the image can be improved by increasing the number of signal averages. This is done by increasing the number of RF pulses to knock the protons out of alignment. The scan time is directly proportional to the number of signal averages, sometimes termed number of excitations (NEX). While doubling the signal averages will double the acquisition time, the increase in the signal obtained will be the square root of 2, or only a 40% increase.

The T1 and T2 relaxation rates affect the SNR. The time between RF pulses to move the protons out of

Table 1.1.

Relationship of image parameters to signal-to-noise ratio (SNR), resolution, and imaging time

Increase Parameters	SNR	Resolution	Acquisition Time
FOV	+	−	nc
NEX	+	nc	+
Slice thick	+	−	nc
Gap	+	−	nc
TR	+	nc	+
TE	−	nc	nc
Matrix size	−	+	+
Bandwidth	−	nc	nc
Magnet strength	+	nc	nc

nc, no change.

longitudinal alignment is termed TR (repetition time). Changing TR will affect the T1-weighting. Since T1 is relatively short, a T1-weighted image has a short TR and a short TE. To improve T2-weighting, the TR is long to allow for a longer TE.

As can be seen from above, the relationship between signal-to-noise, resolution, and acquisition is complex. Changing one element affects the others. A table is given to illustrate these direct features (Table 1.1).

To develop protocols, a very thorough understanding is needed of these interrelationships. Protocol development is beyond the scope of this text. However, familiarity with these basic principles is needed in order to maximize the protocol for the individual patient. This is more challenging in veterinary patients, which can vary tremendously in size. The ultimate goal is to maximize these relationships to provide the best possible image in a clinically viable acquisition time. While it seems counterintuitive, the smaller patient may require thicker slices to maintain sufficient SNR. Another counterintuitive imaging principle is the need to reduce the matrix to improve visualization because of its effects on SNR.

Image sequences occur as two main types. The first is the SE sequence. This is the most commonly used sequence for T1-weighted, proton density, or T2-weighted images. The variables of interest include TR and TE. SE sequences use a 90° RF pulse, followed by one or more 180° refocusing pulses.

A subset of SE sequences includes the inversion recovery (IR) sequences. IR sequences can be used to null any substance, but are most commonly used to null out cerebral spinal fluid, termed the fluid attenuation inversion recovery or FLAIR sequence, or fat, using the short tau inversion recovery or STIR sequence. An IR sequence is a 180° prepulse; time is allowed such that the tissue to be nulled has its vector in the horizontal magnetization plane. Then, the 90° RF pulse will only affect those tissues that were not at the zero or horizontal magnetization plane. Another way to null fat is through fat saturation. These sequences consist of multiple 90° RF pulses that have relatively short TR.

The other basic type of sequence acquisition is the gradient echo (GE or GRE) sequence. The basic sequences are varied by adding de-phasing and re-phasing gradients at the end of the sequence. The variables include TR and TE, but there is also the variable of flip angle. Generally, flip angles of less than 90° are used. GE sequences can be used to acquire images rapidly and are often used for breath holding techniques and visualization of moving structures, including the cardiovascular system. GE sequences generally have less contrast than SE sequences. Lower field MR units often rely on GE sequences due to short TR and TE, permitting short imaging duration. The lack of standard T1 and T2 contrast can limit the utility of these sequences in multiple anatomical regions.

Sequence Selection

Patrick R. Gavin

It is not the intent of this text to go through all the various imaging sequences that could be utilized with MR. These sequences are often explained similar to a recipe in a cookbook. Just as there can be an exhaustive number of recipes to cook with any given list of ingredients, the same is true for the number of imaging sequences.

Imaging sequences are generally either SE sequences or GE sequences. The majority of imaging protocols for conventional clinical MR imaging use SE sequences. GE sequences do have some specific uses. Low field magnets are often heavily dependent on GE sequences to provide shorter examinations with relatively thin sections. However, many GE sequences suffer from lack of contrast or increased magnetic susceptibility artifacts. Because of these limitations, this author favors traditional SE sequences over GE sequences. GE sequences and their specific use(s) will be highlighted throughout the book, but the coverage in this book is not exhaustive.

Standard clinical imaging sequences most commonly utilize T2-weighted sequences, STIR sequences, and T1-weighted sequences. T1 sequences are fundamental in contrast studies with the administration of a paramagnetic gadolinium-based contrast agent.

Other sequences that are commonly utilized are the FLAIR sequence, the GE sequence for the detection of hemorrhage, and heavily T2-weighted images for the visualization of fluid structures, including the subarachnoid CSF columns, the biliary system, or the fluid containing inner ear structures of the cochlea and semicircular canals.

T2 SEQUENCE

T2-weighted sequences are often the bulwark of imaging protocols. When performed with fast SE techniques, reasonable imaging time is achieved and it produces images in which both fat and fluid are seen as relatively high signal intensity. Some systems use T2-weighted fat suppression to further increase conspicuity of fluid, and have the advantage of negating the need to additionally acquire STIR images. Bright fluid in images is desirable as most pathologic abnormalities have an increased fluid signal. The fluid can be from either intracellular fluid, in the case of cellular abnormalities including neoplasia or granulomatous conditions, or intercellular fluid from diseases such as abscessation or edema.

T1 SEQUENCE

T1-weighted sequences are generally utilized with contrast agents. The T1-weighted precontrast study is "always" necessary. One cannot definitively assess contrast enhancement without the pre-enhanced study, and a shortcut eliminating this sequence can lead to serious misinterpretation. In T1-weighted images, fat is hyperintense and fluid is hypointense. Following the administration of contrast, abnormal tissue often has an increased vascular supply leading to increased signal intensity. In some cases there are breaks in tissue structure, such as the blood–brain barrier, that allow the contrast agent to leak into the tissue and change the relaxation of the tissue leading to increased signal intensity. It must be remembered that the gadolinium contrast agent is not visualized. The only element that can be visualized at this time is the element hydrogen. Therefore, the gadolinium-based agents affect the relaxation of the protons in the molecules. This fact needs to be remembered, as the amount of contrast required for the paramagnetic effect on the proton relaxation is not as concentration dependent as iodine-based contrast agents for CT.

If a T1-weighted image (prior to the administration of gadolinium) has hyperintensity in tissues that are not related to fat, then paramagnetic substances must be present. The only paramagnetic substances within the body are iron and manganese. Since the amount of manganese present is in a very small degree, the only reasonable element that could be present would be iron. For iron to be bright on T1-weighting, it requires a degradation of iron through normal processes until it reaches extracellular methemoglobin. The various stages of the iron degradation process that can be seen in MR images will be given with examples utilizing the brain. Again, since T1-weighted images result in high signal intensity with fat, it is often preferable to perform T1-weighted images with fat suppression. However, following the administration of contrast, it is possible that the lesion can have a relaxation time similar to that of fat and its signal can be nulled. Therefore, it is advisable to always have some postcontrast studies used without fat suppression to make certain that lesions are not lost.

STIR SEQUENCE

The STIR sequence is a workhorse sequence as it allows for a T2-weighted type of image with uniform loss of the fat signal. The IR sequence is an easily performed study utilizing a 180° prepulse, prior to the 90° excitation pulse. The relaxation time of fat is known for all magnet strengths. Therefore, it is easy to set the time of inversion (TI) for a specific magnetic field strength, which will ensure uniform and generalized suppression of the fat signal. STIR sequences should always be performed prior to the administration of contrast. It is possible that contrast enhancement could change the relaxation time of the tissues similar to fat, and again the tissue's signal will be nulled on a STIR sequence if performed after contrast administration. STIR sequences are utilized as they display normal vascular or other fluid-filled structures as bright on a generalized dark background. Typically, pathologic changes in tissue are easily detected as "stars" in a dark sky.

FLAIR SEQUENCE

The FLAIR sequence is similar to the STIR sequence except it uses an inversion time to get null fluid signal. In general, the FLAIR is utilized in the brain and gets rid of the usually hyperintense fluid signal from the cerebral spinal fluid. Therefore, lesions that are periventricular are easier to detect as increased signal intensity, adjacent to a black or darkened cerebral spinal fluid. The atten-uation appearance of cerebral spinal fluid is somewhat dependent on time of inversion as well as other factors specific to MR unit. With some protocols, one is capable of detecting abnormal cerebral spinal fluid from its appearance on the FLAIR sequence. The abnormal signal appearance could be due to increased protein content and/or cellularity or associated CSF flow.

This sequence can be useful when applied to other fluids. A FLAIR sequence can be used to get a T2-weighted image of a urinary bladder tumor. Since urine is basically acellular and with no proteins, the TI for CSF can be used. The nulling out of fluid from conditions such as hydrothorax allows darkening of the effusion while still allowing visualization of T2-weighted image characteristics of the thoracic wall and organs. IR times for such studies vary due to many parameters, but essentially all fluid, including urine, synovial fluid, thoracic and abdominal effusions, or cerebral spinal fluid can be nulled with the FLAIR technique.

GRADIENT ECHO SEQUENCE

GE techniques are the most commonly used sequence for rapid studies, and as such are often utilized for localization sequences. In the brain, its most common clinical application is to verify the presence of hemorrhage. GE sequences are very sensitive to magnetic field inhomogeneities. Therefore, the iron concentration within hemorrhagic tissue is detected as a magnetic field inhomogeneity. Unfortunately, this same degree of inhomogeneity can cause massive image artifacts from small metallic implants including BBs, steel bird shot, the wire around microchip placement, or simple anatomical tissue differences including the frontal sinuses (air) next to the brain. Other than the benefit of detecting hemorrhage, the overall tissue contrast is poor with GE sequences, even though T1- and T2-weighted GE sequences are available. Therefore, this author tends to limit them to the detection of hemorrhage in studies of the CNS. GE sequences are commonly used in the thoracic and abdominal studies to minimize motion artifact.

In the subsequent chapters, we will utilize a few additional sequences for the visualization of specific structures. These are often heavily T2-weighted images that allow the visualization of structures including vascular structures, the equivalent of an MR myelogram, or the fluid in the semicircular canals and cochlea.

SECTION 4
Artifacts

Patrick R. Gavin

The goal of all imaging modalities is to aid in visualization of normal anatomy and disease states. Unfortunately, all imaging modalities have some artifacts that can mimic pathologic change and lead to misdiagnosis. MR is no different. Knowledge of the common MR artifacts and the ability to distinguish artifactual change, which may be mimicking pathologic change from a true pathologic abnormality, are critical to accurate interpretation of MR images.

HARDWARE ARTIFACTS

Some artifacts come from the magnetic field inhomogeneity. The artifacts can be intensity, spatial, or both. An artifactual bending of the spine may be seen when at the edge of the main magnetic field (Figure 1.1). The patient should be repositioned in the gantry if this is creating a diagnostic dilemma.

Artifacts can also occur from defects in the RF shielding. The shield could be faulty but often these artifacts are from transient breaks in the shielding and most often are seen if someone enters the magnet room during a sequence. This type of "zipper" artifact can be avoided by waiting until the end of a sequence to enter the room (Figure 1.2).

The advantage of MRI over CT is its ability to visualize the body in any plane. As mentioned, the three common planes are (1) transverse (axial), (2) dorsal (coronal), and (3) the sagittal plane. The images are made from different slices within these planes, which are formed from the three magnetic gradients used. When understanding the orientation gradients, it is useful to assume that the patient went into the bore of the magnet head first and supine for the imaging study. One of the gradients is selected for the slice selection to provide the desired plane. In this scenario, the gradient in the Z direction is used for transverse or axial slices, the X direction is used for sagittal slices, and the Y direction is used for coronal or dorsal slices. All gradients can be modified depending on the patient positioning. For instance, if the patient is in the right decubitus position, then the Y gradient would be used for the sagittal slices of the body.

The other two gradients map the signal in the two dimensions of the slice plane. The signal is mapped according to its phase and frequency. The frequencies of the signals are similar to the range frequencies of different radio stations. Think of the phase as a time zone. There could be an FM 101.1 station in Denver, Colorado, and a station with the same frequency in Los Angeles, California. Then, if one were to realize that the time zones are a continuum from east to west, this allows for many more time zones than the current artificially drawn time zones for a 24-h clock. The number of frequencies and the number of phases are often 256, but can go much higher.

PHASE AND FREQUENCY ARTIFACTS

Some artifacts are propagated in the frequency direction while others are propagated in the phase direction. Therefore, a prior knowledge of the direction of these encodings is needed to determine the image artifact. Some institutions print this information in the images. It is always part of the DICOM header information that can be assessed if one can access this file. It is often simpler to find some ubiquitous motion artifact from flowing blood, for example, that will be propagated in the phase direction. By changing the background of the image, one can readily depict this in the background (Figure 1.3). Motion artifact can be from gastrointestinal motion, respiratory motion, blood flow, or patient motion. Attempts to limit some of this motion can be made by gaiting the acquisition to the respiratory or cardiac cycles. This form of image acquisition will prolong the study to a degree and may limit its clinical utility. Therefore, some motion is generally an accepted consequence of MRI.

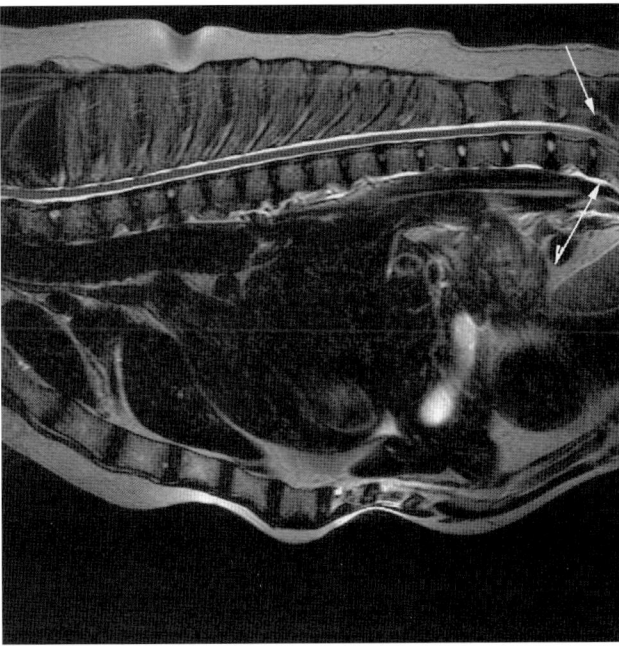

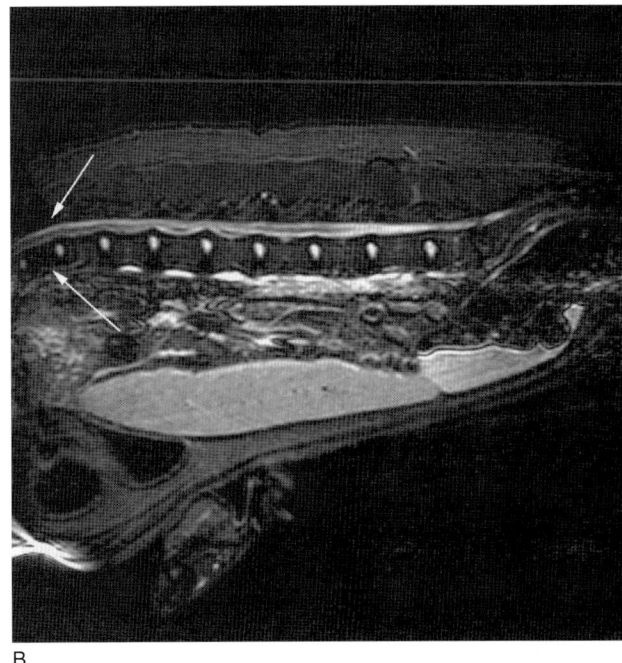

A

B

Figure 1.1. (A) T2-weighted sagittal imaging. Arrows show the bending of the field at the edge of the field of view. This is from magnetic inhomogeneity at the periphery of the imaging volume. (B) Sagittal STIR sequence of the lumbar spine of the same patient showing bending at the opposite end of the patient from the same affect.

The signal from flowing blood is often accentuated following the administration of contrast due to the increased signal intensity of the blood with the contrast agent. Pseudolesions can be seen that would mimic pathologic change. Swapping the phase and frequency encoding directions allows one to ascertain, with certainty, if this is artifactual or real (Figure 1.4).

CHEMICAL SHIFT ARTIFACT

Another artifact that can be confused with pathologic change is a chemical shift artifact. This artifact is a mis-mapping that occurs at water–fat interfaces and in the frequency direction. The artifact is often easily recognized in abdominal studies, but in other areas can mimic pathologic change (Figure 1.5). The same ability to swap the phase and frequency encoding directions and to change the direction of the chemical shift artifact helps clarify the existence of the artifact versus pathologic change (Figure 1.6).

FOLD-OVER OR ALIASING ARTIFACT

Fold-over or aliasing is another artifact that occurs in the phase direction. This artifact occurs when a portion of anatomy is outside the selected image field of view. This anatomy can be wrapped around to the opposite side of the image as a mirror image into the area of interest. This can confuse the interpretation (Figure 1.7). Field of view should be large enough to encompass

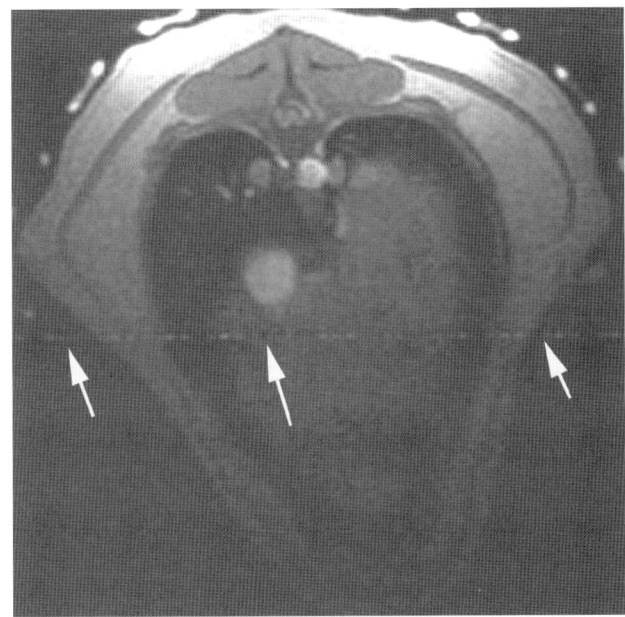

Figure 1.2. Zipper artifact: T2-weighted transverse image with a horizontal zipper artifact (arrows).

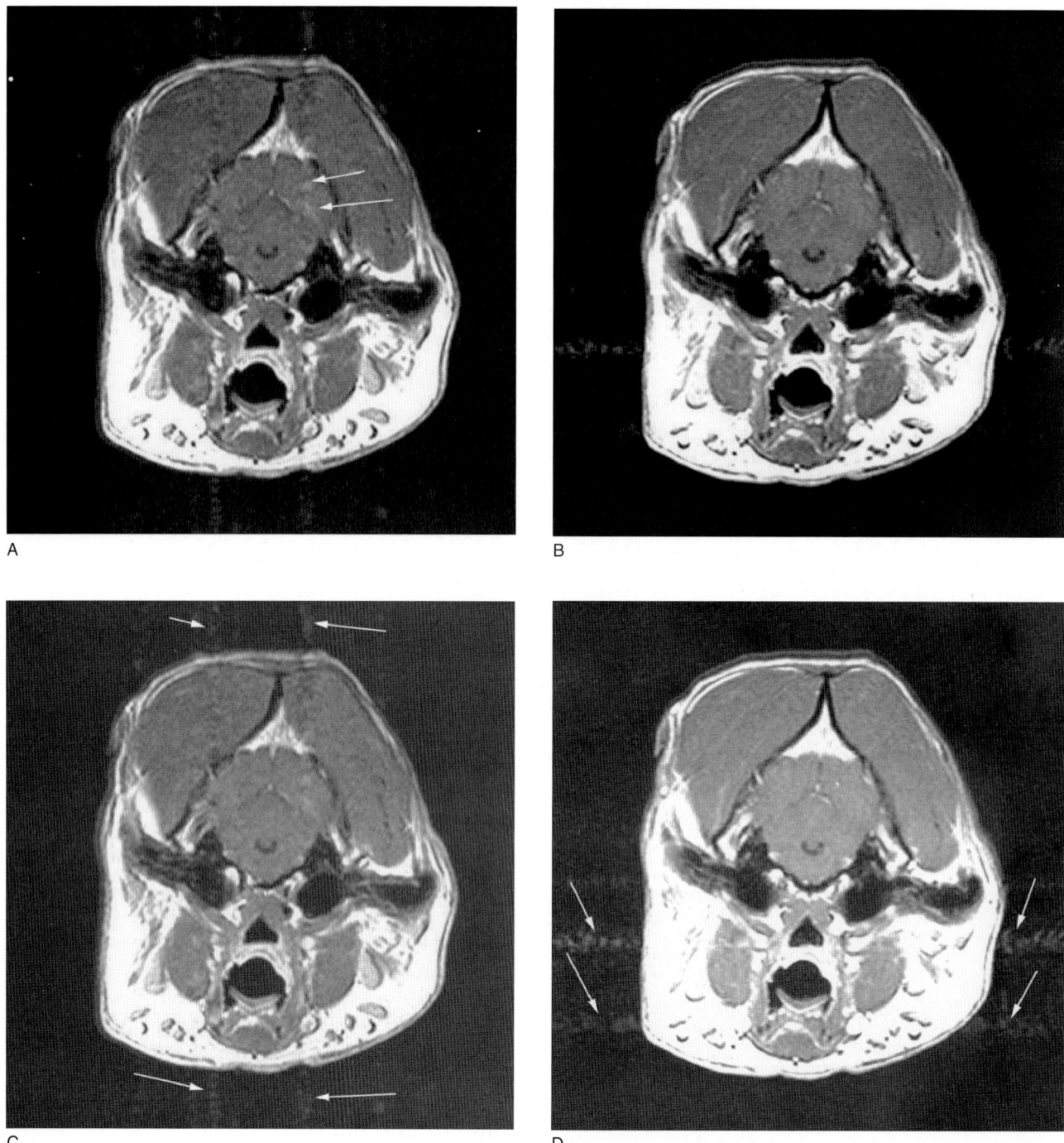

Figure 1.3.   Motion artifact. (A) Apparent small lesion in the left occipital cortex on T1 postcontrast. (B) Lesion gone. (C) Brightened background and phase is ventral to dorsal and flow artifact is seen in alignment with the "lesion." (D) Brightened background with phase left to right.

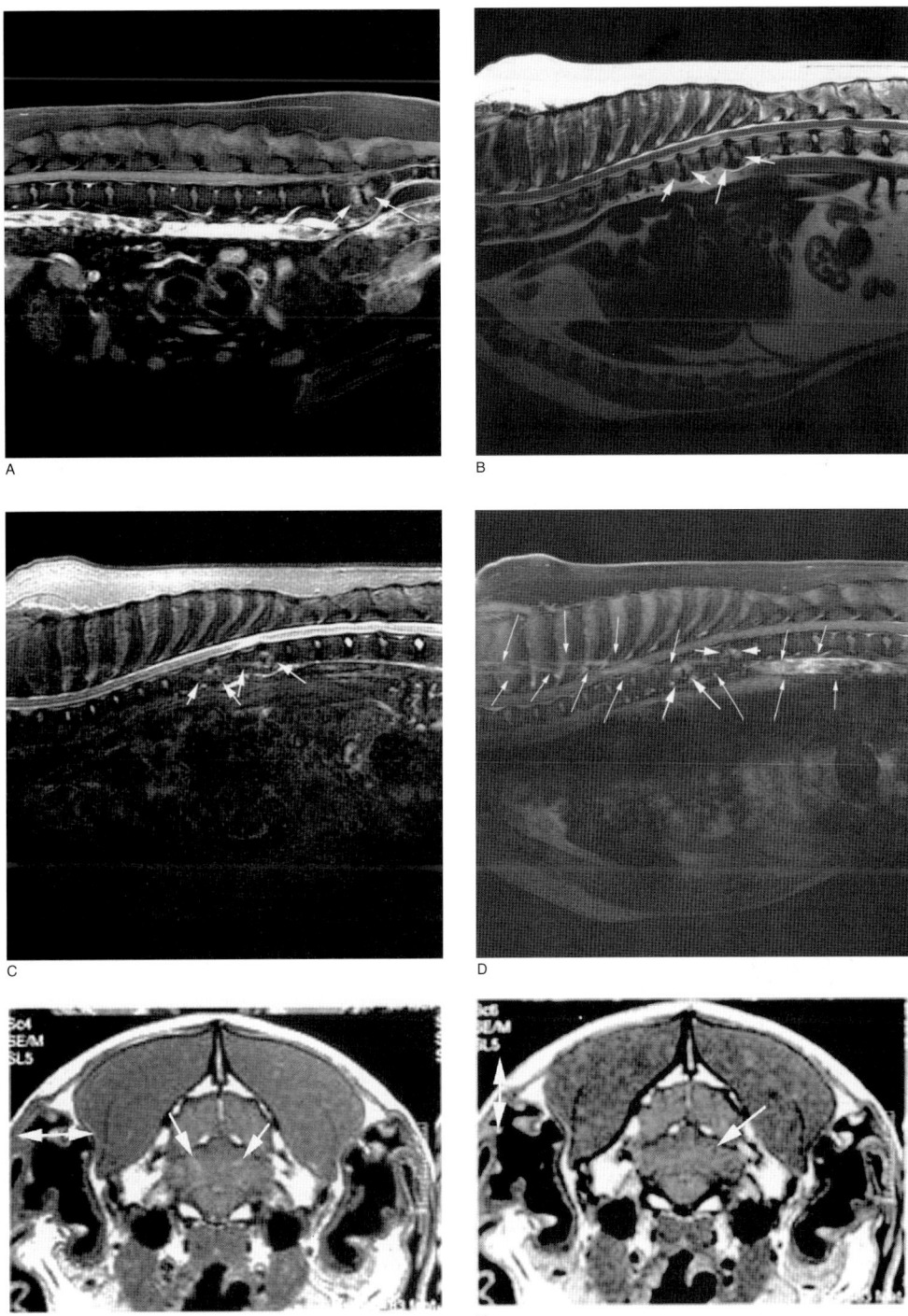

Figure 1.4. (A) STIR sagittal sequence of the lumbosacral spine showing the presence of hyperintensity of the endplates at L7-S1. (B) T2-weighted sagittal image of the thoracic spine showing hyperintensity of the endplates at two sites. (C) STIR sequence of the same location as (B). Hyperintensity is somewhat obscured due to flow artifact from the aorta. Phase direction is in the foot-to-head direction such that the aortic signal is bleeding into the spine at this site. (D) Contrast enhancement T1-weighted sequence with fat suppression. The aortic signal can readily be seen bleeding through the spine, spinal cord, and the dorsal spinous processes of the first few thoracic vertebrae. This type of flow artifact could be prevented by changing the phase direction, but then the entire aortic signal would have motion artifact into the spinal cord. Therefore, foot-to-head direction as in this case is greatly preferred, but one must be cognizant of the artifact. (E), (F) T1 postcontrast images of a brain. Brain: phase is going in the direction of the arrows on the left-hand side of the image. The phase is left to right in this image and the arrows point to hyperintensities within the cerebellum. These are flow artifacts, probably from the internal carotid artery, and as in part (F) these hyperintensities are not present when the phase direction is changed to a ventrodorsal direction. Any time contrast enhancements cannot be substantiated on multiple planes, they should be suspect. If one needs to prove the presence of artifacts, the change in phase direction with a repeating of the sequence, as in this case, can be helpful.

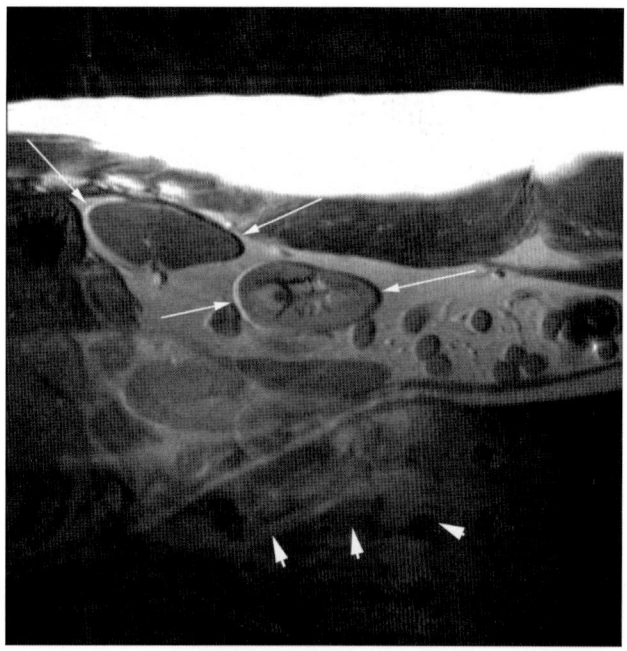
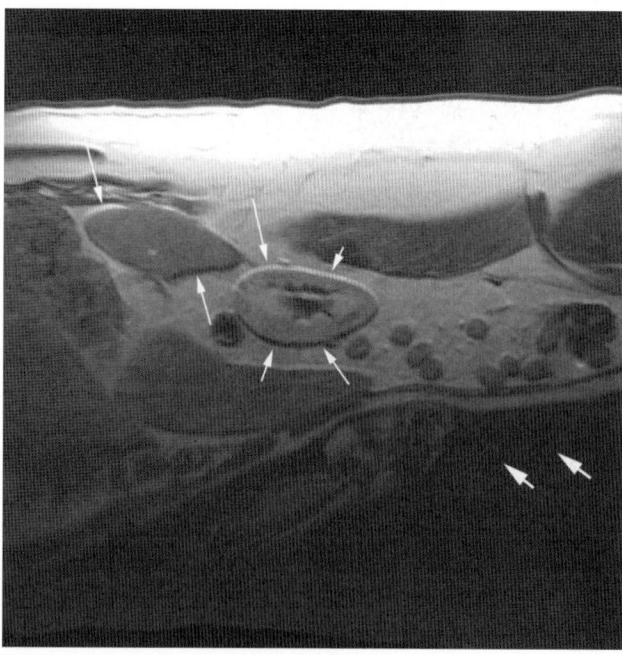

A

B

Figure 1.5. (A) Phase direction is ventrodorsal, which means the frequency direction is foot to head. This chemical shift artifact can readily be seen as the black line at the posterior aspect of the spleen and the white line at the cranial aspect. This chemical shift artifact occurs due to the water signal from the spleen interacting with the abdominal fat signal. When the phase direction is changed, as in (B), to a ventrodorsal orientation, the change in direction of the chemical artifact is readily seen.

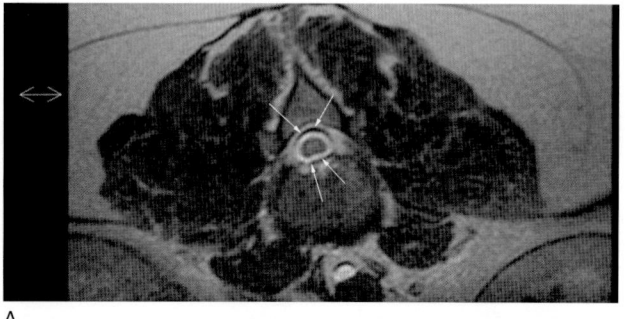
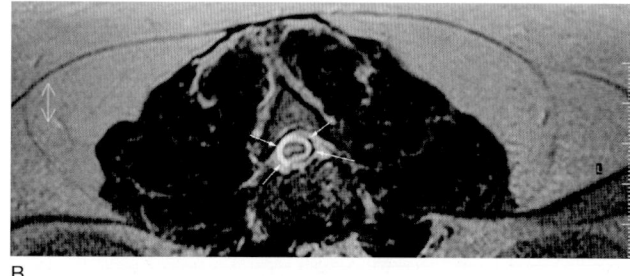

A

B

Figure 1.6. (A) Chemical shift artifact in the spinal column. The phase direction is in the direction of the arrows on the left-hand side of the image, in a left-to-right direction. Therefore, the chemical shift is of a ventrodorsal nature. There is a decreased signal intensity at the dorsal aspect of the subarachnoid space, which is artifactual and slightly brighter ventrally, which is also artifactual. (B) The phase direction is ventrodorsal and the frequency direction is left to right. Now, there is a black line at the left-hand side of the subarachnoid space and a bright line at the right side. These are both artifactual due to the chemical shift between the water of the subarachnoid space and the epidural fat. This type of chemical shift artifact is often seen in large dogs due to the amount of epidural fat. This should not be mistaken as a dural lesion.

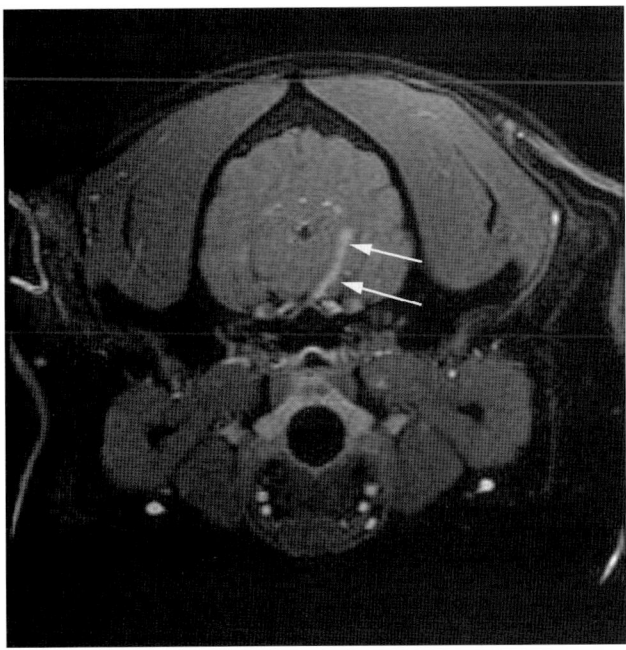 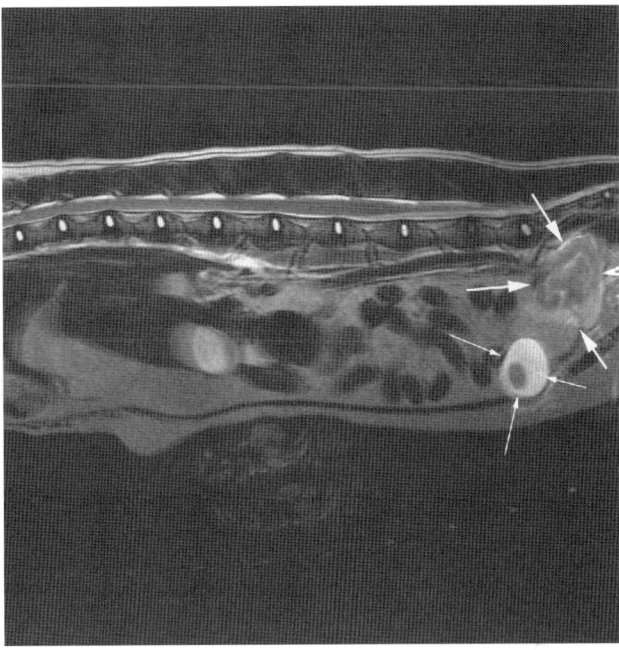

A   B

Figure 1.7. (A) Fold-over or aliasing artifact of the pinna of the ear superimposed over the brain. These artifacts can be negated by a slight increase in the field of view to include the pinnae. One should also try to keep the pinnae close to the surface of the head when imaging to help alleviate this problem while maintaining a relatively small field of view. (B) Aliasing artifact where the head is being superimposed over the caudal portion of the abdomen. The small arrows show the eye and the larger arrows the brain, superimposed over the region of the urinary bladder. While the eye makes it relatively easy to see this fold-over, if one was at a different sagittal plane, the artifact could be easily misinterpreted for a pathologic lesion. One of the best ways to prevent these confusions is to always obtain sequences in multiple planes, and be able to confirm lesions on more than one sequence and more than one plane.

the anatomy visualized or techniques for fold-over suppression need to be employed to avoid this artifact. Unfortunately, many of these suppression techniques result in increased scan time. Therefore, where possible, fold-over suppression should not be used to either reduce acquisition time or improve signal-to-noise levels. Since fold-over is in the phase direction, the phase must often be set in a certain direction to prevent blood flow related artifacts within the area of interest. For instance, in sagittal images of the lumbar spine, it is preferred to have phase oriented in a foot-to-head direction and, thus, the frequency going anterior to posterior. If one were to have the phase encoding direction going ventral to dorsal, the blood flow artifact from the aorta would superimpose on the spinal cord leading to erroneous interpretation. In this instance, the phase must be oriented foot to head and fold-over suppression is needed to prevent wrap-around artifact.

TRUNCATION ARTIFACT

Truncation artifact occurs when the number of phase encoding steps is decreased in relation to the frequency

encoding steps to save time. With excessive reduction in phase encoding steps there may be a mis-mapping of the image in the phase direction. Truncation artifacts can make conditions such as a dilated central canal within the cervical spinal column or the appearance of a syringohydromyelia appear in an image when, in fact, none exists. Often, this artifact is readily seen and ignored when the change is only seen on one plane and cannot be confirmed on an orthogonal view (Figure 1.8).

MAGNETIC SUSCEPTIBILITY ARTIFACT

One of the more sizable artifacts is from magnetic susceptibility. This artifact occurs when magnetic material is present within the patient. Ferrous metal is especially problematic, including BBs and steel bird shot. Other sources of this artifact can come from the spring on the identification microchips, orthopedic devices, or small bits of metal left behind from a surgery. It is

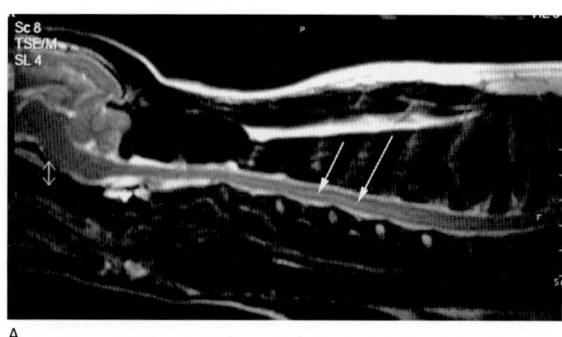 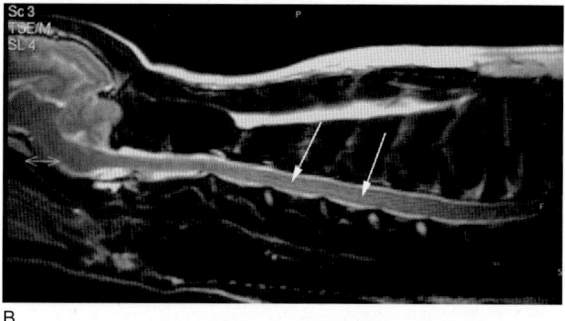

A   B

Figure 1.8. (A) Truncation artifact. Truncation artifacts create a mis-mapping of the signal. In this case, the subarachnoid signal is being mis-mapped into the center of the spinal cord making it appear as an enlarged central canal or syrinx. This happens when the phase and coding steps are reduced too much in an effort to save time. By increasing the phase and coding steps, as in (B), the hyperintense signal in the center is negated.

important to appreciate that small metal fragments that are too small to be seen on a conventional radiograph can create very large artifacts in the MR image. Other problem substances come from ingested rocks containing minerals and even from barium sulfate suspension. High concentrations of gadolinium, especially in the urinary tract from excretion of the contrast agent, will result in a dark artifact on T2- and T1-weighted sequences, which is a magnetic susceptibility artifact (Figure 1.9–1.11).

VOLUME AVERAGING ARTIFACT

The signal intensity of the voxel is the average of all the different signal intensities from different tissues within the slice thickness. When a slice "cuts" through areas of disparate intensity or contour, the intensity mapped into the voxel is a misrepresentation of the different structures. This is referred to as volume average or slice thickness artifact. It can greatly affect spatial resolution. This is often seen where the change or difference is of small volume (some disc herniations) or when there is a marked change in contour. The curvature of the calvarium at the frontal sinus and brain interface can make lesions, like a meningioma, appear to cross the bone and occupy the sinus (Figure 1.12). The orthogo-

nal views must be assessed to evaluate partial volume average artifact.

MAGIC ANGLE ARTIFACT

This artifact affects structures of low signal intensity that are oriented at a 55° angle off the main magnetic field. Their true signal is misrepresented as hyperintense on short TE sequences. There are two 55° cones, one positive and one negative within the bore of the magnet. This artifact is common in orthopedic studies, recognized most commonly in tendinous or ligamentous structures. These, in a normal state, have low signal intensity and in diseased states are hyperintense. Thus, this artifact produces lesion in certain orientations, and is avoided by the inclusion of a T2-weighted (long TE) SE sequence in all studies (Figure 1.13).

CROSS-TALK ARTIFACT

This artifact occurs when setting up multiple stacks of images and their fields of view intersect, which results in loss of signal (Figure 1.14). This can be avoided by adding an additional sequence to allow for proper placement of all slices. This is especially a problem in the lumbosacral region.

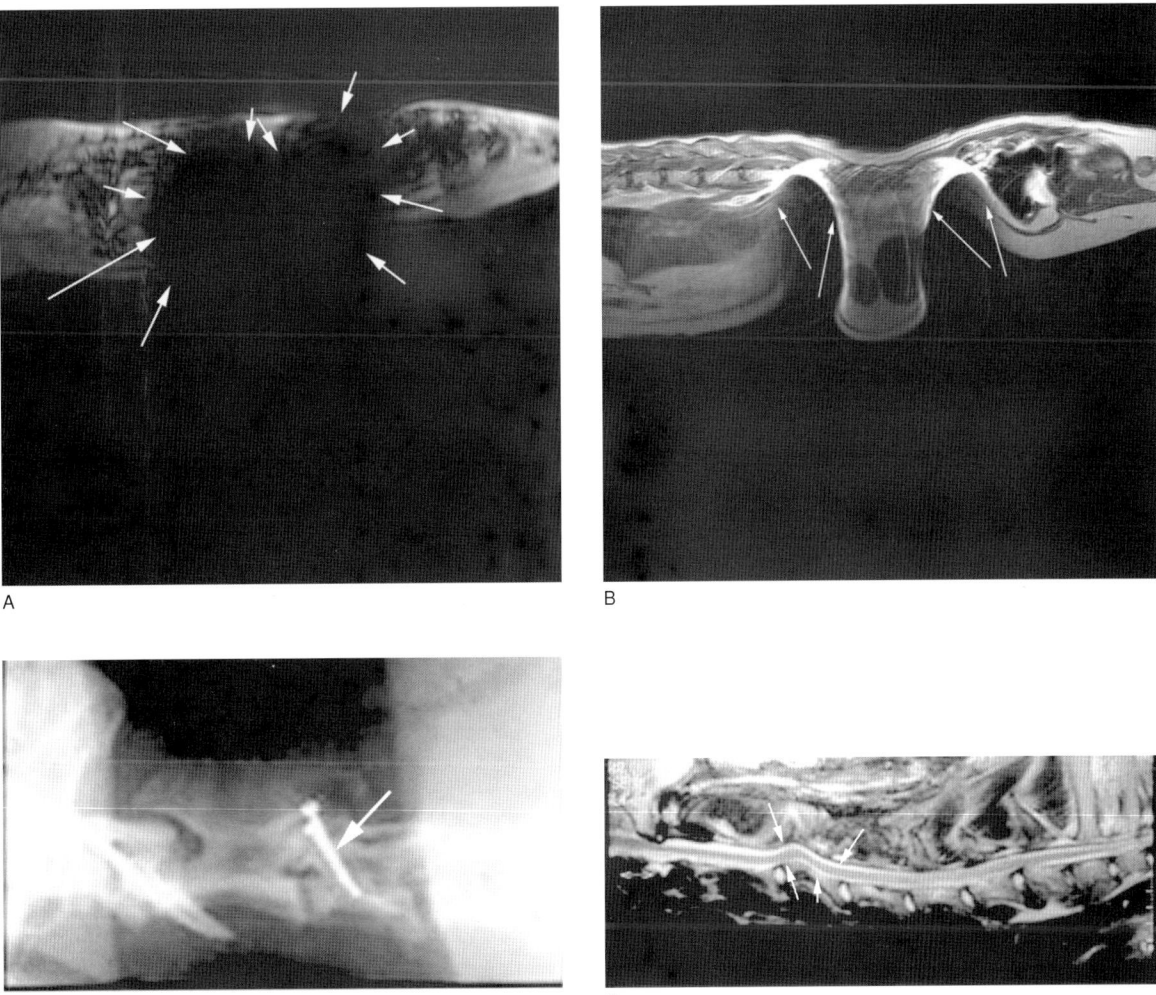

A

B

C

D

Figure 1.9. (A), (B) Artifact from a small BB in the region of the subcutaneous tissues of this cat. A small BB still causes a very large magnetic susceptibility artifact negating visualization of the lumbar spine in this patient. Part (A) is the gradient echo localizer sequence. Gradient echoes are more prone to magnetic susceptibility artifact and a very large black hole can be seen. Part (B) is a T2-weighted sequence showing some visualization of the spine, but marked warping of the image is due to the magnetic susceptibility artifact. (C) Two stainless steel orthopedic screws placed across the facets. While stainless steel creates some magnetic susceptibility artifact, it is nowhere near that seen with the steel of a BB. However, part (D) shows the warping of the image from these stainless steel screws in the facets. The curvature of the spinal cord that appears in C3 is artifactual due to the magnetic susceptibility artifact. (See Color Plates 1.9C,D.)

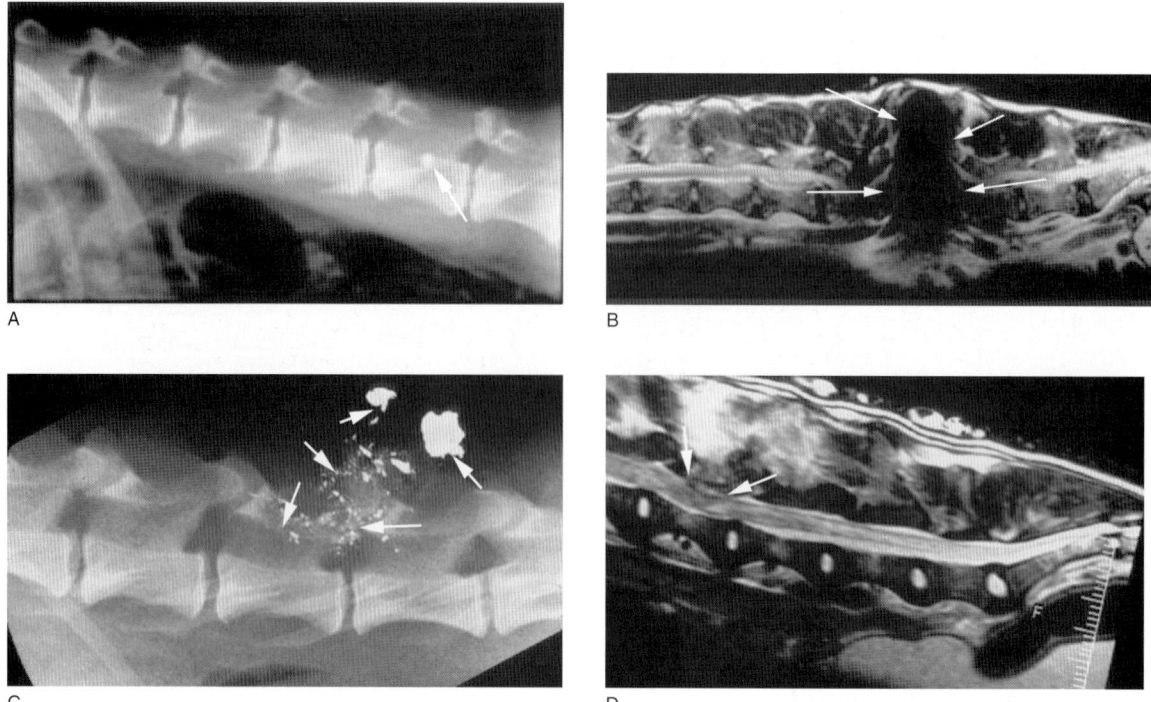

Figure 1.10. This image shows the difference between types of metal and the artifacts that are created. (A) Radiograph showing a small steel shot next to the vertebra. (B) This small piece of steel creates a huge magnetic susceptibility artifact negating visualization of the spine in the L4 through L6 region. Part (C) is a radiograph of an animal that has suffered a gunshot wound. In this case, the metal is lead. While the radiograph shows fragmentation of the lead, the radiograph cannot depict the spinal cord. Numerous small fragments of lead are identified with the arrows. (D) The MR shows that the lead does not create a magnetic susceptibility artifact and the spinal cord can be seen. The arrows point to a small osseous fragment that has been created from the gunshot wound. The hyperintensity on this STIR sequence is hemorrhage and edema from the gunshot wound. (See Color Plates 1.10A–D.)

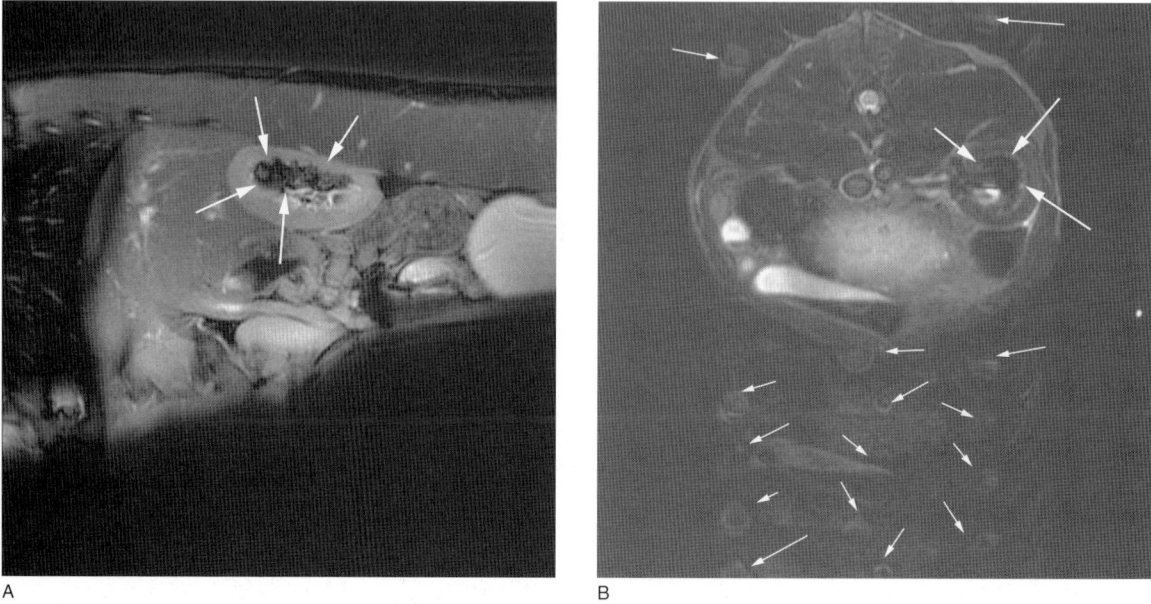

Figure 1.11. (A) T1 fat-saturated postcontrast sagittal image. The very low signal intensity within the renal pelvis is due to the high concentration of gadolinium contrast agent that is being excreted by the urinary system. The concentration is so high that instead of being "enhanced," it actually gets a low signal intensity with this high concentration. (B) T2-weighted sagittal image following the administration of contrast showing the same low signal intensity of the renal pelvis due to the high concentration of gadolinium. This is also commonly seen in the urinary bladder and should not be mistaken for a lesion.

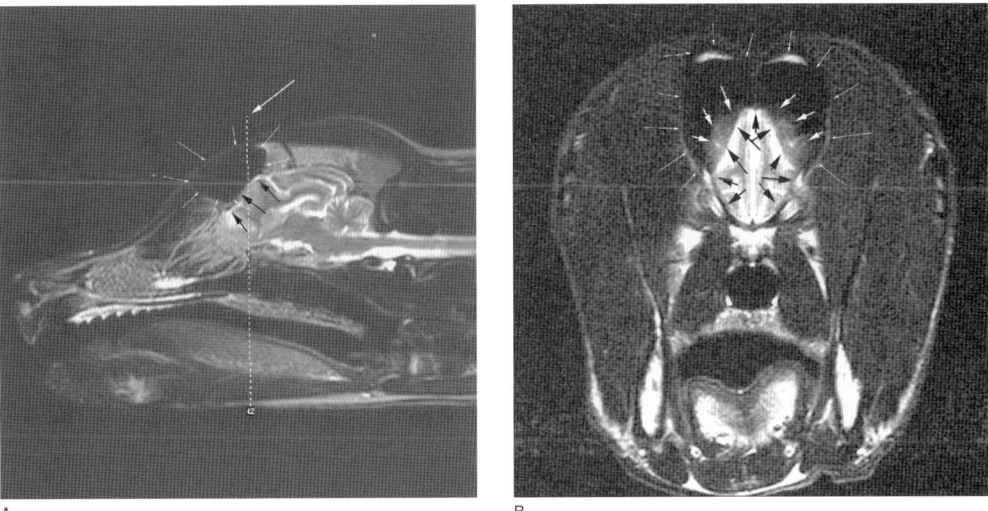

Figure 1.12. Volume averaging artifact. (A) Sagittal T2 image. Dotted line (large white arrow) is the location of (B). The smallest white arrows depict the air-filled frontal sinus. The black arrows point to the periphery of the olfactory bulb of the cerebrum. (B) T2 transverse image. This image is the average of the signals from a 4 mm slice thickness, 2 mm on either side of the dotted line in (A). The smallest white arrows depict the air-filled frontal sinus. The black arrows point to the periphery of the olfactory bulb of the cerebrum. The larger white arrows indicate the volume averaging of the brain and frontal sinus in this 4-mm-thick section.

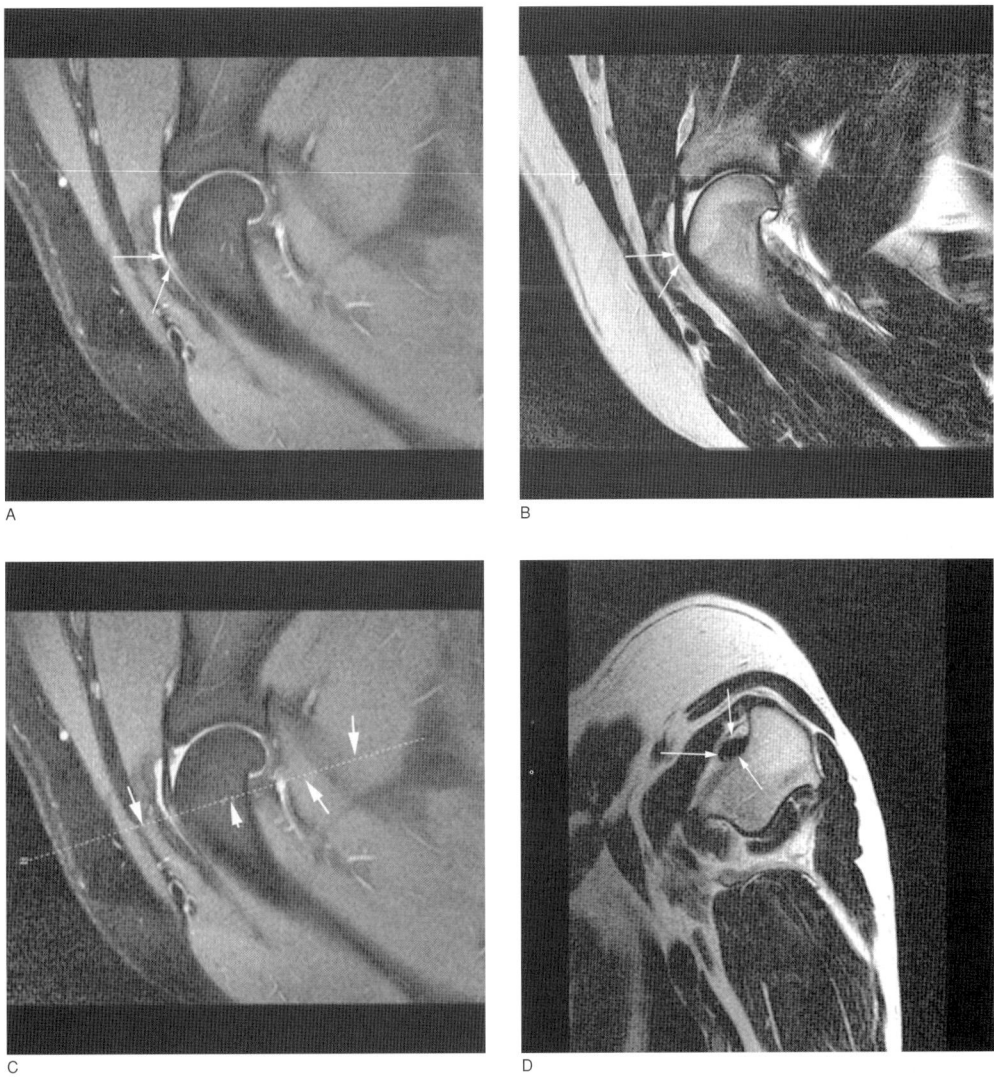

Figure 1.13. Magic angle artifact. (A) Proton density fat-saturated image with hyperintensity in the biceps tendon (arrows). (B) T2 image of same slice as in (A) with normal intensity of the tendon (arrows). (C) Same image as (A) showing location of (D). (D) Transverse T2 image of the biceps tendon with uniform signal.

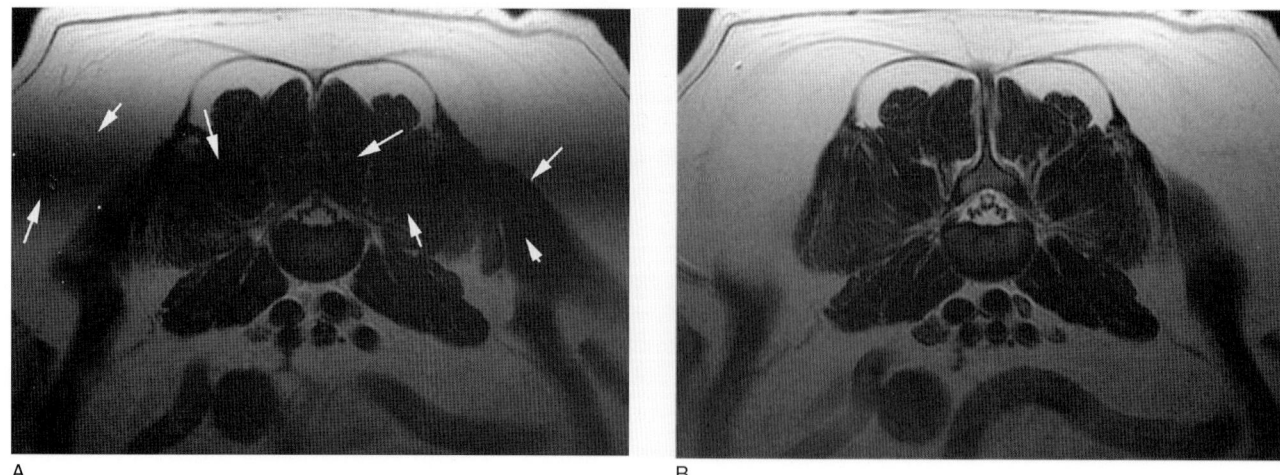

A   B

Figure 1.14. Part (A) shows the lack of signal homogeneity due to cross-talk when multiple stacks intersect each other. This commonly occurs at the lumbosacral area due to the change in the angulation. The transverse images should be perpendicular to the spinal canal. This can result in intersection between the images through the caudal lumbar area and those through the lumbosacral junction. The homogeneity of the signal can be seen in (B) where this problem was eliminated by a separate series of slices through the lumbosacral area with no intersection of neighboring slices.

Equipment Consideration and Selection

Patrick R. Gavin

The main component of the magnetic resonance unit is obviously the magnet. The main magnetic field is called the B_0 field. Within the magnet are gradient coils needed to produce a GE in the X, Y, and Z directions or a gradient in B_0. Within the gradient coils are RF coils that provide the RF energy needed to rotate the nuclear spins by $90°$ or any other value selected by the sequence. The strength of the gradient coils determines the ability of an MR unit to change the magnetic field per unit distance. The strength of the gradient coils will have the largest contribution to end-plane resolution. The RF coil, besides an emitting RF coil, is also a receiving coil capable of detecting the signal from the spins within the body.

Most modern magnets are self-shielded with an opposing magnetic field such that they do not need to be magnetically shielded. All magnets do, however, need to have some form of RF shielding. This shield not only prevents RF pulses from radiating out from the magnet, but also prevents RF signals from television, radio, cell phones, etc. from being detected by the imager.

MRI requires powerful computers since every component is under the control of the computer. The computer controls the shape and amplitude of the gradient fields, and the strength and duration of the RF pulses. The computer also provides the necessary method to convert the received RF energy into an image.

The imaging magnet is the most expensive component. Permanent magnets are present as smaller field units. These magnets must be pure and uniform. Permanent magnets have the advantage of not requiring cryogens. They are heavy but their main drawback is their field strength. Most higher field MR units are superconducting magnets. A superconducting magnet keeps the temperature close to zero kelvin by immersing it in liquid helium. Once electrical current is initiated in the coil, it will continue so long as it is maintained at this temperature. Liquid helium is at $-269°$ C or $4°$ above absolute zero. Large volumes of liquid helium are required, which is also costly with regard to maintenance. In initial designs, the liquid helium was surrounded by liquid nitrogen to decrease helium consumption. Currently, cryo-coolers are used to maintain the liquid helium temperature and have eliminated the need for liquid nitrogen. Early magnets required approximately four refills per year of liquid helium. Current machines can be filled less than yearly and some every ten years.

The gradient coils within the main magnet are fundamental to image creation. While the "body coil" can be used for a receiver coil, often specialized RF detector coils designed specifically for certain body areas are utilized to receive the image. There are numerous types of coils. Some of these are volume or quadrature coils with the antenna coils running at right angles to each other to better capture the signal. Other coils are linear coils. Linear coils are often flexible to allow for contouring of the coil to the patient. Circular coils are commonly used for extremity work. The depth of penetration of a circular coil is equal to its radius. One of the more useful coils for veterinary imaging is a multi-element spine coil. Multiple element spine coils allow for the entire patient's spine to be imaged without physically repositioning the patient. This can greatly speed the imaging process while providing various fields of view for proper examination of the spinal column.

SAFETY

Safety is of critical importance with MRI. The safety issues are related to dangers associated with ferromagnetic objects near the magnet. Ferromagnetic objects that are often forgotten include pagers, cell phones, hoof knives, scissors, and other sharp or heavy objects. Obviously, items such as ferrous oxygen tanks, standard ECG machines, etc. can become flying, and potentially lethal, projectiles inside an MR suite. All personnel entering an MRI suite should be given instructions on MR safety. Of special concern are those people that would rarely need to enter the suite, including maintenance personnel.

Some safety issues of extreme importance that are much less commonly experienced by veterinary radiologists deal with patients having pacemakers or aneurysmal clips being exposed to the magnetic field. This is less common in veterinary medicine; however, pacemakers are a definite contraindication. Typical orthopedic appliances may cause an artifact, but do not create a hazard for the patient. Similarly, small objects that are ferrous, including BBs, "gold beads," and steel shot used for water fowl hunting, all create large imaging artifacts but actually create no problem for the patient. They will not become dislodged or move significantly within tissue, but will create a large artifact and may prevent imaging in an area of interest. Similarly,

the small wire used in identification crystals can also create an artifact. The veterinary profession will need to find a better site for implantation of these crystals, other than the neck of small dogs and cats, as the popularity of MR continues. Cervical spinal studies can be compromised by these identification chips in small and toy breeds. These chips must occasionally be removed to allow for proper evaluation of the study.

The amount of energy absorbed during an examination is of concern. However, for the time utilized in veterinary imaging due to the anesthetic concerns, the amount of energy for MR studies has not been a problem to date. If medically indicated and anesthesia concerns can be answered, there is no reason why pregnant patients and neonates cannot be imaged with conventional MR units.

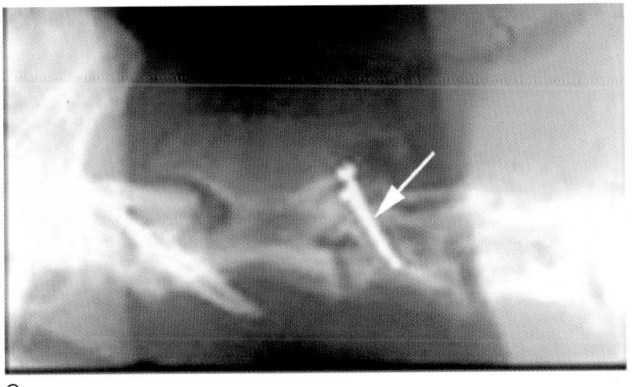

C

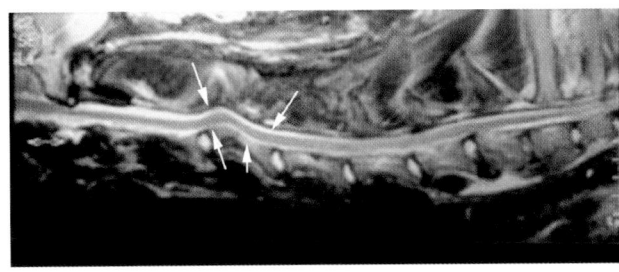

D

Plate 1.9.

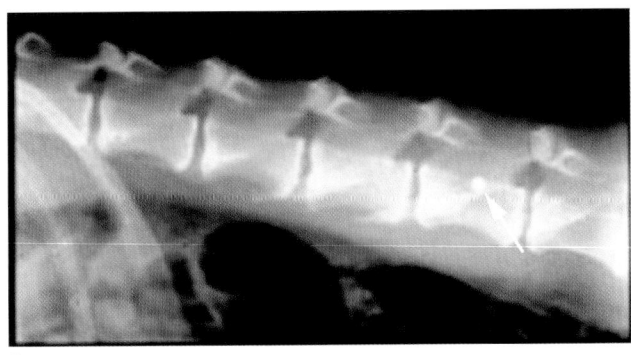

A

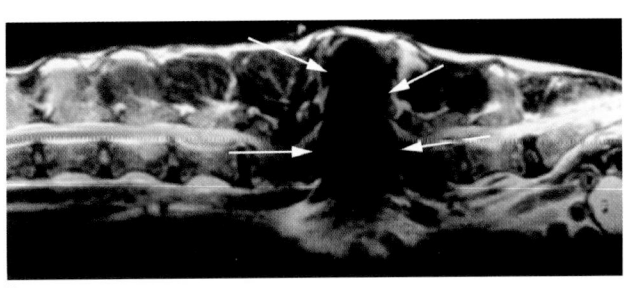

B

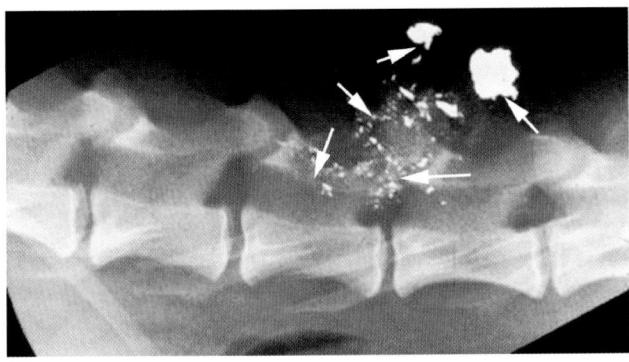

C

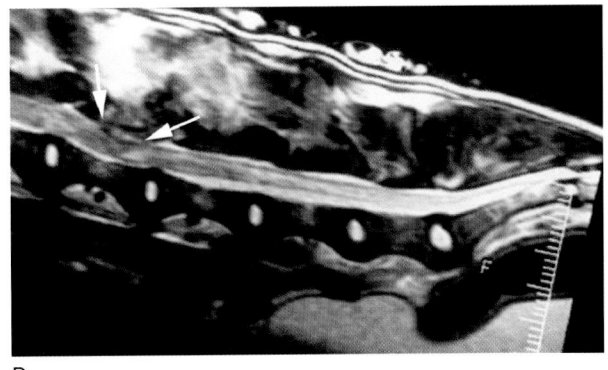

D

Plate 1.10.

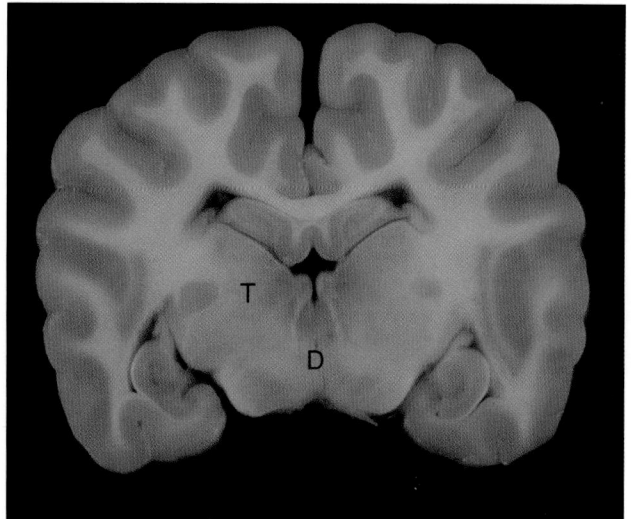

B

Plate 2.9.

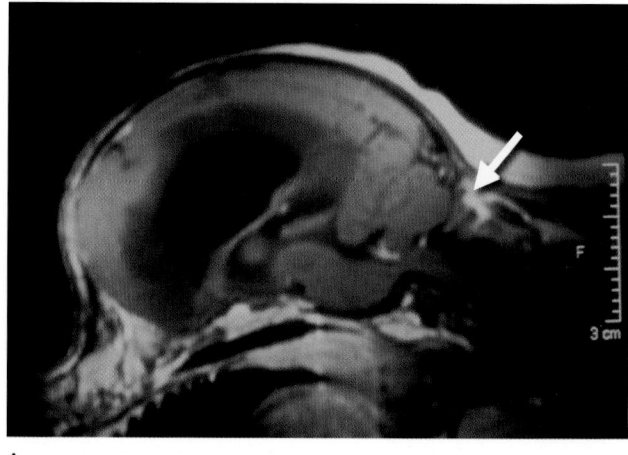

A

Plate 2.189.

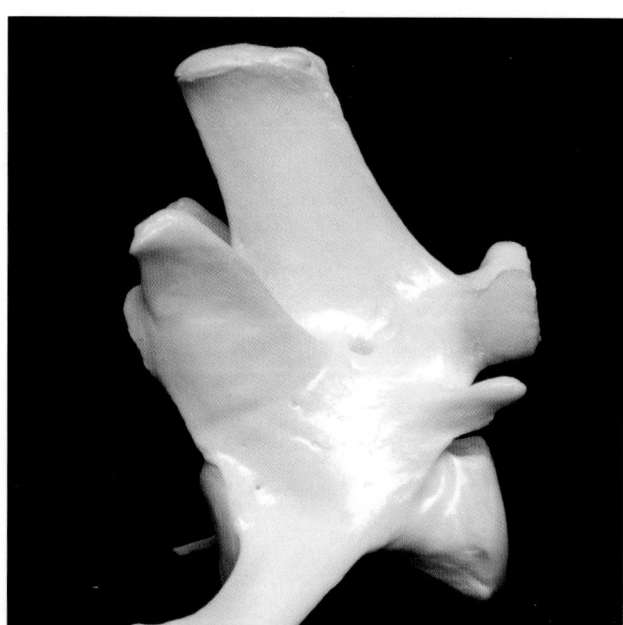

H

Plate 2.111.

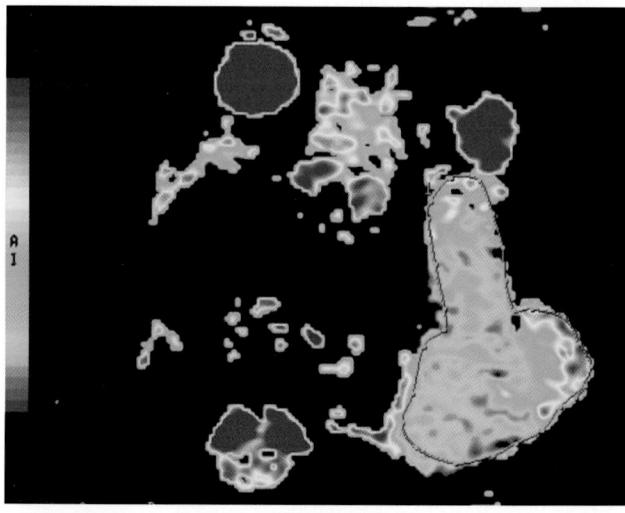

B

Plate 7.6.

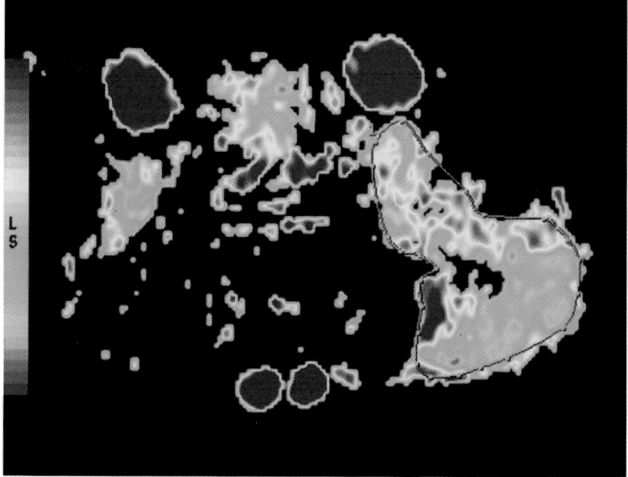

C

Plate 7.8.

CHAPTER TWO

VETERINARY CLINICAL MAGNETIC RESONANCE IMAGING

SECTION 1

Diagnosis of Intracranial Disease

Rodney S. Bagley, Patrick R. Gavin, and Shannon P. Holmes

One of the initial clinical uses of magnetic resonance (MR) imaging in animals was in the diagnosis of intracranial disease. Intracranial disease may affect the function or anatomical structure of the intracranial nervous system, and MR imaging has proven extremely helpful in identifying diseases that result in anatomical abnormalities of the brain, cranial nerves (CNs), and associated anatomical structures. As with all anatomical imaging modalities, knowledge of both normal MR appearance of anatomical structures as well as the MR appearance of pathological alterations of the nervous system is imperative for this imaging modality to be clinically useful and the images accurately interpreted. The initial portions of this chapter will review important normal anatomical characteristics of the intracranial nervous system structures, followed by a discussion of the appearance of the representative intracranial disease processes when viewed with MR imaging. Additionally, key individual caveats to populational generalizations will be noted.

NEUROANATOMICAL CONSIDERATIONS

The intracranial nervous system primarily includes what is generically referred to as the "brain" as well as the associated structures such as the skull, meninges, and blood vessels. Additionally, neuronal extensions and connections of these intracranial structures important for functions in and around the head are formed into discrete peripheral nerves referred to as CNs. CNs are analogous to the spinal nerves in that they have cell bodies either within CN ganglia or in localized intraparenchymal regions of the brain referred to as a nucleus. The following overview of neuroanatomy is intended not as an extensive treatise but rather as an introductory overview of important structural considerations to consider when interpreting intracranial MR images from dogs and cats. Depending upon the strength of the magnet, slice orientation, and other imaging parameters, the appearance of the anatomical components of the intracranial nervous system may be more or less apparent, and therefore, more or less discretely identifiable. The relative signal intensity of intracranial elements may also vary based on sequences used, individual sequence characteristics, and viewing parameters. All imaging appearances are relative in comparison to some "standard" tissue's imaging appearance and can be manipulated at the time of the imaging study and digitally manipulated for viewing. It is important to determine the "standard" of reference when describing image characteristics. As an MR image provides, in essence, a view of in vivo anatomy, it is necessary for the evaluator of clinical MR images to have a working knowledge of intracranial neuroanatomical structures.

SUPRATENTORIAL NERVOUS SYSTEM

The supratentorial region anatomically includes the cerebral hemispheres, basal nuclei, diencephalon, and rostral portion of the mesencephalon (Beitz and Fletcher 1993; deLahunta 1983; Jenkins 1978; King 1987). This region may also be referred to as the prosencephalon or forebrain. The anatomical structures reside rostral to the division of the intracranial contents formed by an approximate imaginary line extending parallel to the tentorium cerebelli (Figure 2.1). Structures in this supratentorial region are responsible for many functions requiring or associated with consciousness, awareness, behavior, sensory recognition, and coordinated responses of the body.

The cerebral hemispheres (also referred to as the telencephalon) are made up of neuronal cell bodies (gray matter) and supporting cells as well as white matter (axonal processes of neurons). The gray matter of the cerebral cortex has been divided into six cellular layers; however, these layers are not always discernable in dogs and cats. The cerebral cortex is located between the white matter and the pia mater (i.e., the innermost layer of the meninges).

The surface of the cerebral hemispheres resembles collections of interwoven tubular structures (Figure 2.2). The convex portions of the cerebral hemispheres are referred to as gyri, and the depressions between the convex portions are referred to as sulci. There are numerous gyri and sulci of the cerebral hemisphere. The number, location, configuration, and pattern of gyri and sulci, however, are anatomically diverse and inconsistently present between breeds and even between

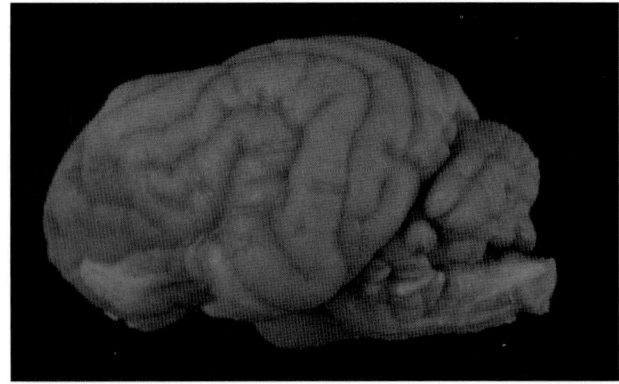

Figure 2.2. Lateral view of the formaldehyde-fixed brain from a normal dog. The gyri and sulci of the cerebral hemisphere are apparent.

individuals within a breed. Each cerebral hemisphere is divided into four regions based on associated functions. These are the frontal, parietal, temporal, and occipital cortex.

The white matter of the cerebral hemispheres, or corona radiata, consists of axonal projections from nerve cell bodies. These white matter tracts can be association axons (axons from one cortical area to another in the same hemisphere), commissural axons (axons that cross from one cortical area to an area in the opposite hemisphere), or projection axons (axons that project to nuclear areas in the brain stem and spinal cord). Projection axons to and from the cerebral hemispheres are found as collections of tracts referred to as the internal capsule.

As a general rule, cerebral cortical elements are used as a "standard" tissue imaging appearance to which other anatomical structures, and intracranial pathologies, are compared. Therefore, these cortical or compacted neuronal elements often are relatively "isointense." Neural elements with similar tissue characteristics such as, for example, cerebral hemisphere cortical tissue or brain stem tissue, tend to have similar imaging characteristics. This is one reason why concentrations of neurons such as in individual nuclei may not be easily distinguished from surrounding tissue elements in individual instances.

Standard MR imaging sequences have been discussed previously in Chapter 1. As image acquisition may influence anatomical appearance, it is important to assess MR images in light of these influences. The more standardized imaging appearances of intracranial structures using more universally accepted MR sequences will be described here as a starting point for MR image interpretation. The appearance of these structures in individual animals may vary somewhat, however, due to both individual animal and MR imaging influences.

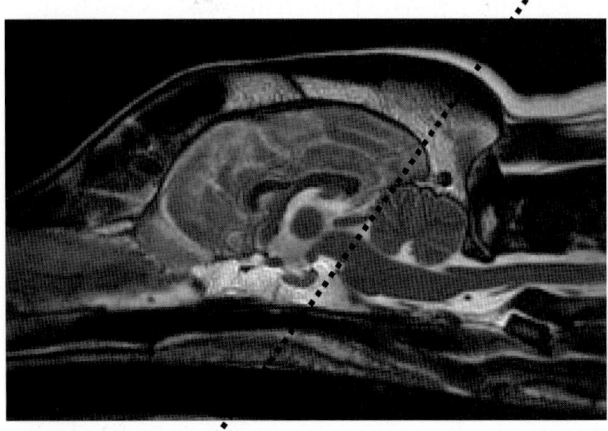

Figure 2.1. Sagittal, T2-weighted MR image of a dog brain. The dotted line represents an imaginary anatomical division between the supra- and infratentorial structures at the level of the tentorium cerebelli.

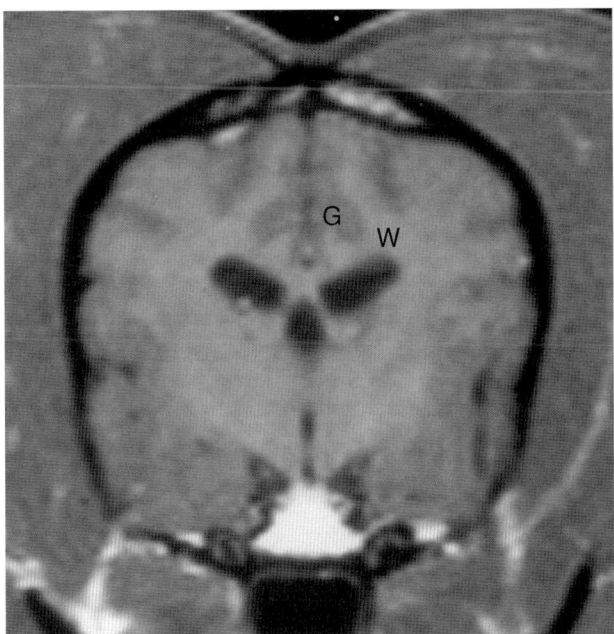

Figure 2.3. Transverse T1-weighted MR image at the level of the third ventricle. The cerebral white matter (W) is slightly hyperintense in this study compared with cerebrocortical gray matter (G).

The white matter of the cerebral hemisphere tends to appear isointense to mildly hyperintense relative to the cerebral hemisphere cortical signal on T1-weighted sequences (Figures 2.3 and 2.4). With T1-weighted sequences, cerebral cortical tissue and cerebral white matter tissue may be indistinguishable. White matter on T2-weighted sequences tends to appear isointense to hypointense relative to cerebral cortical signal, and obviously hypointense relative to cerebrospinal fluid (CSF) signal (Figure 2.5). Similarly, white matter signal with proton density weighting tends to be relatively hypointense compared to cortical tissue (Figure 2.6). The proton density image usually provides the most obvious distinction between gray and white matter of the cerebral hemispheres.

In the supratentorial region, the most rostral intracranial structures are associated with the olfactory bulb (Figure 2.7). Progressing caudally from this region, the next most identifiable structures include the rostral extensions of the lateral ventricles and the caudate nucleus (Figure 2.8). Ventral and medial to the frontal cortex of the cerebral hemispheres at approximately this level are the basal nuclei (sometimes referred to as the basal ganglia). These structures are important for certain types of movements in association with the cerebral cortex and brain stem.

The diencephalon is the portion of the brain caudal to the basal nuclei and rostral to the mesencephalon (Figures 2.9 and 2.10). The thalamus and hypothalamus are located within the diencephalon. The pituitary gland or hypophysis is located immediately ventral to this area (Figure 2.11). The caudal pituitary or neurohypophysis contains extension axons

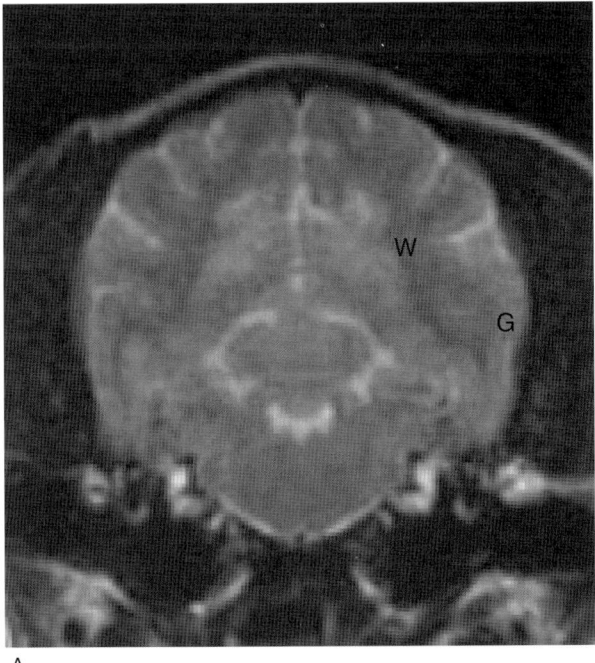

A

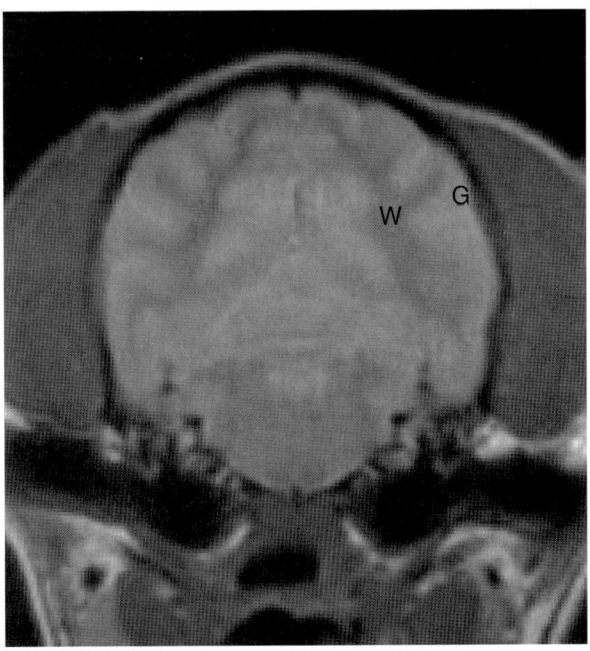

B

Figure 2.4. Transverse T2-weighted (A) and proton density (B) MR images at the level of the cerebellum and brain stem. The cerebral white matter (W) in this study is hypointense relative to cerebrocortical gray matter (G).

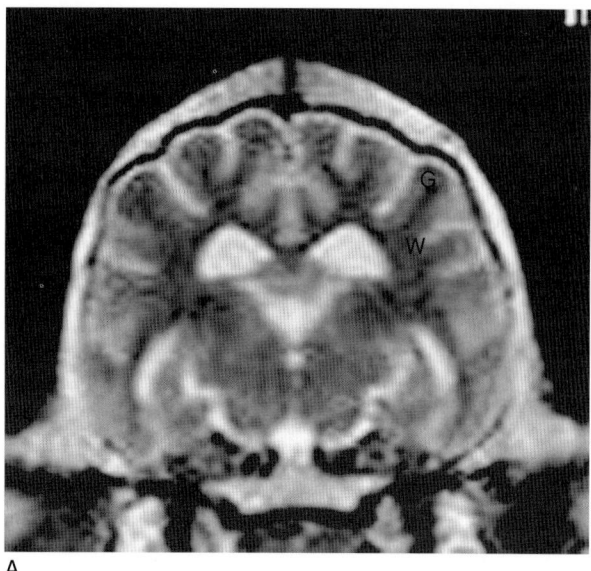
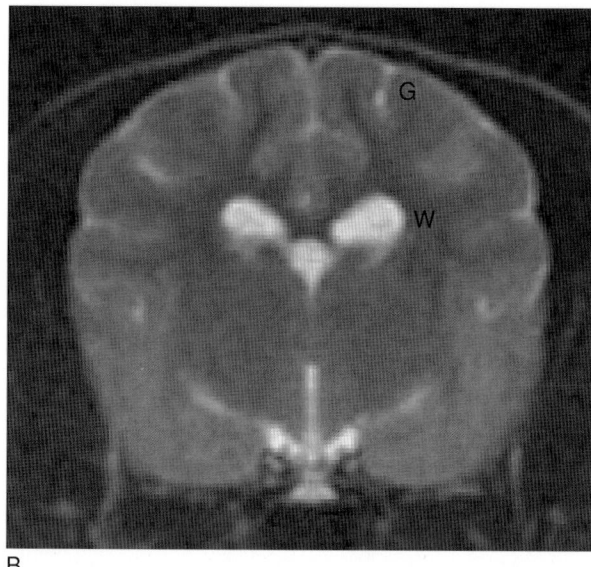

A   B

Figure 2.5.   Transverse T2-weighted MR images from two separate dogs ((A) and (B)) at the level of the geniculate bodies (A) and the thalamus (B). The cerebral white matter (W) in these studies is hypointense relative to cerebrocortical gray matter (G).

from the hypothalamus. The rostral pituitary (adenohypophysis) is responsible for the production of many endocrine hormones such as ACTH (adrenocorticotropic hormone) and thyroid stimulating hormones. There may be an associated focal hyperintense signal present

in the normal pituitary, the origin of which is debatable but may, in fact, be from various neurotransmitters (Figure 2.11).

The thalamus has been equated to a "relay or train station" and is an area where projections to and from the cerebral hemispheres synapse or traverse. In the sagittal image, the circular interthalamic adhesion is readily apparent with a discretely circular shape. Ventral in the thalamus and immediately dorsal to the pituitary is the hypothalamic region. The hypothalamus is associated with many rudimentary functions of life, such as eating, drinking, water homeostasis, body temperature, and reproductive functions. This area is responsible for production of many of the endocrine hormones that have global body effects. The pituitary gland functions in association with the hypothalamus in many endocrine functions via either the production (anterior pituitary) or release (posterior pituitary or neurohypophysis) of hormones and metabolically active elements.

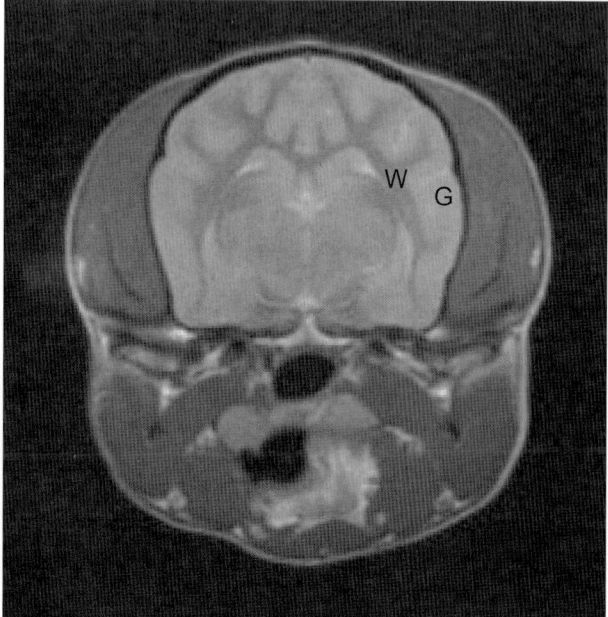

Figure 2.6.   Transverse proton density MR image from a dog at the level of the geniculate region. The cerebral white matter (W) in these studies is hypointense relative to cerebrocortical gray matter (G).

INFRATENTORIAL NERVOUS SYSTEM

The infratentorial structures include much of what is commonly referred to as the brain stem (Beitz and Fletcher 1993; Jenkins 1978; King 1987) (Figures 2.12–2.16). The cerebellum resides in this region dorsal to the brain stem. For this discussion, the brain stem

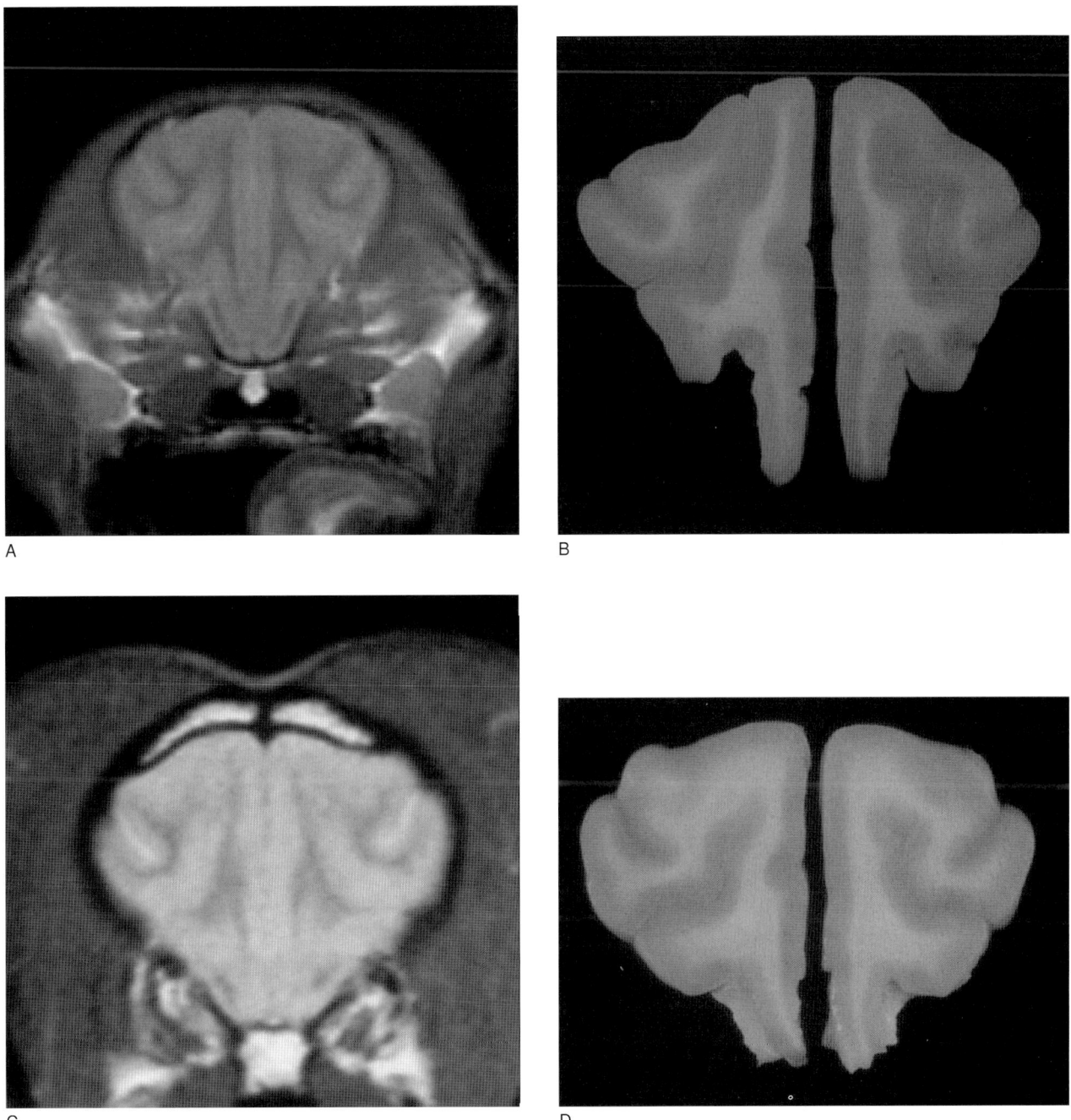

Figure 2.7. Transverse proton density MR images from a dog at the level of the olfactory bulb (A) and slightly more caudal (C). Associated gross brain structures at similar levels ((B) and (D)) are provided for comparison.

includes part of the mesencephalon (midbrain), the metencephalon (pons), and the myelencephalon (medulla oblongata). Many of the CN nuclei (CNs III through XII) and neurons responsible for important vital functions, such as wakefulness and respiration, reside in the brain stem.

The vestibular system (CN VIII and its connections) works in close association with the cerebellum with regard to posture. A portion of the cerebellum (flocculonodular lobe) is primarily responsible for vestibular-associated functions such as balance in the equilibrium. The vestibular system has an important influence over body, head, and eye posture.

The CNs are nerve projections to and from neurons in brain stem nuclei and structures in the head and neck (deLahunta 1983; Evans and Kitchell 1993; Jenkins

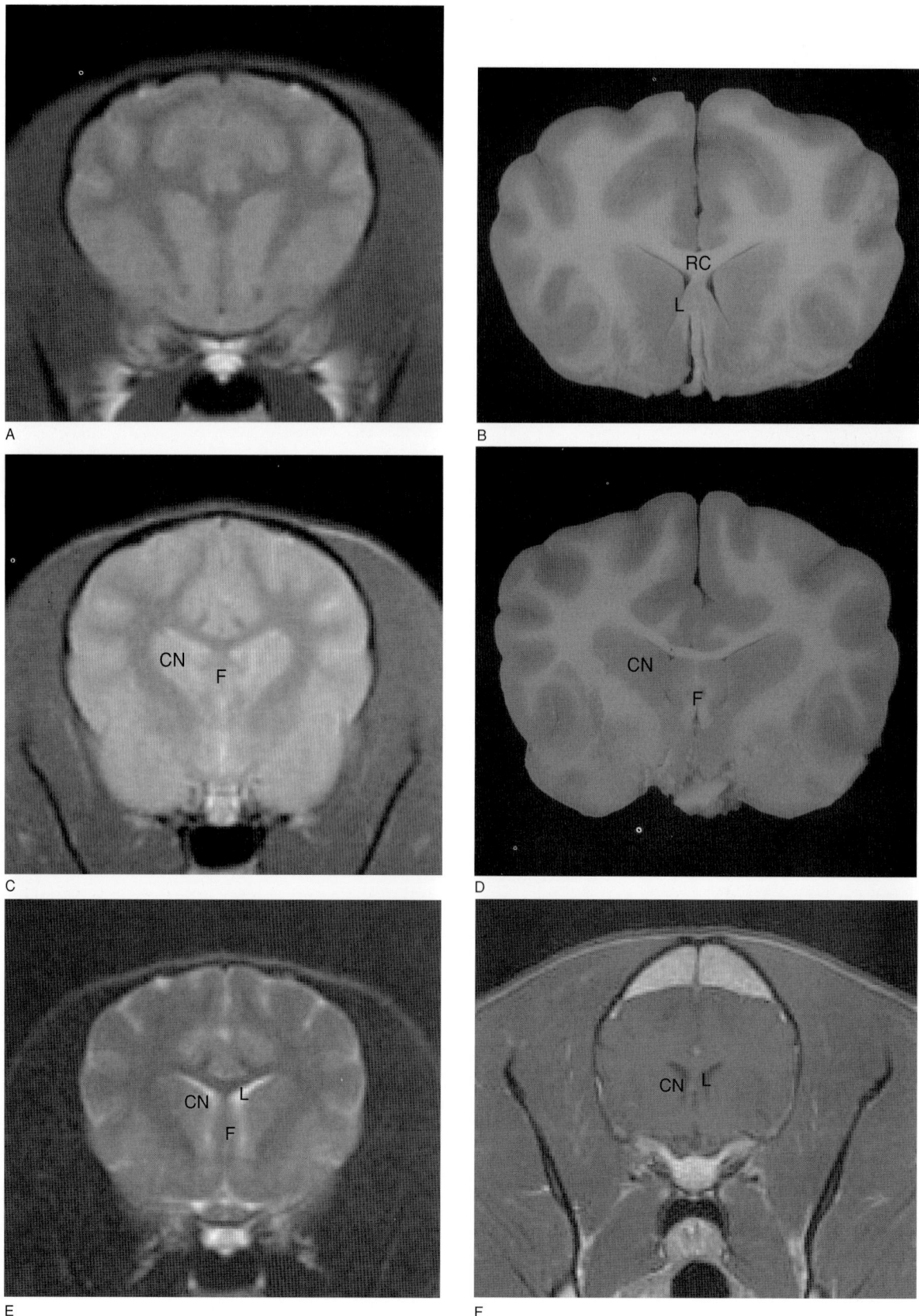

Figure 2.8. Transverse proton density MR images from a dog at the level of the rostral commissure (A) and slightly more caudal at the level of the caudate nucleus (C). Associated gross brain structures at similar levels ((B) and (D)) are provided for comparison. Transverse T2-weighted (E) and T1-weighted image (F) at a similar level for comparison (CN, caudal nucleus; F, fornix; L, lateral ventricle; RC, rostral commissure).

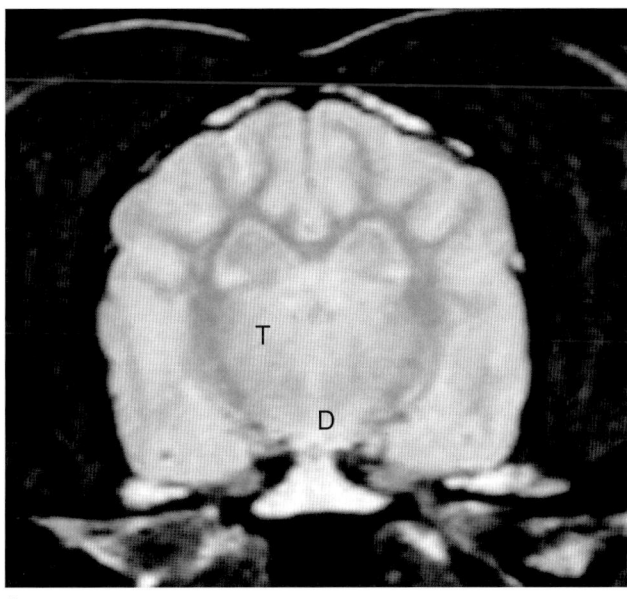

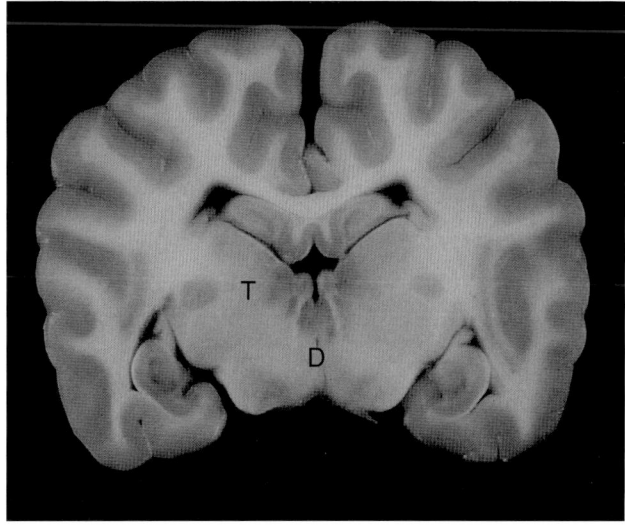

A   B

Figure 2.9. Transverse proton density MR image (A) and gross brain image (B) from a dog at the level of the thalamus (T, thalamus; D, diencephalon). (See Color Plate 2.9B.)

1978; King 1987)(Figure 2.17). There are 12 pairs of CNs ordered I through XII. CNs I (olfactory nerve important for smell) and II (optic nerve important for vision) are functionally associated with the supratentorial structures. CNs III through XII have cell bodies that reside within or adjacent to (in ganglia) the brain stem. Afferent or sensory information from some CNs is projected into the intracranial nervous system.

Information flowing to and from the cerebral cortex, thalamus, and other components of the supratentorial structures travels through the brain stem to and from brain stem nuclei and the spinal cord. The brain stem contains functional systems such as the vestibular system and the reticular systems that have important roles in extensor tone and maintenance of body position relative to the influence of gravity. Brain stem structures also have significant roles in gaiting and walking.

INDIVIDUAL CRANIAL NERVES

The CNs are similar to other peripheral nerves except that the cell bodies associated with these nerves are either within intracranial nervous system or in ganglion in close proximity to the head (Figures 2.18–2.20). CNs provide for numerous special functions such as sight, hearing, taste, and smell. These nerves are also important for sensation and proprioception from the head region and provide motor innervation to many of the muscles of the head and face. The vestibular system

(including CN VIII) plays a significant role in balance and equilibrium in relationship to gravity.

Cranial Nerve (CN) Olfactory Nerves

CN I is, in reality, a constellation of multiple nerve fibers and synapses (deLahunta 1983; Evans and Kitchell 1993). The first-order neuron is a bipolar neuron in the caudodorsal olfactory epithelium in the nose and functionally acts as chemoreceptors. The distal (toward the nose) portion of these cells consists of ciliated processes (numbering 6–8) that penetrate the olfactory mucous membranes. Unmyelinated axons from these cells project caudally to penetrate the cribriform plate and synapse on neurons (brush or mitral cells) in the olfactory bulbs.

Cranial Nerve II (CN II) Optic Nerve

CN II is one of the components of the visual system (deLahunta 1983; Evans and Kitchell 1993). Nerve fibers originate in the retina and form CN II proper as the discrete optic nerve, which travels from the retina caudally toward the brain, entering the skull in the optic canal of the presphenoid bone. Depending upon the species, a majority (75% in dogs; 65% in cats) cross at the optic chiasm immediately rostral to the pituitary. The remaining fibers remain ipsilaterally. Visual fibers then continue dorsally and caudally in the optic tract to synapse in the lateral geniculate nucleus of the

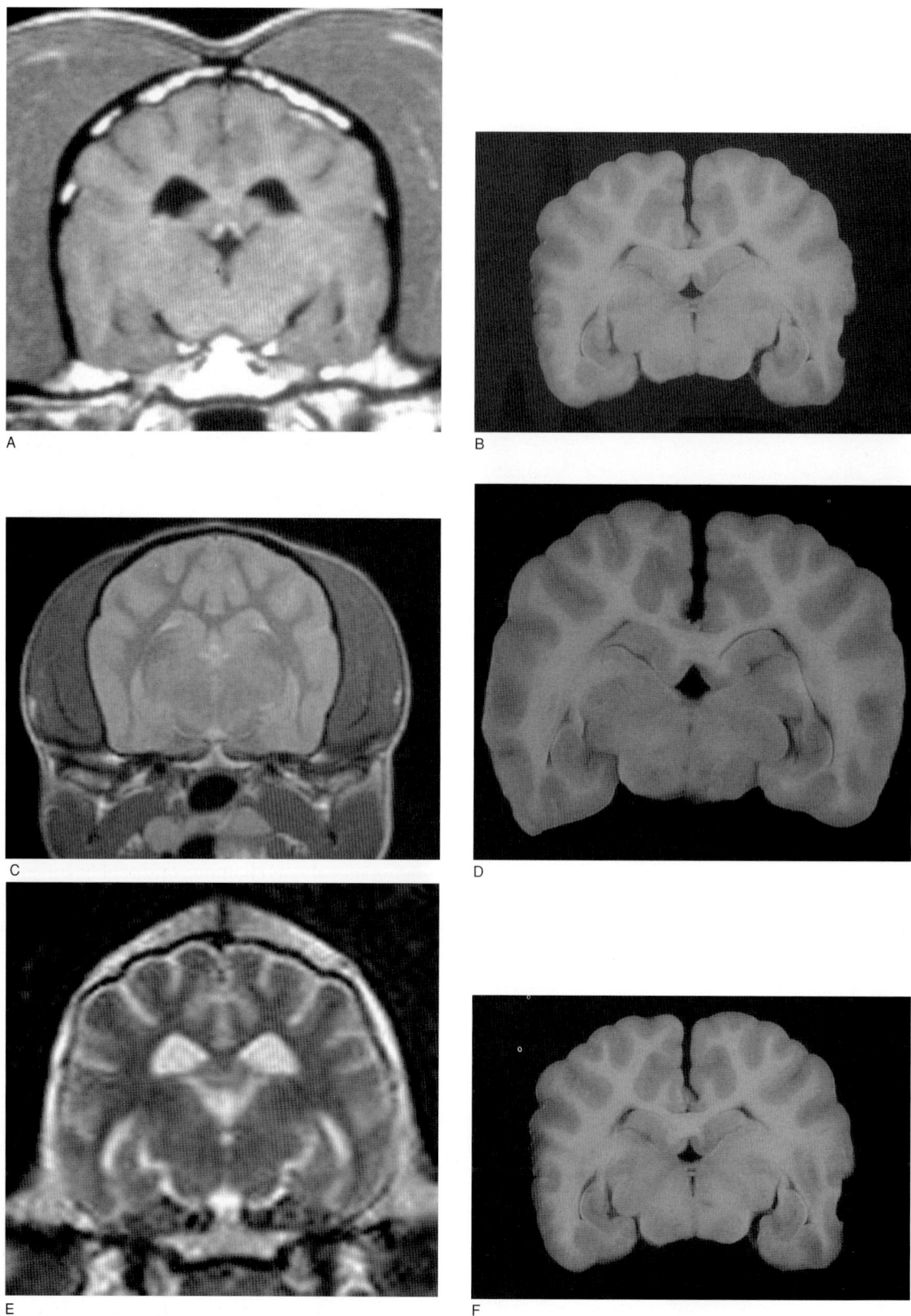

Figure 2.10.   Transverse T1-weighted MR image (A) and gross brain image (B) from a dog at the level of the caudal thalamus and geniculate bodies. Transverse proton density MR image (C) and gross brain image (D) from a dog at the level of the caudal thalamus and geniculate bodies. Transverse T2-weighted MR image (E) and gross brain image (F) from a dog at the level of the caudal geniculate bodies and rostral mesencephalon.

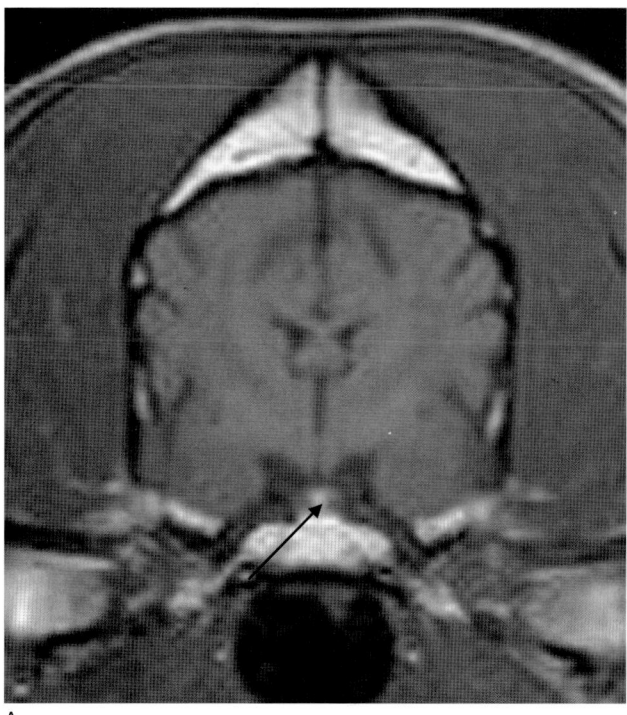

A

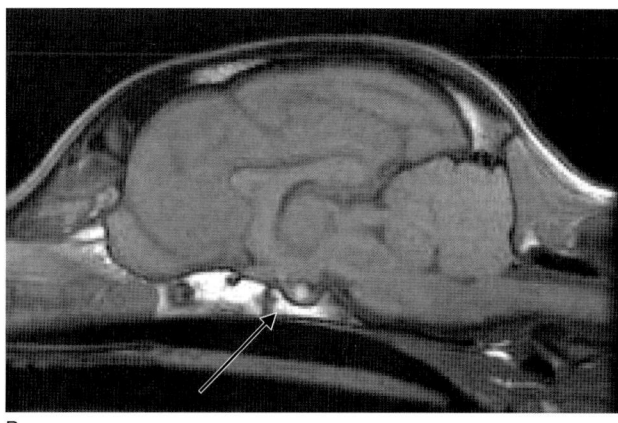

B

Figure 2.11.   Transverse (A) and sagittal (B), T1-weighted images prior to intravenous contrast administration from a dog showing the focal, hyperintense signal from the pituitary (arrows).

thalamus. From here, visual fibers travel further caudally in the optic radiations to synapse in the visual cortex of the occipital hemisphere.

Cranial Nerve III Oculomotor Nerve

The oculomotor nerve has two main functions, movement of the eye and pupillary constriction (deLahunta 1983; Jenkins 1978; King 1987). The extraocular muscle motor nucleus of CN III is located in the rostral mesencephalon at the level of the rostral colliculus. The cell bodies of the parasympathetic division of this nerve associated with pupillary constriction are found in the parasympathetic nucleus of CN III, which is found medial to the associated motor nucleus. Axons pass ventrally through the tegmentum, exit the brain stem on the lateral side, course rostrally lateral to the hypophysis close to the cavernous sinus to exit the skull in the orbital fissure. The nerve divides near the orbit into a dorsal and ventral branch. The dorsal branch innervates the dorsal rectus and the levator palpebrae muscles. The ventral branch travels near, lateral to, and slightly ventral to the optic nerve. The fibers of this branch innervate the ventral and medial rectus and the ventral oblique muscles. These fibers also terminate on the ciliary ganglion, which supplies postganglionic parasympathetic innervation to the iris.

Cranial Nerve IV Trochlear Nerve

The trochlear nerve is unique in that it is the only CN in which 100% of its axons decussates, or crosses, and this nerve is the only CN that exits the dorsal aspect of the brain stem (deLahunta 1983; Jenkins 1978; King 1987). The trochlear nucleus is located in the caudal mesencephalon at the level of the caudal colliculi. The axons course dorsally and caudally to exit the brain stem just caudal to the caudal colliculus. The nerve crosses midline and travels ventrally and in close proximity to the cavernous sinus. Axons exit the skull in the orbital fissure to innervate the dorsal oblique muscle of the eye.

Cranial Nerve VI Abducent

The abducent nucleus is located in the rostral medulla oblongata adjacent to midline ventral to the floor of the fourth ventricle at the level where the caudal cerebellar peduncles merge with the cerebellum (deLahunta 1983; Jenkins 1978; King 1987). This nerve carries only motor (somatic efferent) fibers to some extraocular muscles. The axons pass ventrally through the reticular formation and exit the brain stem through the trapezoid body lateral to the pyramids. This nerve travels close to the cavernous sinus on the floor of the skull and leaves the skull through the orbital fissure. Cranial VI innervates

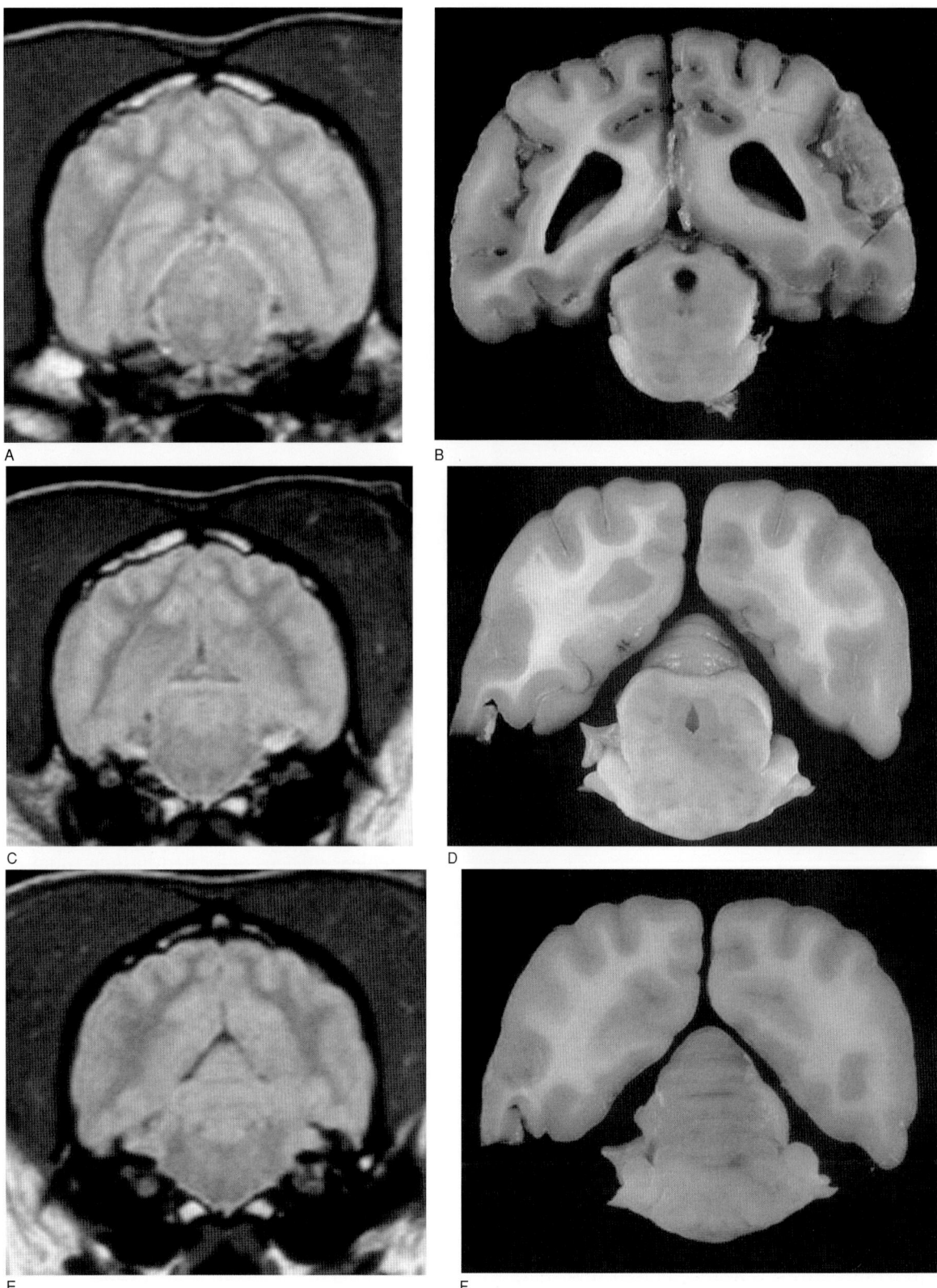

Figure 2.12.   Transverse proton density MR image (A) and gross brain image (B) from a dog at the level of the more rostral mesencephalic aqueduct. Transverse proton density MR image (C) and gross brain image (D) from a dog at the level of the caudal colliculus. Transverse proton density MR image (E) and gross brain image (F) from a dog at the level of the slightly caudal to the mesencephalic aqueduct at the level of the more rostral aspects of the cerebellum.

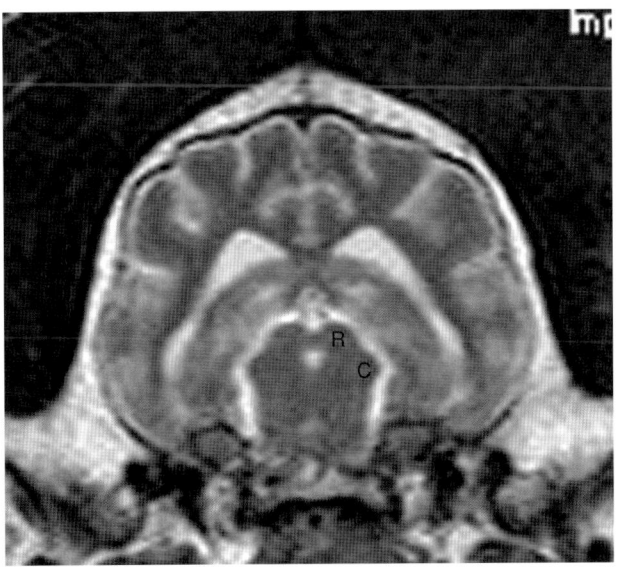

G

Figure 2.12. (*Continued*) Transverse T2-weighted MR image (G) at the level of the rostral and caudal colliculi.

the lateral rectus and retractor bulbi extraocular muscles.

Cranial Nerve V Trigeminal Nerve

CN V, the trigeminal nerve, as the name suggests, contains three main branches or divisions (deLahunta 1983; Jenkins 1978; King 1987). The three major branches of this nerve are the ophthalmic, the maxillary, and the mandibular nerves. The ophthalmic and maxillary branches provide afferent sensory information, and the mandibular nerve is responsible for both sensory and motor functions. The trigeminal nerve, therefore, has both a larger sensory nucleus, and a more discrete motor nucleus found in the brain stem region. The sensory nucleus extends from the mesencephalon to the caudal medulla into the cranial spinal cord. The motor nucleus is found in the rostral brain stem at the level of the rostral cerebellar peduncle.

The motor portions of this nerve originate in the motor nucleus, exit the lateral and slightly ventral aspects of the brain stem, and travel through the trigeminal canal in the petrosal bone to exit the skull through the oval foramen. The cell bodies of the ophthalmic and maxillary nerves are present in the trigeminal ganglion, which lies in the trigeminal canal. Nerve fibers traveling toward these cell bodies from peripheral structures in or around the eye enter the skull through the orbital fissure. Nerve fibers traveling toward these cell bodies from peripheral structures in or around nose and muz-

zle areas enter the skull through the rostral alar canal (externally) and the round foramen (internally).

Cranial Nerve VII Facial Nerve

CN VII supplies innervation to the facial muscles, to the lacrimal and salivary glands, to the middle ear and the blood vessels of the head, and to the palate and the rostral two-thirds of the tongue associated with branches of the trigeminal nerve (deLahunta 1983; Jenkins 1978; King 1987). Neurons supplying innervation to the muscles of facial expression are located in the facial nucleus in the brain stem. This nucleus lies caudal to the trapezoid body and the attachment of the caudal cerebellar peduncle. The axons pass dorsomedially to midline near the floor of the fourth ventricle, where they pass rostrally over the nucleus of CN VI in the genu (knee) of the facial nerve. These fibers then course ventrolaterally through the medulla and emerge from the brain stem through the trapezoid body next to CN VIII. The facial nerve courses through the facial canal in the petrosal bone, and exits the skull through the stylomastoid foramen. The facial nerve runs through the middle ear before branching in the petrosal bone.

In the petrosal bone, the major petrosal nerve exits initially, prior to the geniculate ganglion, to innervate the lacrimal glands. The chorda tympani branch next exits and projects to the tongue, salivary glands, and stapedius muscle. The facial nerve proper then exits the stylomastoid foramen, courses ventral to the external ear canal, and gives rise to three branches: (1) the auriculopalpebral branch, which innervates the eye and ear muscles; (2) the dorsal buccal branch to the muscles of the maxilla; and (3) the ventral buccal branch to the muscles of the maxilla and mandibular areas. These branches of the facial nerve innervate the muscles of the ear, eyelids, nose, cheeks, lips, and caudal portion of the digastricus muscle.

Cranial Nerve VIII Vestibulocochlear Nerve

CN VIII has two main divisions: vestibular and cochlear. These serve to maintain the position of the head in space (vestibular) and function in hearing (cochlear) (deLahunta 1983; Jenkins 1978; King 1987).

Vestibular Division

The vestibular division of CN VII is responsible for maintenance of the head and other structures relative to gravity. The receptors for both the vestibular

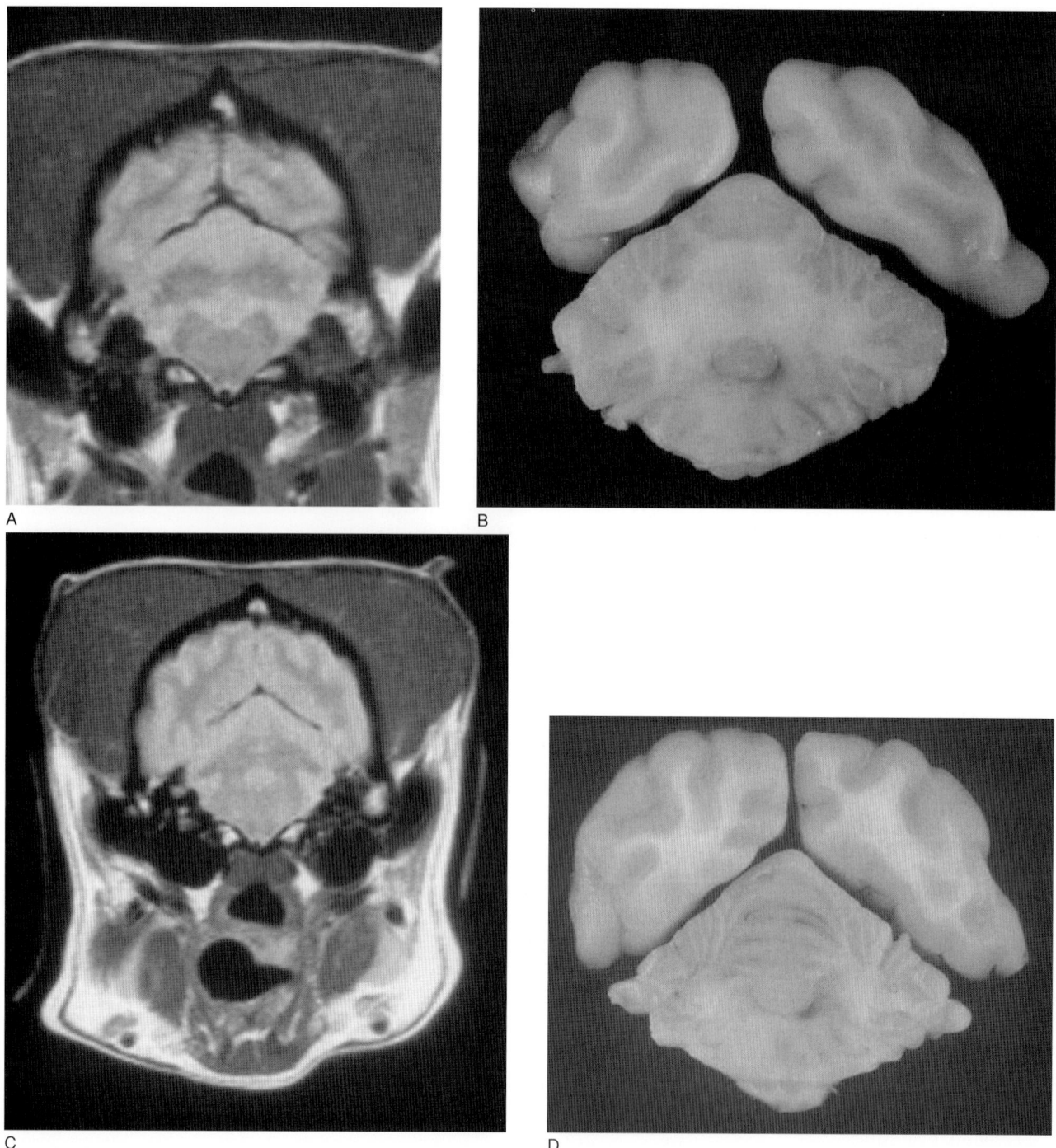

Figure 2.13.   Transverse proton density MR image (A) and gross brain image (B) from a dog at the level of the mid cerebellum. Transverse proton density MR image (C) and gross brain image (D) from a dog at the level slightly more caudal to (A) and (B).

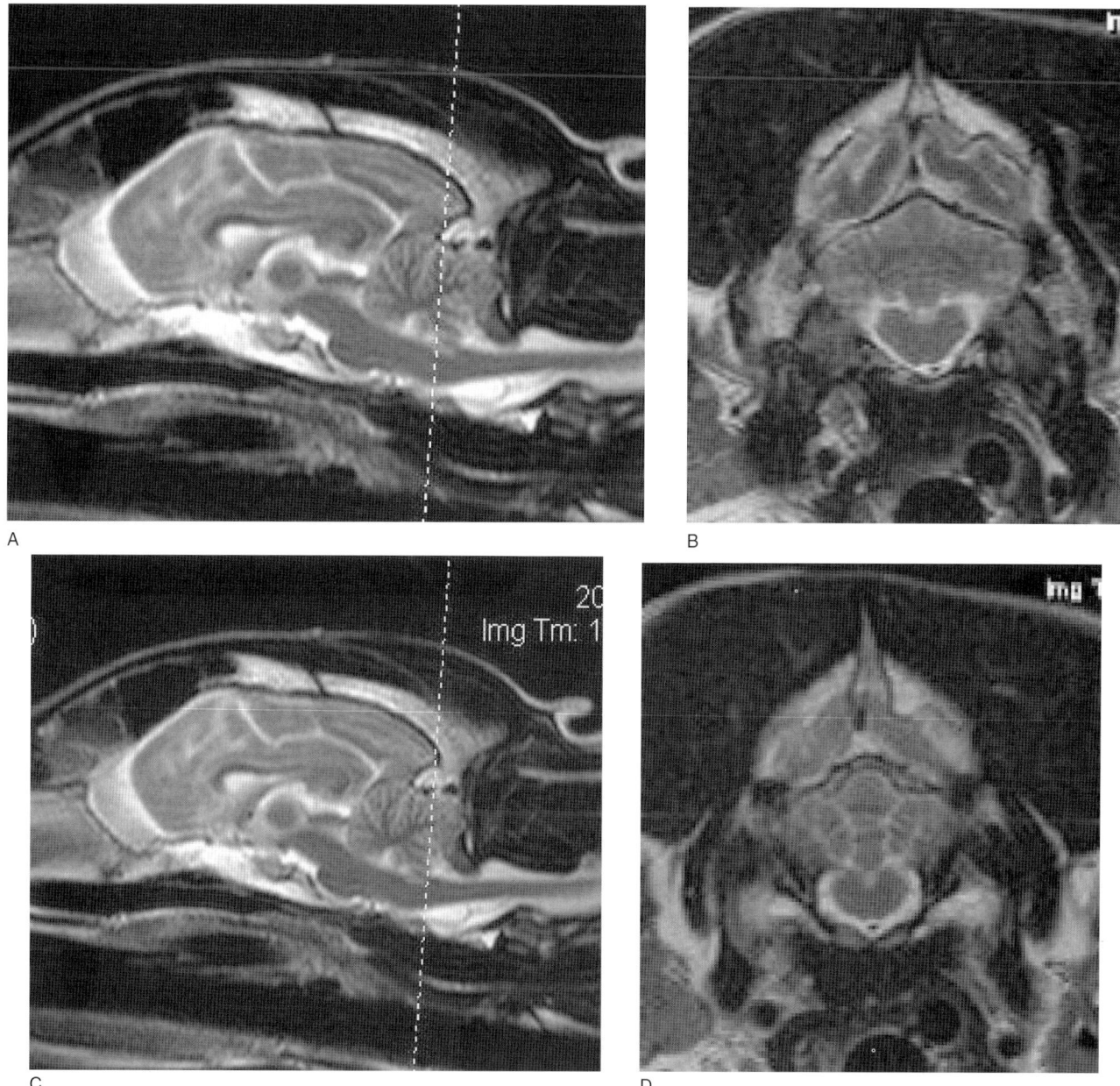

Figure 2.14.   Sagittal (A) and transverse (B) T2-weighted MR images from a dog at the level of the mid to caudal cerebellum. Sagittal (C) and transverse (D) MR images from a dog at a level slightly more caudal than (A) and (B).

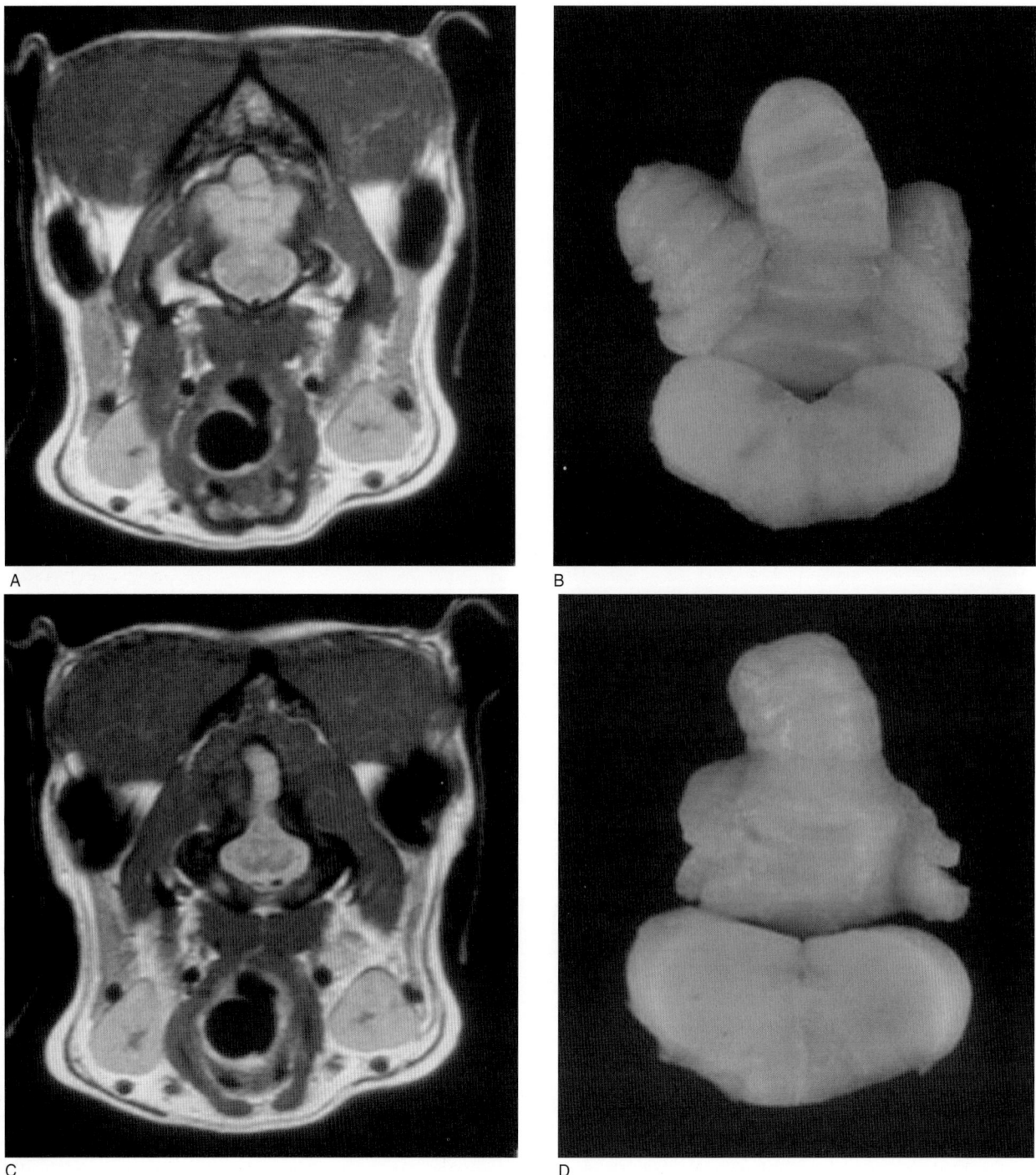

Figure 2.15. Transverse proton density MR image (A) and gross brain image (B) from a dog at the level of the caudal cerebellum. Transverse proton density MR image (C) and gross brain image (D) from a dog at the level slightly more caudal to (A) and (B).

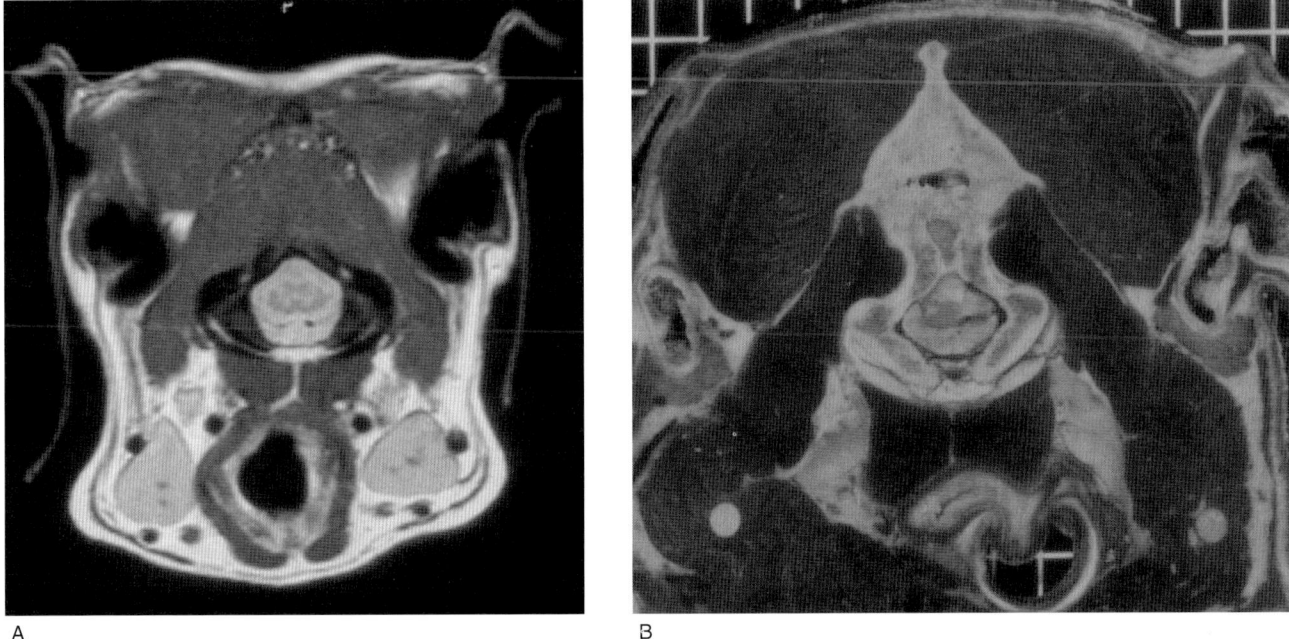

Figure 2.16. Transverse proton density MR image (A) and gross full slice head image (B) from a dog at the level of the foramen magnum.

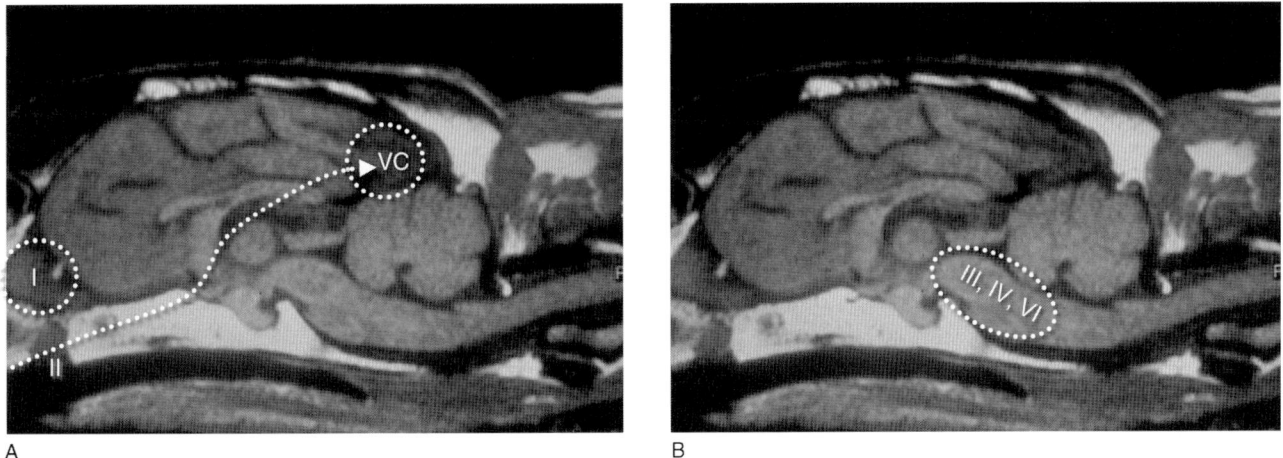

Figure 2.17. Sagittal T1-weighted MR imaging showing the approximate locations of the nuclei associated with the various CNs (A) CN I (I) and CN II (II). The dotted line represents the central path of the visual fibers to the level of the visual cortex (VC) in the occipital lobe. (B) Approximate location of the nuclei of CNs III, IV, and VI (circle III, IV, VI).

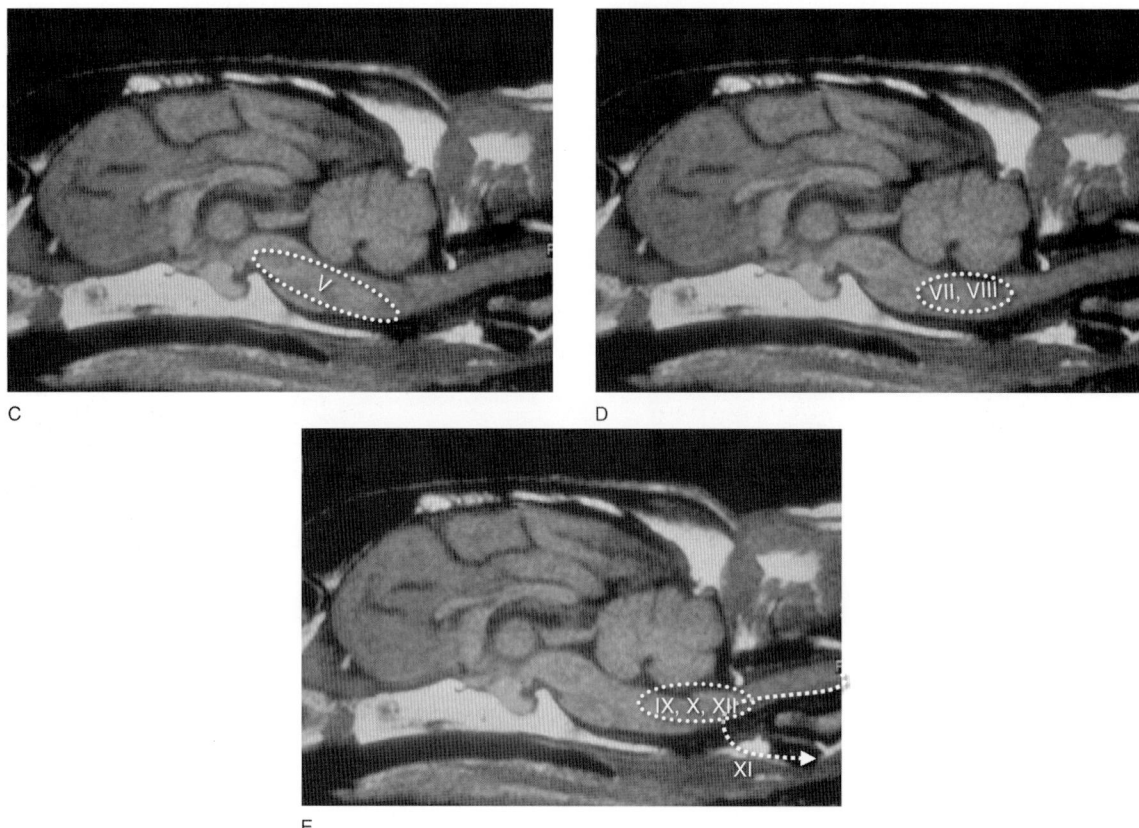

Figure 2.17. (*Continued*) (C) Approximate location of the nuclei of CN V. (circle V) (D) Approximate location of the nuclei of CNs VII and VIII (circle VII, VIII). (E) Approximate location of the nuclei of CNs IX, X, and XII (circle IX, X, XII) and the course of CN XI (dotted line XI).

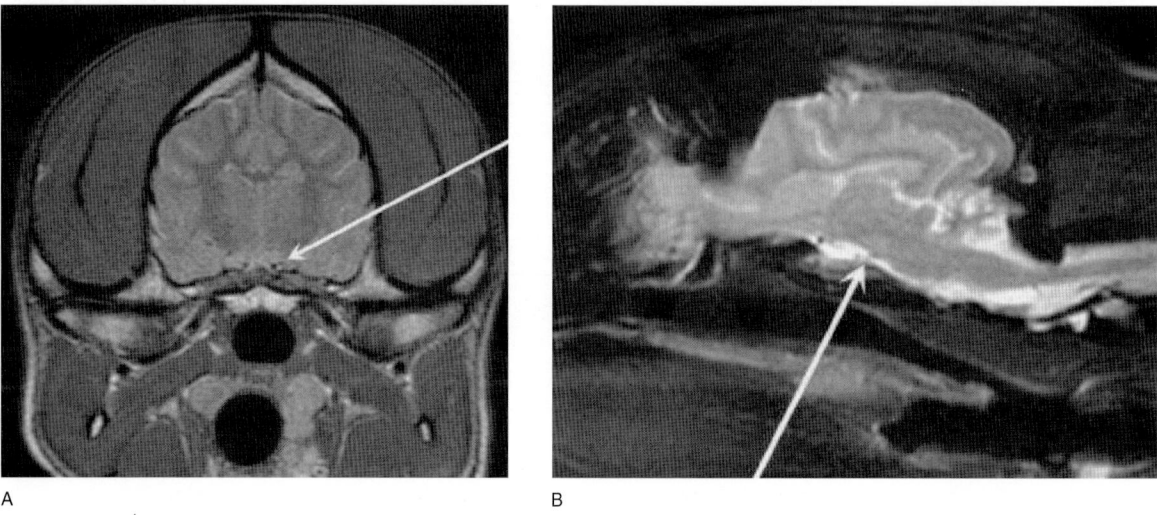

Figure 2.18. Transverse proton density (A) and parasagittal (B) T2-weighted MR images from a healthy dog showing the approximate location of the oculomotor nerve (CN III) (arrows).

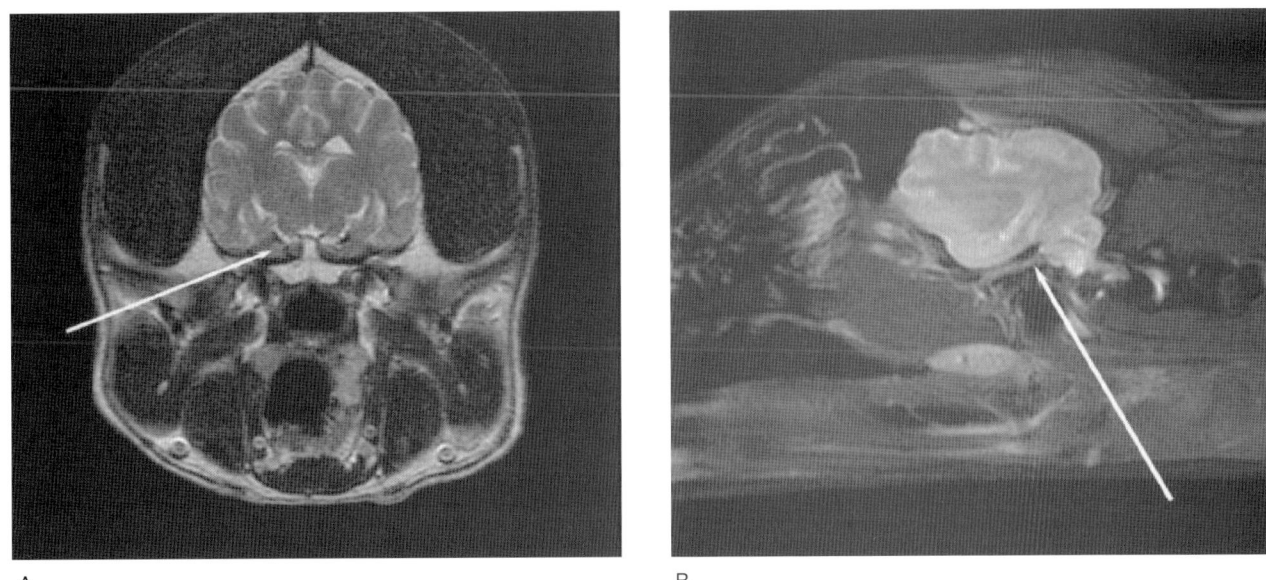

Figure 2.19. Transverse (A) and parasagittal (B) T2-weighted MR images from a healthy dog showing the approximate location of the trigeminal nerve (CN V) (arrows).

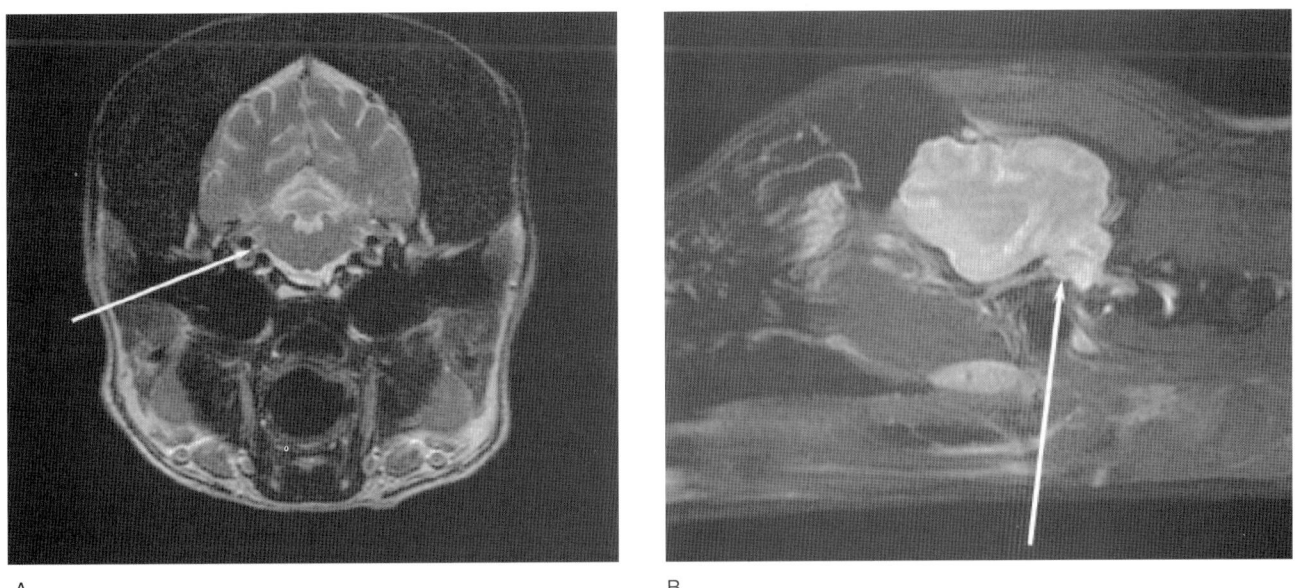

Figure 2.20. Transverse (A) and parasagittal (B) T2-weighted MR images from a healthy dog showing the approximate location of the vestibular cochlear nerve (CN VIII) (arrows).

and cochlear portions of CN VIII are contained within the inner ear structures. Vestibular receptors are contained within the membranous labyrinth. There are three semicircular ducts containing a fluid substance called endolymph. During movement of the head, the endolymph flows in the semicircular ducts to stimulate the hair cells.

The maculae within the peripheral vestibular apparatus are important in sensing gravitational forces via the force of gravity affecting the statoconia.

The dendritic zone of the vestibular division of CN VIII is in synaptic relationship with the hair cells. The axons from these cells course through the internal acoustic meatus with those of the cochlear division. The cell bodies are located in the vestibular ganglion. The axons enter the brain stem at the cerebellomedullary angle at the level of the trapezoid body and the attachment of the caudal cerebellar peduncle. After entering the brain stem, the majority of these axons terminate in the vestibular nuclei. Some enter the cerebellum directly through the caudal cerebellar peduncle and terminate in the fastigial nucleus and flocculonodular lobe of the cerebellum. While there are central and peripheral vestibular components, it should be remembered that CN VIII never actually projects beyond the limits of the skull.

Axons from the vestibular nuclei also project to the cerebellum via the caudal cerebellar peduncle to terminate in the flocculus of the cerebellar hemisphere and the nodulus of the caudal vermis (flocculonodular lobe) as well as the fastigial nucleus.

Cochlear Division

The cochlear division of CN VIII is important for auditory stimulus recognition (deLahunta 1983; Jenkins 1978; King 1987). Receptors of the cochlear division of CN VIII are located in the cochlear duct within the ear. The dendritic zone of the cochlear portion of CN VIII is in synaptic relationship with the base of the hair cells. The cell bodies are located in the modiolus at the origin of the spiral lamina, forming the spiral ganglion. The axons course through the internal acoustic meatus where they join the vestibular division of CN VIII. These axons terminate on cell bodies in the cochlear nucleus that bulges on the lateral side of the medulla.

Cranial Nerve IX Glossopharyngeal Nerve

The glossopharyngeal nerve provides motor and sensory innervation to the pharynx, as well as parasympathetic functions for salivation and taste sensation (deLahunta 1983; Jenkins 1978; King 1987). The cell bodies

of the motor (visceral efferent) fibers are located with CN X and CN XI in the nucleus ambiguus, an ill-defined column of neurons in the ventrolateral medulla oblongata. CN IX emerges from the medulla lateral and caudal to CN VIII. The nerve courses through the jugular foramen and the tympanooccipital fissure to innervate the stylopharyngeus and other pharyngeal muscles.

Cranial Nerve X Vagus Nerve

The vagus nerve is important for motor and sensory innervation of the pharynx and provides a major component of the parasympathetic innervation to the esophagus and the gastrointestinal tract (deLahunta 1983; Jenkins 1978; King 1987). Other functions of the vagus include taste sensation and salivation. Motor cell bodies (visceral efferent) of this nerve are similarly located in the nucleus ambiguus as are those for CN IX. The axons of CN X traverse the skull through the jugular foramen and tympanooccipital fissure. Some fibers join the pharyngeal plexus and innervate the muscles of the palate, pharynx, and cervical esophagus. Some leave the vagus nerve in the cranial laryngeal muscle to innervate the cricothyroid muscle, with the recurrent laryngeal nerve and its caudal laryngeal branch innervating all the other muscles of the larynx, cervical, and cranial esophagus. In cats, these latter axons have been noted to arise from the caudal nucleus ambiguus and course to the vagus by the internal branch of the accessory nerve. Cell bodies from the nucleus ambiguus innervate the entire length of the esophagus.

Cranial Nerve XI Spinal Accessory Nerve

The spinal accessory nerve provides motor innervation to the trapezius as well as portions of the sternocephalicus and brachiocephalicus muscles (deLahunta 1983; Jenkins 1978; King 1987). Spinal accessory nerve (visceral efferent) axons project from the caudal nucleus ambiguus and emerge from the ventrolateral aspect of the medulla with the visceral efferent fibers of CN X. The cranial roots join to form the internal branch. The internal branch passes laterally and joins the external branch to form the accessory nerve. Other visceral efferent cell bodies of the external branch are located in the motor nucleus of the accessory nerve in the lateral portion of the ventral spinal cord gray matter from the first (C1) to possibly the seventh (C7) cervical spinal cord segments. The axons leave the spinal cord laterally as roots of the accessory nerve. The external branch passes through the foramen magnum. This nerve enters the jugular foramen and leaves the tympanooccipital fissure. Here the internal branch leaves the accessory nerve and joins the vagus nerve. The external branch then forms the accessory nerve to innervate the trapezius as well as portions of the sternocephalicus and brachiocephalicus muscles.

Cranial Nerve XII Hypoglossal Nerve

The hypoglossal nerve provides motor function to the muscles of the tongue (deLahunta 1983). Cell bodies of these motor (somatic efferent) axons are located in the hypoglossal nucleus in the medulla oblongata, adjacent to midline on floor of the fourth ventricle. Axons of this nerve cross the lateral aspect of the olivary nucleus in the brain stem, and emerge as numerous longitudinal small roots lateral to the pyramids. These roots merge at the small hypoglossal canal to form CN XII proper. This nerve innervates the extrinsic muscles of the tongue (styloglossus, hyoglossus, and genioglossus), the intrinsic muscles of the tongue, and the geniohyoideus. A few cell bodies of neurons to the intrinsic lingual muscles are located in the caudal area of the facial nucleus. Each genioglossus muscle is innervated by neurons from both hypoglossal nuclei.

NON-NEURAL INTRACRANIAL ELEMENTS

In addition to neural elements, the intracranial nervous system also contains a number of non-neural elements that are intimate with components of the nervous system. These non-neural elements may contribute to the imaging appearance of the intracranial system and, in some instances, these normal structures may be misconstrued for pathological abnormalities. In other instances, these non-neural structures may contain pathology that secondarily affects the intracranial neural elements.

The Skull

The components of the skull surround the majority of the intracranial neural elements. Some of the neural elements, such as the CNs, traverse the skull through foramen and fissures. The olfactory elements traverse the cribriform plate in the rostral calvarium. The brain stem becomes contiguous with the spinal cord at the foramen magnum.

Cortical (compact or dense) bone tends to be hypointense on both T1- and T2-weighted sequences (Figure 2.21). Other elements of the skull bones such as fat, blood vessels, and air, may influence the imag-

ing appearance of these structures. For example, diploic (spongy or cancellous bone) cavities often appear relatively hyperintense, most likely due to the fat signal in these bones. This hyperintense signal may be more obvious on the T1 sequences compared to T2 sequences. These regions of bone are most noticed in the sagittal crest, zygomatic arch, as well as the frontal, parietal, temporal, occipital, sphenoid, and petrous temporal bones. It is important to not overinterpret these regions as pathologic based on the hyperintense signal.

Air-filled sinus structures are hypointense on both T1 and T2 sequences (Figure 2.22). Not all breeds and species, however, have air-filled frontal sinuses (Figure 2.23). The lining of these cavities (mucoperiosteum) is normally not visible, however, may become apparent in pathological state, especially following intravenous contrast (gadolinium) administration.

The Meninges

The meninges are the "covering tissues" of the central nervous system (CNS) (deLahunta 1983; Jenkins 1978; King 1987). There are three layers of the meninges: the dura, arachnoid, and pia mater extending from outer to inner surfaces respectfully. The dura mater is the most external layer, which is primarily a fibrous tissue of collagen matrix. The arachnoid is usually intimate in ventral or medial contact with the dura. The space present ventral or medial to the arachnoid (subarachnoid space) is where CSF is present. The pia is a thin tissue layer that is intimate with the outer surface of the nervous tissue. The pachymeninx refers to the dura mater. The leptomeninx or leptomeninges refers to the arachnoid and pia mater as a function unit. These meningeal structures are also found encircling the spinal cord.

An invagination of the meninges is located between the dorsal cerebral hemispheres. This is the falx cerebri (Figure 2.24). Portions of the meninges may also be found more centrally around or within the ventricular system (tela choroidea).

The normal meninges are usually not apparent on standard T1 and T2 sequences. Also, normal meningeal tissue does not enhance following contrast administration as a general rule.

Ventricular System and CSF

The brain normally contains areas that are devoid of cells but filled with CSF (Beitz and Fletcher 1993; deLahunta 1983; Jenkins 1978; King 1987). These areas are collectively known as the ventricular system (Figures 2.25 and 2.26). From rostral to caudal, beginning in the cerebral hemispheres, the components of this

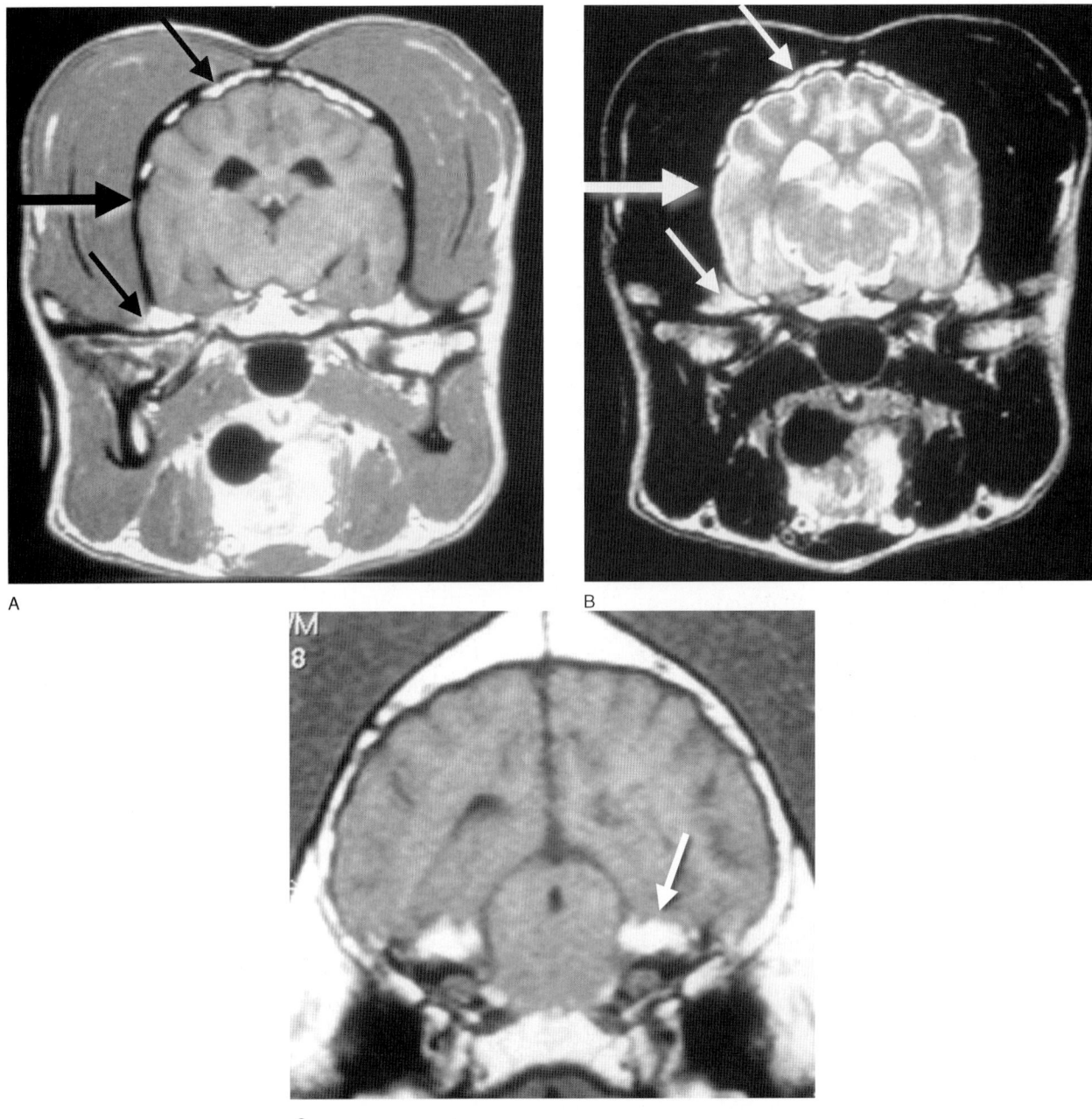

Figure 2.21. Transverse T1-weighted (A) and T2-weighted (B) MR images from a dog at the level of the caudal thalamus and geniculate bodies. Note the hyperintense signal from fat in bone marrow (small arrows) and the hypointense signal from cortical bone (larger arrows). Transverse T1-weighted MR image from a dog at the level of the colliculi (C). Note the hyperintense signal from fat in pertous temporal bone (arrow).

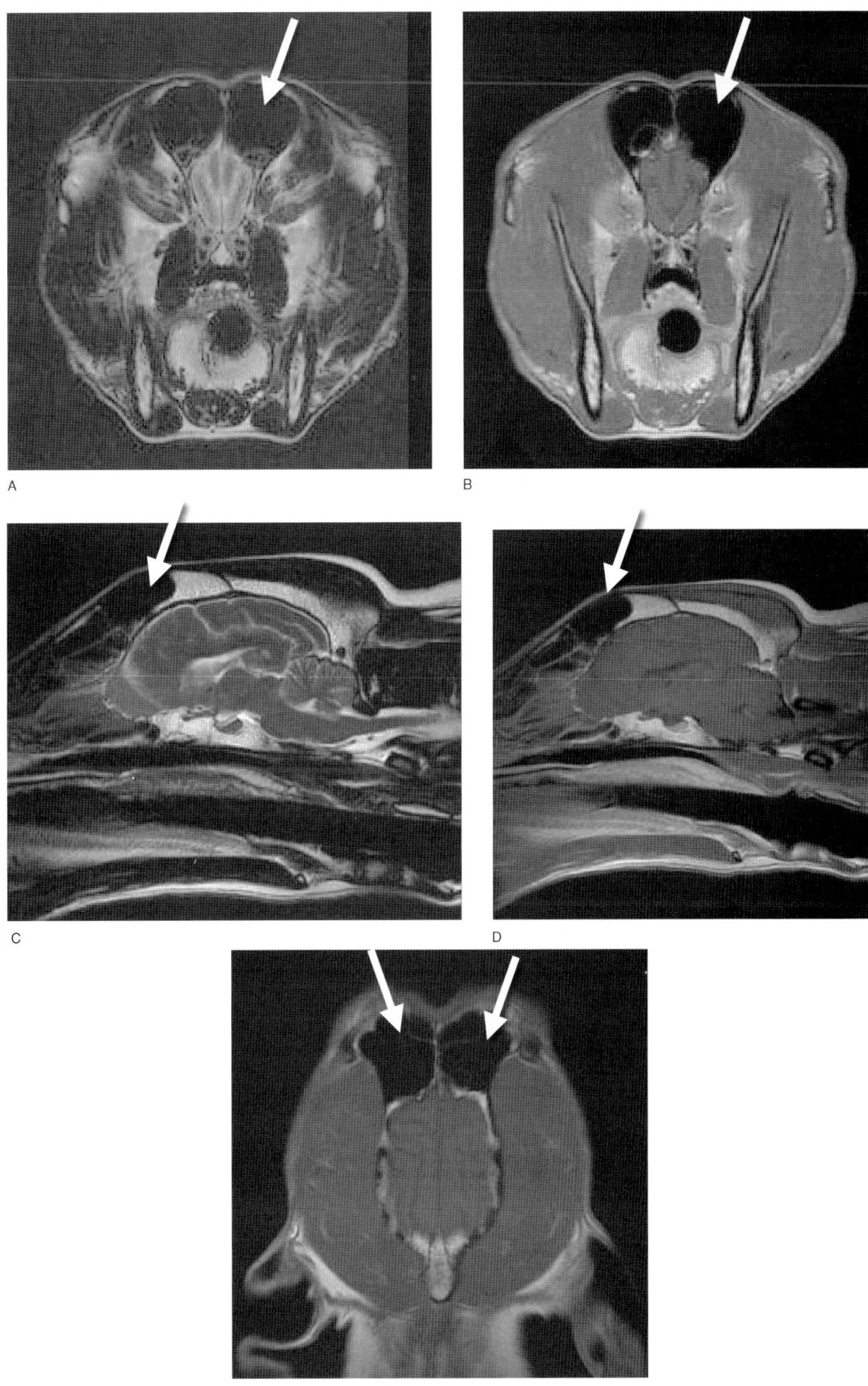

Figure 2.22. Transverse T2-weighted (A) and T1-weighted (B) MR images from a dog at the level of the frontal sinus. Note the hypointense signal from air in these cavities (arrows). Sagittal T2-weighted (C) and T1-weighted (D), and dorsal T1-weighted (E) MR images from a dog with an air-filled frontal sinus.

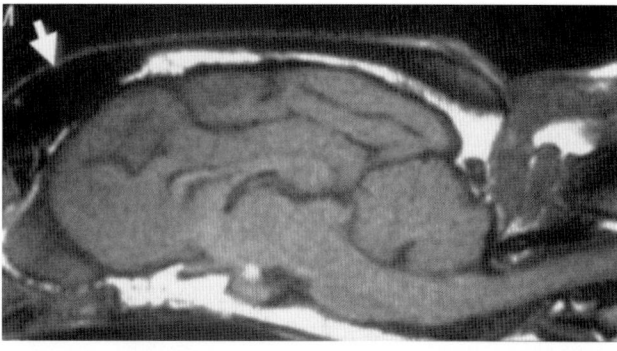

A

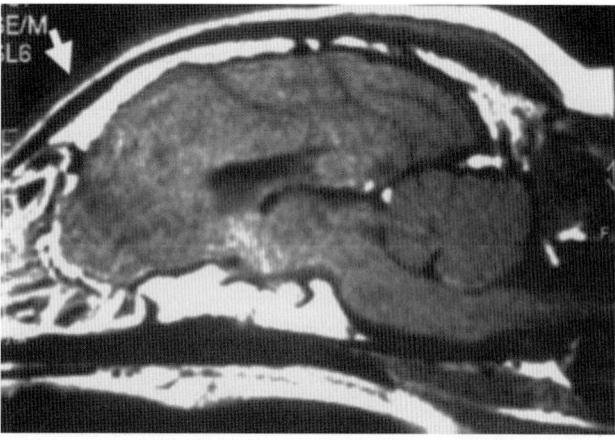

B

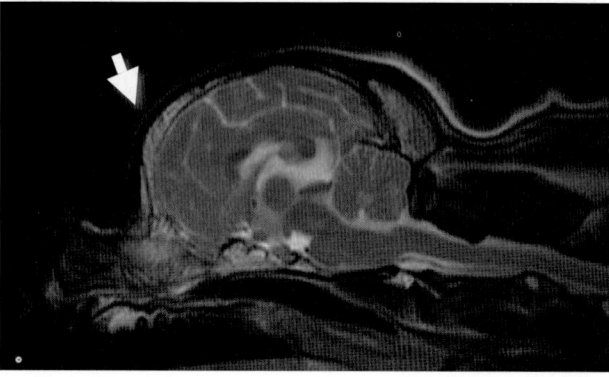

C

Figure 2.23. Sagittal T1-weighted MR images from two separate dogs, one with (A) and without (B) and air-filled frontal sinus. Sagittal T2-weighted MR image (C) from a brachycephalic dog breed without an air-filled frontal sinus (arrow).

system include the lateral ventricles, the third ventricle, the mesencephalic aqueduct, and the fourth ventricle. The lateral ventricles are somewhat C-shaped structures within the cerebral hemispheres. There is an extension of the lateral ventricle into the olfactory

bulb. The third ventricle is present in a circular pattern around the thalamus. The mesencephalic aqueduct is the relatively smaller connection between the third and fourth ventricle in the mesencephalon. The fourth ventricle is present between the brain stem (ventrally) and the cerebellum (dorsally). The fourth ventricle is continued into the spinal cord via the central canal. The ventricular system is lined by specialized columnar cells with microvilli known as ependymal cells. These cells are important as a partial barrier between the CSF and the brain parenchyma, and also play an important role in production of CSF. In some areas of the ventricular system, there are concentrations of a vascular structure and an associated ependymal lining known as the choroid plexus. This tissue also has an important role in CSF production, and pulsations in these structures may result in the movement of CSF.

CSF originates from the choroid plexus of the lateral, third, and fourth ventricles, directly from the brain by way of the ependymal lining of the ventricular system, directly from the brain by way of the pial–glial membrane covering the external surface, and from the blood vessels of the pia and arachnoid (deLahunta 1983). Flow of CSF is dependent on the pulsation of the blood (systole and diastole) in the choroid plexus. With each pulsation, CSF pressure increases aided by the cilia of the ependymal cells. CSF flow occurs in both directions (cranial and caudal), but primarily flows caudally in dogs. The pressure exhibited by the CSF contributes to intracranial pressure (ICP).

The major site of CSF absorption is in the arachnoid villus within a venous sinus or a cerebral vein (deLahunta 1983). The villus is a prolongation of the arachnoid and the subarachnoid space into the venous sinus. Collections of these villi are known as arachnoid granulations. The venous endothelium acts like a ball valve (from transient transcellular channels that develop for the passage of fluid) so as to be open when CSF pressure exceeds the venous pressure (the normal relationship). If venous pressure rises above CSF pressure, the villi will collapse. Directional flow, therefore, is always from CSF to blood.

Normal CSF has a relatively hypointense signal on T1 sequences and a relatively hyperintense signal in T2 images compared to surrounding neural elements. The ependymal lining of the ventricles is normally not apparent on both sequences, and is normally not enhanced following contrast administration. Normal choroid plexus, however, does contrast enhance following intravenous contrast administration.

The blood-CSF barrier exists at the choroid plexus and consists of two cell layers separated by a thin basement membrane. This is a semi-permeable

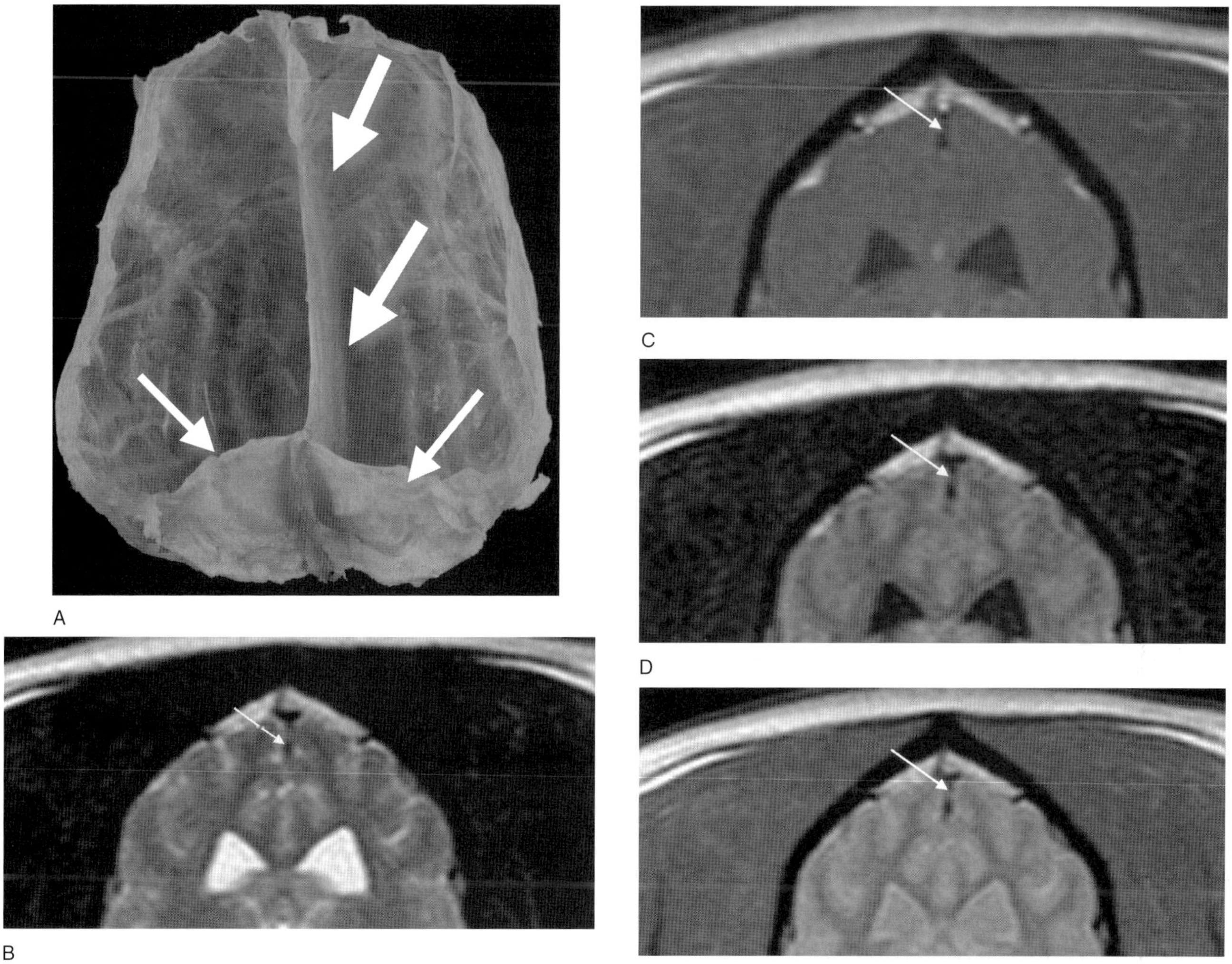

Figure 2.24. Pathologic specimen (ventral view (A)) of the dural meninges from a dog. The falx (larger arrows) and membranous tentorium cerebelli are shown (smaller arrows). (The top aspect of the photo is rostral.) Transverse T2-weighted (B), T1-weighted (C), FLAIR (D), and proton density (E) MR images of a dog's brain. The falx cerebri is shown by the arrow.

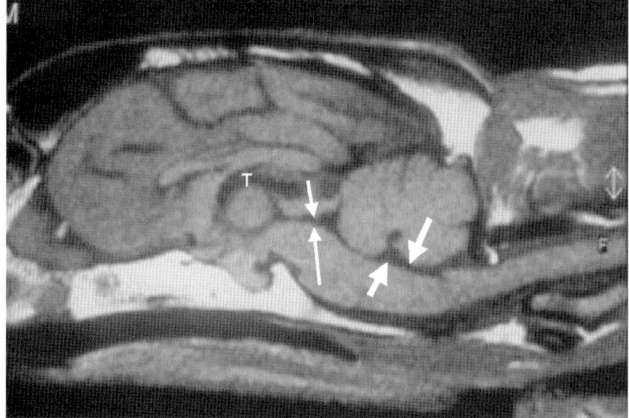

Figure 2.25. Sagittal T1-weighted MR image from a dog. The third (T), mesencephalic aqueduct (smaller arrows), and the fourth ventricle (larger arrows) are shown.

membrane between the CSF and the plasma. The CSF-extracellular fluid (ECF) barrier occurs over the outer surface of the brain and in the ventricles. This barrier is formed primarily by the ependymal cells. On the surface of the brain, a pial–glial membrane is present to limit exchange from the CSF and the nervous system parenchyma.

Importantly, there is also a barrier between the vascular system and the brain parenchyma, termed the "blood brain barrier" (BBB). This barrier exists between the plasma and the ECF and consists of non-fenestrated, tightly joined endothelial cells of the blood vessel, surrounded by a relatively complete layer of astrocyte foot processes. The BBB plays an important role in preventing the free exchange of various substances within the vascular system and brain cells.

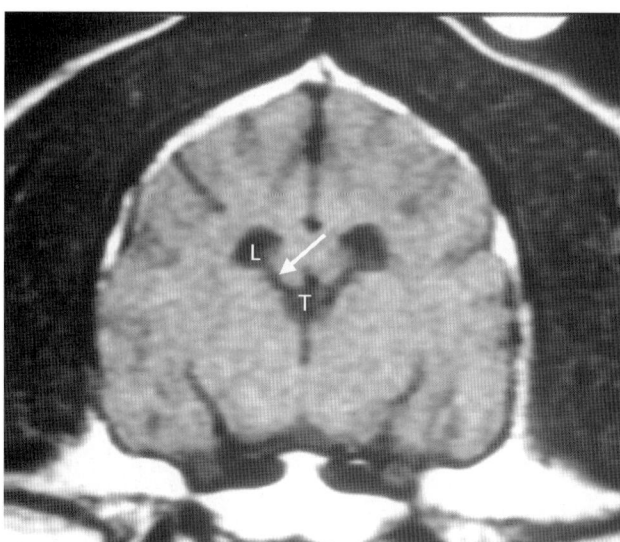

Figure 2.26. Transverse T1-weighted MR image from a dog at the level of the thalamus. The interventricular foramen (arrows) is shown between the lateral (L) and the third (T), ventricle.

Intracranial Blood Flow

Blood flows to the brain from the heart, aorta, brachiocephalic trunk, and carotid arteries. There are species differences in the anatomical arrangement of vessels responsible for cerebral perfusion from the carotid level. In dogs, blood flows into the circle of Willis from the internal carotid artery (deLahunta 1983; King 1987). In cats, the internal carotid artery is apparently non existent shortly following birth, and blood is directed from the external carotid artery through the maxillary artery to the ventral arterial system (King 1987).

The circle of Willis supplies the majority of arterial blood flow to the cerebral cortex. Blood also reaches the caudal brain stem from the subclavian arteries via the vertebral arteries and ultimately the basilar artery. In cats, blood flow has been suggested to be reversed in the basilar artery and the majority of the blood supply to the intracranial nervous system results from blood flow from the maxillary artery (King 1987). This reversed blood flow in the basilar artery in cats, however, is debatable.

Flowing blood in cerebral vessels that are large enough to be seen can have a variety of appearances based on flow characteristics. Blood in the dorsal sagittal sinus is most often hypointense on T1 and T2 sequences, however the region of the cavernous sinus is often hyperintense on T2 sequences (Figure 2.27).

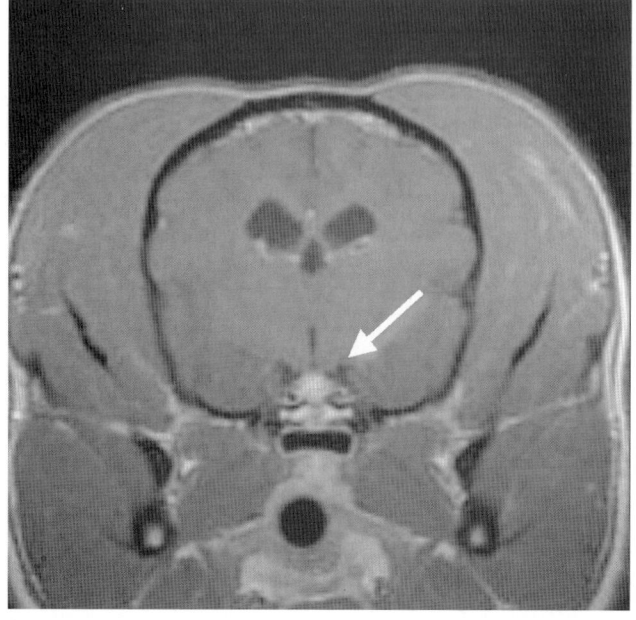
A

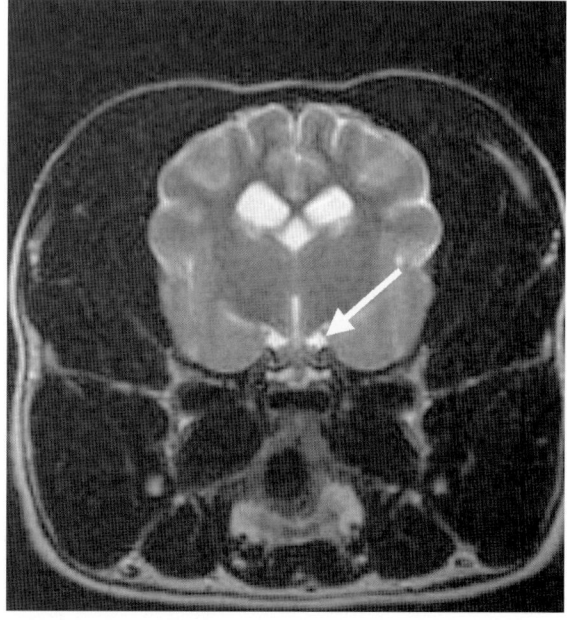
B

Figure 2.27. Transverse T1-weighted following intravenous contrast administration (A) and T2-weighted (B) MR images from a dog at the level of the thalamus. The cavernous sinus region (arrows) is relatively hypointense in the T1-weighted image, and relatively hyperintense in the T2-weighted image.

IMPORTANT AND DEFINABLE LANDMARKS

It only takes a comparison of a standard brain atlas or anatomical textbook brain views to determine that appearance of the intracranial nervous system structures as imaged with MR (using magnetic strengths commonly employed for diagnostic imaging) is not as distinct as with pathologically prepared specimens. It is also apparent that most brain atlas publications are taken from a single individual, whereas the spectrum of anatomical nuances between individuals may be relatively large. In pathologically prepared specimens, only the surface of the specimen is viewed, whereas, with clinical MR imaging the appearance is based on the magnetic properties of all the tissues contained within the slice thickness. Therefore, when imaging anatomical diverse individuals, it is not unreasonable to expect some individual "normal" anatomic variations. In some instances these "normal" variations in anatomy occur without apparent associated clinical consequences, whereas in other instances, it has not been established whether these normal anatomical variants have clinical effects (such as seizure activity).

As an example of normal anatomical diversity, the cortical gyral and sulcal patterns of individual dogs may vary so as that individual gyri or sulci may differ in size, shape, location, or may not even exist at all. In addition, Boxers, for example, have a very characteristic "pointed" appearance to their cortex that is easily identifiable. (Figure 2.28). It is important for the evaluator of an individual MR study to become familiar with these various anatomical differences so as to avoid overidentification of these "normal" variations.

While some anatomical differences in appearance of the intracranial nervous system structures when viewed with MR are "real," other differences of appearance are the result of variation in animal positioning in the MR scanner or the result of differences in slice plane angulation (Figures 2.29 and 2.30). Again, the evaluator of individual studies needs to be aware of how animal positioning and slice plane selection influence the "normal" anatomical appearance of an individual patient.

Even with these limitations, some more consistently appearing anatomical structures can be used as anatomical landmarks to aid in localization within the intracranial nervous system. For example, the colliculi (rostral and caudal) and the mesencephalic aqueduct have a reasonably standard anatomical appearance in MR studies of dogs and can be used to identify this region of the intracranial nervous system.

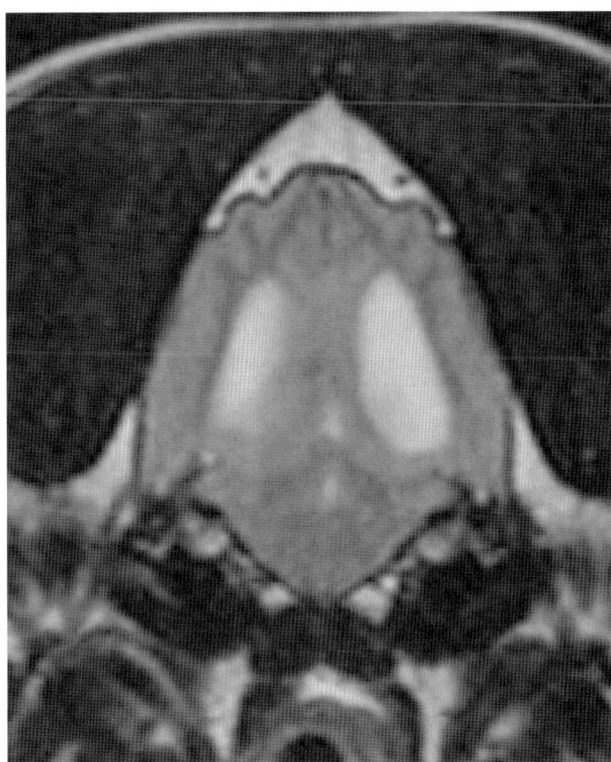

Figure 2.28. Transverse T2-weighted MR image from a boxer dog.

Identification of individual CNs has been somewhat more troublesome, as not all nerves are actually "seen" and the course of the CNs may be varied, traveling in various directions relative to the slice plane. Therefore, normal CNs may be imaged in a variety of transverse or sagittal planes throughout their normal course. While some portions of the nerve may be apparent, the location for where many of the CNs are located is often merely inferred (Figures 2.18–2.20). In some instances normal intracranial structures may be confused for CNs (Figures 2.31 and 2.32).

As many of the CNs enter, exit, or travel ventral and or lateral to the brain stem region, the appearance of many of the CNs may be influenced and even obscured by the associated vascular and other non-neural anatomical elements. For example, the cavernous sinus is a venous vascular structure that surrounds the pituitary region, and in which or immediately adjacent to a number of the CNs travel (Figure 2.27). This structure often appears hyperintense on T2-weighted sequences and hypointense on T1-weighted sequences. Normal CNs associated with this sinus are often not detectable until they become pathologically enlarged.

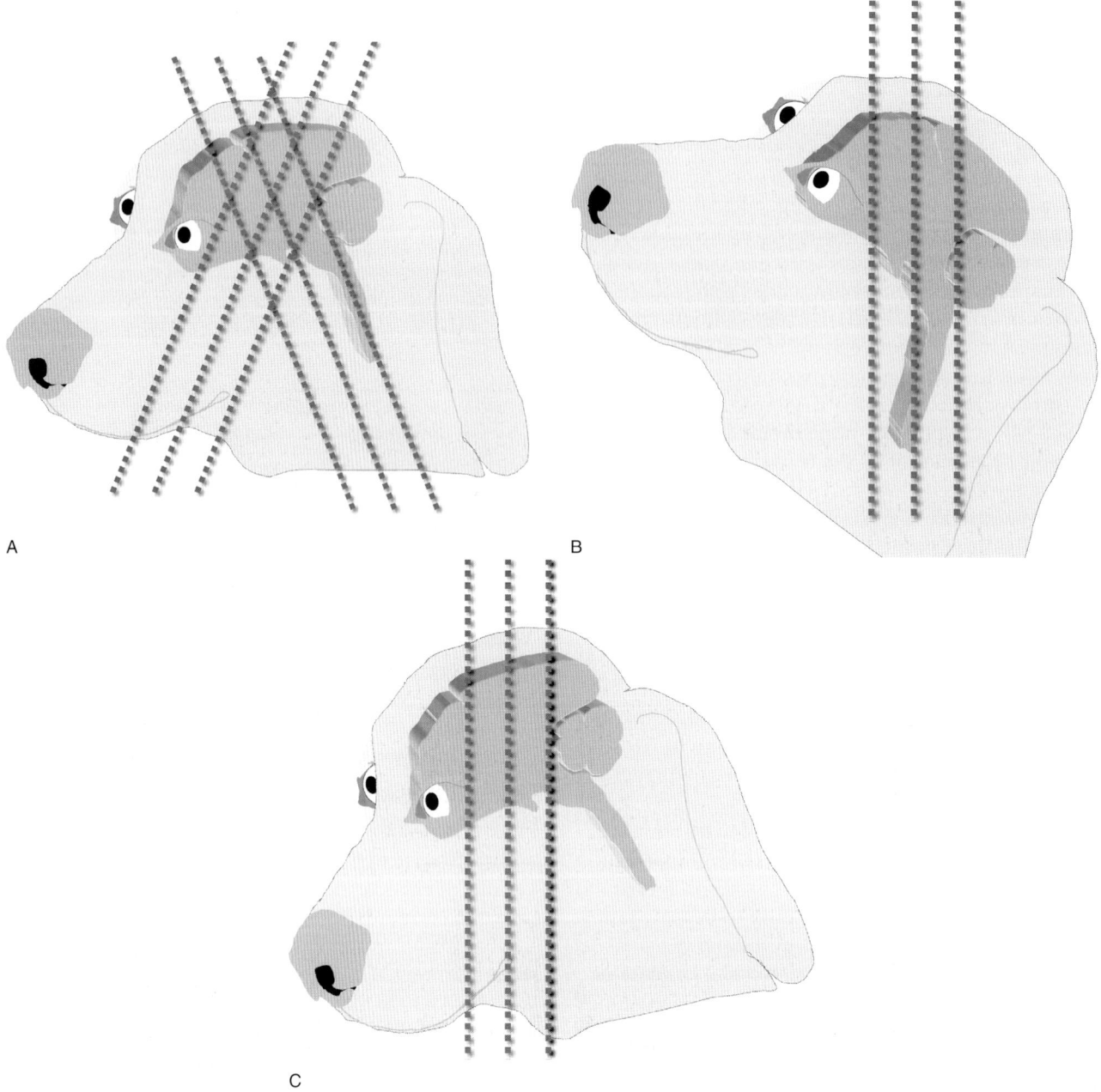

Figure 2.29. (A) Schematic relationship of direction of slice plane. (B), (C) Schematic representation of possible effects on anatomical images of differing animal head positions within the MR gantry.

DIAGNOSIS OF PATHOPHYSIOLOGICAL CONDITIONS OF THE INTRACRANIAL NERVOUS SYSTEM

Intracranial disease can alter normal physiological relationships in numerous ways. These include, but are not limited to, physical invasion and/or destruction of neurons, metabolic alterations in neuronal or glial cells, impairment of vascular supply to normal tissue (ischemia or hypoxia), impairment of autoregulation, hemorrhage, irritation (seizure generation), obstruction of the ventricular system, edema formation, production of physiologically active substances, and increased ICP (Bagley 1996b). These processes may initiate and perpetuate each other. Regardless of the pathophysiologic effects, intracranial disease that results in structure

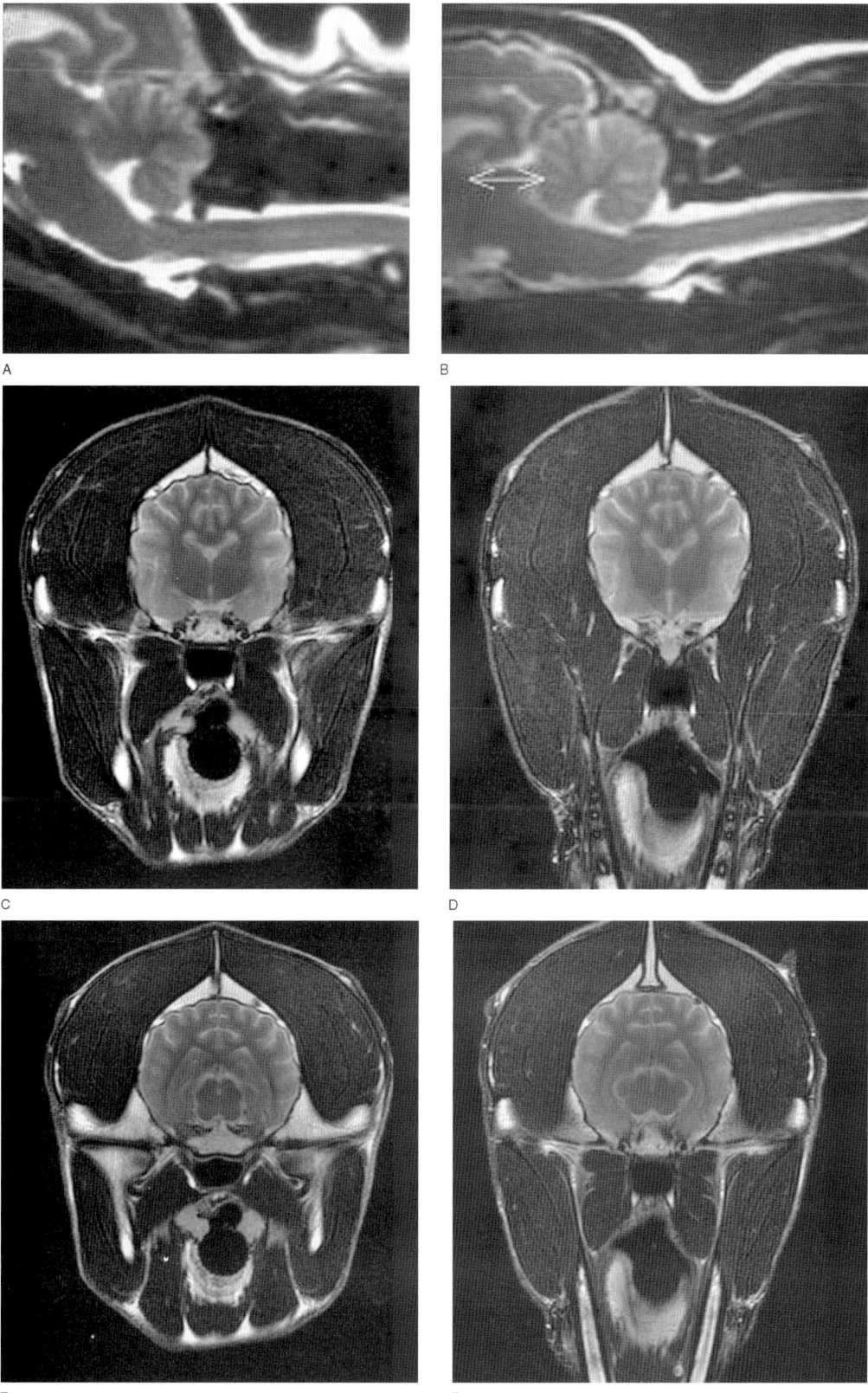

Figure 2.30. (A), (B) Sagittal T2-weighted MR images from two dogs positioned differently at the time of MR imaging. (C), (D) Transverse T2-weighted MR images from the same dog at the level of the thalamus at slightly differing transverse plane angulations. Note the subtle alteration in the appearance of the anatomical structures. (E), (F) Transverse T2-weighted MR images from the same dog at the level of the mesencephalon at slightly differing transverse plane angulations. Note the subtle alteration in the appearance of the anatomical structures. In (F) the caudal aspects of the geniculate bodies are more obvious.

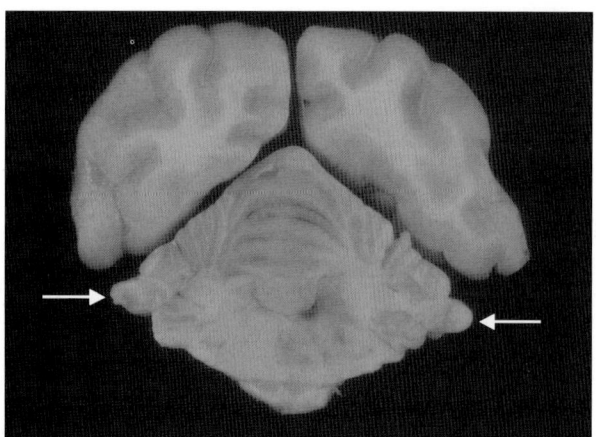

Figure 2.31. Transverse anatomical specimen of a dog's brain showing the lateral extension of the cerebellum (arrows) (flocculus or paraflocculus) that is often confused on MR interpretations with either the seventh or eighth CNs.

alterations can add to the overall volume of a component of the intracranial tissues. This additional volume can subsequently expand or displace normal anatomy. This distortion of anatomy is often referred to as "mass effect," and is common with many intracranial structural anatomical alterations (Figure 2.33).

CEREBRAL EDEMA

Many intracranial diseases result in, or are associated with, brain edema. With acute injury, brain edema becomes maximal between 24 and 48 h after injury, but

may persist for a week or more (Figure 2.33). Brain edema has been categorized as either vasogenic, cytotoxic, or interstitial based upon cause and anatomic areas of involvement (Fishman 1975; Reulen 1976). Any or all of these types of edema may be present in an animal with brain disease.

Cytotoxic edema (intracellular edema) results from failure of cellular energy with resultant failure to extrude sodium from within the cell. Intracellular water increases and cells swell. This edema most often results in disease processes such as toxicity, ischemia, or hypoxia.

Interstitial edema is increased water content of the periventricular white matter due to movement of CSF across the ventricular walls in instances of hydrocephalus. Periventricular white matter is reduced due to the disappearance of myelin lipids secondary to increases in white matter hydrostatic pressure or decreases in periventricular white matter blood flow (Rosenberg et al. 1983).

Vasogenic edema is the most common form of edema associated with CNS neoplasia. This type of edema results from vascular injury secondary to physical disruption of the vascular endothelium or functional alterations in endothelial tight junctions. Differences in transmural pressure gradients result in extravasation of fluid from cerebral vessels to the ECF spaces of the brain (Rosenberg et al. 1983). These abnormalities allow for fluid to move from the vascular to perivascular spaces. Areas of the brain where ECF is normally enlarged provide a natural conduit for fluid movement. Increases in intravascular pressure due to loss of autoregulation, vascular obstruction, or hypertension

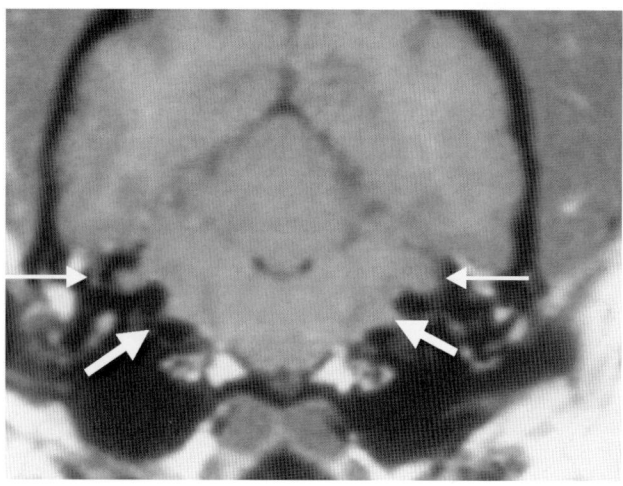
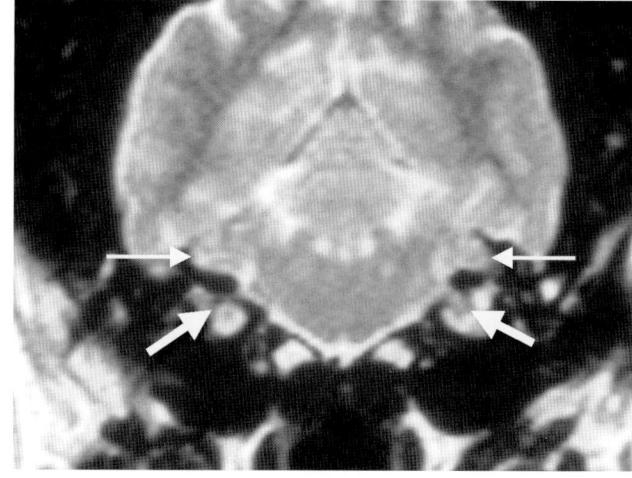

A B

Figure 2.32. Transverse T1-weighted (A) and T2-weighted (B) MR images from a normal dog showing the distinction between the lateral extension of the cerebellum (smaller arrows) and the eighth CN (larger arrows).

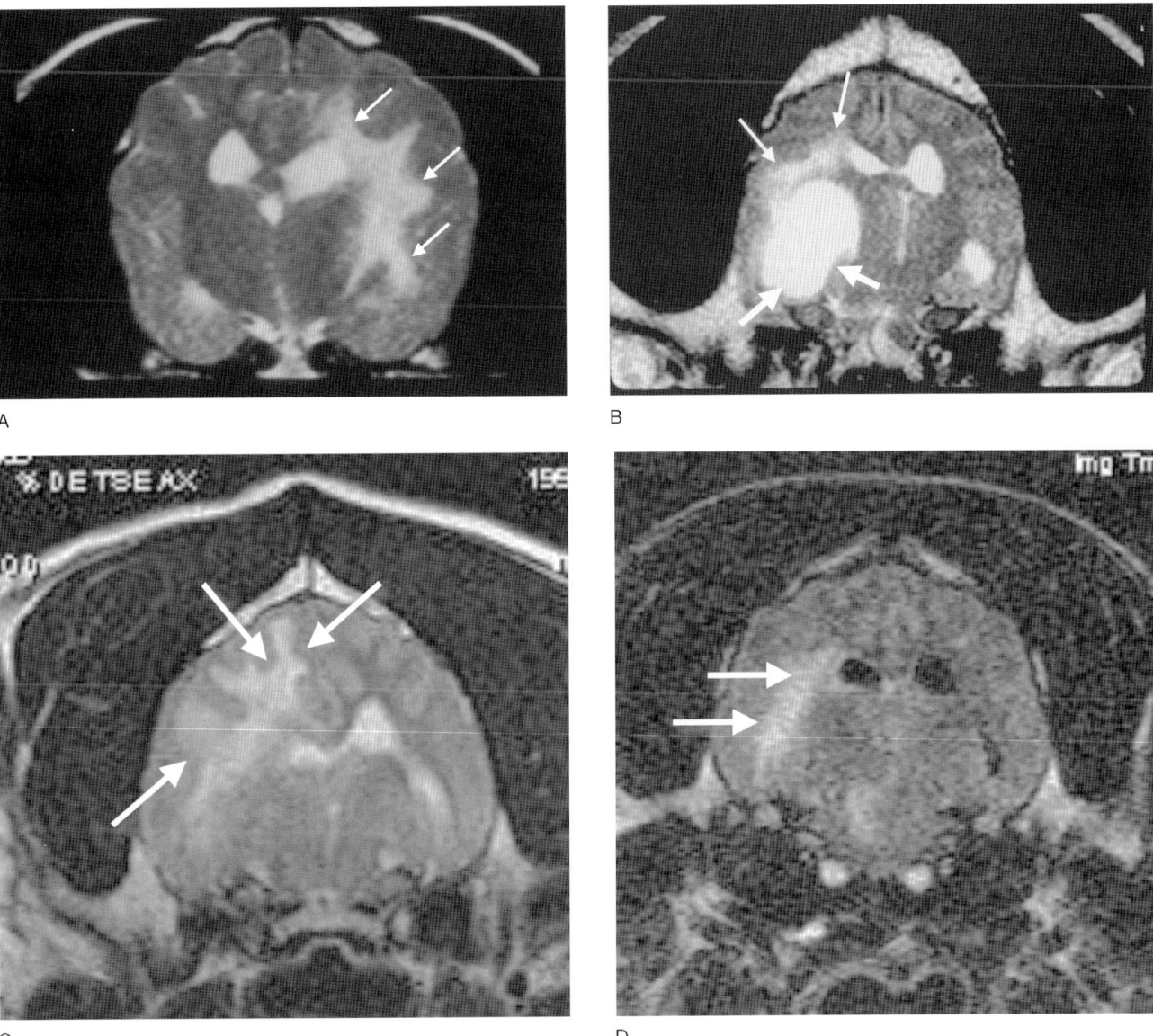

Figure 2.33. Transverse T2-weighted (A) MR image at the level of the thalamus in a dog showing edema and mass effect (arrows). Transverse T2-weighted (B) MR image at the level of the thalamus in a dog showing a glioma (larger arrows) and associated edema and mass effect (smaller arrows). Transverse T2-weighted (C) and FLAIR (D) MR images at the level of the thalamus in a dog showing edema and mass effect (arrows). Edema persists as a hyperintense signal in the FLAIR image (arrows).

(Cushing's response, cerebral ischemic response) may perpetuate edema formation. Vasogenic edema migrates away from areas of vascular disruption via bulk flow. Fluid movement depends upon a balance between the opposing forces of capillary hydrostatic pressure and tissue resistance pressure. Vasogenic edema usually spreads readily through the white matter, possibly because of the orderly arrangement of nerve fibers found there. Also, the movement of this type of edema may be related to low capillary density and

blood flow in normal white matter. Deep white matter of the affected cerebral hemisphere is preferentially affected.

Edema, as a general rule, appears hypointense relative to neural parenchyma on T1 sequences, and hyperintense relative to neural parenchyma on T2 sequences. It has been suggested that vasogenic edema tends to travel long white matter which is why edema may outline the cerebral white matter of the corona radiate in some instances. This provides for a "crown-like" or spiked appearance of the edema within the cerebral white matter (Figure 2.33).

INTRACRANIAL VASCULAR DISEASE

Primary cerebrovascular disease is increasingly being identified in animals as a cause of acute intracranial deterioration. Diseases of the cerebral vasculature may result from excessive blood flow through cerebral vessels (hypertension), transmural extravasation of blood, ischemia, thrombosis, and embolization. Hypertension, associated with a variety of diseases in animals such as renal disease and hyperadrenocorticism, can result in increases in cerebrovascular hydrostatic forces leading to intracranial hemorrhages. Disorders of coagulation (coagulopathies, DIC) and platelet function (thrombocytopenia and thrombopathies) can also result in cerebral hemorrhage. Diseases that predispose one to hypercoagulability, such as glomerulonephritis, may result in intramural emboli and subsequent thrombosis of cerebral vessels. Bacteremias (endocarditis) may result in septic embolization of intracranial vessels. Vessel wall integrity can be disrupted by neoplastic infiltration or inflammatory diseases, including vasculitis syndromes, and can result in thrombosis and hemorrhage. Less commonly, arteriovenous malformations and aneurysms have been reported in dogs. All of these intracranial vascular abnormalities may predispose one to cerebral hypoxia and ischemia, as well as intracranial hemorrhage.

Cerebrovascular disease primarily results in ischemia, infarction, and hemorrhage (Figures 2.34–2.43). Other secondary consequences include edema formation, mass effect, and increases in ICP. Ischemic damage, regardless of cause, results in endothelial cell damage predisposing to thrombosis, necrosis, and hemorrhage. One of the most devastating effects of severe intracranial vascular disease is intracranial hemorrhage. Hemorrhage into and around the brain can result in an associated inflammatory reaction, increases in overall intracranial volume, and increases in ICP. Intraventricular and subarachnoid bleeding is irritating to local nervous tissue and may result in inflammation (meningitis, myelitis, or encephalitis). If bleeding is substantial enough hematomas may subsequently form, altering CNS volume/pressure relationships and potentially increasing ICP and decreasing cerebral blood flow. While the initial hematoma will create a certain degree of pressure, clinical signs may worsen as the hematoma is resorbed ("ages"). This was originally thought to result from the hyperosmolar environment of the resorbing hematoma increasing the movement of fluid (water) into the hematoma, actually increasing its volume; however, this is not always found. Increasing hematoma volume may ultimately cause worsening clinical signs as compared to those associated with the initial hemorrhagic event.

Intracranial hemorrhage can have some of the most variable MR imaging appearances of any pathologic alteration. The MR appearance of hemorrhage will depend on the time frame of when the hemorrhage occurred relative to when the animal was imaged, the field strength of the magnet, the imaging sequences obtained, the oxygen content of the blood (arterial vs. venous), and the location of the hemorrhage (parenchymal vs. extradural vs. subdural). In some instances an obvious fluid line interface can be present. Simplistic guidelines for interpretation of hemorrhage have been established (Table 2.1); however, the spectrum of appearance of hemorrhage is much more complex.

With MR, hemorrhage less than 12–24 h old will not be differentiated from vasogenic edema. In the circulating blood, hemoglobin alternates between the oxyhemoglobin state and the deoxyhemoglobin state. The heme iron in both oxy and deoxy is in the ferrous (Fe^{2+}) state. When hemoglobin is removed from the high-oxygen environment of the circulation, the heme iron undergoes oxidative denaturation to the ferric state ($Fe3+$), forming methemoglobin. Continued oxidative denaturation forms ferric hemochromes (hemosiderin). As red blood cells (RBCs) break down, the various forms of hemoglobin have changing paramagnetic properties influencing the appearance of the clot in the various images (T1- and T2-weighted). The appearance of the varying stages of hemorrhage also depends upon the strength of the magnet. Table 2.1 is a rough guide to the appearance of parenchymal hematomas imaged with a 1.5 T MR system.

The use of gradient echo imaging helps identify hemorrhage due to the magnetic susceptibility artifact of the iron concentration. The signal intensity will be hypointense with a "blooming" or artifactual enlargement of the hemorrhagic area.

SEIZURES

Seizure activity is a common sequelae to intracranial disease. Seizure activity may result in anatomical changes in intracranial nervous elements. Often, there are associated focal (possibly coalescing) hyperintense

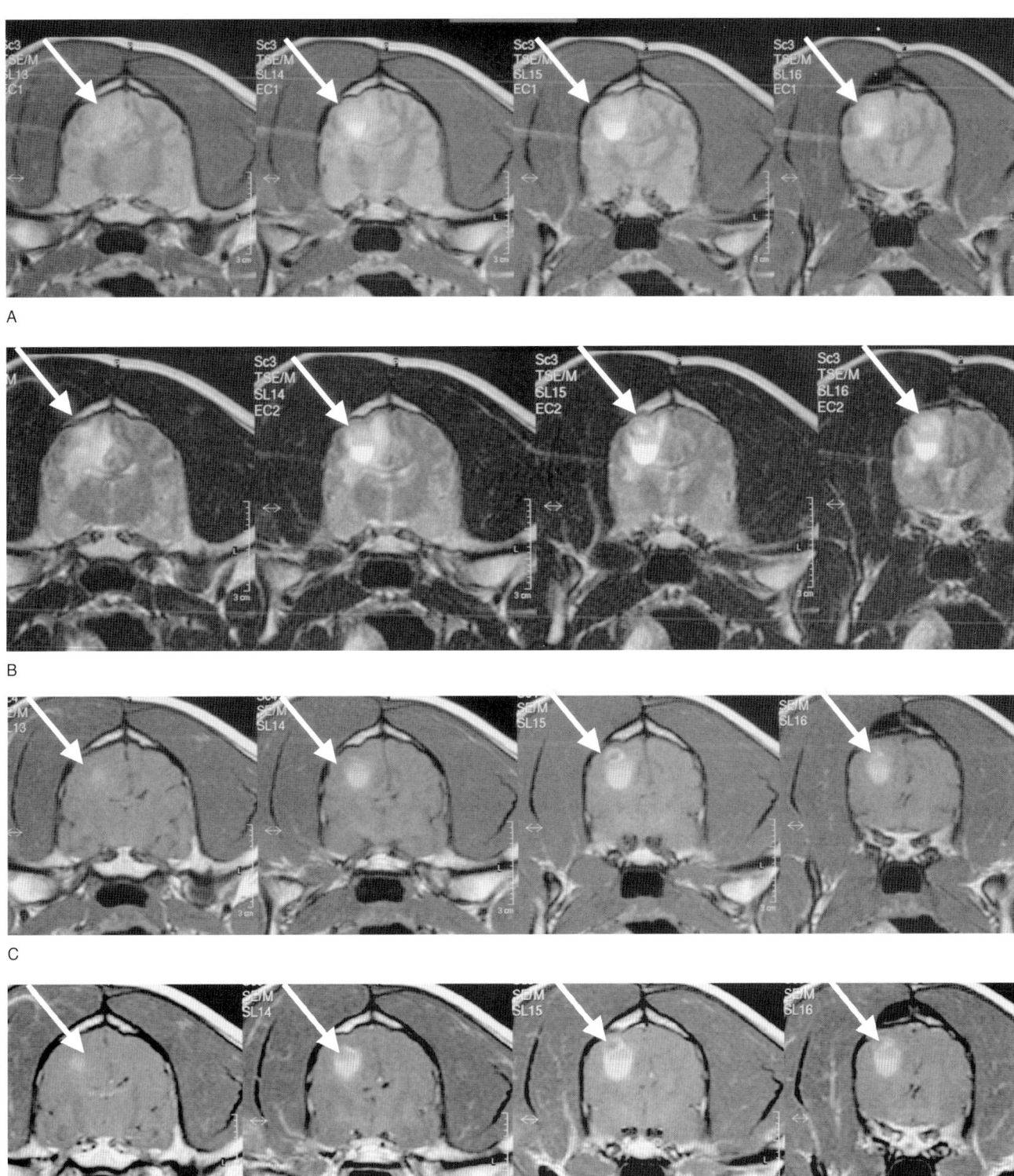

Figure 2.34.   Transverse proton density (A), T2-weighted (B), T1-weighted before (C), and following intravenous contrast administration (D) MR images from a dog with an intracranial hematoma (arrows).

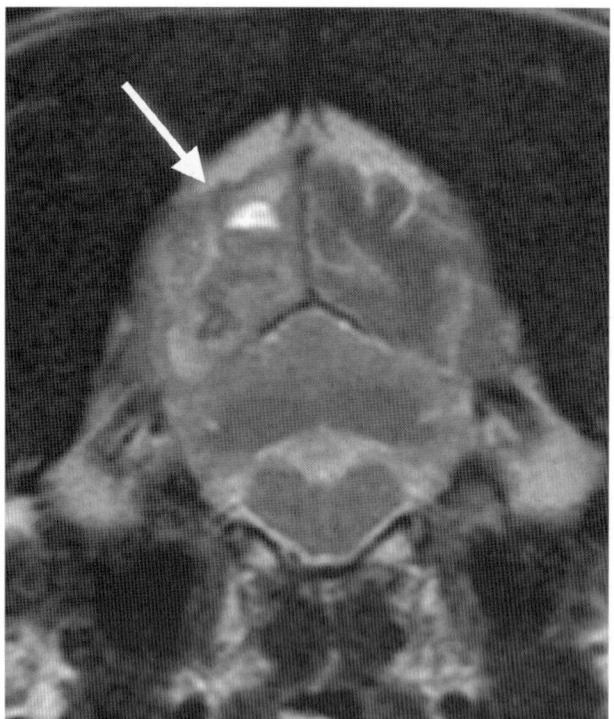

A

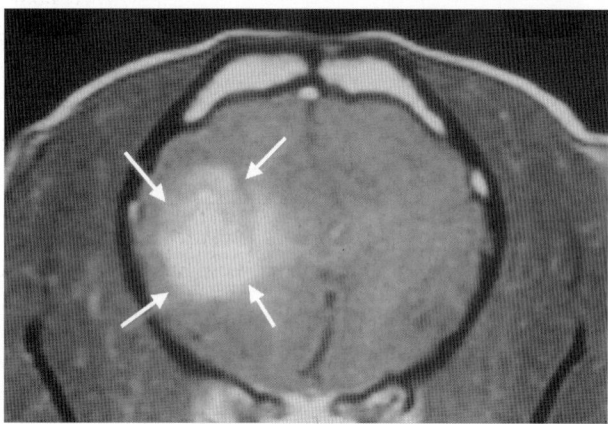

B

Figure 2.35. Transverse T2-weighted (A) and T1-weighted (B) before contrast administration MR images from two dogs with intracranial hematomas (arrows).

regions on T2 sequences following seizure activity (Figure 2.44). The exact nature of the pathologic changes in these regions is not known; however, these changes may represent focal edema, vascular change, neurotransmitter accumulation, or some other chemical change. These regions of abnormal signal may resolve in the days or weeks following seizures. These abnormalities are usually more obvious if seizures are prolonged or frequent over a shorter time span. With chronic seizure activity, permanent anatomical changes

may result in neural tissues that may be apparent on MR imaging sequences.

VENTRICULAR OBSTRUCTION (ALSO SEE SECTION "HYDROCEPHALUS" IN THIS CHAPTER)

Hydrocephalus can result from obstruction of the ventricular system, irritation of the ventricle (from inflammation or hemorrhage), increased size of the ventricles due to loss of brain parenchyma (hydrocephalus ex vacuo), be present without an obvious cause (congenital), or rarely, be the result of overproduction of CSF associated with a choroid plexus tumor. Ventricular obstruction can occur due to intraventricular or extraventricular obstruction.

With most T1-weighted sequences, normal CSF will be hypointense relative to neural and specifically cortical elements. With T2 sequences, normal CSF will appear hyperintense. With FLAIR sequences (used to suppress signal from normal CSF), CSF will usually be black.

Ventricular size, however, is difficult to quantitate. As a general rule, T2 sequences may slightly overrepresent ventricular size. Additionally, ventricular size does not consistently correlate with clinical abnormalities. Therefore, apparently enlarged ventricles may not be associated with clinical dysfunction. Finally, ventricular size is not always correlated with intraventricular pressure, the latter of which is also an important cause of clinical dysfunction. In some instances, especially in the acute situation, intraventricular pressure may be pathologically elevated while ventricular size remains within normal limits. Occasionally, the contour of the ventricle can provide a clue to the associated intraventricular pressure.

Generalized ventricular enlargement suggests congenital ventricular dilation or obstruction at the level of the lateral apertures or foramen magnum, or diffuse parenchymal loss (Figures 2.45–2.47). Focal ventricular enlargement suggests focal obstruction or parenchymal cell loss. It is not uncommon to have bilateral lateral ventricle enlargement that is asymmetric. Animals with asymmetric appearance of the ventricles should be critically evaluated for focal obstruction of or impingement on the ventricular system due to mass effect. Hemorrhage into the ventricular system can occur with head trauma, hypertension, and bleeding disorders. Blood products are irritating to the ependyma, and result in associated inflammation.

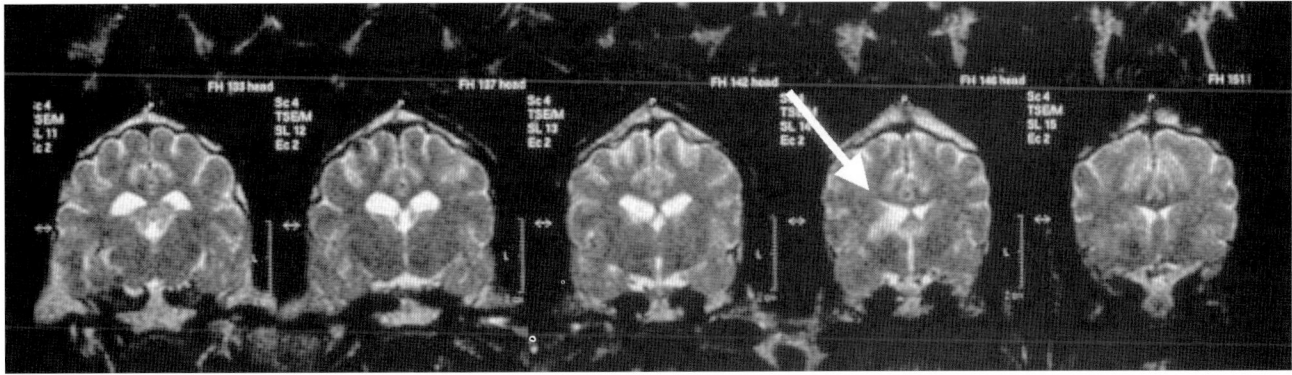

A

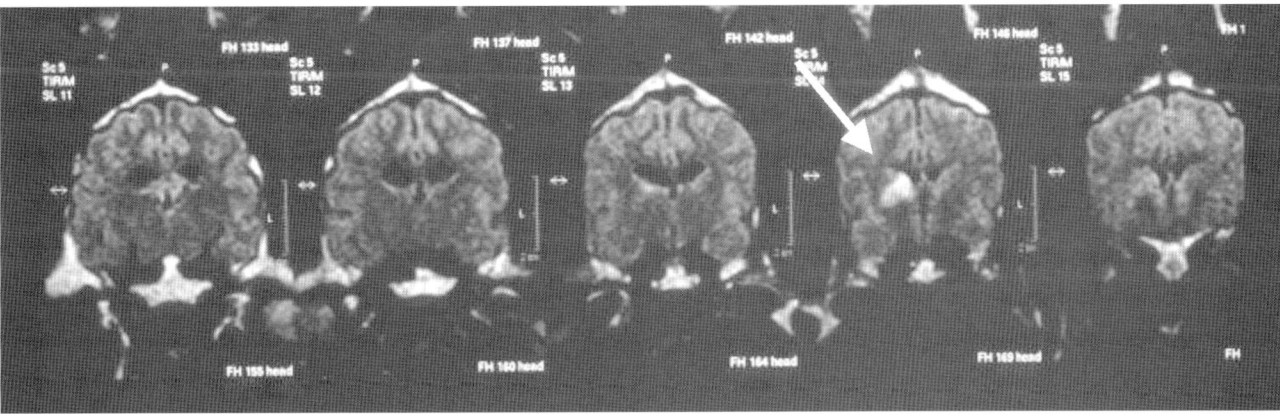

B

C

Figure 2.36. Transverse T2-weighted (A), proton density (B), and FLAIR (C) MR images from a dog with an intracranial infarction (arrows).

If the ventricular system is obstructed, CSF will be trapped behind the level of obstruction. This may also be referred to as a non-communicating hydrocephalus (deLahunta 1983). As some inadequate amounts of CSF may pass the level of the obstruction, this may not always be the most appropriate description of the pathophysiological state. CSF that is trapped in this way will often have significant elevations in protein content. This elevation of protein content may alter the appearance of

the CSF signal, more so on the FLAIR and T1 sequences. In these situations, the CSF signal can appear relatively hyperintense compared to the relatively hypointense normal CSF (Figures 2.45C and 2.47).

Anatomically smaller areas of the ventricular system are common sites of obstruction. These include the interventricular foramen and the mesencephalic aqueduct. Obstruction can result from tumor, granuloma, hemorrhage, or inflammation. Rarely, abnormalities of

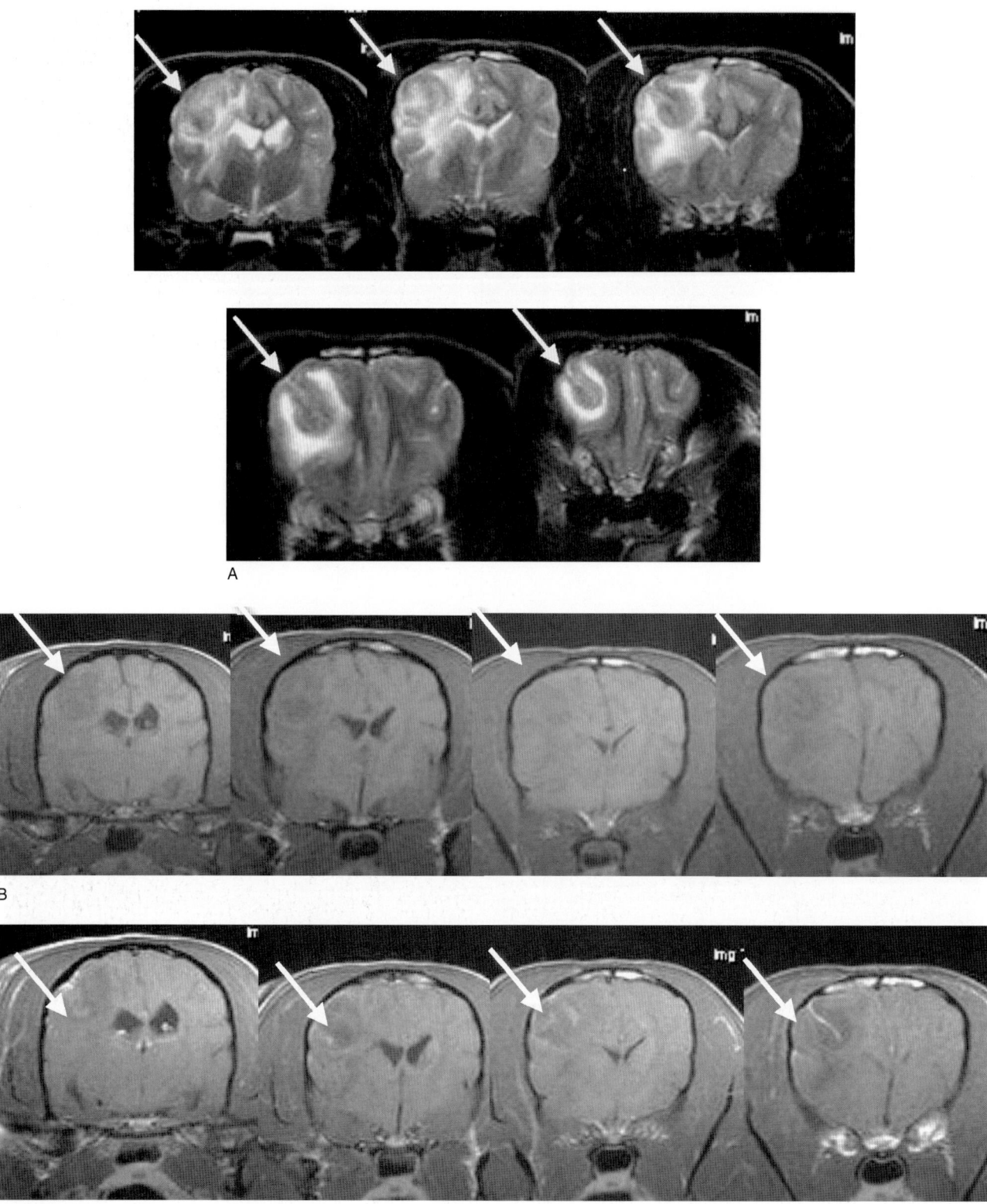

Figure 2.37. Transverse T2-weighted (A), T1-weighted before (B), and after (C) intravenous contrast administration MR images from a dog with acute intracranial infarction (arrows).

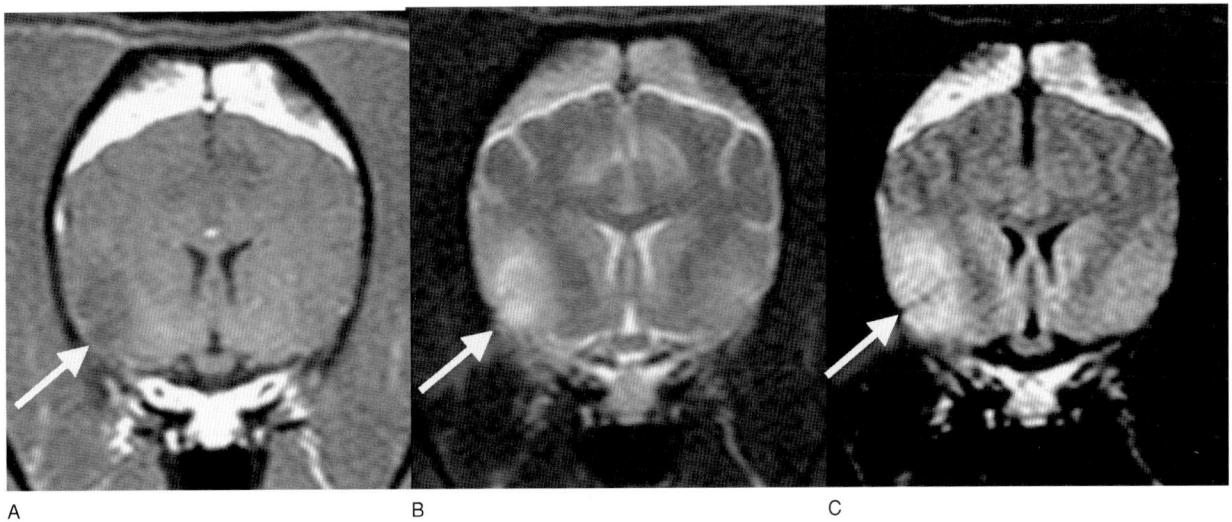

Figure 2.38. Transverse T1-weighted (A), T2-weighted (B), and FLAIR (C) MR images from a dog with intracranial infarction (arrows).

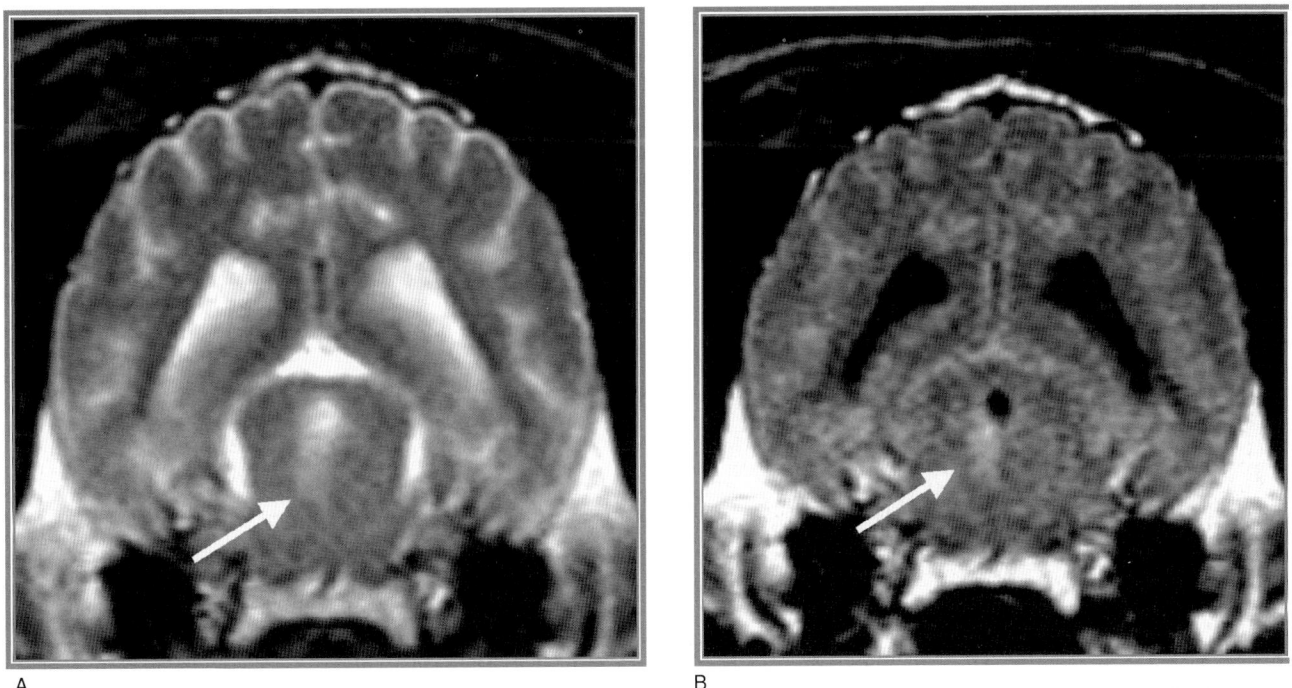

Figure 2.39. Transverse T2-weighted (A) and FLAIR (B) MR images from a dog with acute intracranial infarction (arrows).

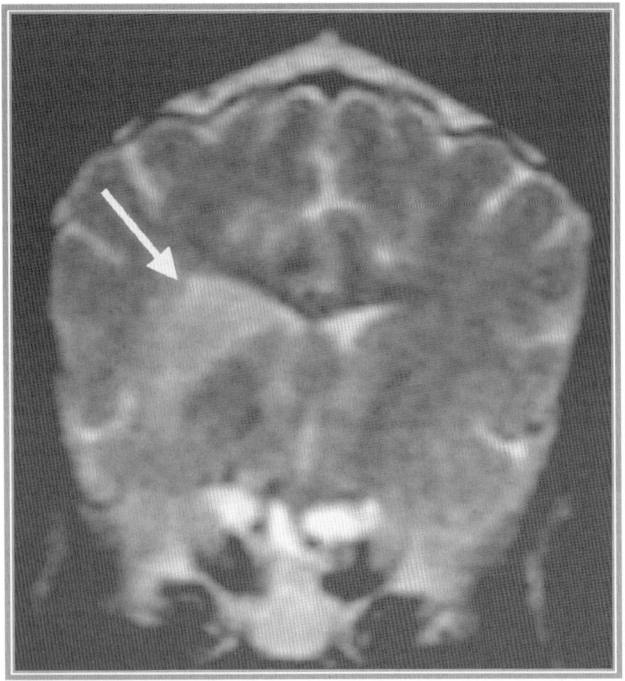
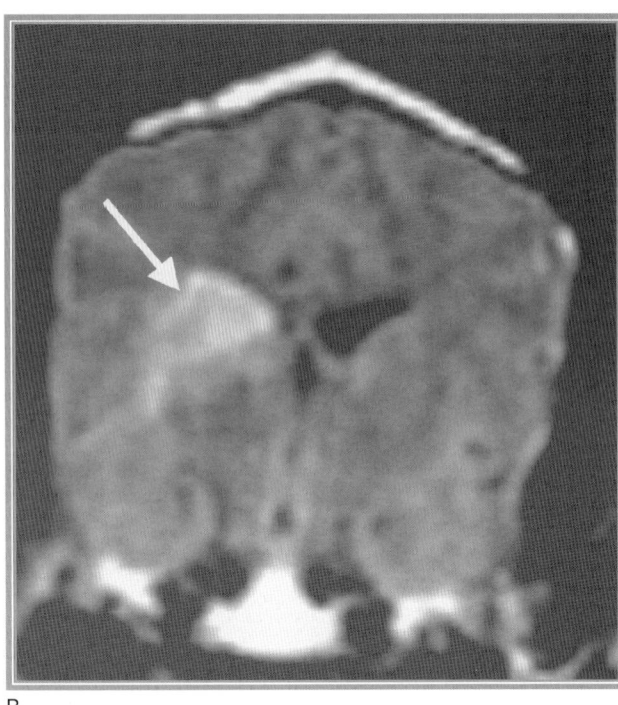

A   B

Figure 2.40.   Transverse T2-weighted (A) and FLAIR (B) MR images from a dog with acute intracranial infarction (arrows).

ependymal cilia function can result in ventricle dilation, probably due to poor or absent CSF flow; immotile cilia syndrome and Kartagener's syndrome are the examples.

Hydrocephalus can result in clinical signs due to loss of neurons or neuronal function, alterations in ICP, and associated pathophysiological effects of intracranial disease. Interstitial edema, for example, is increased water content of the periventricular white matter due to movement of CSF across the ventricular walls in instances of hydrocephalus. Periventricular white matter is reduced due to the disappearance of myelin lipids secondary to increases in white matter hydrostatic pressure or decreases in periventricular white matter blood flow. Increased CSF pressure may contribute to intracranial disease through alterations in ICP. The periventricular white matter may have a relatively hyperintense appearance in these instances. Additionally, when CSF is trapped in a region of the ventricle, the lining of the ependyma can be enhanced following intravenous contrast administration (Figure 2.47).

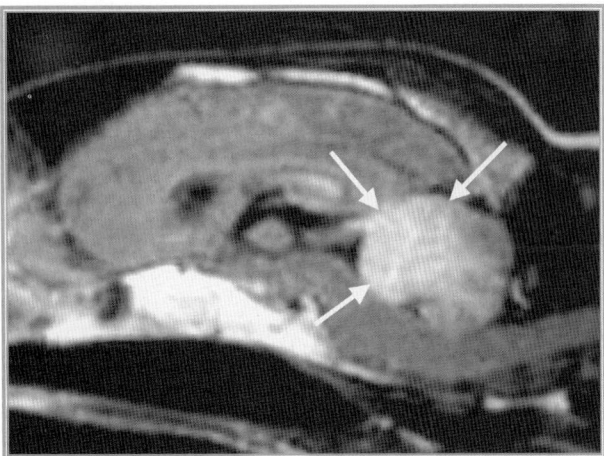

Figure 2.41.   Sagittal, FLAIR MR image from a dog with cerebellar infarction (arrows).

INCREASES IN INTRACRANIAL PRESSURE

Intracranial pressure (ICP) is the pressure exerted between the skull and the intracranial tissues. As the skull is relatively inelastic compared to the other intracranial tissues, ICP is determined primarily by changes in intracranial tissue volume and the compensatory ability of these tissues to accommodate for volume changes.

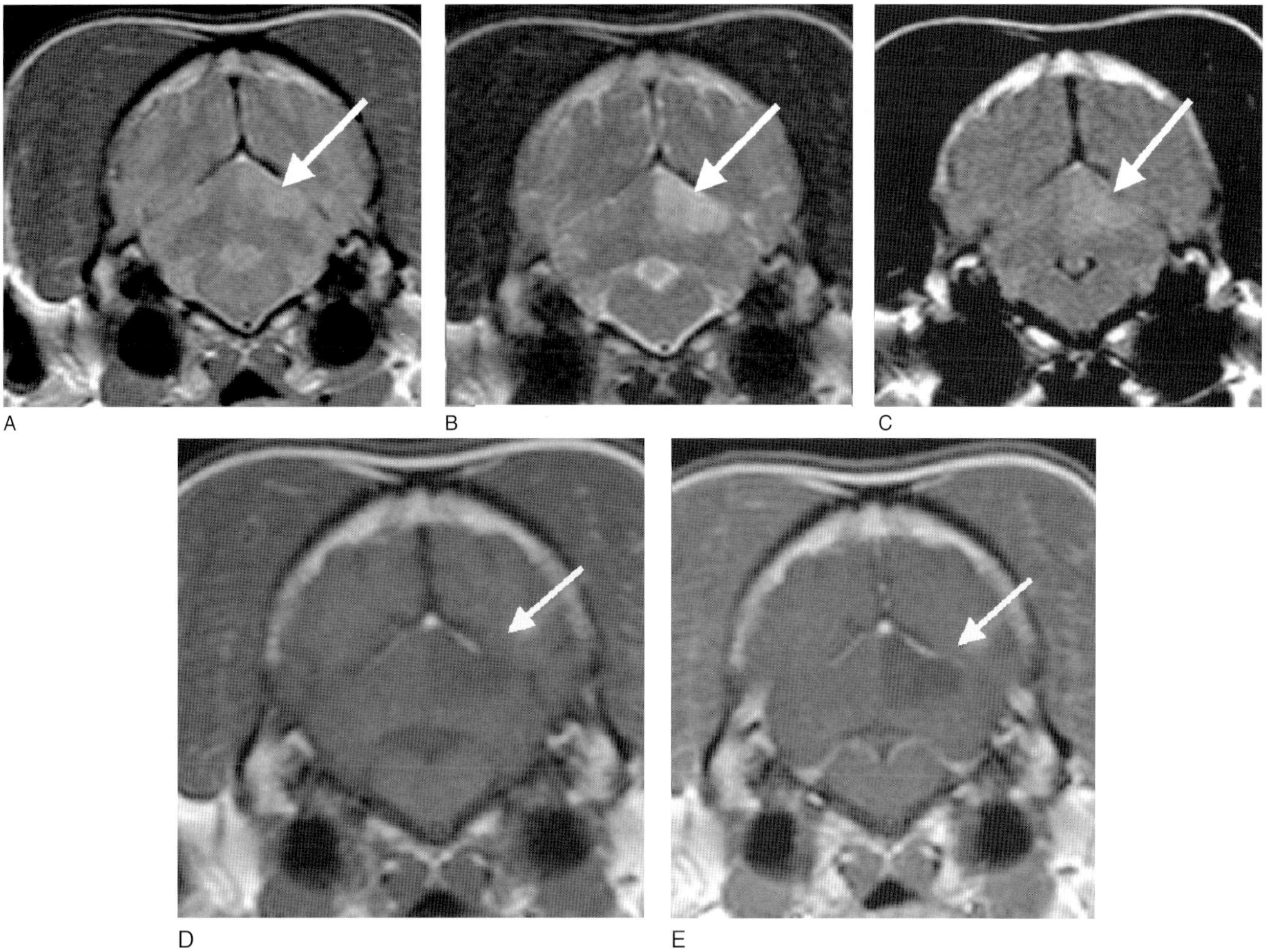

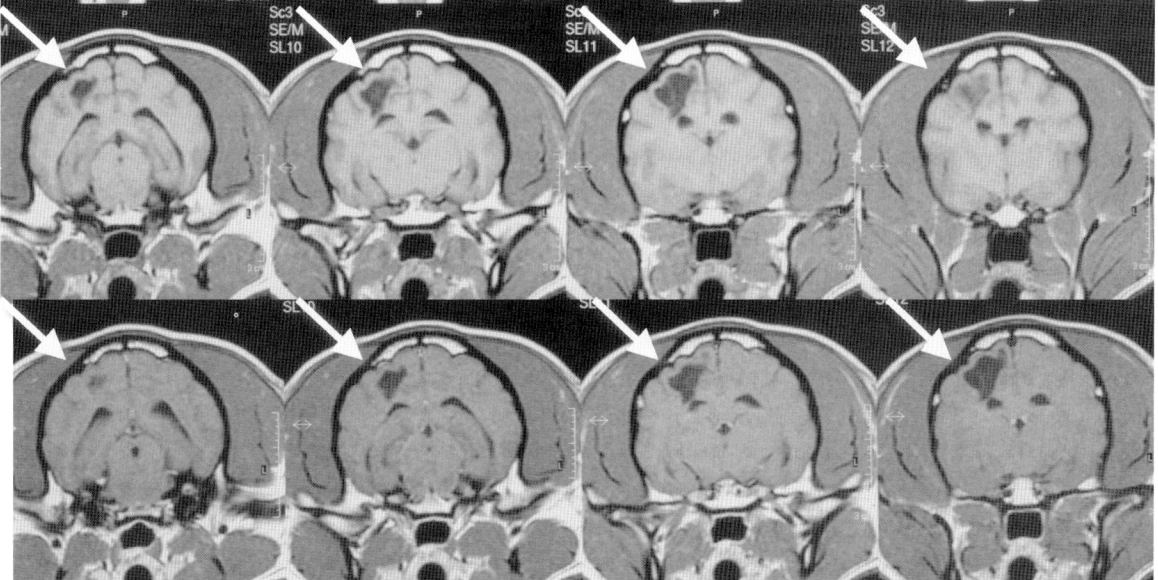

A   B   C

D   E

Figure 2.42.   Transverse proton density (A), T2-weighted (B), FLAIR (C), T1-weighted before (D), and following intravenous contrast administration (E) MR images from a dog with cerebellar infarction (arrows).

Figure 2.43.   Transverse T1-weighted MR images from a dog with chronic intracranial infarction and associated porencephaly (arrows).

Table 2.1.
Parenchymal hematoma[12]

Stage	Time	Hemoglobin	T1	T2
Hyperacute	<24 h	Intracellular Oxyhemoglobin	Hypo	Hyper
Acute–subacute	1–3 days	Intracellular Deoxyhemoglobin	Hyper	Hypo
Early	3+ days	Intracellular Methemoglobin	Hyper	Hypo
Late	7+ days	Extracellular Methemoglobin	Hyper	Hyper
Chronic	14+ days	Extracellular Hemichromes	Hypo	Hyper
		Intracellular Hemosiderin	Hypo	Hypo

Increases in ICP cannot be determined, per se, with standard MR imaging as this is a physiological rather than anatomical measurement. As ICP increases, the pressure within the intracranial space decreases cerebral blood flow. With decreased cerebral perfusion, neuronal ischemia, hypoxia, dysfunction, and ultimately neuronal death result. These pathologic changes may result in anatomical abnormalities in neural elements, and these anatomical abnormalities may result in abnormal appearances with MR imaging.

TERMINAL EFFECTS OF COMPARTMENTALIZED ICP INCREASES—BRAIN HERNIATION

As intracranial volume continues to increase beyond the limits of compensation, ICP may increase so precipitously that shifts of brain parenchyma, termed brain herniation, will occur (Kornegay et al. 1983). Coma and severe neurological impairment are noted. Unfortunately, in many instances, brain herniation becomes a terminal event.

Five major types of brain herniation have been described: rostral or caudal transtentorial, subfascial or cingulate gyrus, foramen magnum, and herniation through a craniotomy defect (Fishman 1975; Kornegay et al. 1983). Of these, caudal transtentorial, subfascial, and foramen magnum occur most commonly (Figures 2.45E and 2.48). Clinical signs of caudal transtentorial herniation are frequently the result of pressure distributed downward through the midbrain

with subsequent compression of the oculomotor nerve. With unilateral herniations, an ipsilateral dilated pupil, unresponsive to light stimulation, may be seen. Monitoring for clinical signs of this type of herniation, therefore, should include periodic pupillary evaluations. If unilateral mydriasis is noted in this setting, immediate and aggressive attempts to decrease ICP should be instituted.

Foramen magnum herniation may occur quickly and results in respiratory arrest due to associated pressure on the respiratory centers in the caudal brain stem. Foramen magnum herniation is often fatal, and surgical attempts at decompression after this type of herniation have not been helpful in affected dogs.

Herniation of intracranial tissues is usually readily apparent with MR imaging if the evaluator is familiar with the normal anatomical appearance of the associated brain structures prior to herniation. Acutely, herniated tissue may be isointense relative to its normal appearance. As the tissue becomes vascularly compromised, the herniated tissue may appear relatively hyperintense. If this tissue becomes edematous and eventually necrotic, the appearance of the tissue will reflect the associated tissue pathology (edema, hemorrhage).

DIAGNOSIS OF SPECIFIC INTRACRANIAL DISEASES

MR imaging can be used as an aid in the ante mortem diagnosis of many diseases of intracranial structures. While some disease processes have distinct imaging appearances, many diseases have more characteristic,

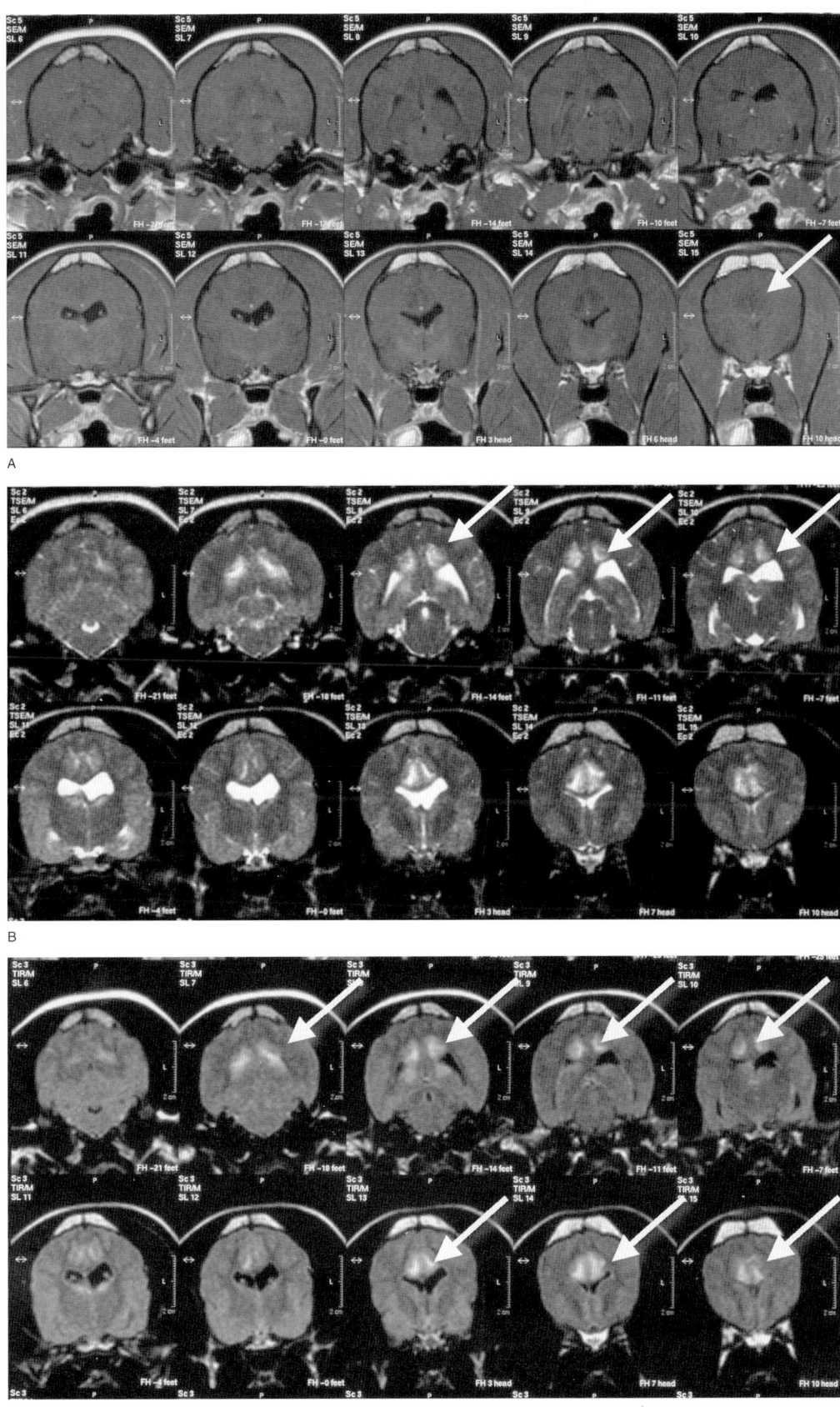

Figure 2.44. Transverse T1-weighted (A), T2-weighted (B), and FLAIR (C) MR images from a dog with idiopathic epilepsy imaged within 24 h of seizure activity. Note the hypointense regions (T1-weighted study) and the hyperintense regions (T2-weighted and FLAIR studies) (arrows).

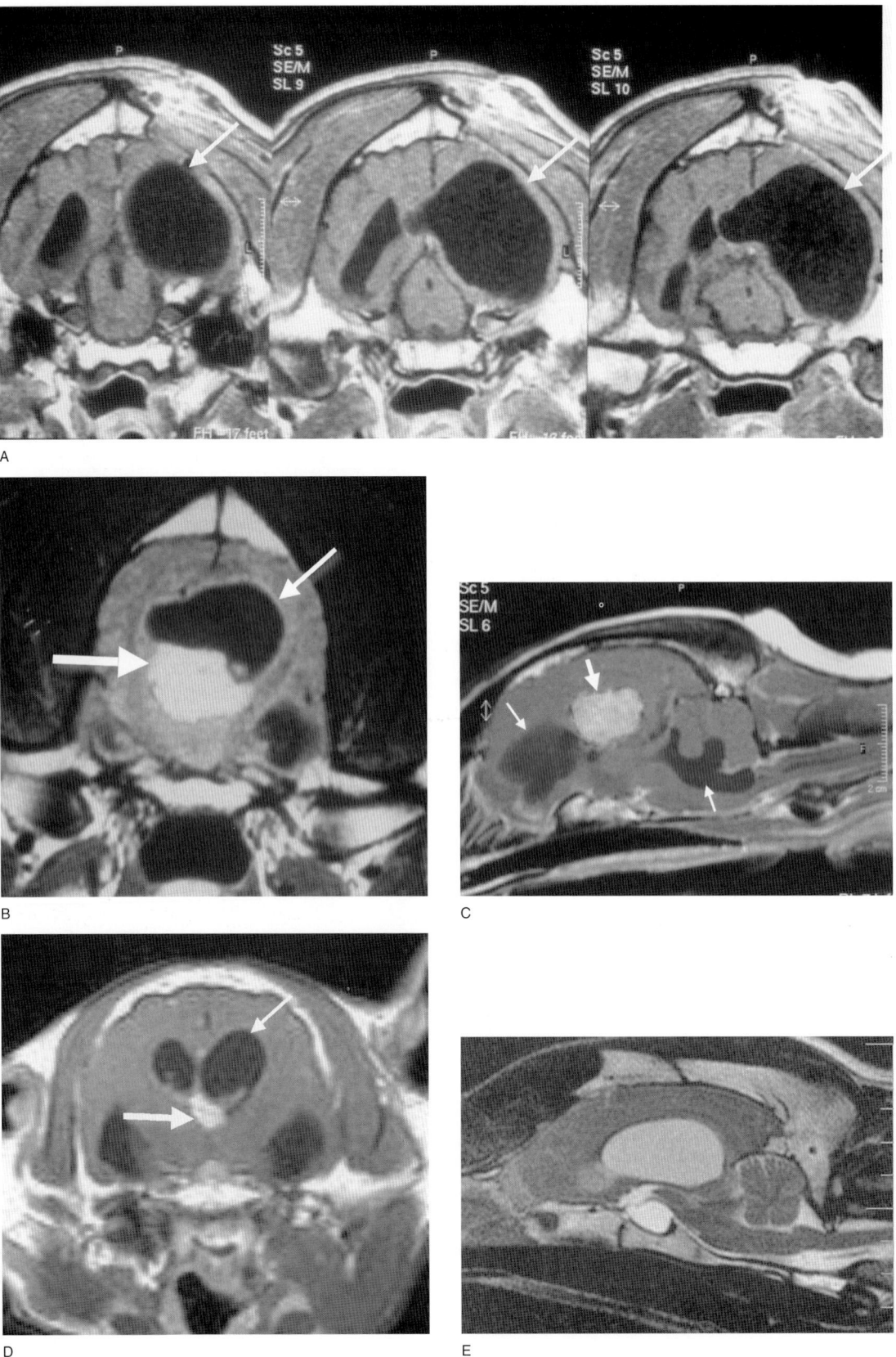

Figure 2.45.   Transverse T1-weighted MR images before (A), and following intravenous contrast administration (B), (C) from three separate dogs and one cat (D) with ventricular obstruction (small arrows). In (B) and (C) there are intraventricular masses (choroid plexus tumors) (larger arrows). Image (A) is ventricular obstruction following intracranial surgery. Sagittal T2-weighted MR image (E) from a dog with obstruction of the ventricles at the level of the third ventricle.

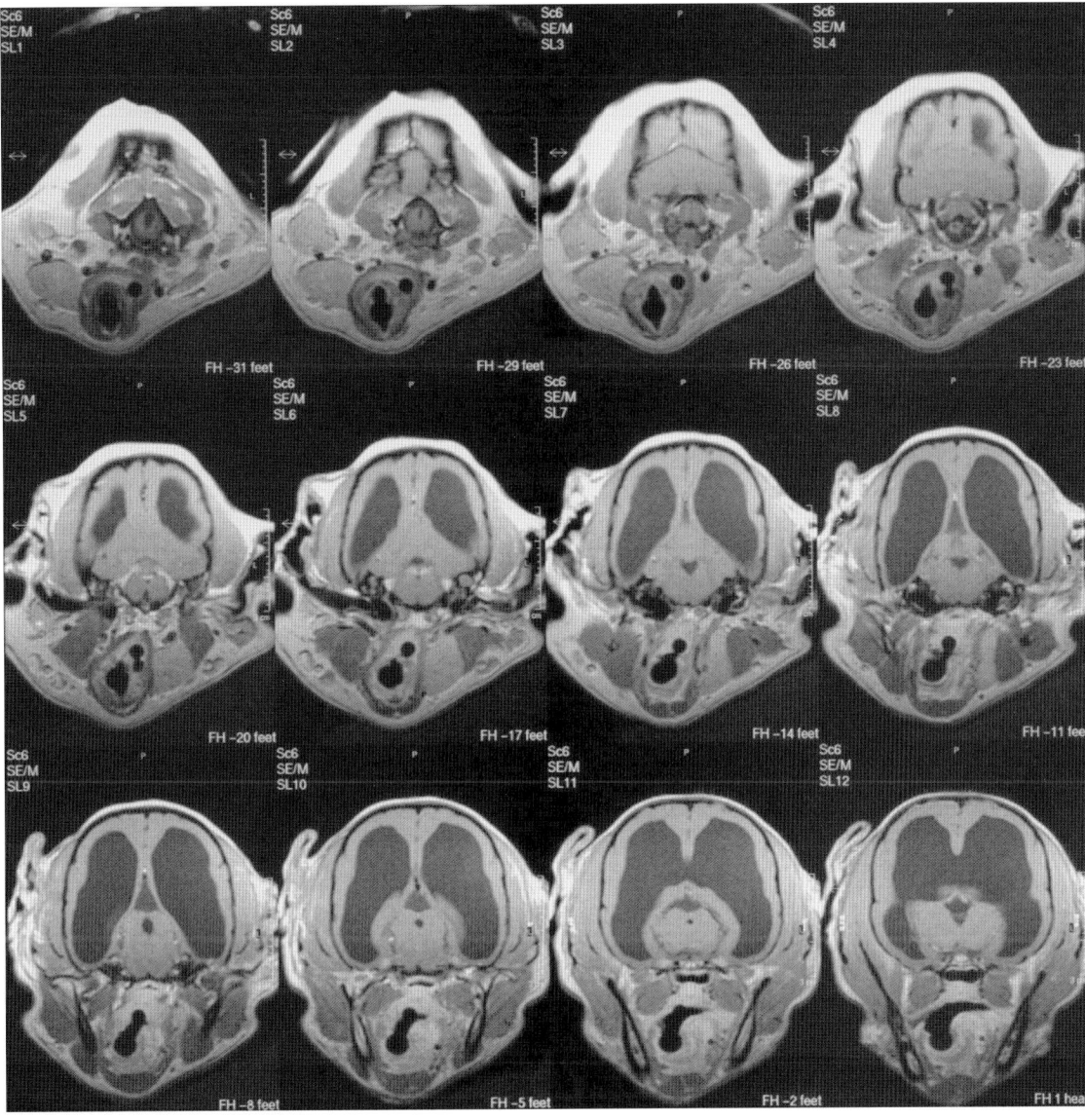

A

Figure 2.46. Transverse T1-weighted MR images before intravenous contrast administration from a dog with congenital hydrocephalus (A).

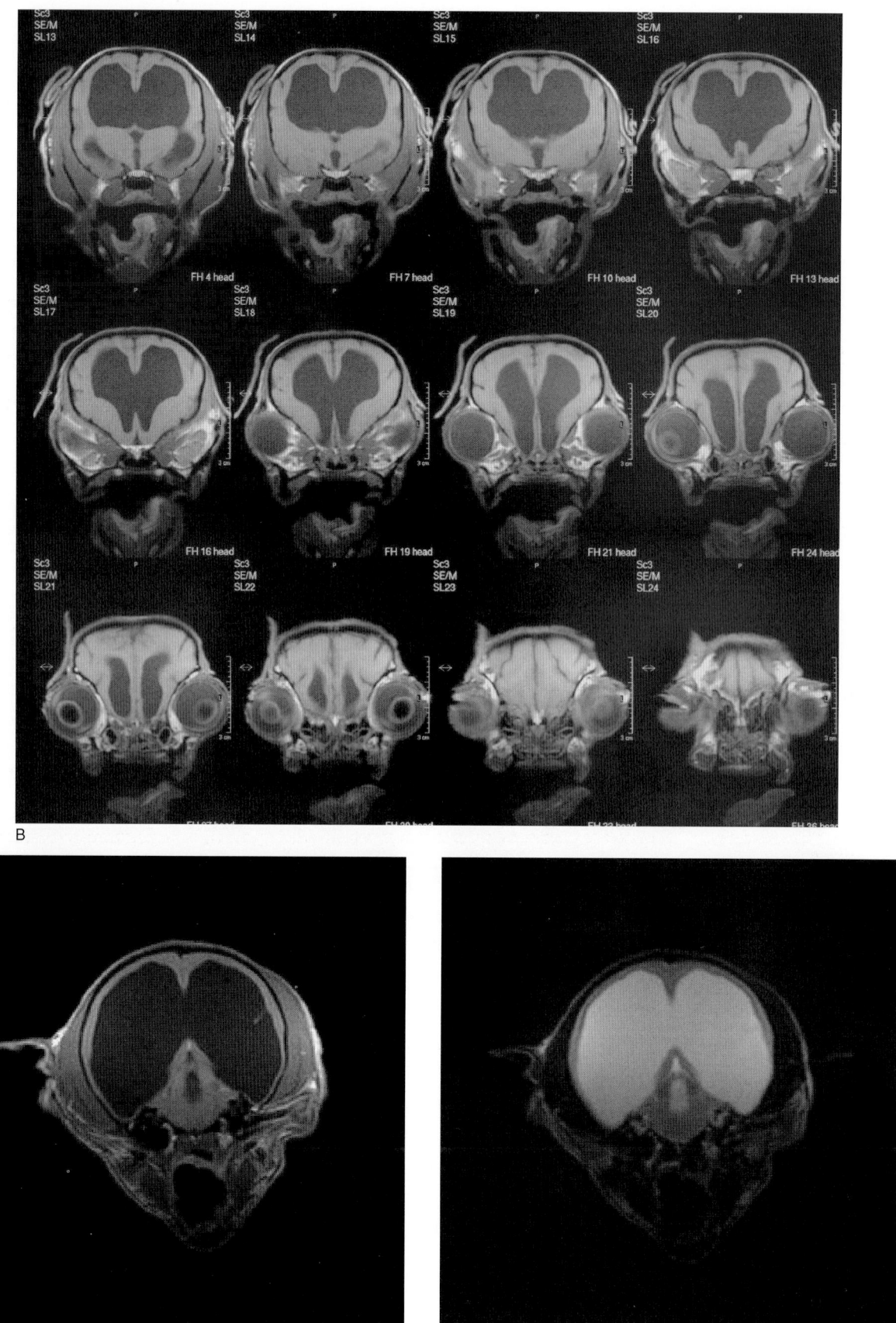

Figure 2.46. (*Continued*) Transverse T1-weighted MR images before intravenous contrast administration (B) from a dog with congenital hydrocephalus. Transverse T1-weighted (C) and T2-weighted (D) MR images from a dog with presumed congenital hydrocephalus.

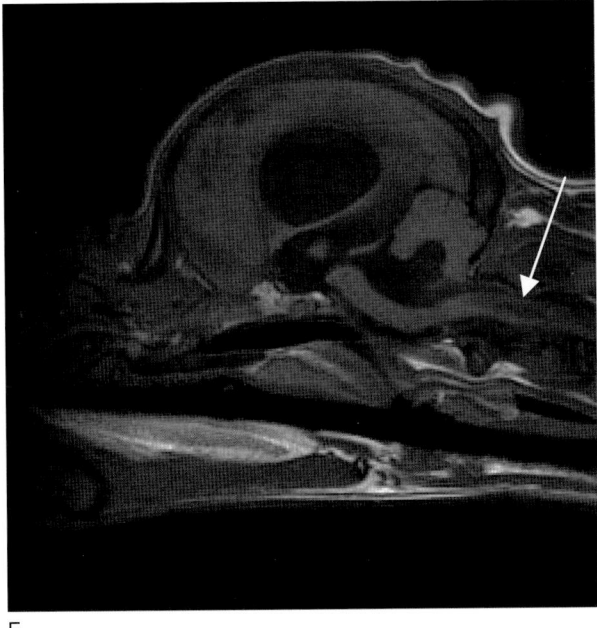 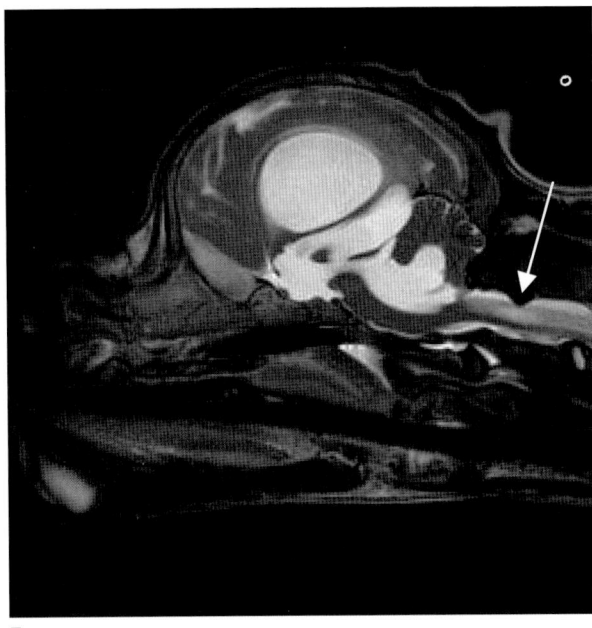

E   F

Figure 2.46. (*Continued*) Sagittal T1-weighted (E) and T2-weighted (F) MR images from a dog with hydrocephalus and syringomyelia (arrow).

but less absolute, imaging characteristics. This is in part due to the fact that many different disease processes result in similar associated pathophysiological alterations (such as edema), and these associated pathophysiological processes contribute to the MR appearance of the disease. For example, as numerous intracranial disease

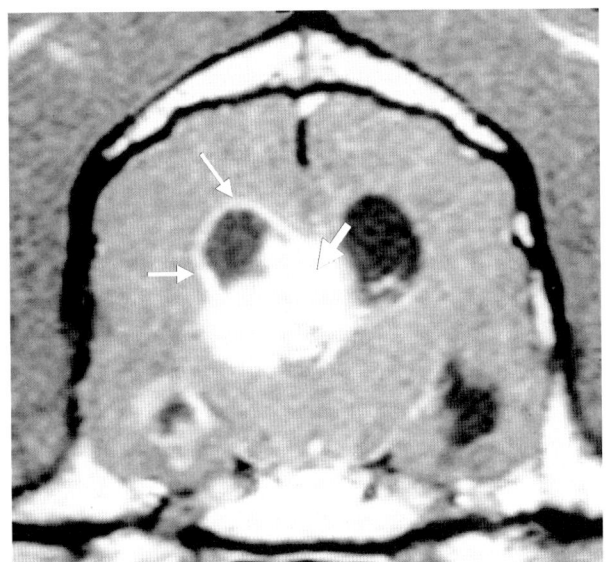

Figure 2.47. Transverse T1-weighted MR image following intravenous contrast administration from a dog with ventricular obstruction due to an intraventricular mass (choroid plexus tumors) (larger arrows). Note the hyperintense signal from the lining of the ventricle (small arrows).

processes result in associated edema (either intra- or extracellular edema), the appearance of many of these same disease processes is hyperintense in T2 images (Figure 2.33). This, in turn, is also why T2-weighted images are a good general screening sequence for a variety of intracranial diseases. In fact, many intracranial disease processes alter water content either focally or diffusely and therefore, are apparent on T2-weighted sequences. These same changes may not be apparent in T1-weighted images. FLAIR sequences are used subsequently to accentuate these T2-weighted alterations due to the nulling out of the normal CSF signal from the brain tissues.

Degenerative Diseases

Many primary degenerative intracranial diseases of dogs and cats are inherited or congenital, and occur primarily in young animals. The majority of these diseases result in neurologic dysfunction without alterations in gross anatomical structure of the brain. Therefore, advanced intracranial imaging studies, such as MR imaging, are invariably normal in affected animals. If the degenerative process results in atrophy or loss of intracranial cells and structural elements, this atrophy may be evident with MR imaging. For example, with some cerebellar diseases, the cerebellum is hypoplastic or becomes atrophied. A smaller than normal or absent cerebellum compared to an age-matched control animal might be found in MR evaluations of these

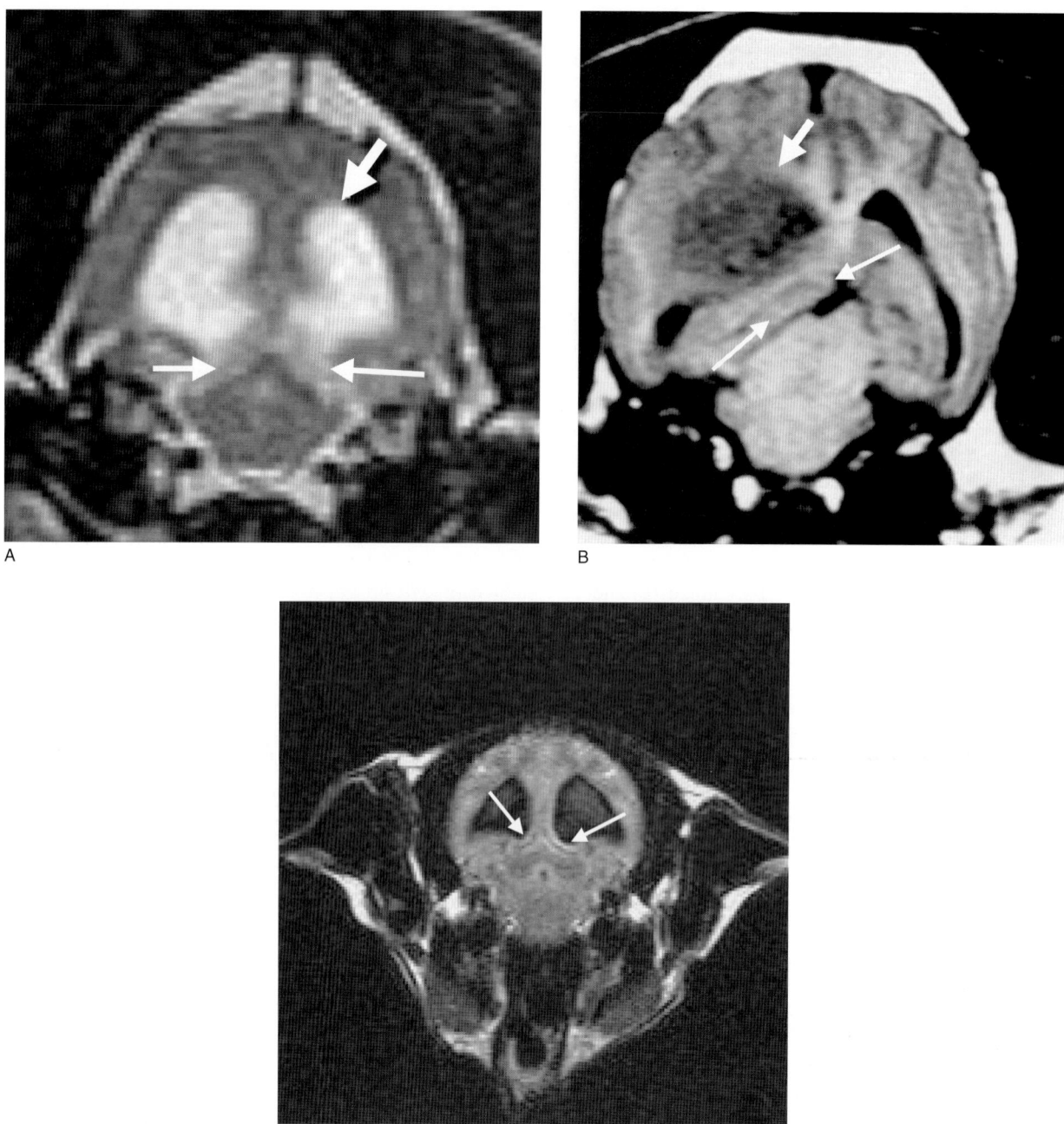

Figure 2.48. (A) Transverse T2-weighted MR image from a dog with bilateral caudal transtentorial herniation (smaller arrows) and associated ventricular obstruction (larger arrow). (B) Transverse T1-weighted MR image from a dog with unilateral caudal transtentorial herniation (smaller arrows) and associated intra-axial mass (larger arrow). Transverse (C) FLAIR MR images from a cat with bilateral caudal transtentorial herniation (arrows).

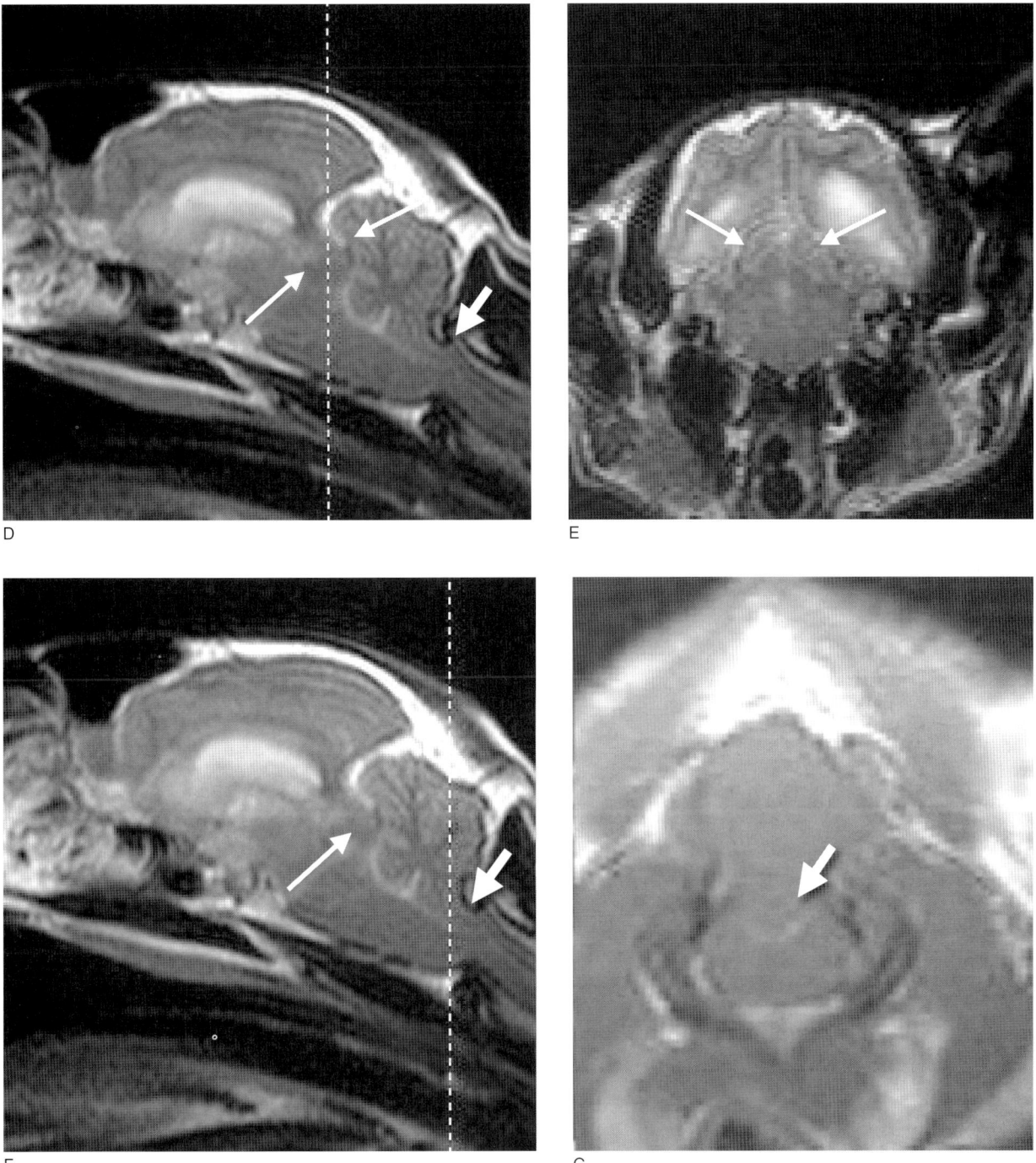

Figure 2.48. (*Continued*) Sagittal (D) and transverse (E) T2-weighted MR images from a cat with both bilateral caudal transtentorial herniation (smaller arrows) and associated foramen magnum herination (larger arrow). The dotted line represents the level of the transverse imaging plane at the region of the caudal transtentorial herniation. Sagittal T2-weighted (F) and transverse (G) T1-weighted MR images from the same cat with both bilateral caudal transtentorial herniation (smaller arrows) and associated foramen magnum herination (larger arrow). The dotted line represents the level of the transverse imaging plane at the region of the foramen magnum herniation.

animals. In some instances, the cerebellum will be reduced to a fluid-filled cyst.

Other diseases may result in diffuse alterations in either white matter or gray matter of the brain (Vite et al. 2001). Some degenerative diseases in dogs, such as those similar to Leigh's syndrome in humans, may show bilateral hyperintense lesions (T2-weighted sequences) on MR imaging of the intracranial structures. These abnormalities may be present in various regions of the intracranial structures, but often involve the supratentorial (thalamic) structures. Similar types of MR abnormalities may be seen with other metabolic-based encephalopathies such as electrolyte abnormalities (e.g., sodium) and thiamine deficiency (see Section "Metabolic Encephalopathies" in this chapter).

Otherwise normal older animals (usually older than 10–12 years of age depending upon the breed) if evaluated with MR imaging may show decreased size of the cortical layers of the hemispheres and resultant increases in cerebral ventricular dimensions. There may also appear to have more prominent sulci (possibly the result of smaller than normal gyri). It is important to recognize that a degree of ventriculomegaly is a "normal" age-related change within the intracranial structures, most likely the result of cortical atrophy with increasing age. Occasionally in MR images of older animals there will be concurrent increased signal intensity in T2-weighted images immediately adjacent to the ventricular walls (Figure 2.49). This may be an "aging" change in many of these dogs; however, the significance of this finding is under investigation. In still other instances, cortical atrophy may result from diffuse or focal vascular-related cell loss. This may also accompany secondary hypertensive disease affecting the brain cells. Hyperadrenocorticism may also result in brain atrophy, possibly from vascular-based ischemia, secondary hypertension, cerebral vessel disease, or primary cell death.

Older dogs with progressive cognitive decline, which is unusual for the normal aging process, have been suggested to have evidence of brain atrophy on MR evaluations. This has been suggested to primarily be evident as thalamic atrophy with a small appearance of the interthalamic adhesion (Figure 2.49). This same appearance, that is, the decrease in size of the interthalamic adhesion, however, has also been seen in clinically normal older dogs.

Anomalous Disease

Development anomalies such as aplasia, hypoplasia, or dysplasia, may alter the normal intracranial anatomical relationships and be evident as anatomically abnor-

mal regions within the nervous system in MR studies (Jeffery et al. 2003) (Figure 2.50). As an example, with lissencephaly, the cortical gyri may be more prominent and thicker than normal (Dewey et al. 2003). Other types of dysplasia are evident as anatomic abnormalities. In other instances, specific regions of the brain may be malformed or underdeveloped.

Intracranial arachnoid cysts may be congenital in origin, or may result as out-pocketing of the cerebral ventricles specifically in the corpora quadrigemina region. These cystic abnormalities are usually readily apparent with MR imaging; however, it is often difficult if not impossible to distinguish whether the cystic abnormality is a distinct cystic structure (has a wall or lining) or an extension of the third ventricle (Figure 2.51). The borders of these cystic abnormalities may be slightly overestimated on T2 sequences.

Epidermoid and dermoid cysts result from abnormal development of the neural tube (Figure 2.52). These abnormalities are often found in the fourth ventricle and foramen magnum area as irregular, multilobulated, partially fluid-containing structures on MR imaging. Depending upon the cellular constituents of the cyst, complex appearances of signal intensity may be seen ranging from hypo- to hyperintense regions within the abnormality. Generally, these types of abnormalities are relatively hypointense on T1-weighted sequences, and relatively hyperintense on T2-weighted sequences. Contrast enhancement (following intravenous administration of contrast media) may be present heterogeneously within the tissues and/or more uniformly enhanced on the periphery of the cystic structures.

Hydrocephalus

Hydrocephalus can result from obstruction of the ventricular system, irritation of the ventricle (from inflammation or hemorrhage), and increased size of the ventricles due to loss of brain parenchyma (hydrocephalus ex vacuo). Diagnosis of hydrocephalus can be supported by information obtained from a variety of imaging and electrophysiologic modalities.

MR imaging affords evaluation of the ventricular system (Harrington et al. 1996). The ventricular system filled with CSF will appear hypointense (blacker) on a T1-weighted, and hyperintense (whiter) on a T2-weighted imaging sequence. The ability of MR imaging to provide anatomical views in multiple planes without reductions in image quality allows for a more thorough assessment of the ventricular system. Focal dilation of portions of the ventricular system is also readily determined. MR imaging features and considerations

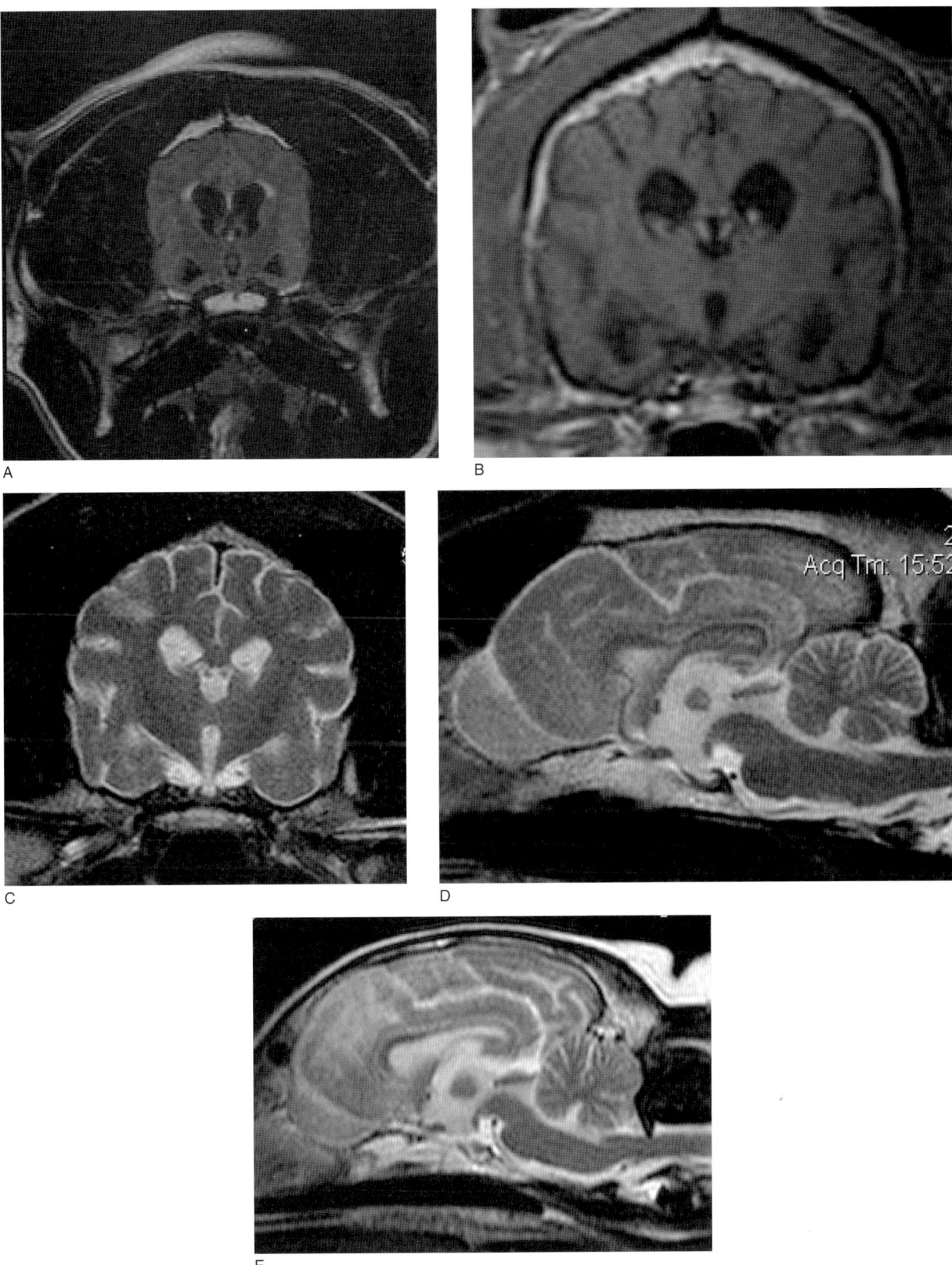

Figure 2.49.   Transverse FLAIR MR image (A) from a dog with periventricular hyperintense signal. Transverse T1-weighted (B), transverse T2-weighted (C), and sagittal T2-weighted (D) MR images from an older dog with cognitive decline. Note the small appearance of the interthalamic adhesion, most evident in the T2-weighted sagittal image. Sagittal T2-weighted image (E) from a clinically healthy older dog with a relatively smaller interthalamic adhesion.

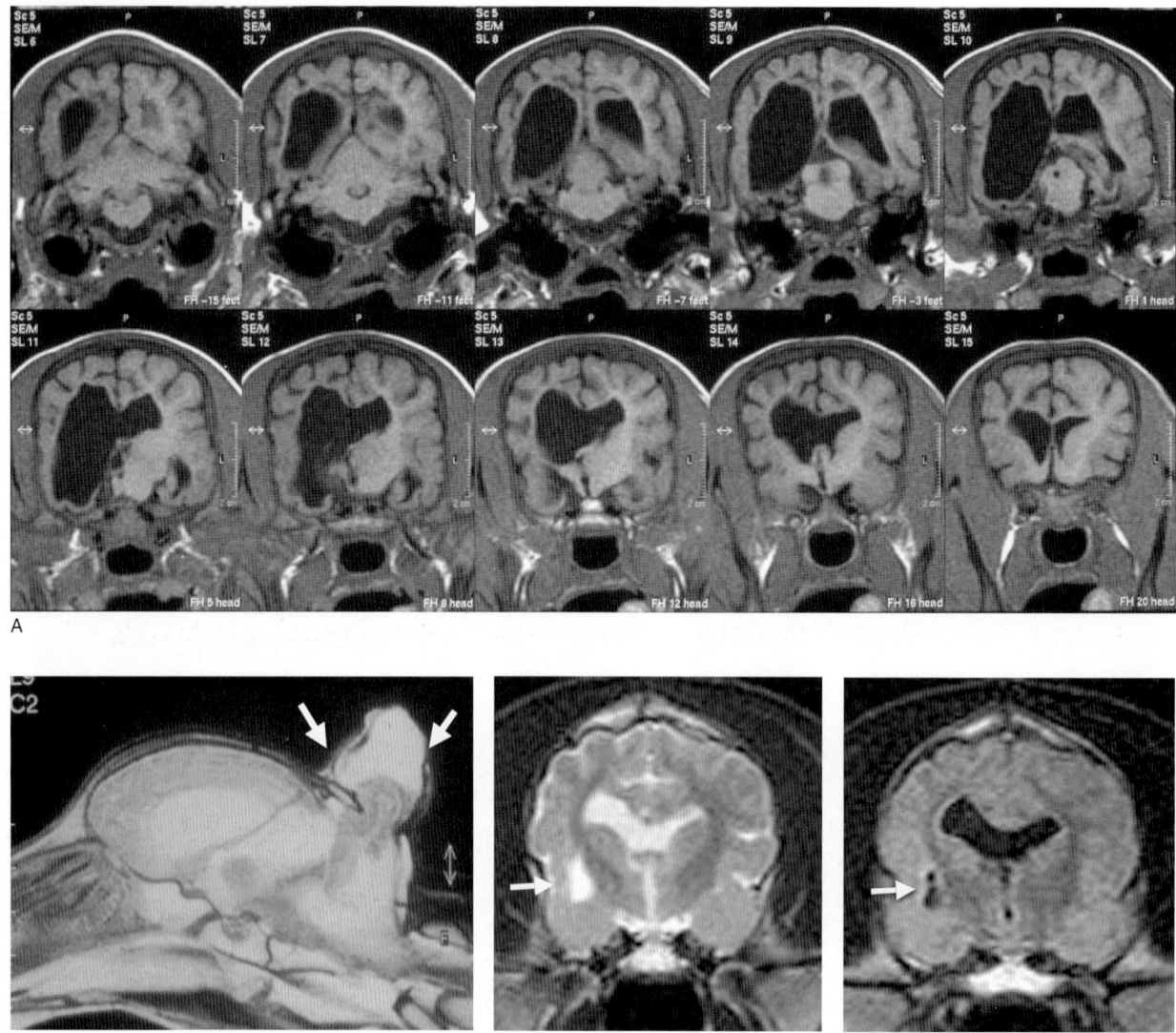

Figure 2.50. (A) Transverse T1-weighted MR image from a dog with congenital supratentorial anatomical defect and associated ventricular enlargement. (B) Sagittal T2-weighted MR image from a sheep with a congenital defect of the dorsal cerebellar region with an associated encephalocele (arrows). Transverse T2-weighted (C) and FLAIR (D) MR images from a dog with congenital supratentorial anatomical defect and porencephaly (arrow).

of hydrocephalus are discussed in Section "Ventricular Obstruction" in this chapter.

Metabolic Encephalopathies

Numerous metabolic abnormalities may alter intracranial functions. Clues to the diagnosis of many of these diseases can be present on routine database blood and urine assessments. A diagnosis of hepatic encephalopathy (HE) is supported by clinical signs and abnormal liver function studies such as bile acids testing. Various ultrasound, scintigraphic, portal angiography, and MR-angiography studies of the liver and abdominal vasculature may show the anatomical vascular abnor-

malities of the liver and portal system. Liver biopsy and direct visualization of the liver and portal system at laparotomy may be used for diagnosis of abnormalities of the portal system and liver parenchyma.

Abnormalities on MR imaging of the brain in animals with HE may be found (Figure 2.53). In some instances, these abnormalities are independent of clinical signs. In our hospital, the most consistent intracranial imaging feature associated with HE is hyperintense signal on T2-weighted sequences from the cerebral white matter and, in some instances, the periventricular white matter. The exact histologic nature of these signal changes is not consistently identified. This abnormality may represent edema. In other

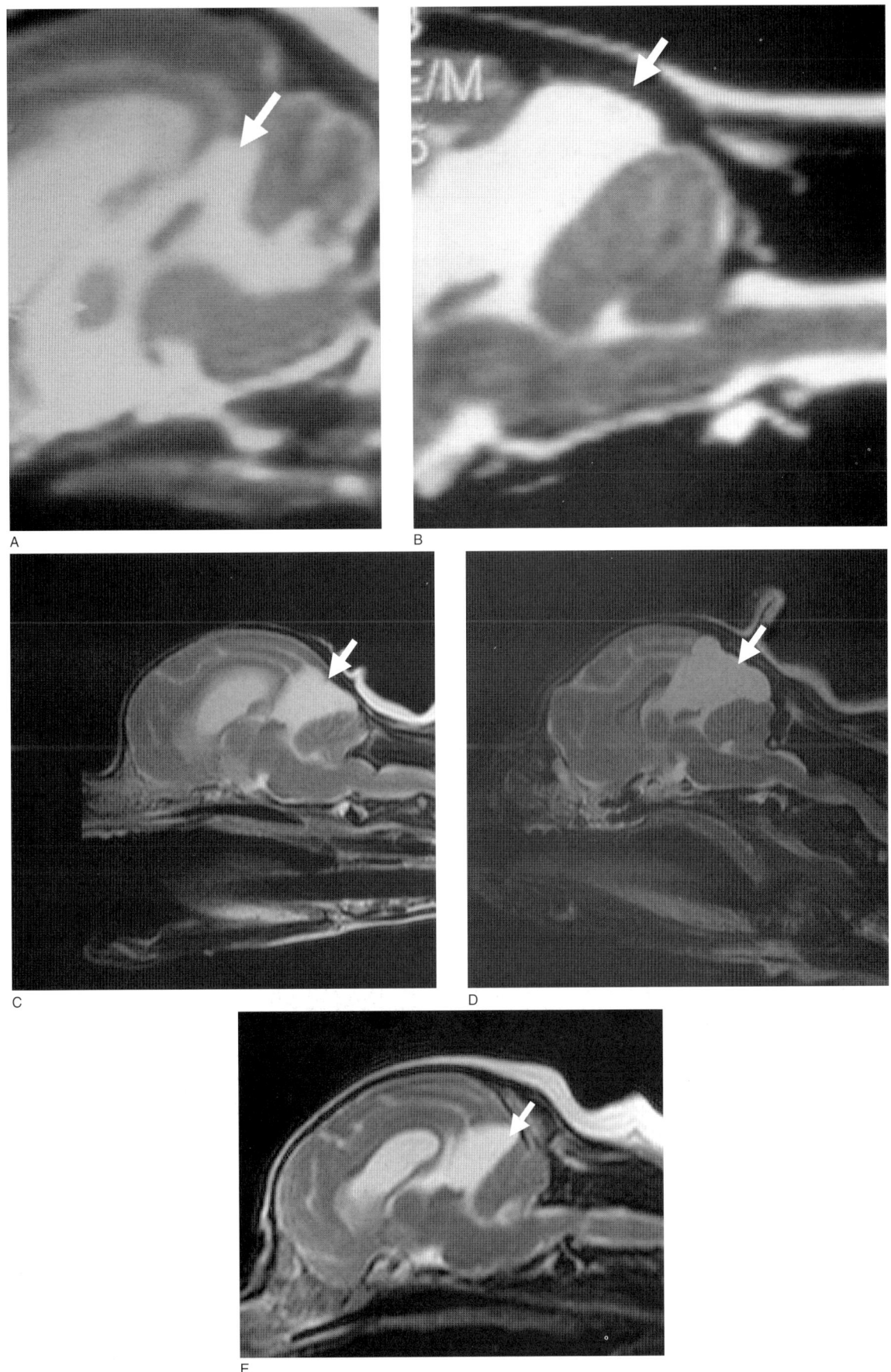

Figure 2.51. Sagittal T2-weighted MR images from five dogs (A)–(E) with cystic intracranial structures (arrows).

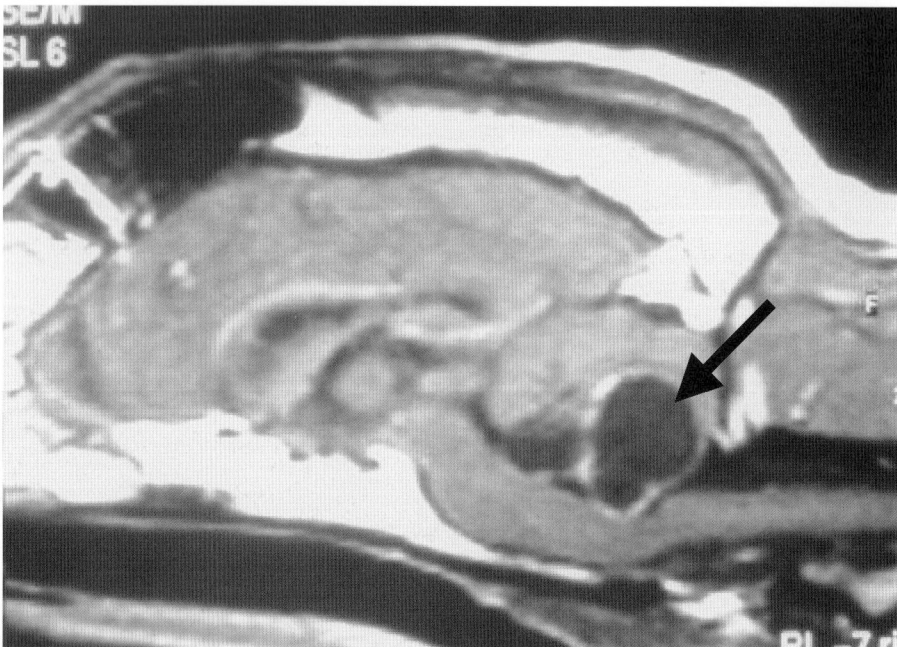

Figure 2.52. Sagittal T1-weighted MR image following intravenous contrast administration from a dog with an epidermoid cyst of the fourth ventricle (arrow).

situations, similar abnormalities are found in animals with HE but also have seizure activity. Therefore, the relationship of these signal changes and seizure activity is not established. Some of these changes are reversible following appropriate medical or surgical treatment for portosystemic shunting. In these latter cases, MR abdominal angiography may additionally be used to identify abnormal portovascular anomalies (see Chapter 4).

Some metabolic abnormalities, such as hypoglycemia, are not associated with any alteration of brain structure on MR. Obviously, if any metabolic derangement results in cerebral edema, ischemia, or hemorrhage, these secondary alterations may be present on MR evaluations of the intracranial space. Abnormalities associated with imbalances of sodium and water in the brain are sometimes associated with more

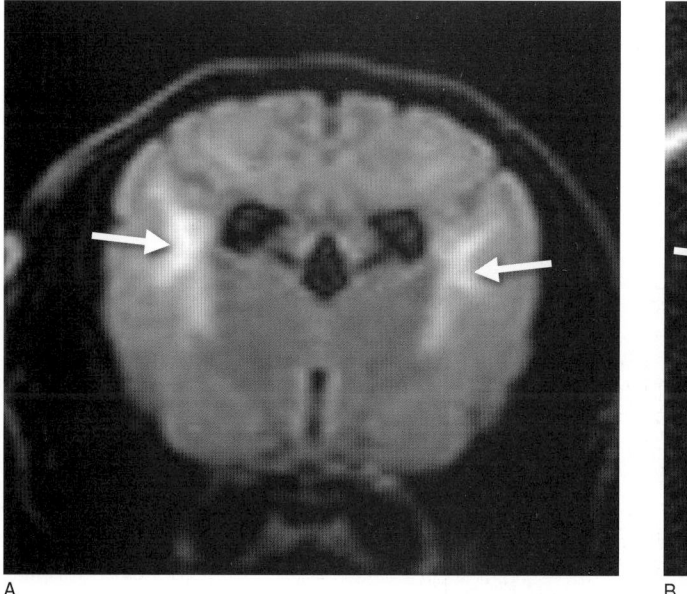

A

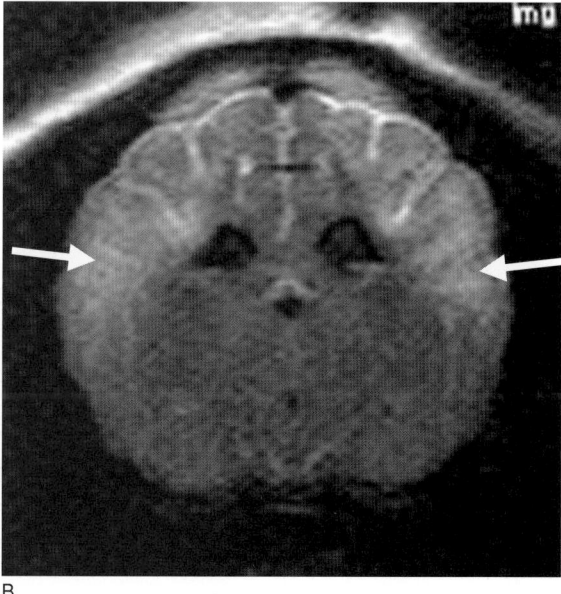

B

Figure 2.53. Transverse FLAIR MR images from two dogs ((A) and (B)) with portosystemic shunt. Note the hyperintense abnormalities bilaterally within the cerebral white matter and grey matter (arrows).

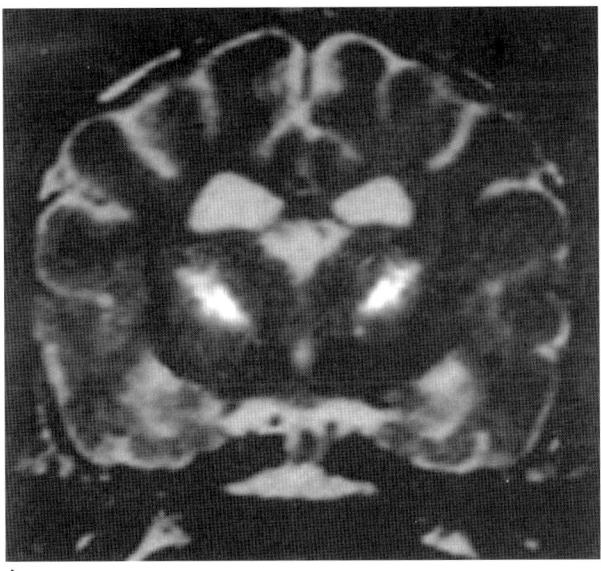

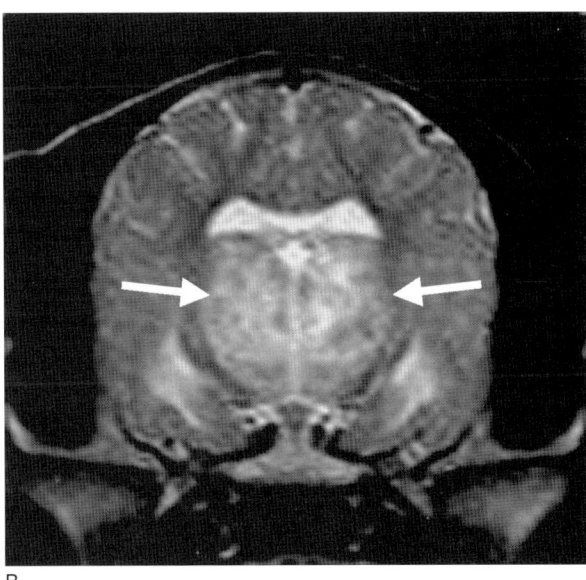

A   B

Figure 2.54. Transverse T2-weighted MR image (A) from a dog with osmotic myelinolysis with increased signal intensity in the thalamus. Transverse T2-weighted MR image (B) from a dog with a metabolic encephalopathy with increased signal intensity in the thalamus.

characteristic MR abnormalities. With MR, these lesions are hypointense in T1-weighted images and hyperintense in T2-weighted images. In dogs, these lesions are often oval in appearance, bilaterally symmetrical, and are present in the thalamus. The degree of T2-weighted MR signal intensity is often correlated with the duration of the abnormality (more hyperintense earlier in the disease).

These lesions are most often found in association with too rapid correction of hyponatremia that may accompany hypoadrenocorticism, or occasionally other diseases associated with persistent hyponatremia, and are referred to in dogs as osmotic myelinolysis (Figure 2.54). While the cellular nature of these abnormalities is not definitively established, these lesions may represent localized edema or demyelination. In human beings this pathologic change is referred to as central pontine myelinolysis. In dogs, however, lesions are characteristically in the thalamus compared to those in the brain stem (pons) in humans. Some of the animals may have associated cerebrovascular disease and evidence of cerebral infarction in MR studies. These lesions may persist on MR imaging for weeks even with associated clinical improvement.

Some endocrine diseases are associated with alterations in the structure or function of the hypothalamus or the pituitary gland (Figure 2.55). The most commonly recognized of these are macroadenomas of the pituitary gland in dogs with hyperadrenocorticism (see

pituitary tumors under neoplasia in this chapter). Persistent, insulin-resistant hyperglycemia may suggest acromegaly from a pituitary tumor, especially in cats. MR imaging of the intracranial structures may reveal a pituitary mass in these animals.

With some of the primary metabolic encephalopathies such as mitochondrial encephalopathies, there is increased CSF lactate and pyruvates in humans; however, this is not established in dogs (Dewey et al. 2003). CSF analysis is usually normal. MR may show bilaterally symmetric, cavitary lesions of brain and spinal cord. With MR, these lesions are hypointense in T1-weighted images and hyperintense in T2-weighted images.

Neoplasia

Neoplastic diseases affecting the intracranial space often alter the anatomical structure of the affected intracranial structures. The diagnosis of an intracranial mass is readily made using advanced imaging modalities such as MR imaging either primarily as due to secondary pathophysiologic structural alterations (mass effect) (Figures 2.56–2.81). Imaging features of primary brain tumor have been reviewed (Tucker and Gavin 1996). While some tumors have more characteristic imaging features, specific neoplastic processes may have diverse imaging characteristics.

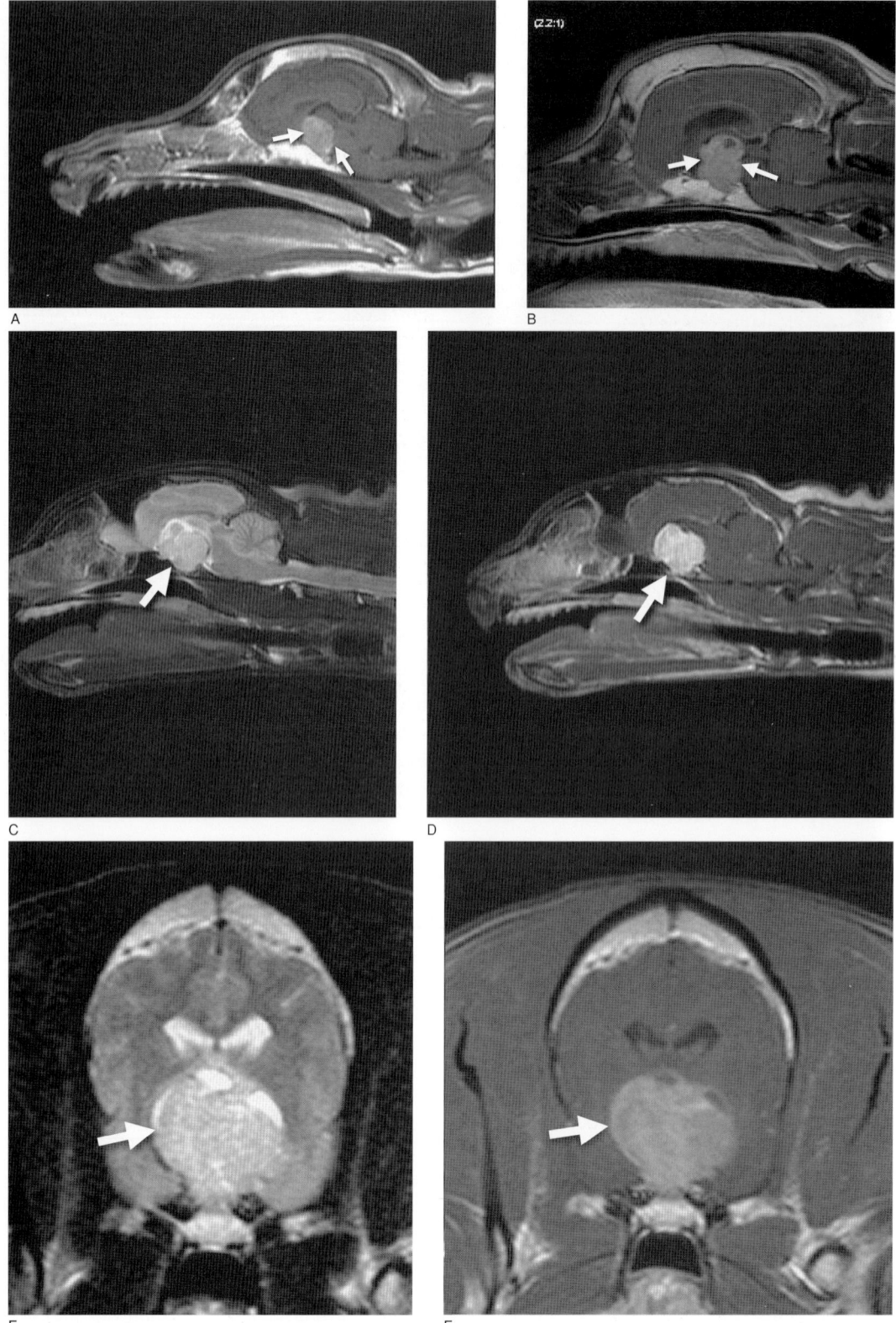

Figure 2.55. (A), (B) Sagittal T1-weighted MR images following intravenous contrast administration from two dogs with a pituitary macroadenoma (arrows). Sagittal T2-weighted (C) and T1-weighted MR images following intravenous contrast administration (D) from a cat with a pituitary macroadenoma (arrows). Transverse T2-weighted (E) and T1-weighted (following intravenous contrast administration) (F) MR images from a dog with a pituitary macroadenoma (arrows).

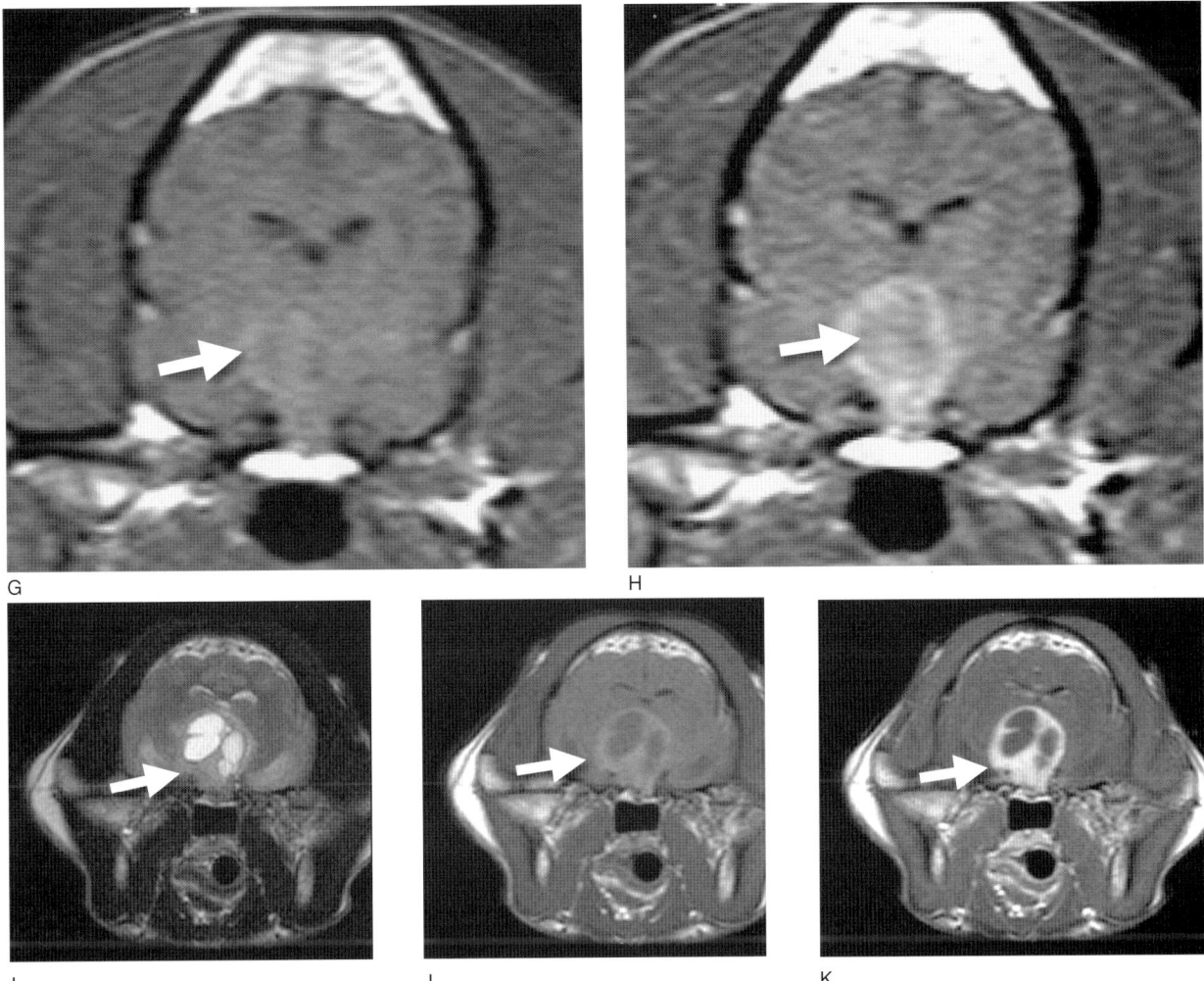

Figure 2.55. (*Continued*) Transverse T1-weighted MR images before (G) and following intravenous contrast administration (H) from a dog with a pituitary macroadenoma (arrows). Transverse T2-weighted (I) T1-weighted MR images before (J) and following intravenous contrast administration (K) from a dog with a pituitary macroadenoma (arrows).

Tumors have a propensity for creating associated cerebral edema (Figure 2.33). This type of edema appears most often as the vasogenic type, as this type of edema is more prominent in, and tends to follow the course of, the cerebral white matter. This gives a spike or crown-like appearance to the lesion.

Meningioma

Meningiomas are the most common brain tumor of both dogs and cats, and often appear as a broad-based, extra-axial (arising outside and pushing into the parenchyma) contrast-enhancing mass on MR imaging (Figures 2.56–2.68). These tumors may contain hem-

orrhagic regions or be mineralized (calcified). Hemorrhage may have a varied appearance with MR depending on the duration of the hemorrhage.

Meningiomas can have a varied appearance in T1- and T2-weighted images (Figures 2.56–2.68). Peritumoral edema can contribute to the imaging appearance as well as associated mass effect. Occasionally, secondary pathophysiologic sequelae are more obvious in images obtained prior to contrast enhancement.

As a general rule, meningiomas are isointense to cortical tissue in T1-weighted MR images prior to contrast administration. In some instances, these tumors are hypointense in T1-weighted images prior to contrast administration. The T2-weighted appearance is often hyperintense. Meningiomas tend to be contrast enhanced

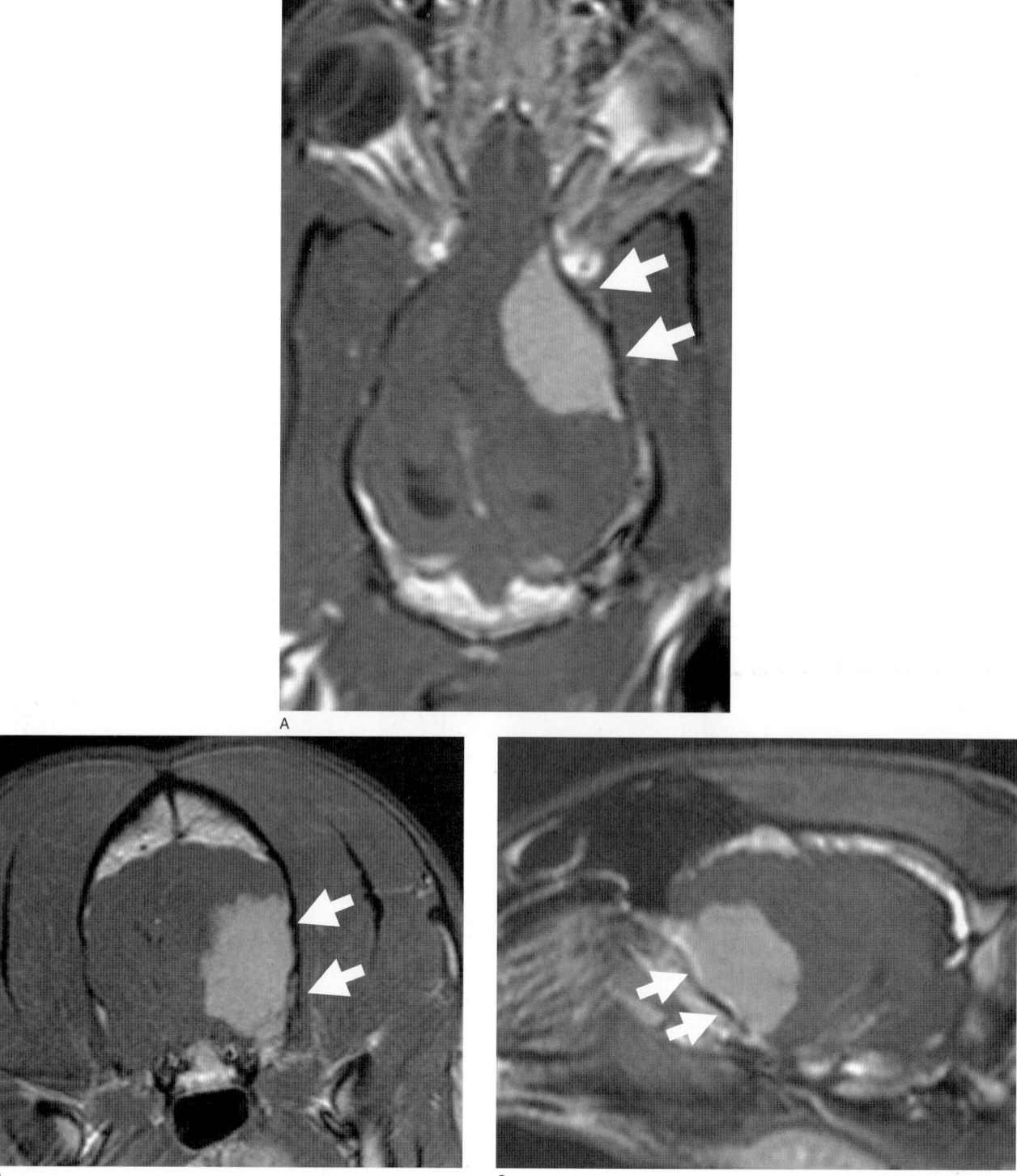

Figure 2.56.   Dorsal (A), transverse (B), and parasagittal (C) T1-weighted MR images following intravenous contrast administration from a dog with a meningioma (arrows).

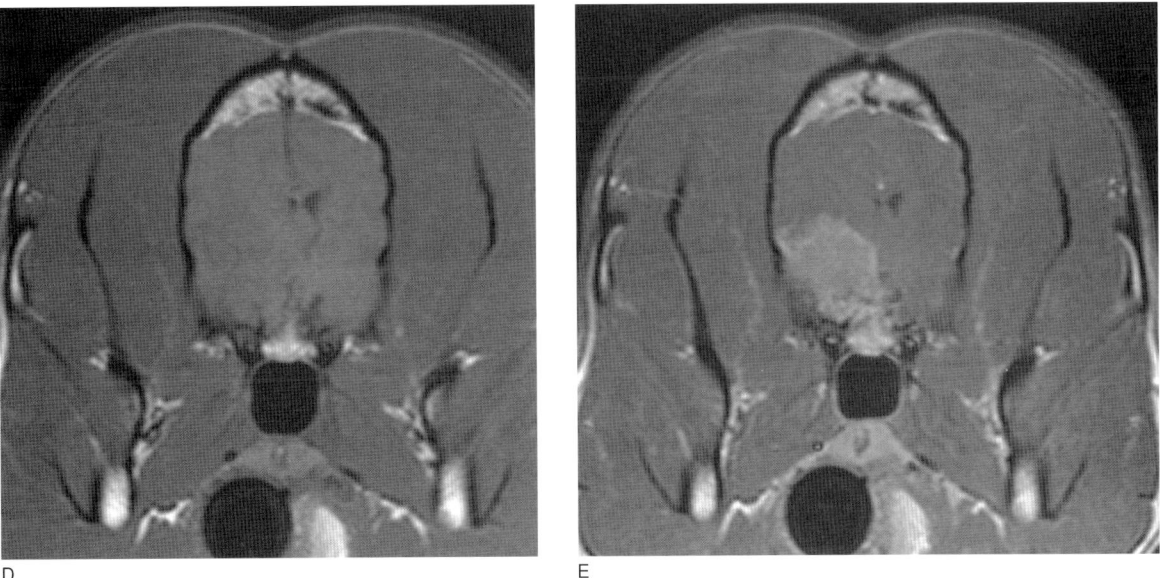

Figure 2.56. (*Continued*) Transverse T1-weighted MR images before (D) and following intravenous contrast administration (E) in a dog with a meningioma.

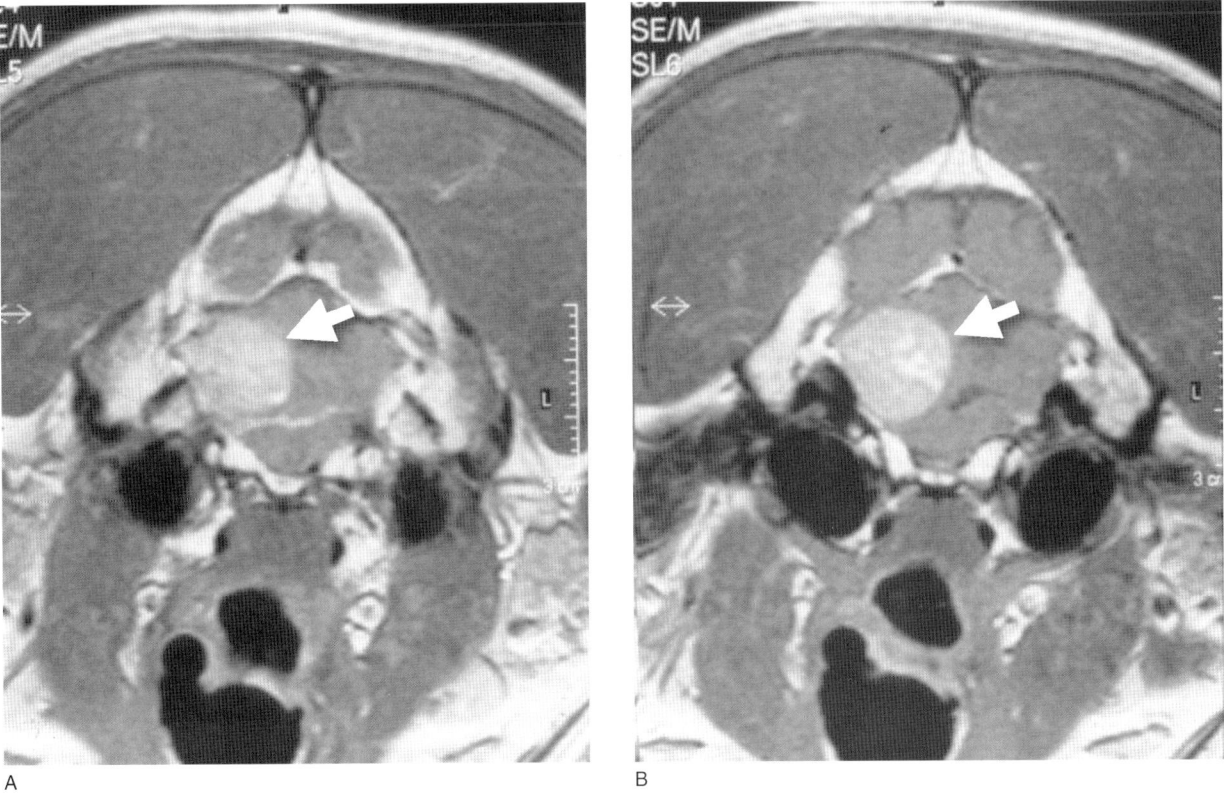

Figure 2.57. Transverse T1-weighted MR images ((A) and (B)) following intravenous contrast administration from a dog with a meningioma (arrows) in the cerebellar region.

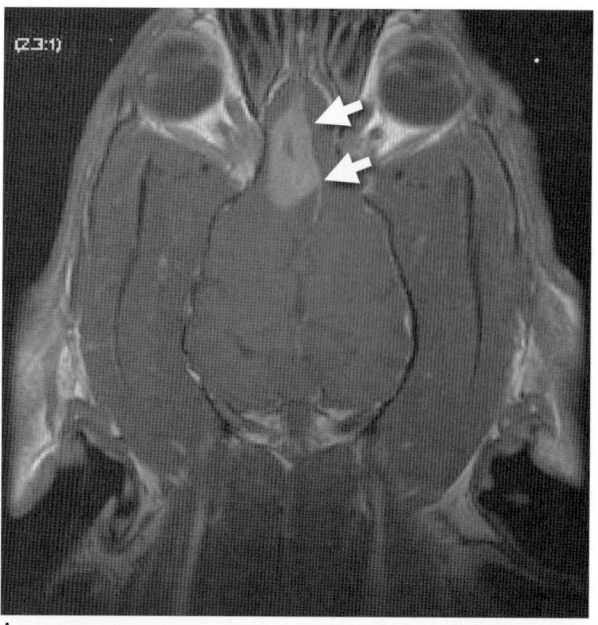

A

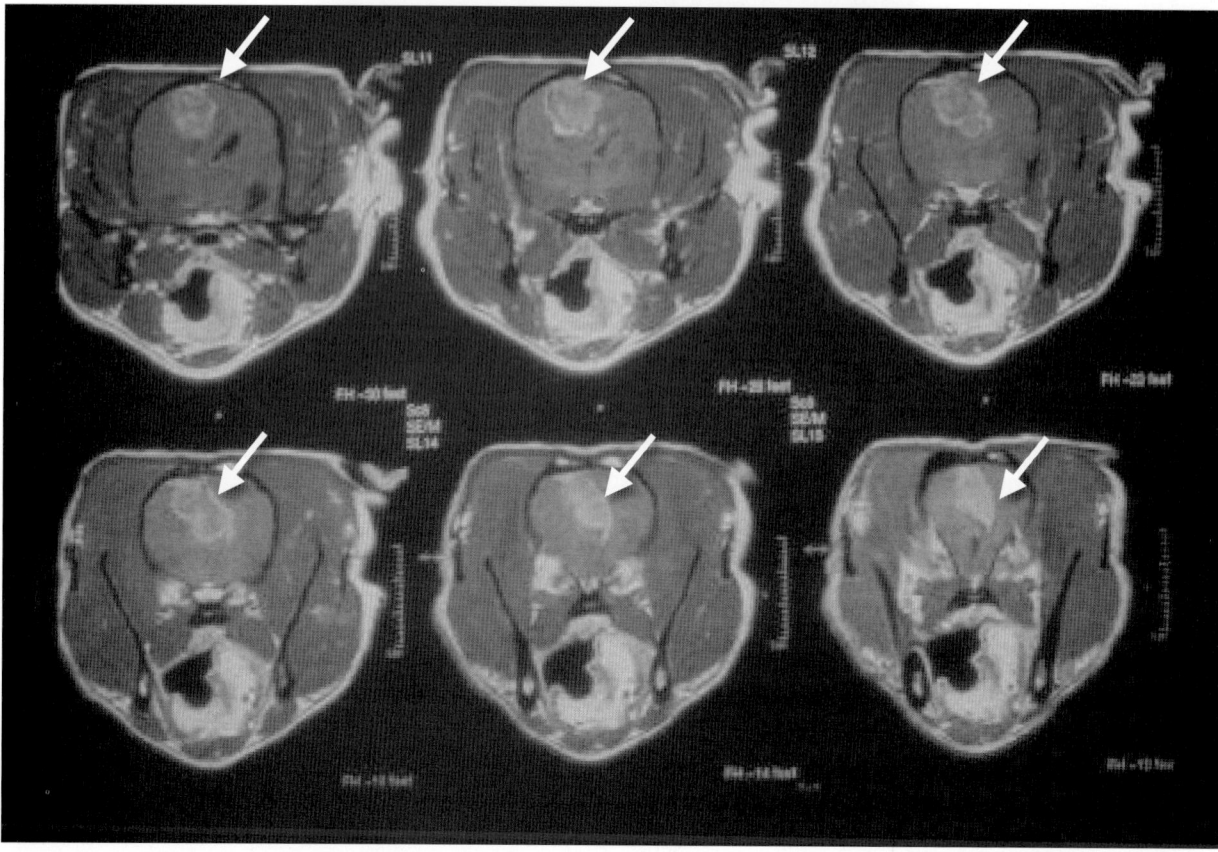

B

Figure 2.58.   Dorsal (A) and transverse (B) T1-weighted MR images following intravenous contrast administration from two different dogs with meningiomas (arrows) in the falx cerebri.

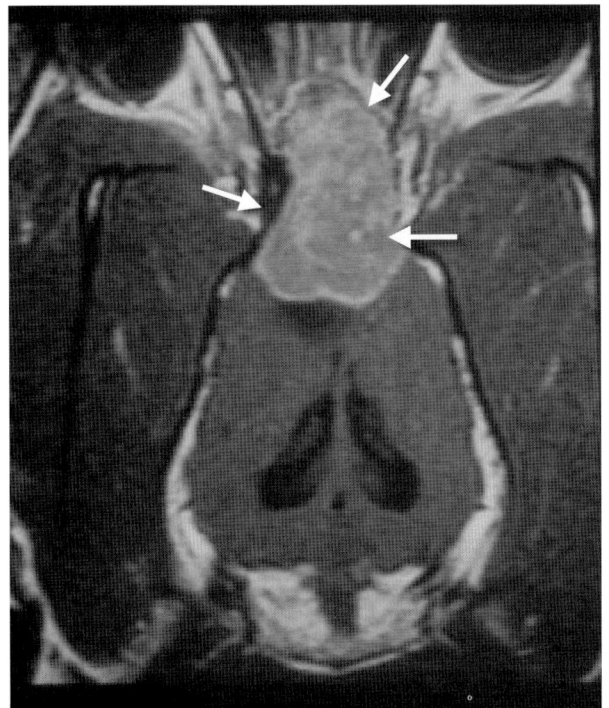

Figure 2.59. Dorsal T1-weighted MR image following intravenous contrast administration from a dog with a meningioma (arrows) of the olfactory region.

following intravenous contrast administration. These tumors tend to displace tissue from a peripheral to central direction. Depending on the slice plane, the largest dimension of tumor may be more peripherally encountered (broad-based). The overlying skull may be hyperplastic (thickened) (Figure 2.64).

There is often a relatively uniform enhancement of these tumors following intravenous contrast administration (Figures 2.56, 2.62–2.64, 2.67, and 2.68). In some instances, there is heterogenous enhancement, more likely centrally compared to peripherally. Occasionally, the dura immediately adjacent to the tumor will have increased enhancement, which is often referred to as a "dural tail sign."

Meningiomas may sometimes be primarily of a cystic character (Figure 2.68). These cystic meningiomas have imaging characteristics of those of a CSF-contain cyst. These tumors tend to be more round or oval, and are hypointense in T1-weighted images, and conversely hyperintense in T2-weighted images. Often there is an associated focal, sometimes plaque-like tissue on the periphery of the cystic lesion that is contrast enhancing. Occasionally, the limiting lining of the cystic cavity may enhance following contrast administration giving a more "ring-like" appearance. Cystic meningiomas are more common in the olfactory bulb regions of the intracranial cavity, but can occur in other regions of the intracranial space.

The tela choroidea (area where pia mater contacts ependyma) may become neoplastic with meningeal tissue. These tissues are located in the floor of each lateral ventricle and in the roof of the third and fourth ventricle. Therefore, meningiomas may arise in an apparent intraventricular location. This is more common in cats (Figure 2.65). Meningiomas are commonly solitary abnormalities in dogs. Cats and, rarely, dogs may have multiple intracranial meningiomas (Figures 2.61 and 2.64).

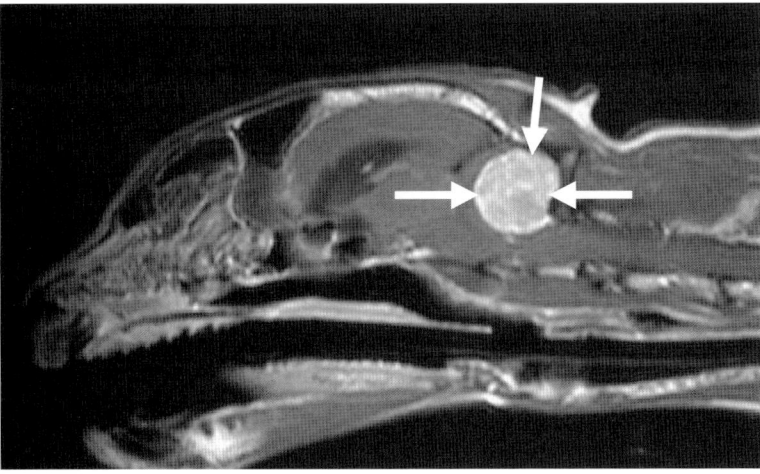
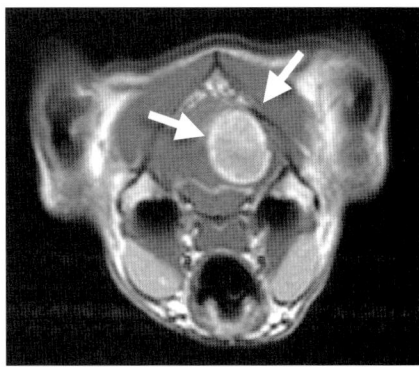

A   B

Figure 2.60. Sagittal (A) and transverse (B) T1-weighted MR images following intravenous contrast administration from a cat with a meningioma (arrows).

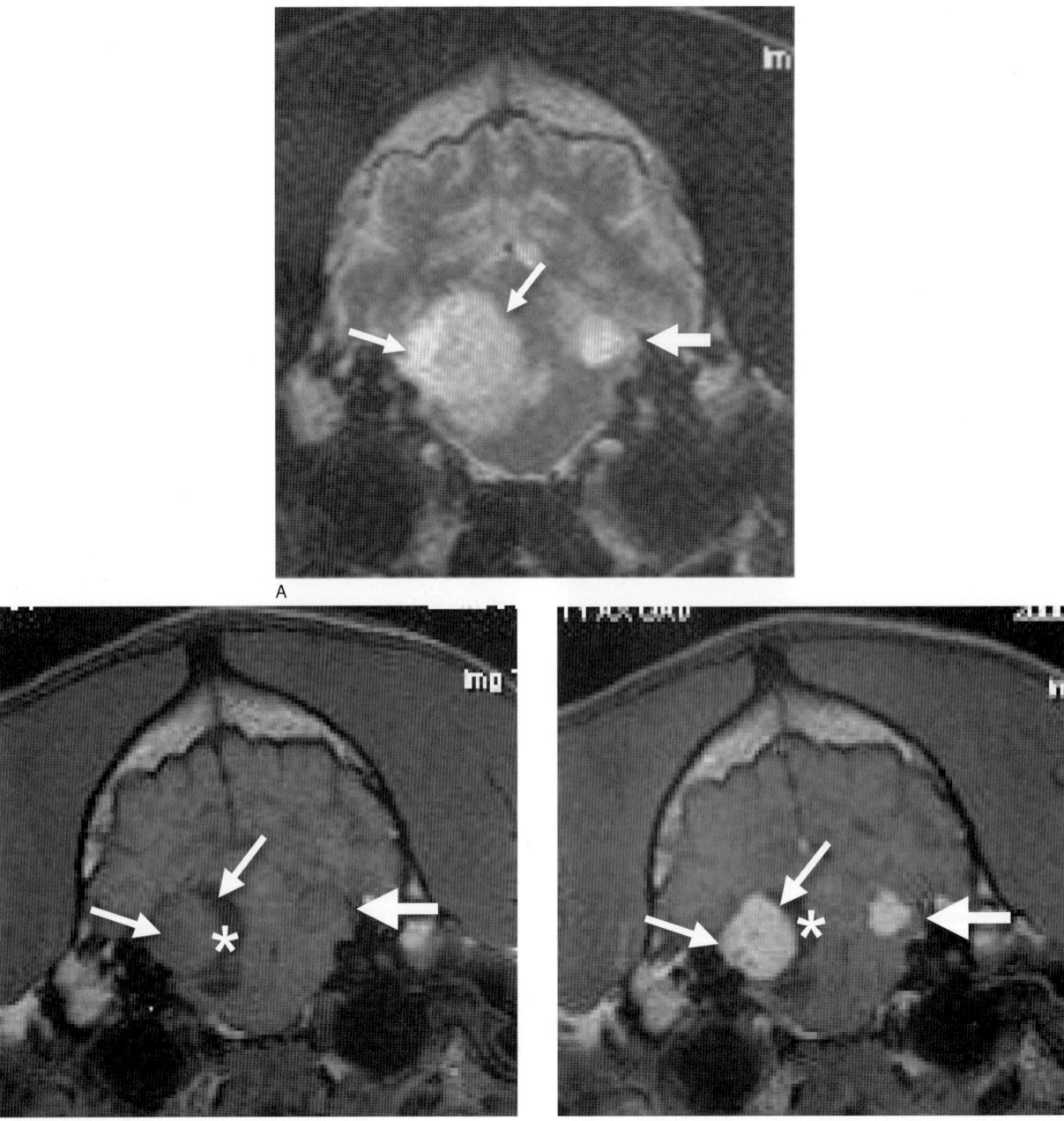

Figure 2.61.   (A) Transverse T2-weighted MR images from a dog with two separate meningiomas (small arrows and larger arrows) of the tentorium cerebelli. Transverse T1-weighted MR images before (B) and following intravenous contrast administration (C) from the same dog. There is also an associated cystic (hypointense) structure with the larger meningioma (*).

Gliomas

Gliomas arise from the supporting cells of the brain parenchyma. These include astrocytes and oligodendrogliocytes. There are varying subtypes within some of these gliomas, ranging from relatively more benign to relatively more malignant varieties. Also, some of these general types of tumors contain multiple cells populations making differentiation into specific diagnoses difficult and inconsistent. Similar to the variety of histologic characteristics of gliomas, the MR appearance of gliomas is varied and enhancement after contrast administration is inconsistent (Figures 2.69–2.73).

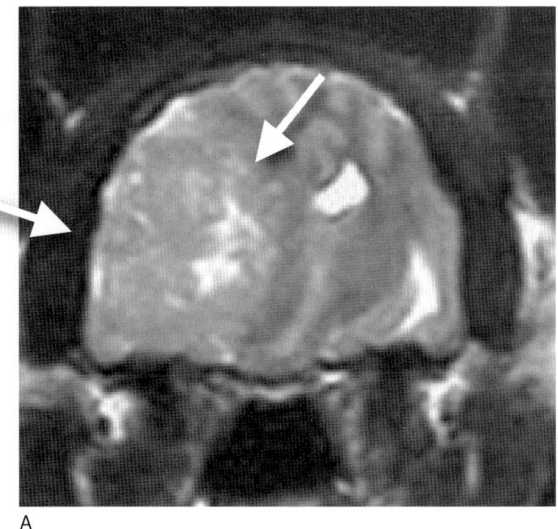
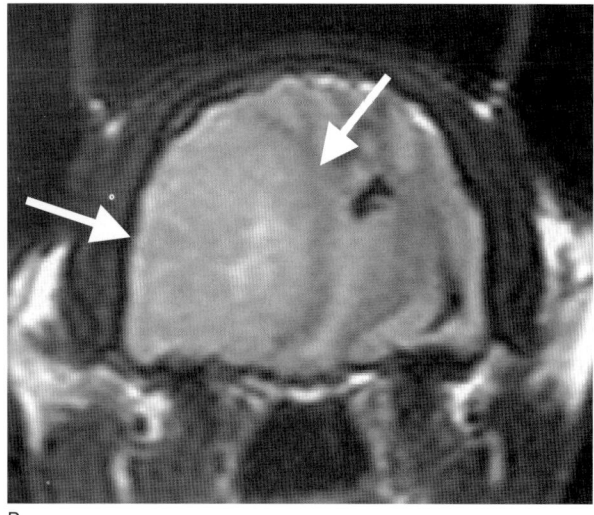

Figure 2.62. Transverse T2-weighted (A) and proton density (B) MR images from a cat with meningioma (arrows).

With MR imaging, gliomas often appear hyperintense in T2-weighted images and hypointense in T1-weighted imaging sequences relative to cerebral cortical tissue. In more advanced tumors, necrosis and hemorrhage may create a heterogenous appearance to the tumor. Diffuse gliomas (throughout the intracranial neural axis) may result in multiple abnormal areas within the intracranial space mimicking an inflammatory process or cerebrovascular disease. Gliomas as a general rule may not be enhanced significantly or even at all following intravenous contrast administration. In some instances, contrast enhancement is present only at the margins of the tumor, providing for the description of a "ring-enhancing" lesion. This type of enhancement pattern while characteristic of gliomas is certainly not pathognomonic for them as other processes including inflammatory disease may appear similarly. In other gliomas, the contrast-enhancement pattern is faint or heterogenous. Additional disease processes such as inflammatory conditions may also have heterogenous or poorly marginated enhancement following contrast administration (Figure 2.74).

Choroid Plexus Tumors

Choroid plexus tumors arise from the choroid plexus tissue (Figures 2.75–2.77). These tumors are also commonly hyperintense in T2-weighted images, and isointense in T1-weighted images. In other instances, these tumors may be hypo- or hyperintense in T1-weighted images. Due to the tissue of origin, these tumor types tend to be located in or around the ventricular system. Obstruction of the ventricle system may result in hydrocephalus in association with these tumors. Because of the concentration of blood vessels within the tumor, these tumors are often markedly enhanced after intravenous contrast administration. Other tumor types, besides choroid plexus tumor, may appear to arise from within the ventricles (Figure 2.78).

Pituitary Tumors

Pituitary tumors may be found in the sella or suprasellar location and expand into the diencephalon

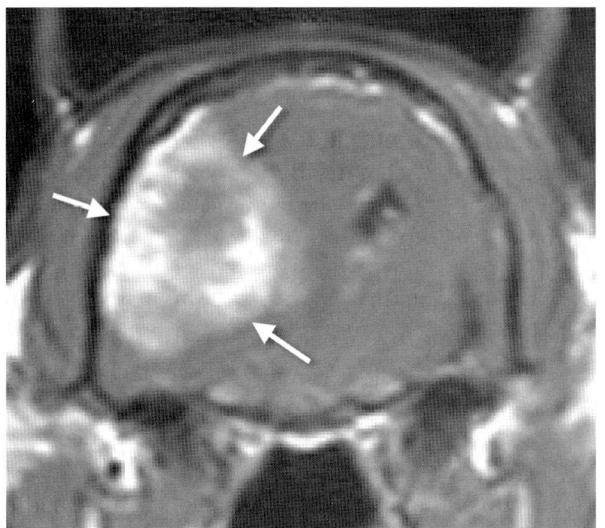

Figure 2.63. Transverse T1-weighted MR image following intravenous contrast administration from the same cat as in Figure 2.62 with a meningioma (arrows).

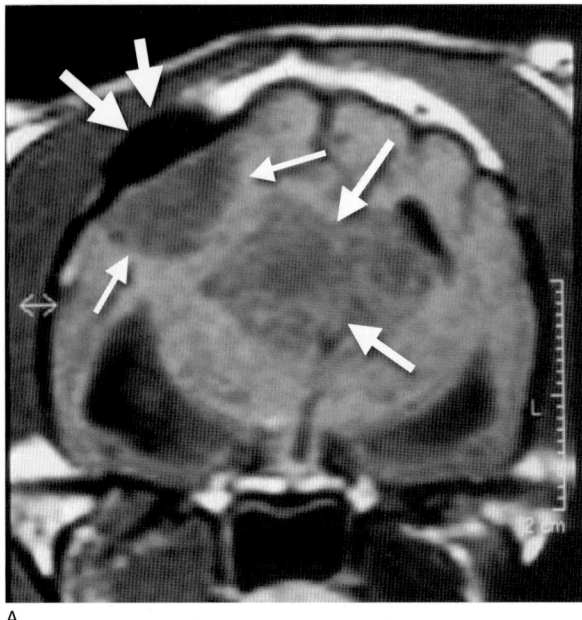

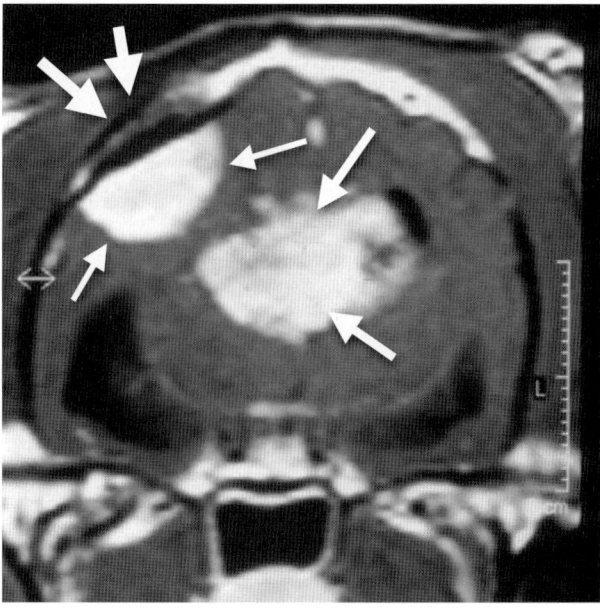

A

B

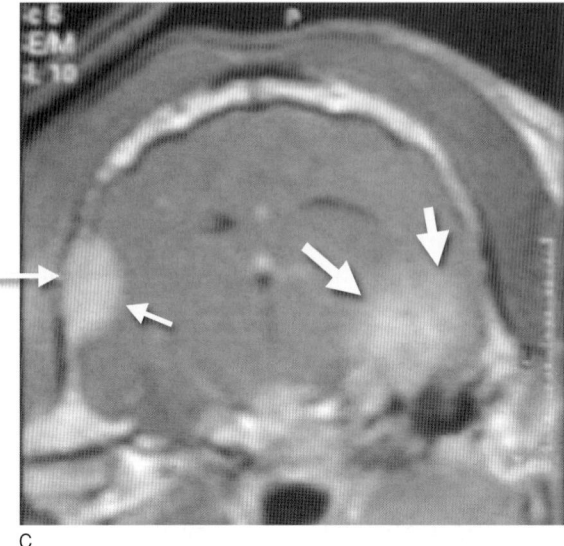

C

Figure 2.64.   Transverse T1-weighted MR images before (A) and following intravenous contrast administration (B) from a cat with two separate meningiomas (small arrows and medium arrows). Note the hyperostosis of the skull overlying the more superficial meningioma (large arrows). Transverse T1-weighted MR image following intravenous contrast administration (C) from a cat with two separate meningiomas (small arrows and larger arrows).

(Figure 2.55). Smaller tumors are more readily seen with MR imaging especially with dynamic contrast studies. Macroadenomas may enlarge dorsally and invade or compress the diencephalon. Macroadenomas are usually hyperintense on T2-weighted sequences, and isointense on T1-weighted sequences. Most macroadenomas are enhanced following contrast administration. As the normal pituitary is naturally enhanced following contrast administration, some adenomas may actually not take up as much contrast as the normal surrounding tissues. Microadenomas, commonly associated with hyperadrenocorticism, may be more difficult to appreciate for similar reasons, that is, the tumor is lost within the normally enhanced pituitary tumor.

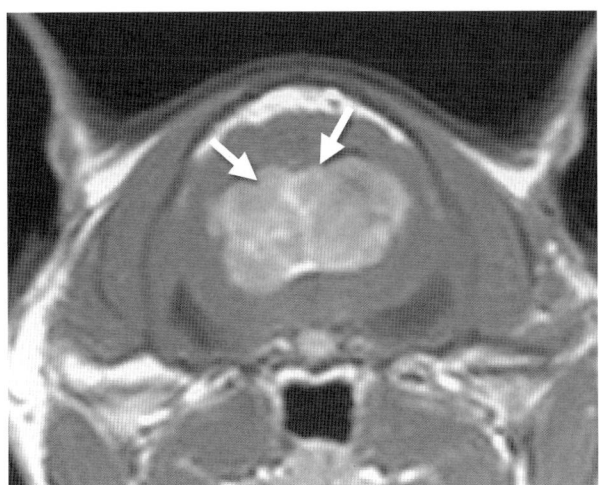

Figure 2.65.   Transverse T1-weighted MR image following intravenous contrast administration from a cat with an intraventricular meningioma (arrows).

Metastasis

Metastatic neoplasia to the brain can also occur (Figure 2.79). As these are generally more aggressive varieties of tumor, they are often apparent on T2-weighted and FLAIR sequences, and are normally contrast enhanced following intravenous contrast administration. Classically, metastatic disease is found primarily at the junction of the gray and white matter in the cerebral hemi-

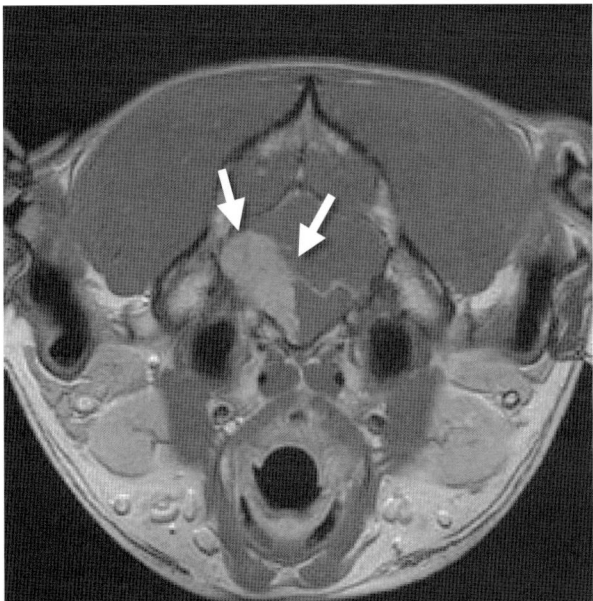

Figure 2.66.   Transverse T1-weighted MR image following intravenous contrast administration from a dog with a meningioma (arrows) along the floor of the skull.

spheres, but obviously can be present at any location in the intracranial space.

Tumors Extending from Local Structures

Neoplastic diseases may also extend into the intracranial cavity from the skull, nasal cavities, ear canals, and other regions in close proximity to the brain. Tumors of the nasal passages may extend caudally through the cribriform plate and invade the olfactory bulb (Figure 2.80). These tumors often have irregular margins and are commonly contrast enhancing. Additionally, there may be a significant amount of associated cerebral edema, primarily in the ipsilateral (to the major lesion) cerebral white matter. Similar appearances may occur, however, with meningiomas in this location (see previous discussion).

Tumors of the skull (multilobular tumors of bone) often will compress the intracranial contents as these tumors expand (Figure 2.81). These tumors obviously have a primary focus of skull bone involvement, which can aid in their differentiation from other types of intracranial tumors.

Nutritional

Thiamine deficiency is the most commonly recognized nutritional abnormality affecting the intracranial structures of animals. Bilaterally symmetrical hyperintense abnormalities may be seen in these nuclear areas, and possibly the cerebellum (in dogs) with MR imaging of affected animals (Garosi et al. 2003). Cats may have similar lesions as well, and may have abnormalities within the colliculi, brain stem, and thalamus. These lesions tend to be hyperintense on T2-weighted sequences and are focal, round to oval, and relatively discrete. Similar lesions may be found in other metabolic encephalopathies.

Inflammatory Diseases

Encephalitis and meningitis may result from both infectious and non-infectious etiologies. Common infectious etiologies in cats include toxoplasmosis, feline infectious peritonitis, cryptococcus, and other as yet unclassified but suspected viral agents. In upto 60% or more cases of encephalitis in dogs and cats, however, an infectious etiology is not identified.

For specific diagnosis, imaging studies such as MR imaging may provide information regarding anatomical lesions associated with primary inflammation (Figures 2.82–2.91). Lesions are often most obvious on T2-weighted or FLAIR imaging sequences as hyperintense

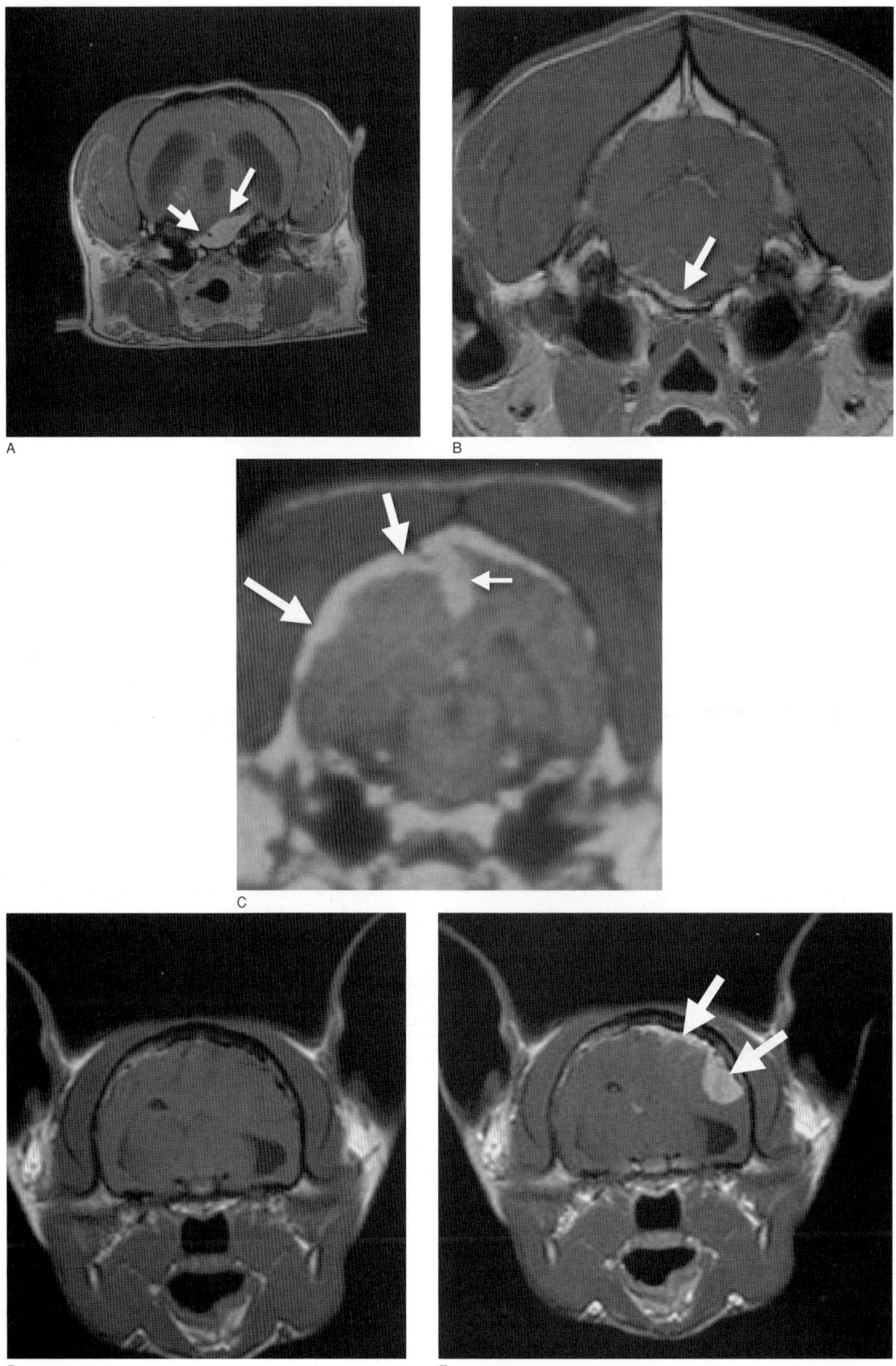

Figure 2.67. Transverse T1-weighted MR images (A)–(C) following intravenous contrast administration from three dogs with a meningioma (arrows) which are more plaque-like in structure. In the third dog (C), the meningioma also involves the falx cerebri (small arrow). Transverse T1-weighted MR images before (D) and following intravenous contrast administration (E) from a cat with a meningioma (arrows) which are more plaque-like in structure (arrow).

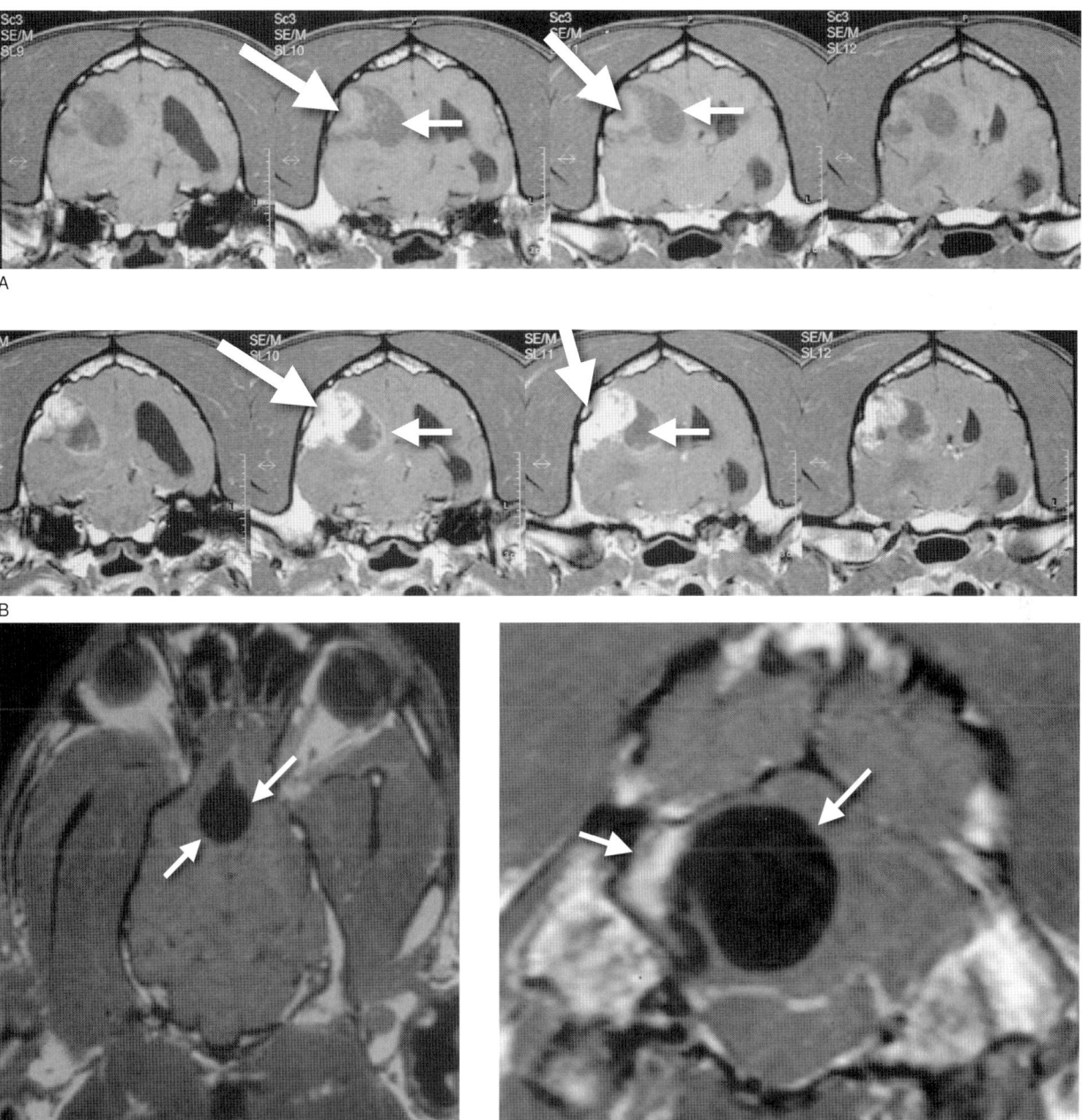

Figure 2.68. Transverse T1-weighted (A) MR images before and following intravenous contrast administration (B) from a dog with a meningioma (larger arrows). Note the associated cystic structure (small arrows). Dorsal T1-weighted MR image (C) before intravenous contrast administration from a dog with a cystic meningioma (arrows) of the rostral falx cerebri. Transverse T1-weighted MR image (D) following intravenous contrast administration from a dog with a cystic meningioma (arrows) of the cerebellar region.

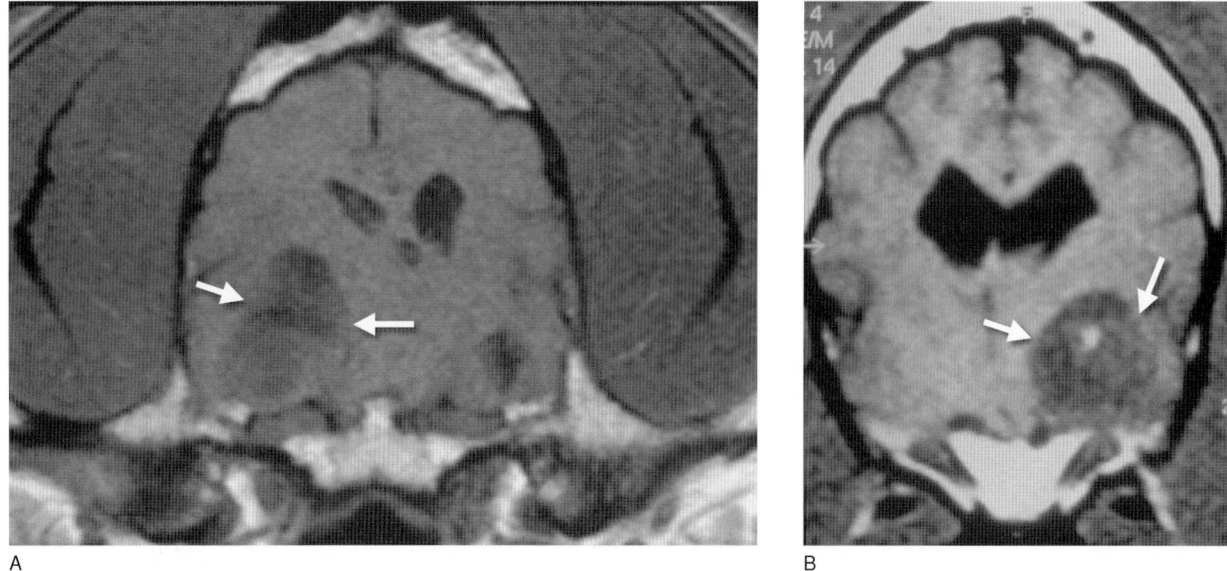

Figure 2.69.   Transverse T1-weighted MR images ((A) and (B)) from two dogs with gliomas (arrows).

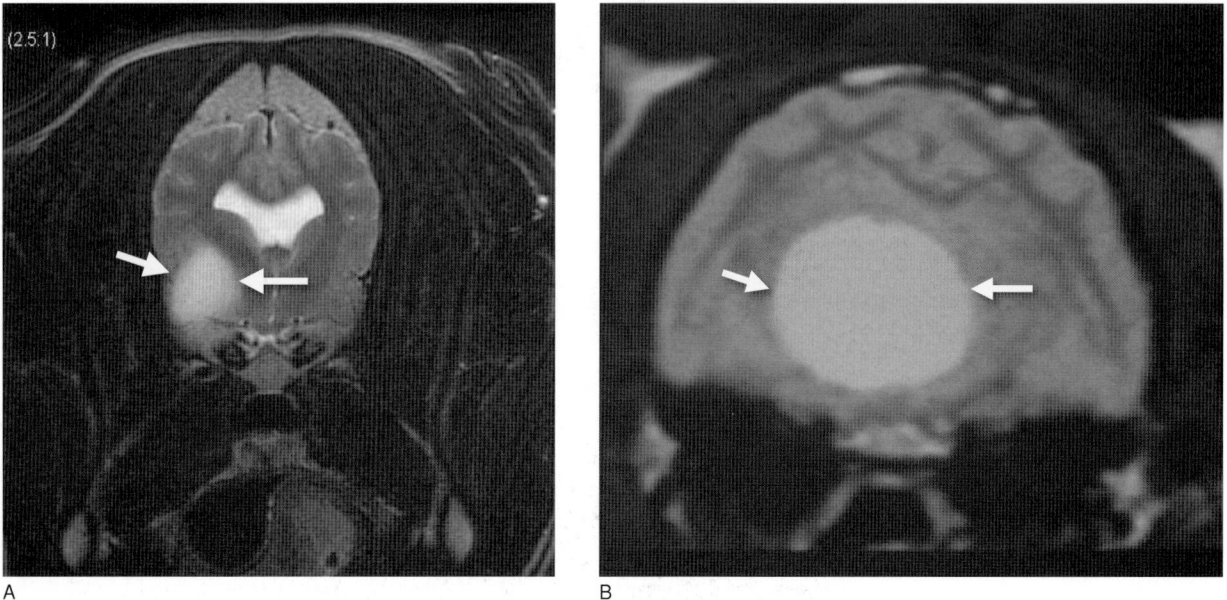

Figure 2.70.   Transverse T2-weighted (A) and proton density weighted (B) MR images from a dog (A) and a cat (B) with gliomas (arrows).

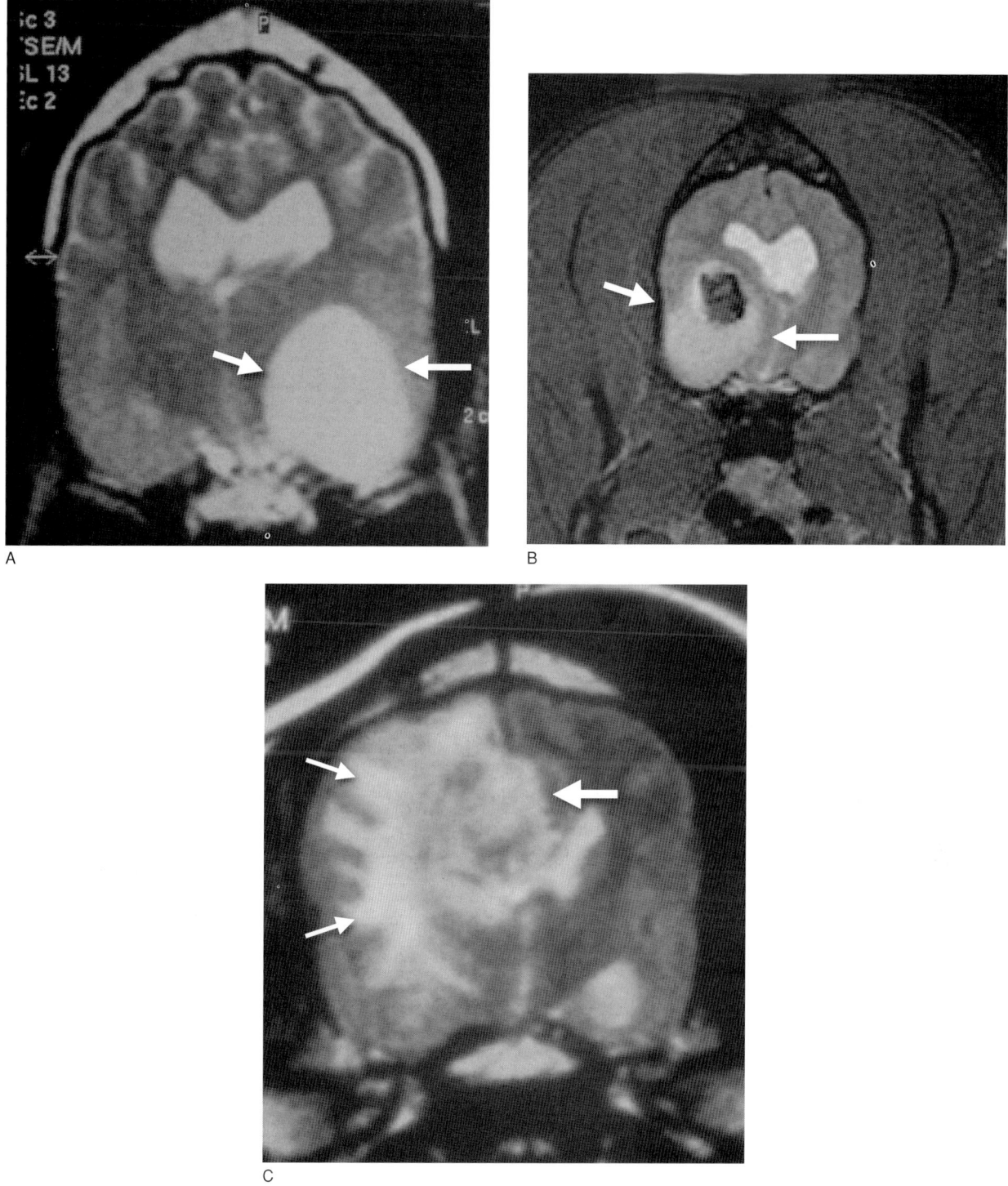

Figure 2.71.   Transverse T2-weighted MR images (A)–(C) from three dogs with gliomas (arrows). Note the associated cerebral edema in dog (C) (smaller arrows).

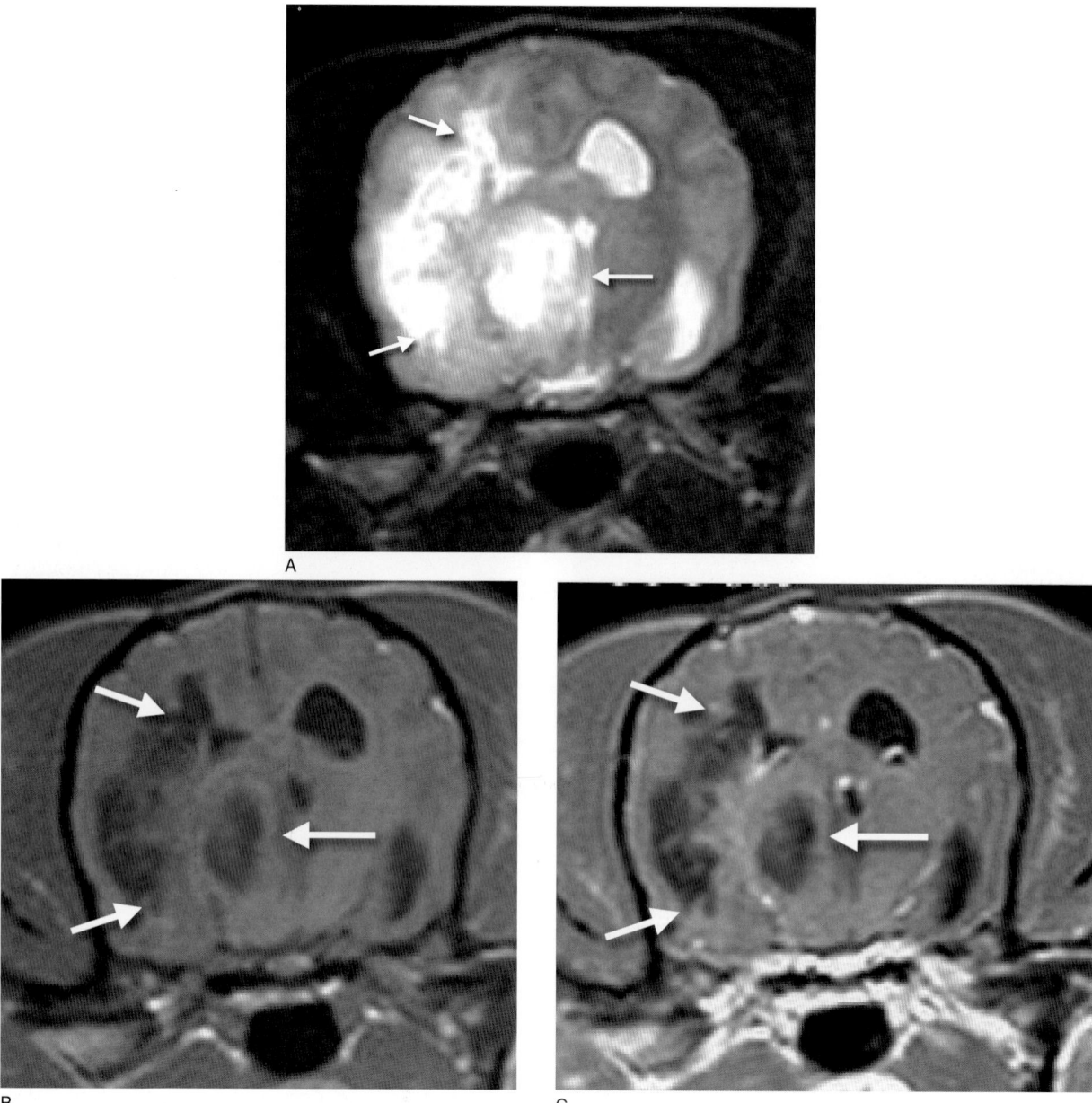

Figure 2.72. Transverse T2-weighted (A) and T1-weighted MR images before (B), and following intravenous contrast administration (C) from a dog with a glioma (arrows).

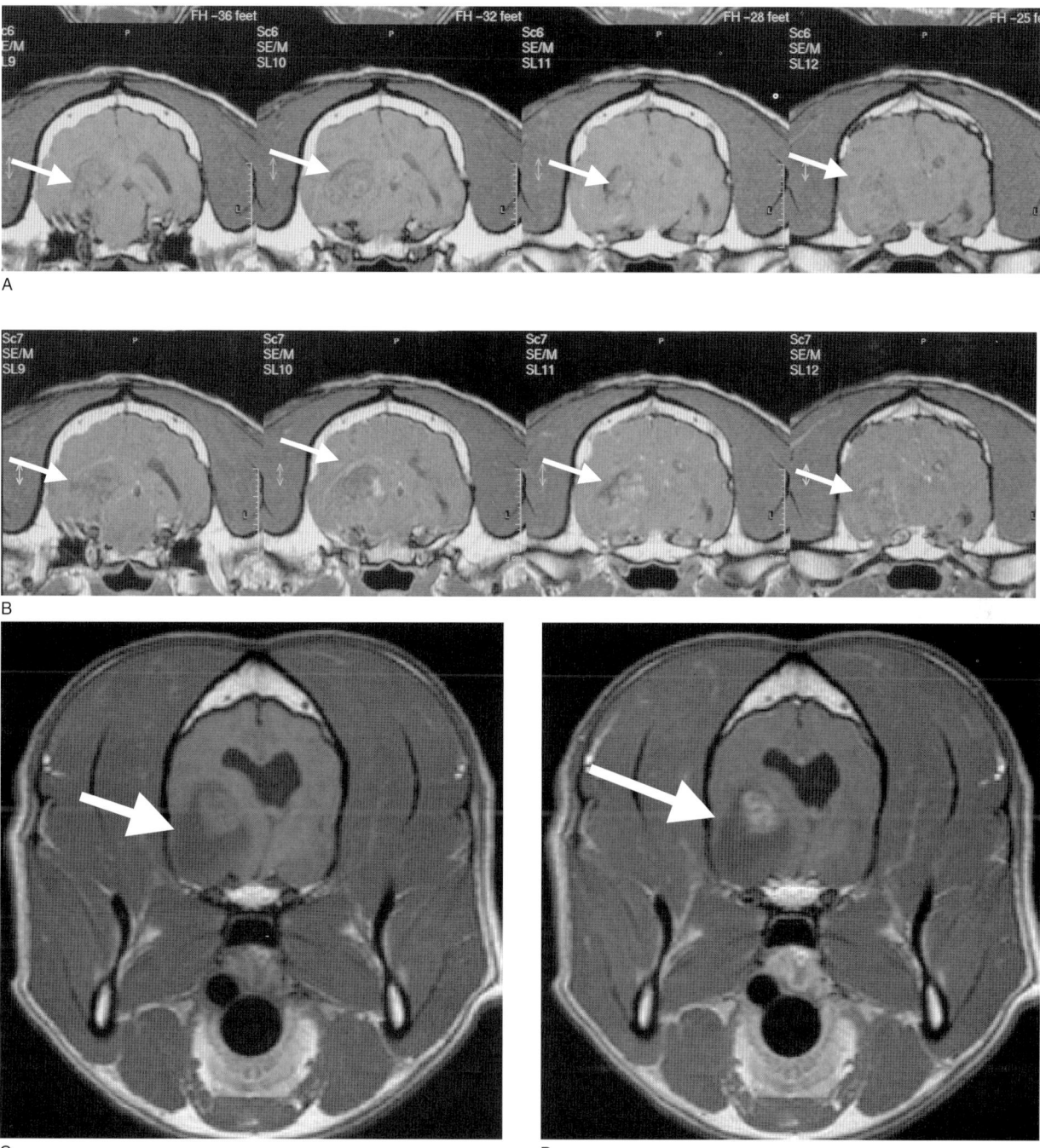

Figure 2.73. Transverse T1-weighted MR images before (A) and following intravenous contrast administration (B) from a dog with a glioma (arrows). Transverse T1-weighted MR images before (C) and following intravenous contrast administration (D) from a dog with a glioma (arrows).

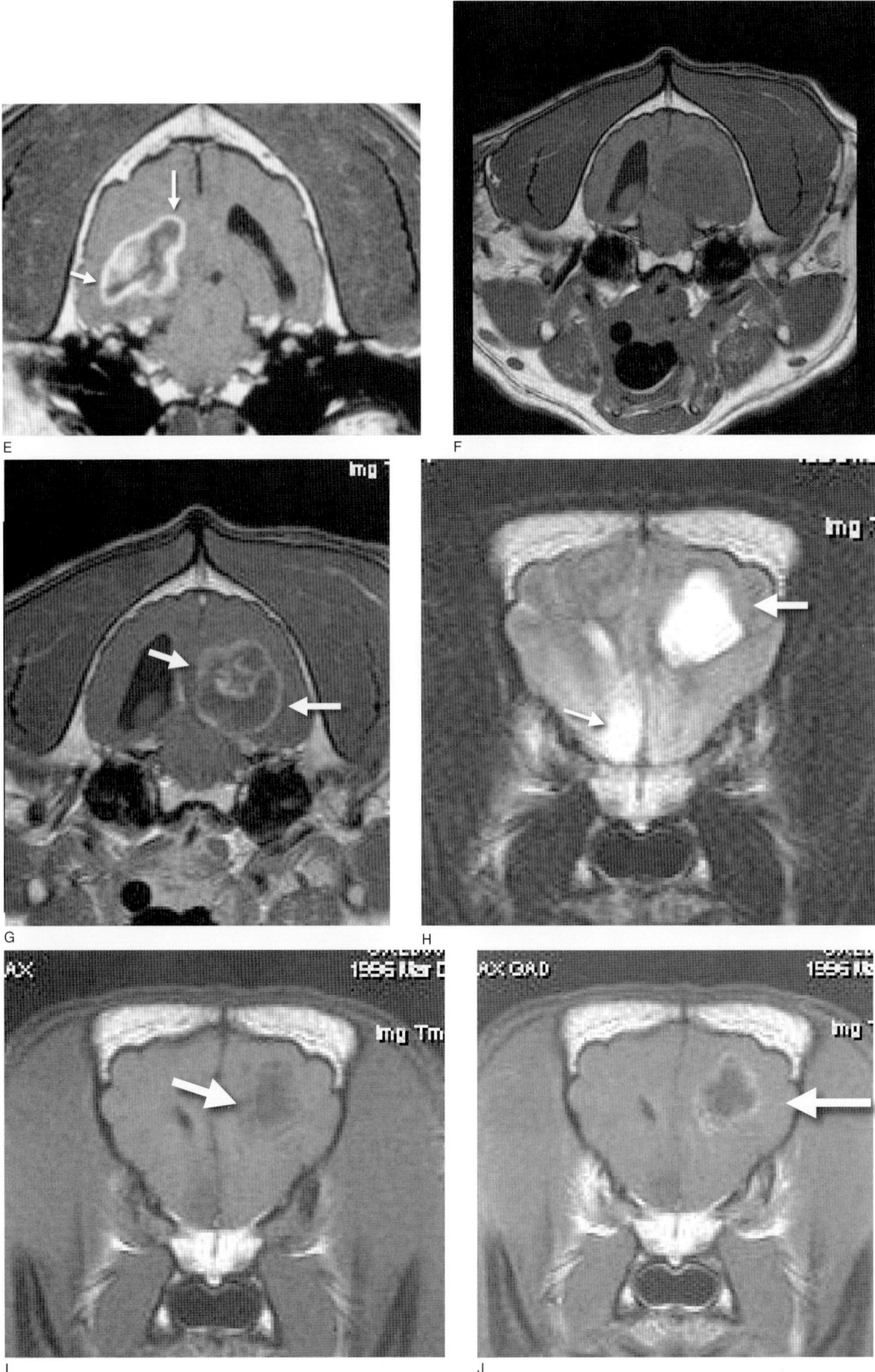

Figure 2.73. (*Continued*) Transverse T1-weighted MR image (E) following intravenous contrast administration from a dog with a glioma (arrows). Note the more peripheral "ring-like" enchancement. Transverse T1-weighted MR images before (F) and following intravenous contrast administration (G) from a dog with a glioma (arrows). Transverse T2-weighted MR image (H) from a dog with a glioma (larger arrows) and an associated focus of edema (smaller arrow). Transverse T1-weighted MR images before (I) and following intravenous contrast administration (J) from a dog with a glioma (arrows).

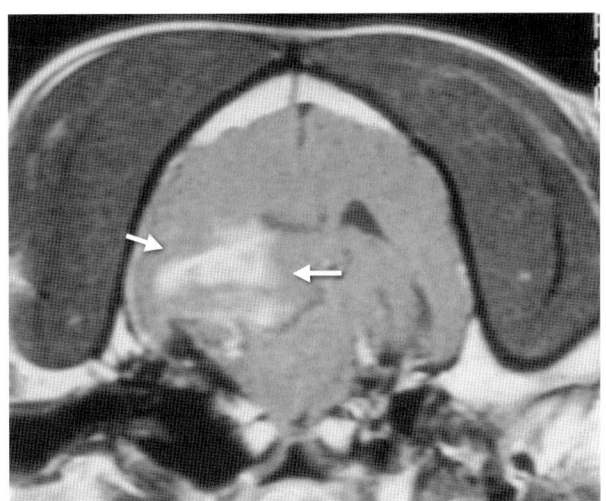

Figure 2.74. Transverse T1-weighted MR image following intravenous contrast administration from a dog with GME (arrows).

regions. Abnormalities are often iso- to hypointense on T1-weighted pre-contrast sequences. In some diseases, such as focal granulomatous meningoencephalitis (GME), focal inflammatory mass lesions can resemble focal neoplastic diseases with similar features on MR sequences (Figure 2.74). Multifocal discrete anatomical lesions may be present within the nervous system, and these lesions may be especially conspicuous after intravenous contrast medium administration suggesting alterations in the BBB or the cerebral vascu-

lature. In some diseases, notably toxoplasmosis, lesions may be seen on T2-weighted and FLAIR sequences, however, are not enhanced following contrast administration. This may also be found in instances of GME (Figure 2.88).

There are a number of CNS inflammatory diseases that occur in specific breeds of animals, referred to as breed-specific encephalitis (Figure 2.87). MR and other advanced imaging studies may show edema, focal mass effect, diffuse hyperintense abnormalities in T2-studies, or focal or multifocal contrast-enhancing lesions. Abnormalities apparent in MR images, however, are not pathognomonic for these diseases.

Infection or inflammation external to the brain can occasionally be extended into the intracranial cavity. Inner/middle ear disease and nasal disease are most often present in these conditions (Figures 2.92 and 2.93). MR imaging can show these foci of inflammation/infection as well as any intracranial extension. Curiously, we have also noted a number of dogs with primary intracranial tumors of the posterior fossa that have associated middle/inner ear disease (Figure 2.94). The relationship of these two abnormalities is unclear, but can be problematic when attempting to determine if the intracranial abnormality is an extension of an ear infection or a second primary disease (such as tumor).

With middle and inner ear (bulla) disease, there is often a hyperintense abnormality within the bulla on proton density or T2-weighted sequences. Contrast enhancement can be variable. In some instances, only the lining of the bulla will be enhanced preferentially.

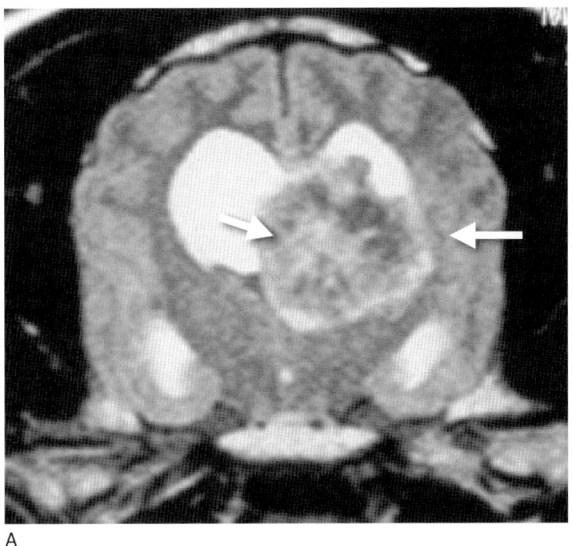
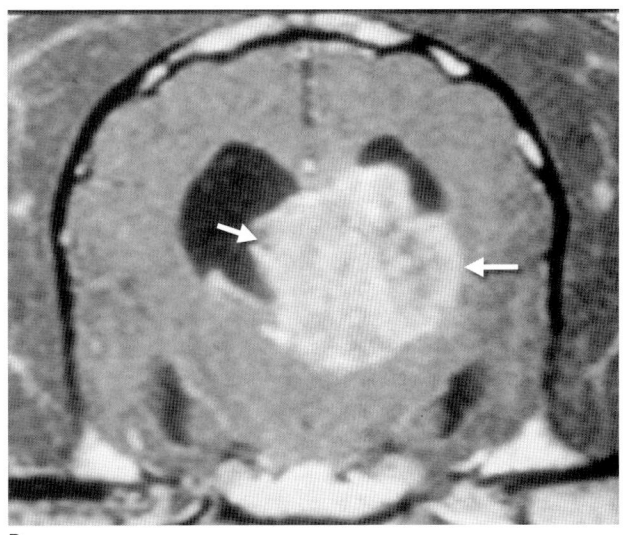

A   B

Figure 2.75. Transverse T2-weighted (A) and T1-weighted MR images following intravenous contrast administration (B) from a dog with a choroid plexus tumor of the lateral ventricles (arrows).

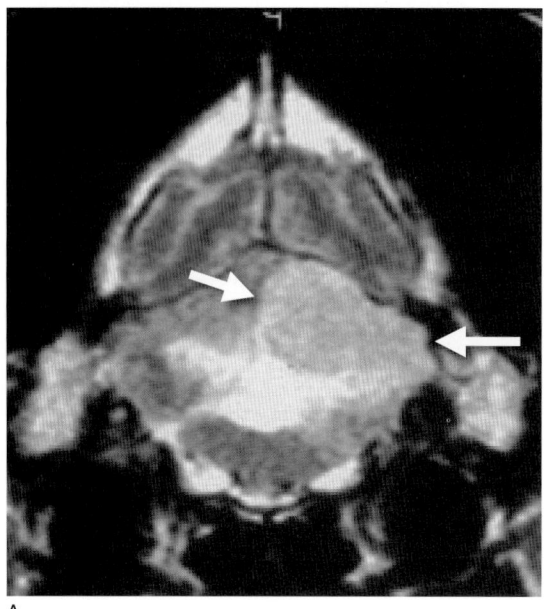
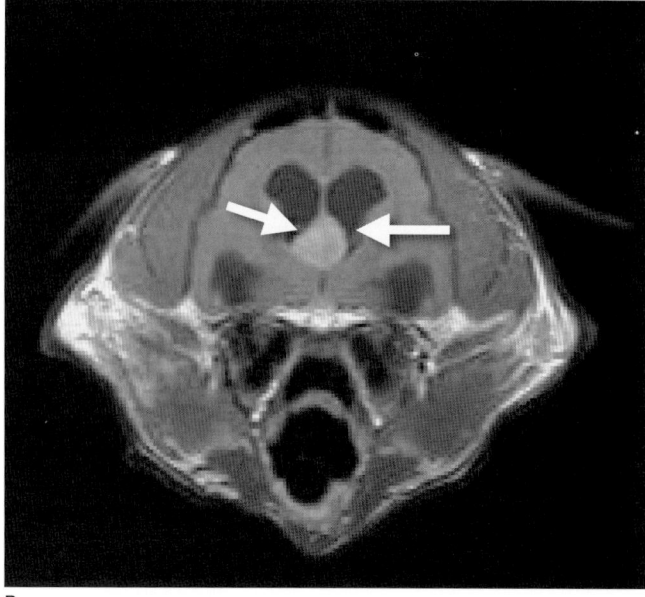

A   B

Figure 2.76. Transverse T2-weighted MR image (A) from a dog with a choroid plexus tumor of the lateral cerebellar pontine angle (arrows). Transverse T1-weighted MR image (B) following intravenous contrast administration from a cat with choroid plexus tumor (arrows) of the third ventricle.

Contrast enhancement of the bulla, however, is not pathognomonic for infection/inflammation, as middle/inner ear tumors may also show contrast enhancement.

Idiopathic Disease

Any disease that does not have a specific etiology is referred to as idiopathic. With some disease processes, even with exhaustive clinical, biochemical, and histologic evaluations over years of observation, no etiology has been established for the disease process. Idiopathic epilepsy, for example, would fulfill these diagnostic criteria. Some dogs with idiopathic epilepsy when imaged with MR following their seizure (usually more than one) will have structural alterations in the intracranial structures (Figure 2.44). Persistent structural alterations in brain tissue due to chronic seizures and associated brain atrophy may also be evident on MR imaging.

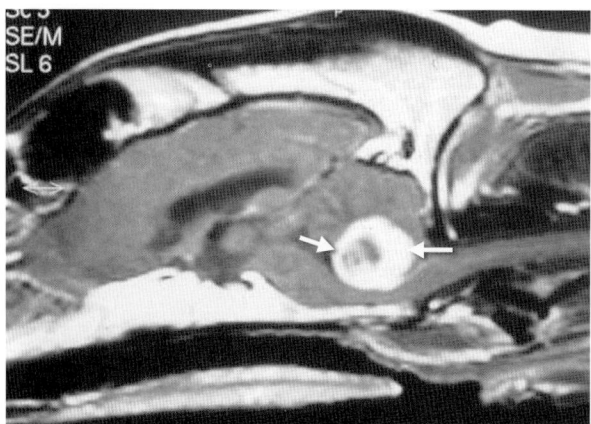

Figure 2.77. Sagittal T1-weighted MR image following intravenous contrast administration from a dog with a choroid plexus tumor (arrows) of the fourth ventricle.

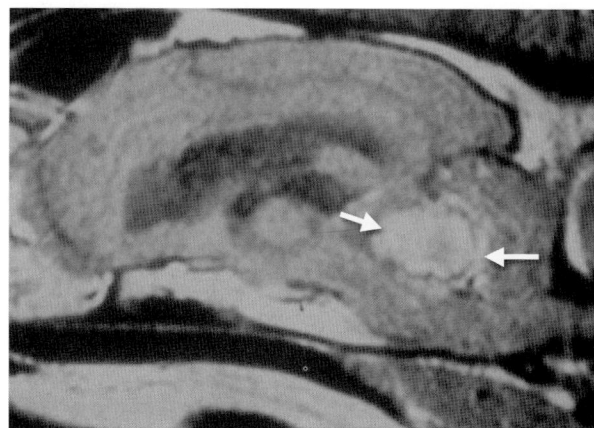

Figure 2.78. Sagittal T1-weighted MR image following intravenous contrast administration from a dog with a cholesteatoma (arrows) of the rostral fourth ventricle.

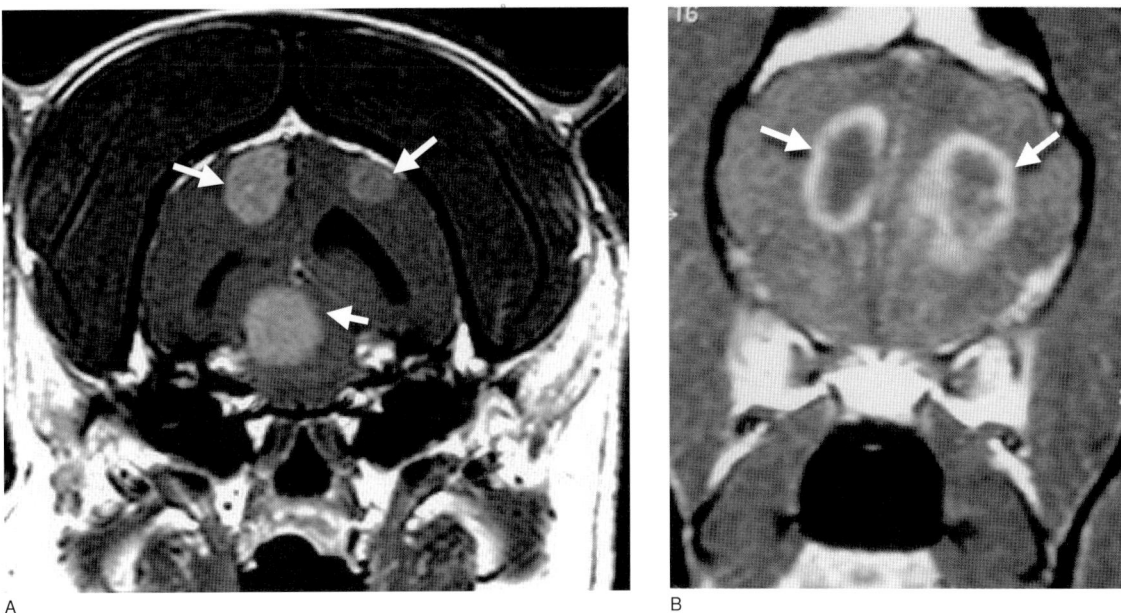

Figure 2.79. Transverse T1-weighted MR images following intravenous contrast administration from two dogs ((A) and (B)) with metastatic neoplasia to the brain (arrows).

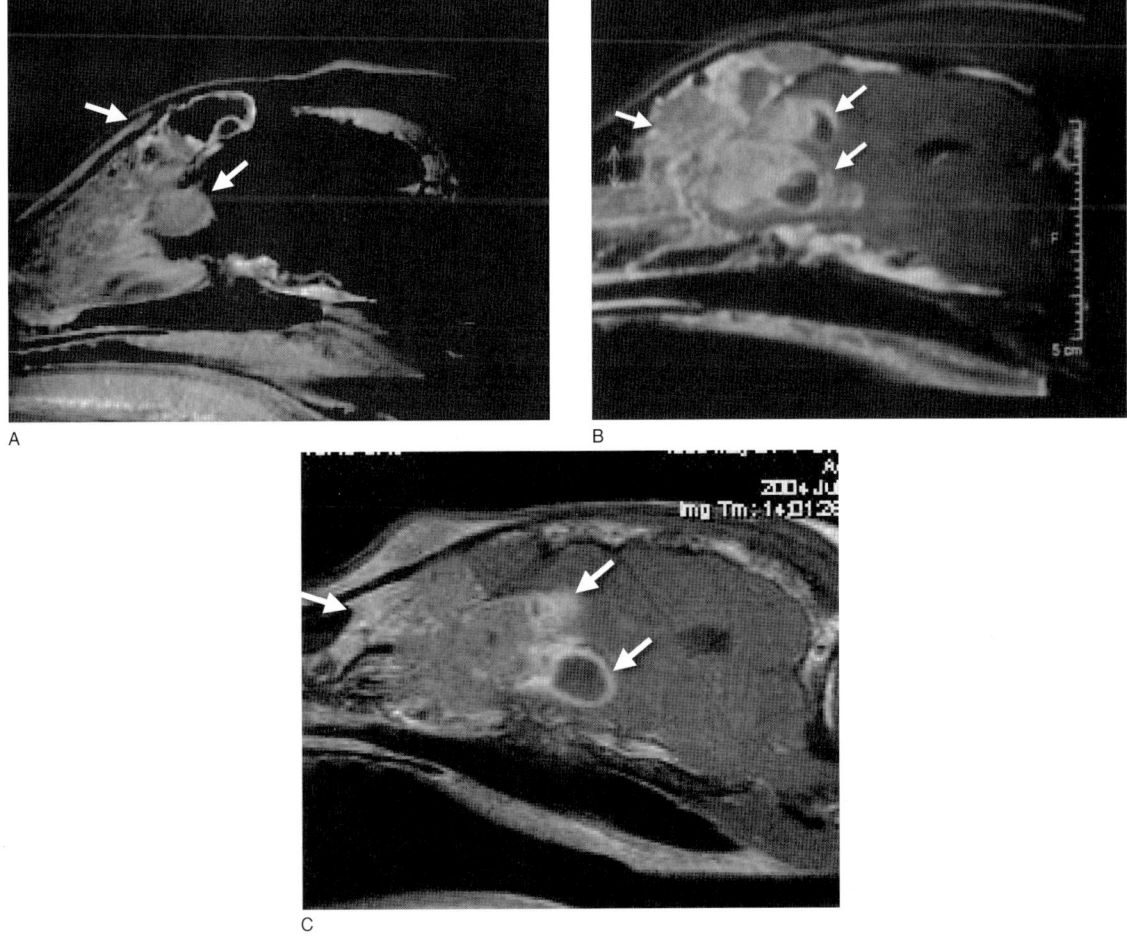

Figure 2.80. Sagittal T1-weighted MR images following intravenous contrast administration from three dogs (A)–(C) with nasal tumors extending into the olfactory region of the brain (arrows).

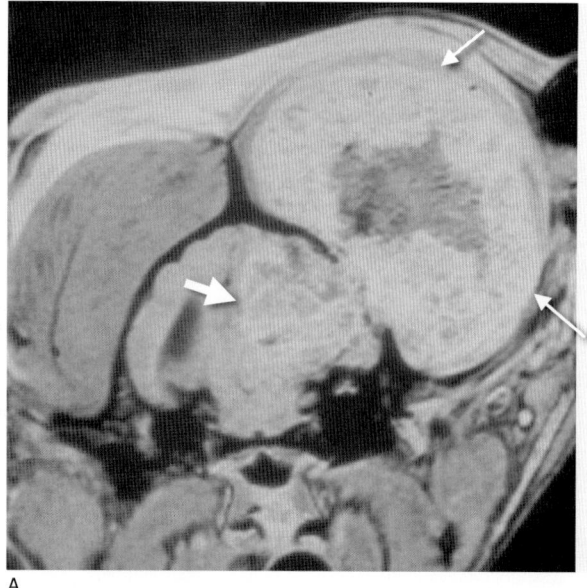

A

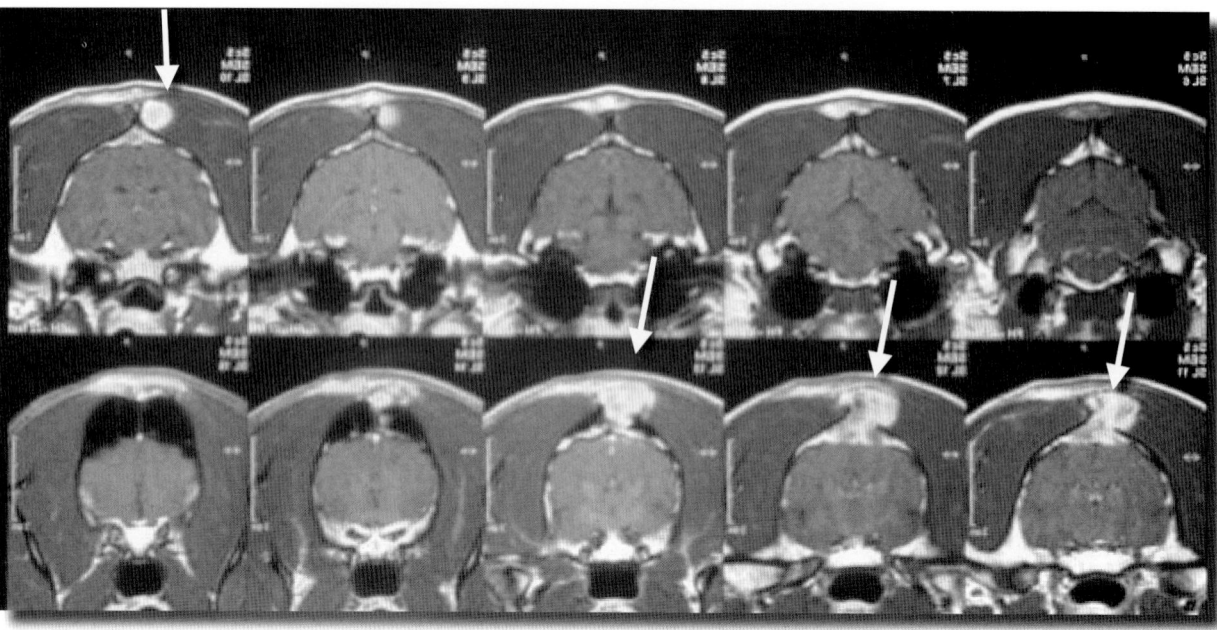

B

Figure 2.81. Transverse T1-weighted MR images following intravenous contrast administration from two dogs ((A) and (B)) with tumors of the skull (arrows).

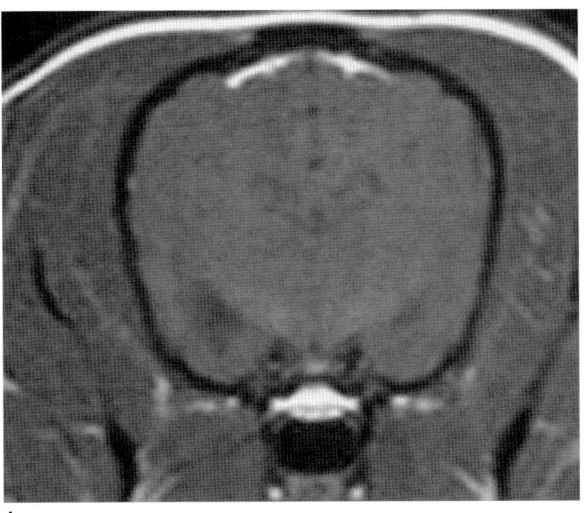 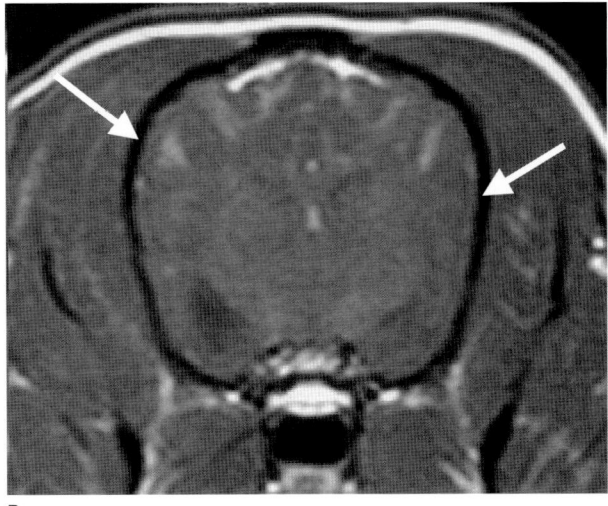

A   B

Figure 2.82. Transverse T1-weighted MR images before (A) and following intravenous contrast administration (B) from a dog with encephalitis. Note the multifocal parenchymal contrast enhancement (arrows).

Trauma

Traumatic injury remains a common cause of brain dysfunction in dogs and cats.

Evidence of cerebral edema or hemorrhage (see the previous discussion in this chapter regarding MR imag-

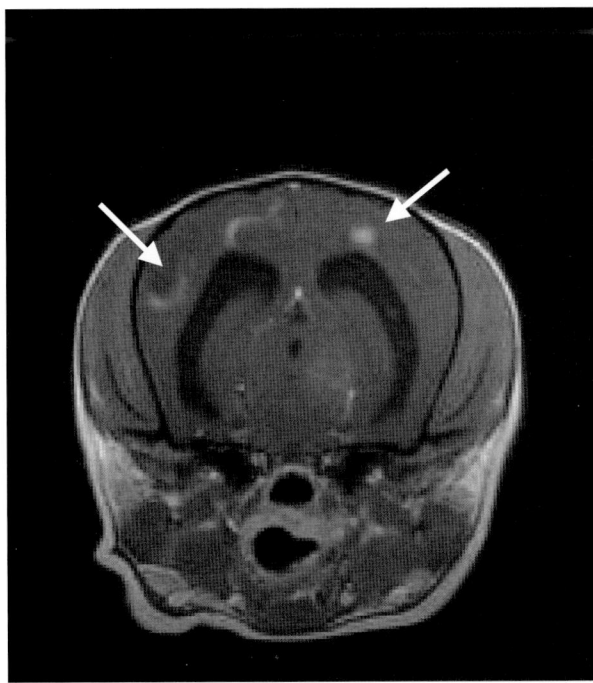

Figure 2.83. Transverse T1-weighted MR image following intravenous contrast administration from a dog with encephalitis. Note the multifocal parenchymal contrast enhancement (arrows).

ing characteristics of hemorrhage) is most often apparent with MR imaging studies (Figure 2.95). Occasionally, a subdural or extradural hematoma or focal intraparenchymal hematoma is found.

With exogenous head injury, there may be associated trauma to the skull (fracture) and associated soft tissues (such as the temporalis muscles). When injury is present in these structures, it can be difficult to determine if the animal had an underlying intracranial disease where in it fell and injured the head, or if the head injury was due to a primary traumatic injury.

Cerebrovascular Diseases

Cerebrovascular disease should be suspected in any animal with acute onset intracranial signs (Thomas 1996). A thorough examination of the body for petechia is important, including the mucous membranes (especially of the penis, prepuce, and vulva) and the retina. Pallor, low-grade heart murmurs, weakness, and tachycardia are hallmark signs of anemia, which may be associated with coagulopathies. These signs may result with significant amounts of bleeding into body cavities. Thoracic auscultation for pleural fluid and abdominal palpation for hemoperitoneum is important. Radiographs and ultrasound may help when the physical examination is unrewarding but large amounts of internal bleeding are suspected. Large amounts of blood can be lost through the gastrointestinal tract and examination of the stool for hematochezia or melena is important.

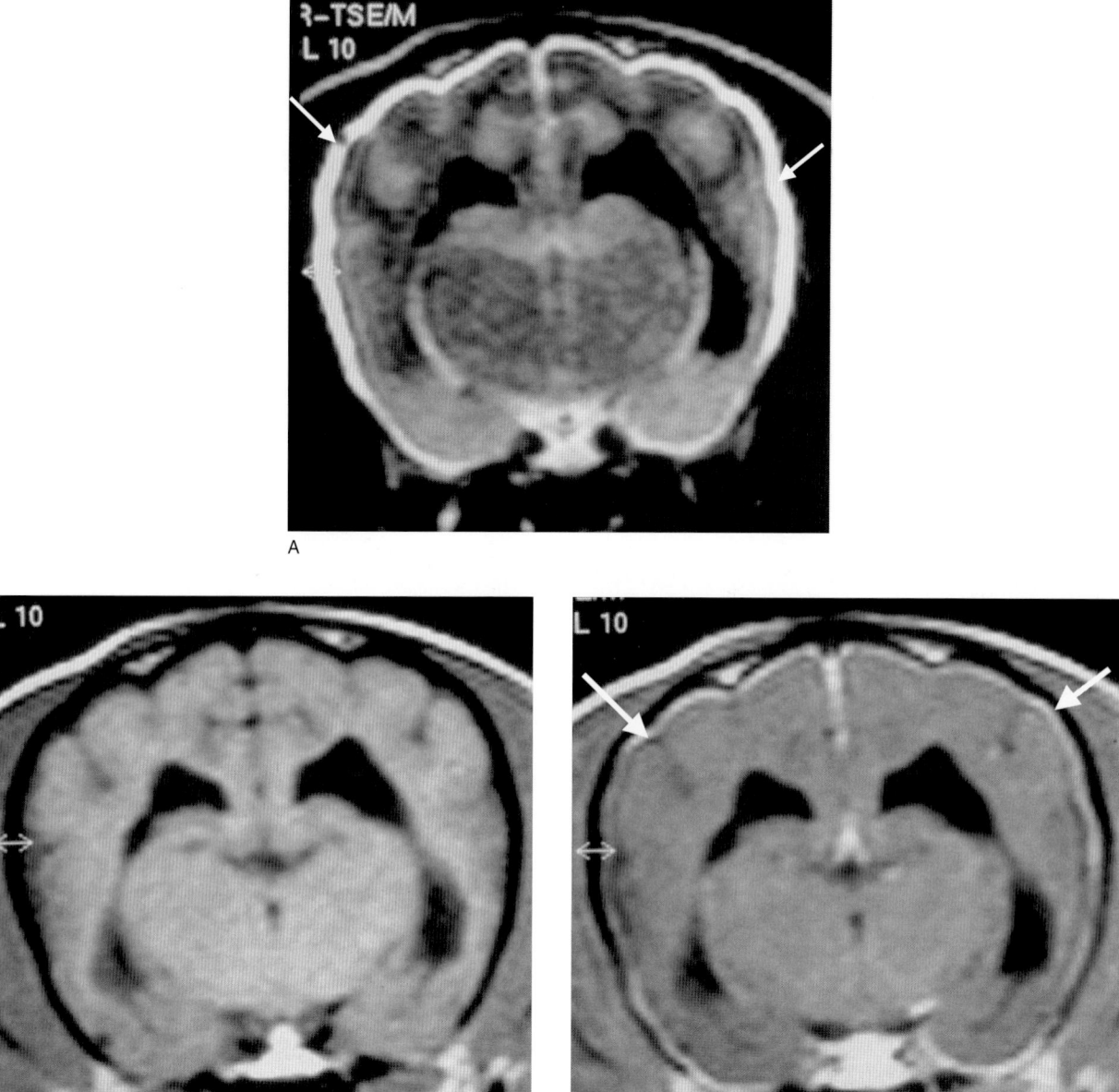

Figure 2.84.   Transverse FLAIR MR image (A) from a dog with meningitis and encephalitis. Note the hyperintense signal on the surface of the brain (arrows). Transverse T1-weighted MR images before (B) and following intravenous contrast administration (C) from a dog with meningitis and encephalitis. Note the contrast enhancement of the surface of the brain (arrows).

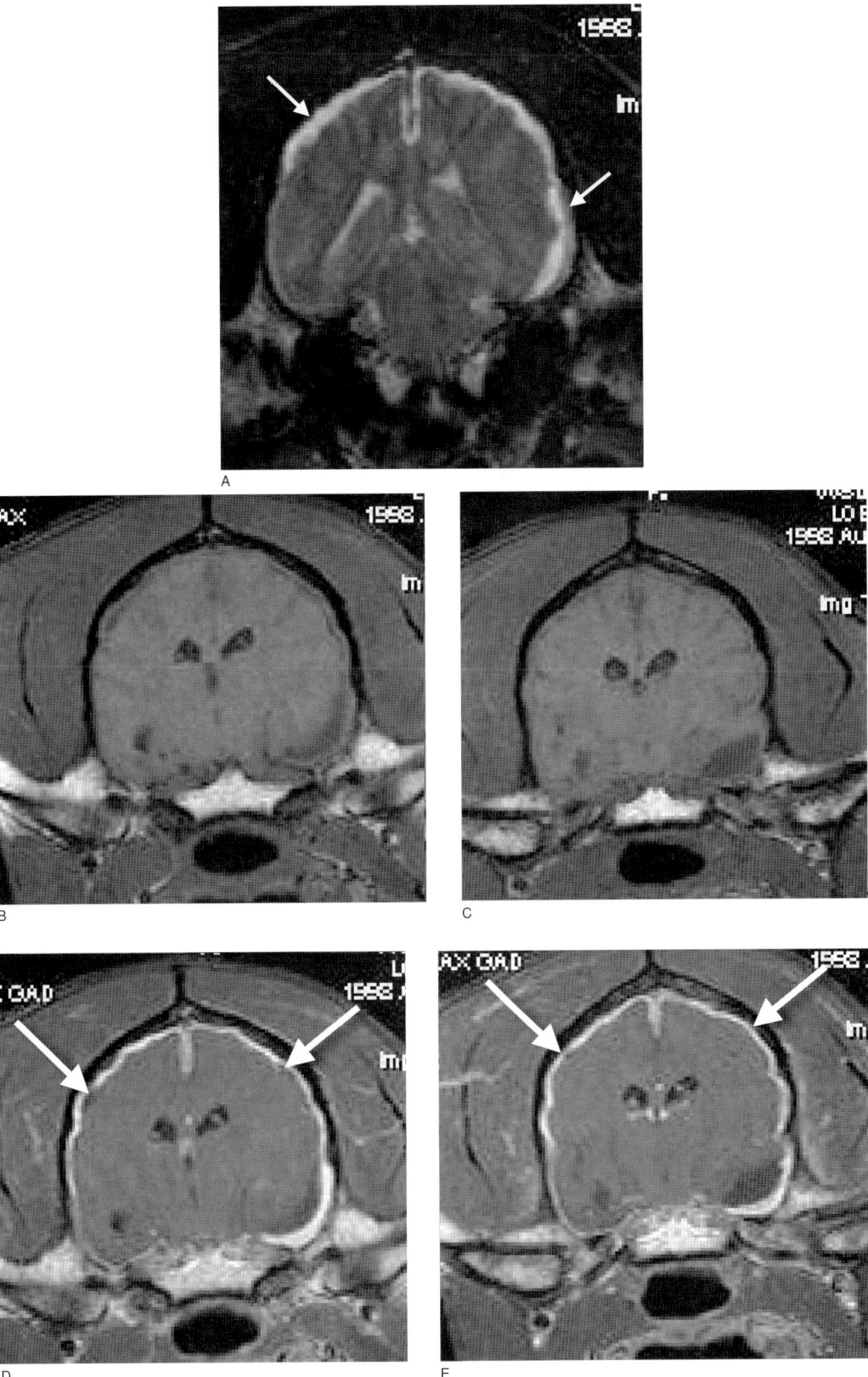

Figure 2.85.   Transverse T2-weighted MR image (A) from a dog with meningitis and encephalitis. Note the hyperintense signal on the surface of the brain (arrows). Transverse T1-weighted MR images before ((B) and (C)) and following intravenous contrast administration ((D) and (E)) from the same dog with meningitis and encephalitis. Note the contrast enhancement of the surface of the brain (arrows).

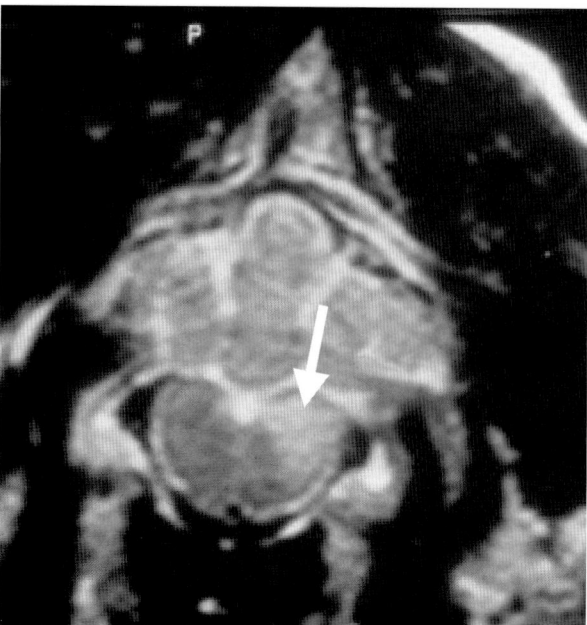

Figure 2.86. Transverse T2-weighted MR image from a cat with meningitis and encephalitis. Note the hyperintense signal within the brain stem (arrows). Final diagnosis was toxoplasmosis.

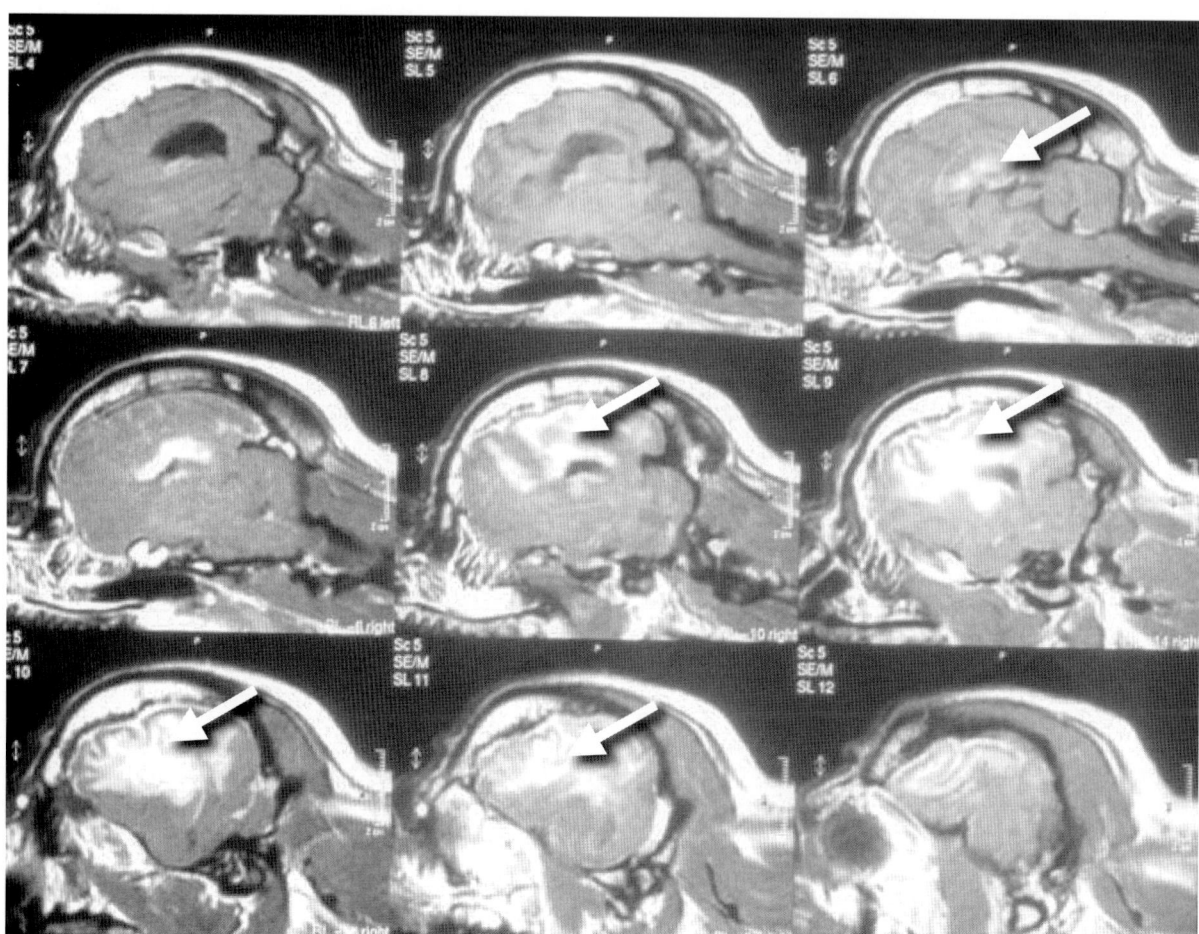

Figure 2.87. Sagittal T1-weighted MR images following intravenous contrast administration from the Pug dog with Pug encephalitis. Note the contrast enhancement of the cerebral cortex of the brain (arrows).

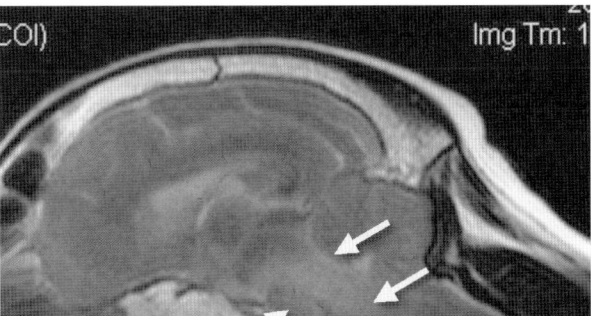

A

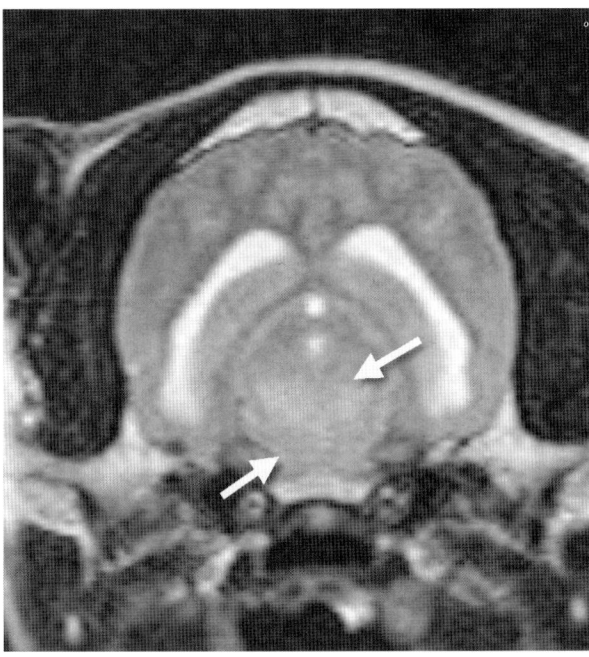

B

Figure 2.88. Sagittal (A) and transverse (B) T2-weighted MR images from a dog with histologically confirmed GME. Note the hyperintense signal within the brain stem (arrows). This lesion did not enhance following intravenous contrast administration.

Besides documenting any hypertension via either direct or indirect methods, complete blood cell count, with special attention to red cell and platelet counts, is often helpful. Specific coagulation testing (bleeding time, PT, PTT, FDPs) is also commonly evaluated. Biochemical evidence of a predisposition to hypercoagulability such as proteinuria should be collected. Diseases associated with hypertension such as renal disease and hyperthyroidism certainly should also be considered.

As cerebrovascular disease often alters the structural integrity of the brain, clarification of the cause of the clinical signs often requires some advanced imaging modality to evaluate brain structure (Figures 2.34–2.42, 2.96, and 2.97). Depending upon the degree of the cerebral disease (i.e., ischemia vs. overt hemorrhage), and the relationship between onset of the disease and the time of imaging, the characteristics of cerebrovascular disease may vary.

With MR imaging, hemorrhage can have a varied appearance, primarily based on the duration of the hemorrhage and alterations in blood hemoglobin (see Table 2.1) (Thomas 1996). As different regions within hemorrhagic focus may contain differing stages of hemoglobin breakdown, a heterogenous appearance to the lesion may be encountered. In addition to the form of hemoglobin present, the signal intensities of a blood clot may vary depending on the operating field strength and the type of sequence used for imaging. Hemorrhage may also vary in appearance depending on the cavity (subdural, intraparenchymal, or subarachnoid) where the bleeding occurred. With MR imaging, cerebrovascular disease may vary from evidence of a focal mass to diffuse or multifocal changes. Often there is evidence of edema, which may be cytotoxic or vasogenic, in the area of the cerebrovascular damage. Therefore, the initial abnormality is usually apparent as hyperintense in both T2-weighted and FLAIR studies. If the animal is imaged acutely (within hours) following the onset of clinical signs, however, smaller lesions may be not apparent. In this situation a gradient echo sequence may reveal abnormalities not previously detectable.

Infarcts can be relatively smaller (lacunar; a few millimeters) to relatively larger (territorial). Smaller regions of infarction are usually more round or spherical in shape. Classically, larger regions of infarction have a wedge-shaped pattern may be encountered with the point of the wedge being directed more centrally. The common sites of infarction are the corona radiata, internal capsule, thalamus, or periventricular white matter of the cerebrum. The white matter of the cerebellum is another common site. In other instances, infarcted regions are more "comet-tail" shaped.

Contrast enhancement following gadolinium administration of the infarcted region will depend on the interval between the time of the vascular damage and the MR examination, the resulting inflammatory response, and the degree of vascular disruption (break in the BBB). Most cases are imaged within 48 h after the insult due to the severity of signs, and therefore contrast enhancement in the majority of the infarcted region is uncommon. When present, contrast enhancement in

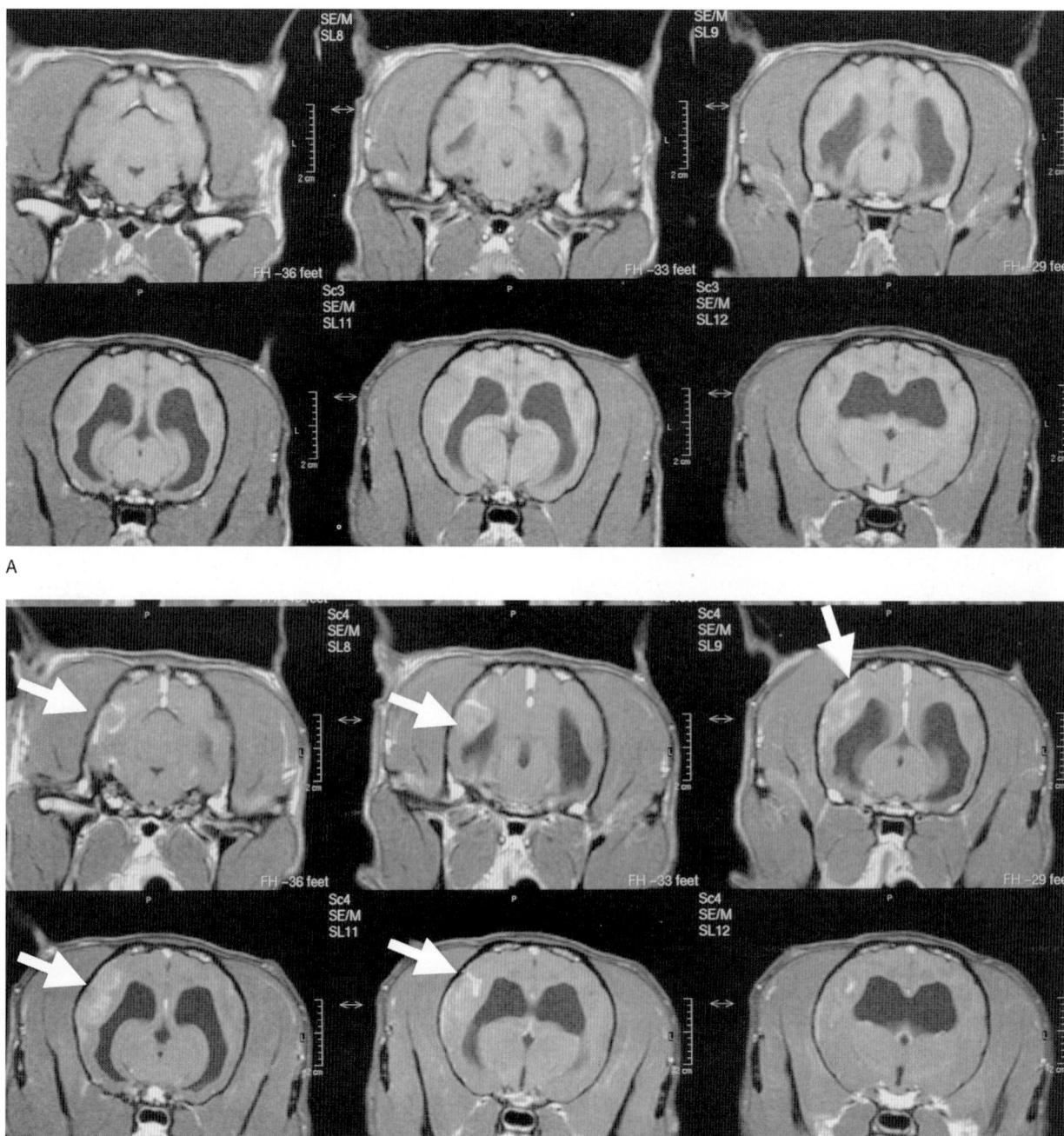

Figure 2.89.   Transverse T1-weighted MR images before (A) and following intravenous contrast administration (B) from a dog with histologically confirmed GME. Note the contrast enhancement within the cerebral hemisphere (arrows).

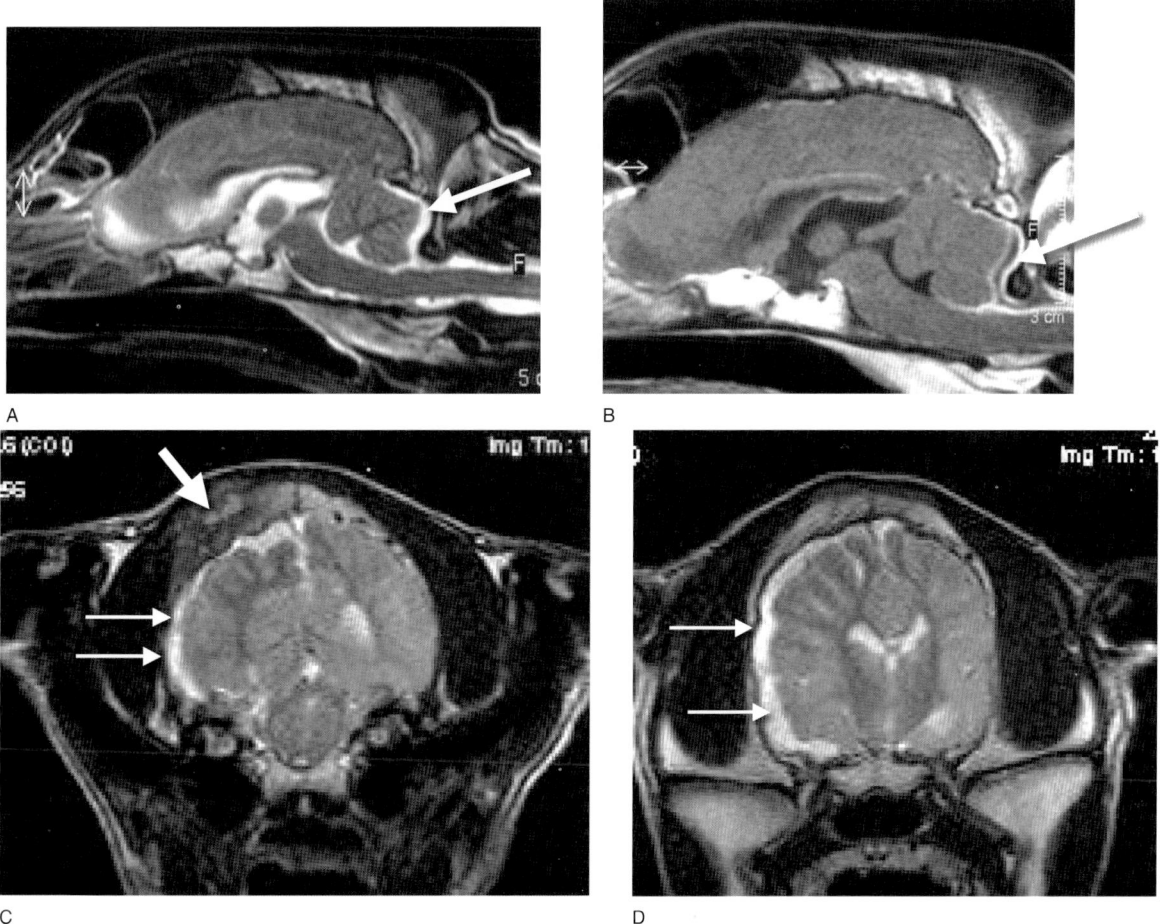

Figure 2.90. Sagittal T2-weighted MR image (A) from a dog with a subdural abscess (arrow) following an attempted cerebrospinal fluid collection. Sagittal T1-weighted MR image (B) following intravenous contrast administration from the same dog with the subdural abscess. Note the contrast enhancement of the surface of the cerebellum (arrow). Transverse T2-weighted MR images at the level of the midbrain (C) and the thalamus (D) from a puppy with a subdural abscess (small arrows) subsequent to a suspected bite wound to the skull (larger arrow).

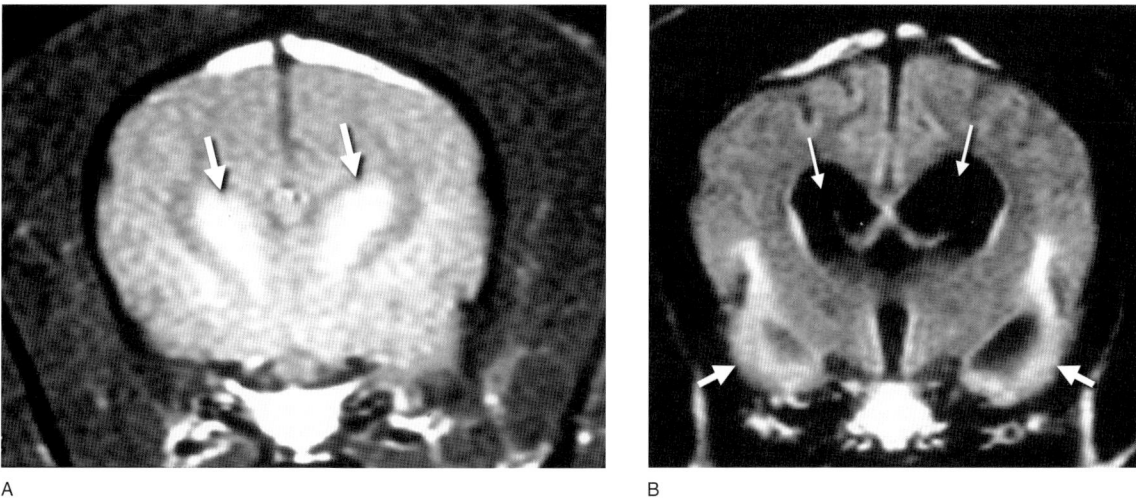

Figure 2.91. Transverse proton density MR image (A) from a dog with encephalitis. The caudal nuclei are bilaterally hyperintense (arrows). Transverse T1-weighted MR image (B) prior to intravenous contrast administration from the same dog as in (A). This image was obtained approximately 1 year after the previous image. Note the dilated ventricles (smaller arrows) and hyperintense signal in the temporal cortex bilaterally (larger arrow).

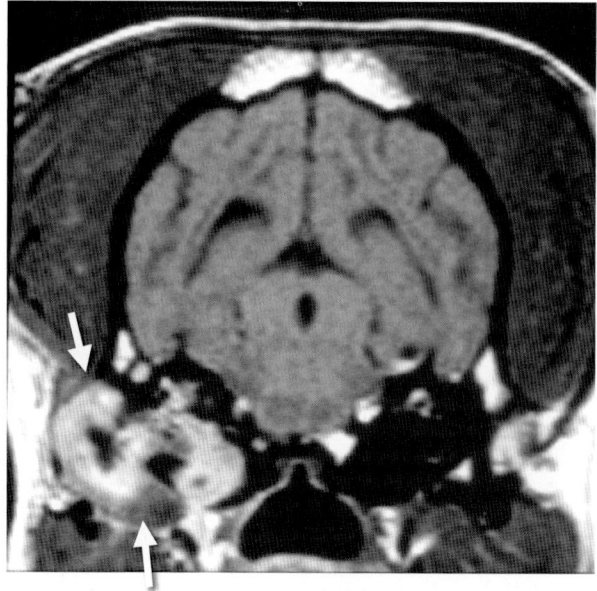

A

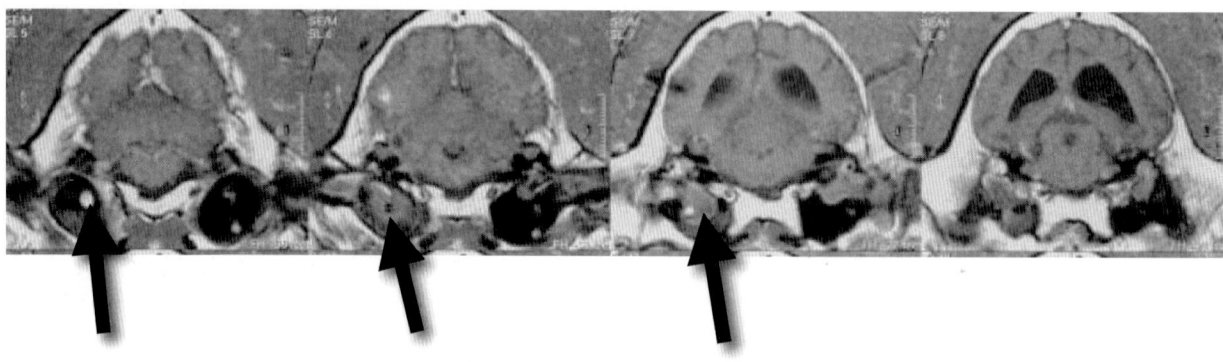

B

Figure 2.92. Transverse T1-weighted MR images from two separate dogs ((A) and (B)) with middle/inner ear infections (arrows).

cerebrovascular lesions is minimal, heterogenous, or peripheral to ring-like. Depending on the imaging characteristics, focal inflammatory brain diseases and some neoplastic processes such as gliomas may have a similar appearance in MR images. It is also important to remember that other pathologic processes (such as tumor or inflammation) may affect cerebral vessels and result in secondary infarction of intracranial nervous tissue.

Diseases of Cranial Nerves

Anatomical abnormalities of the CNs are most often apparent with MR imaging (Figures 2.98–2.100). Tumors and inflammation of CNs often result in enlargement of the affected nerves. Nerves may be more hyperintense on T2-weighted MR sequences, and may enhance following intravenous contrast administration. Occasionally, however, animals with no apparent clinical abnormalities will show contrast enhancement of some CNs, most often the trigeminal nerve. The significance of this contrast enhancement is unknown, and may represent normal variations in blood flow or occult CN pathology.

Surprisingly common, CNs are often infiltrated with diffuse neoplastic diseases such as myelomonocytic leukemia or lymphoma. In these animals, cytologic evaluation of CSF may reveal the neoplastic cells.

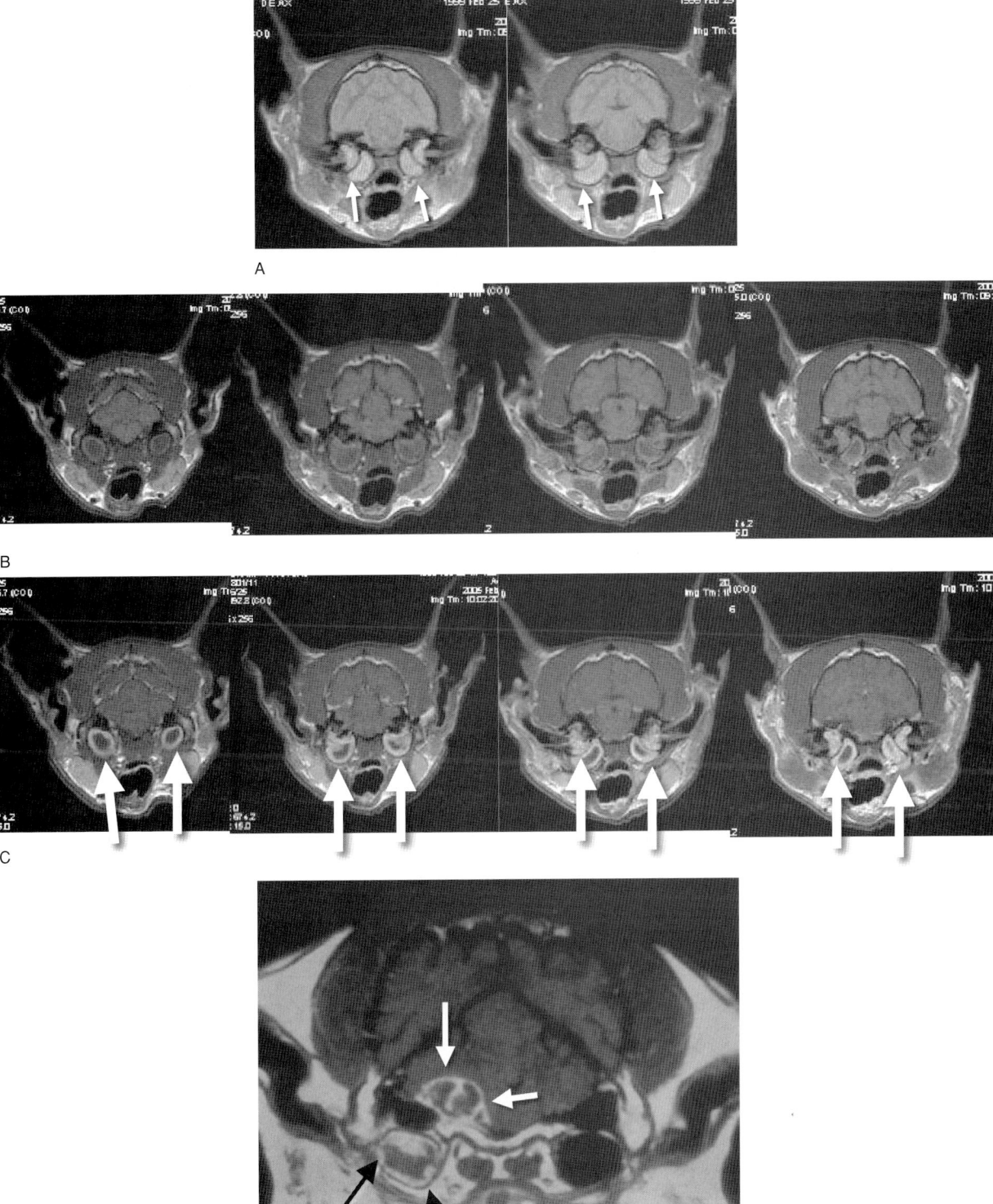

Figure 2.93. Transverse proton density MR image (A) from a cat with bilateral middle/inner ear infection (arrows). Transverse T1-weighted MR images before (B) and following (C) intravenous contrast administration. Note the contrast enhancement of the bulla (arrows). Transverse T1-weighted MR image following intravenous contrast administration from a snow leopard (D). Note the contrast enhancement of the bulla (smaller arrows) as well as within the intracranial cavity (larger arrows).

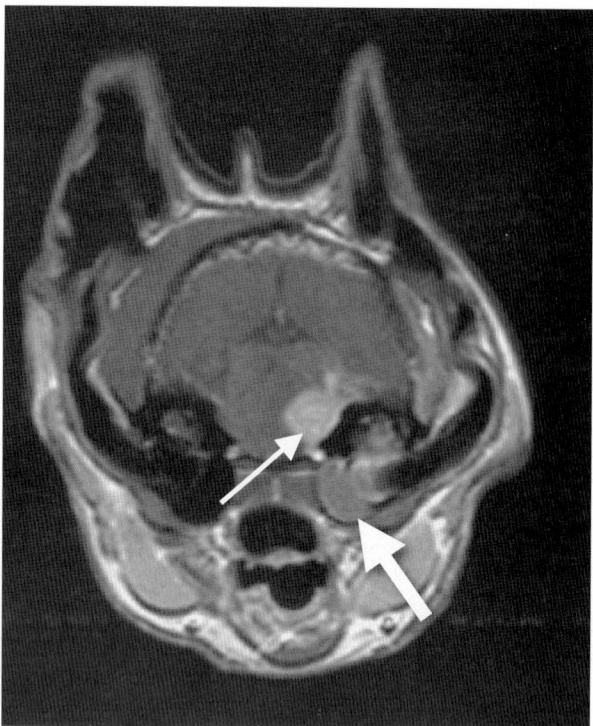

Figure 2.94. Transverse T1-weighted MR image following intravenous contrast administration from a cat with a CN V tumor (smaller arrows). Note the associated fluid signal in the ipsilateral bulla (larger arrows).

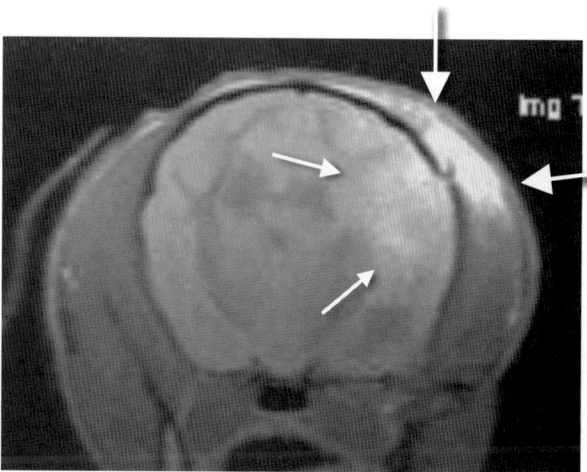

Figure 2.95. Transverse proton density MR image from a dog following intracranial injury. Note the hyperintense abnormalities both within the cerebral hemisphere (smaller arrows) and outside the skull within the temporalis muscle (larger arrows). There is also an associated skull fracture.

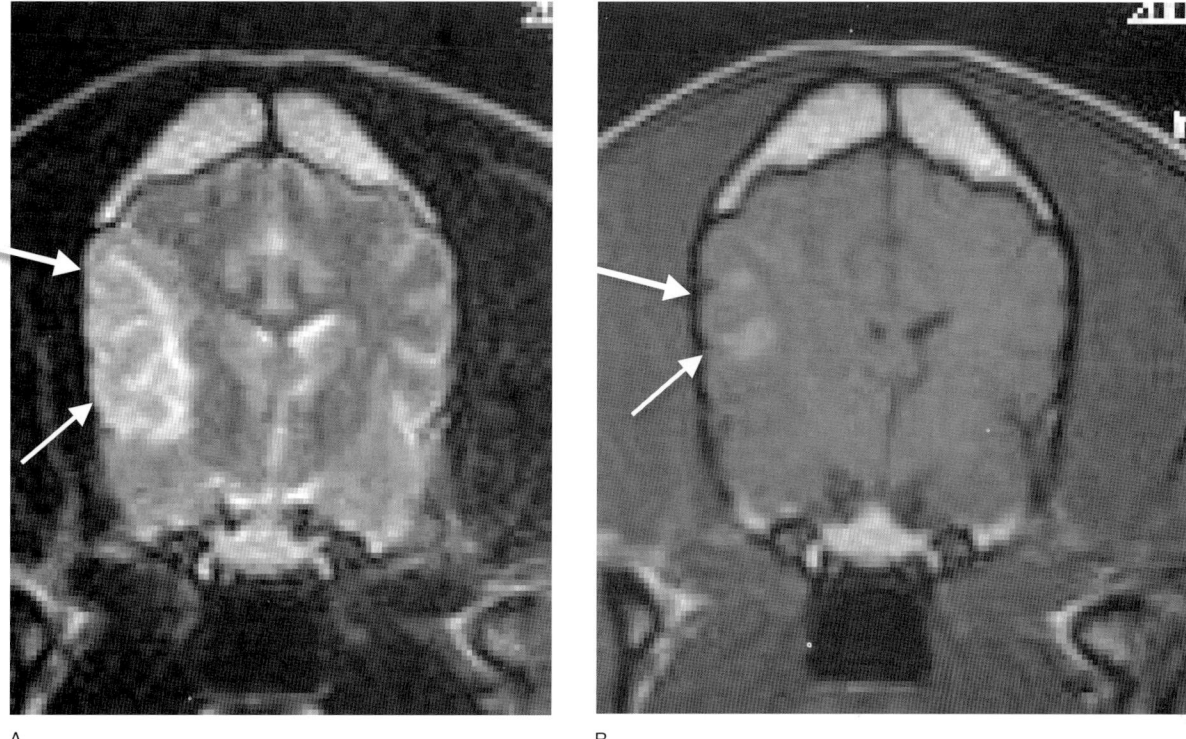

A   B

Figure 2.96. Transverse T2-weighted MR image (A) from a dog with a cerebral infarction (arrows). Transverse T1-weighted MR image following intravenous contrast administration (B) from the same dog as in (A). Note the minimal contrast enhancement present within the lesion (arrows).

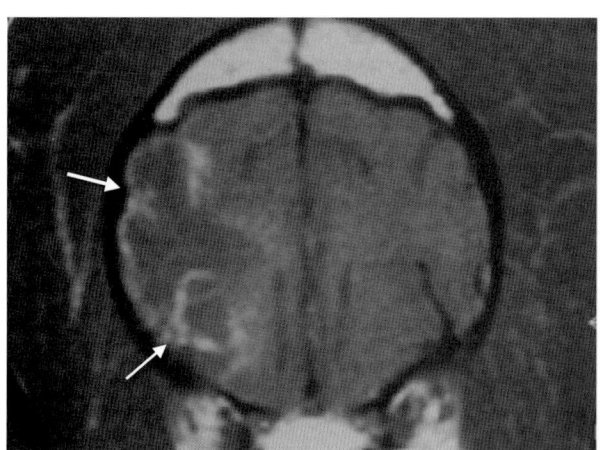

Figure 2.97. Transverse T1-weighted MR image following intravenous contrast administration from a dog with cerebral infarction. Note the contrast enhancement present within the lesion (arrows).

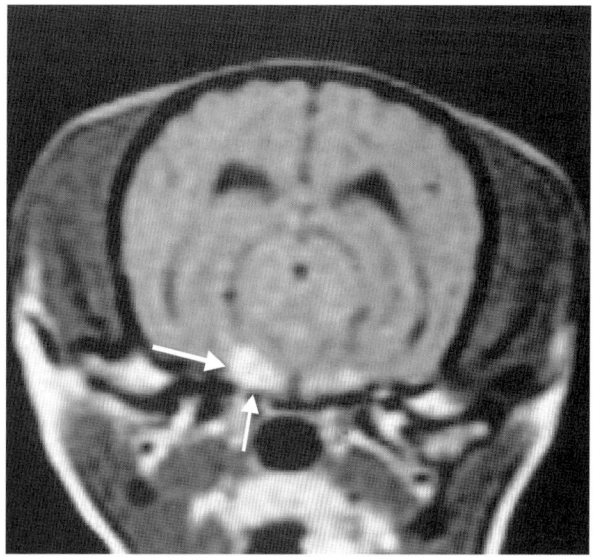

Figure 2.98. Transverse T1-weighted MR image following intravenous contrast administration from a dog with a tumor of the oculomotor nerve (CN III) (arrows).

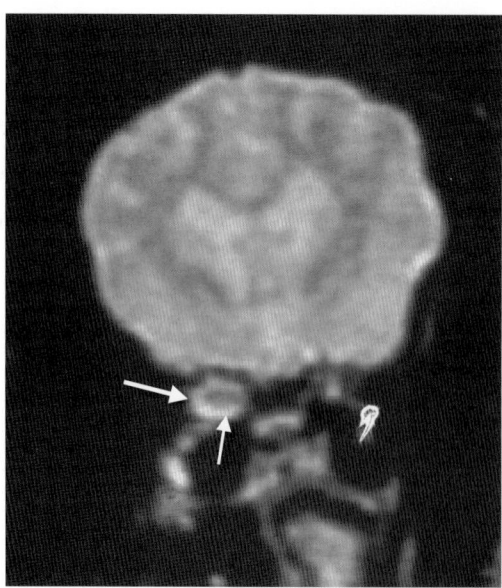

Figure 2.99. Transverse T2-weighted MR image from a dog with an extracranial tumor of the oculomotor nerve (CN III) (arrows).

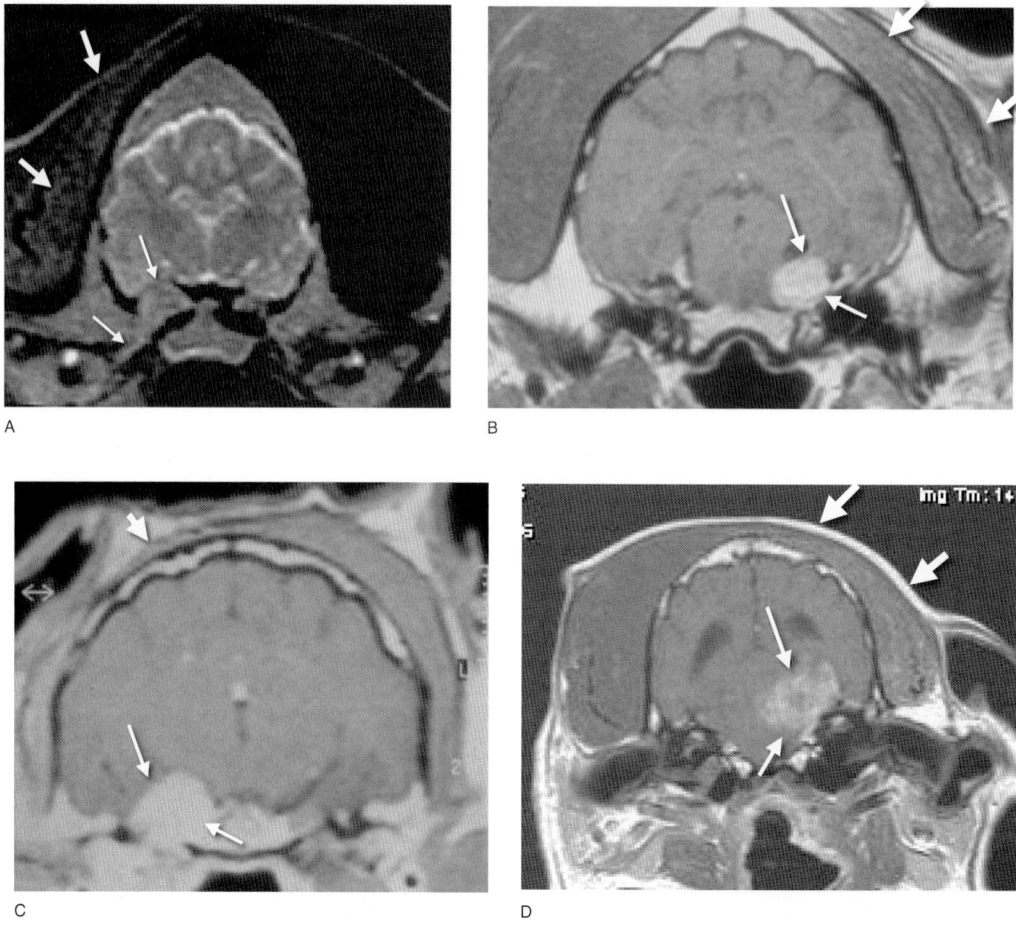

A

B

C

D

Figure 2.100. Transverse T2-weighted MR image (A) from a dog with a tumor of CN V (smaller arrows). Note the atrophy of the ipsilateral temporalis muscle (larger arrows). Transverse T1-weighted MR image (B) following intravenous contrast administration from a dog with a tumor of CN V (smaller arrows). Note the atrophy of the ipsilateral temporalis muscle (larger arrows). Transverse T1-weighted MR image (C) following intravenous contrast administration from a cat with a tumor of CN V (smaller arrows). Note the atrophy of the ipsilateral temporalis muscle (larger arrows). Transverse T1-weighted MR image (D) following intravenous contrast administration from a dog with a tumor of CN V (smaller arrows) with more intracranial extension. Note the atrophy of the ipsilateral temporalis muscle (larger arrows).

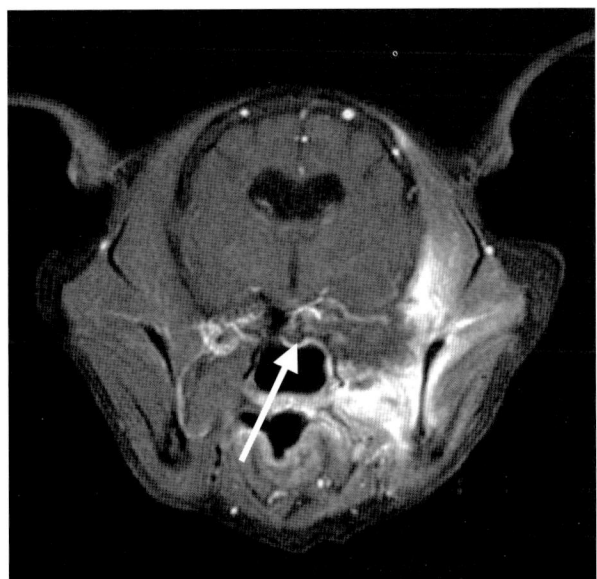

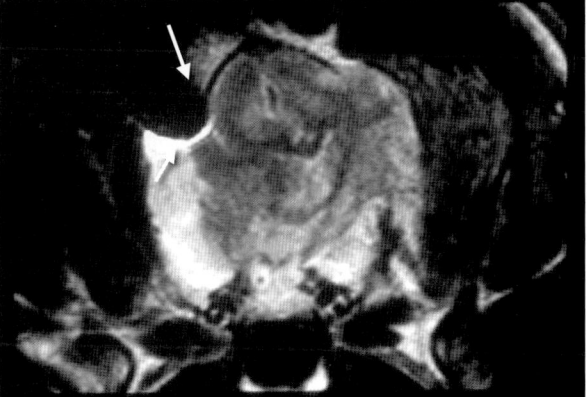

Figure 2.102. Transverse proton density MR image showing a metal artifact (arrows).

Figure 2.101. Transverse T1-weighted MR image following contrast administration with a mass within the cavernous sinus region (arrow).

Lesions of the cavernous sinus may also result in cranial nerve signs (Figure 2.101).

The facial, vestibular, as well as the sympathetic nerves may be affected with disease of the middle and inner ear. MR imaging provides superior anatomical evaluations of the middle and inner ear, and concurrently has an advantage of allowing for anatomical assessment of the brain stem for evaluation of the nuclear regions associated with these CNs. Lesions and associated brain stem structures, however, are often better seen with MR imaging as compared to CT as beam-hardening artifact with the latter commonly obscures structural detail in this area.

INTRACRANIAL IMAGING ARTIFACTS

Artifacts can result in misinterpretation of MR images leading to erroneous diagnoses (Figures 2.102–2.104). While artifacts should always be considered when an unexplained abnormality exists in an MR study, some of the more common artifacts are more readily defined (see Chapter 3).

Certain types of metal obviously create artifacts that can result in inability to interpret the MR image. Metal artifacts can result from metals such as stainless steel

(surgical implants, BBs, other missile projectiles) and gold bead implants (usually used as a possible seizure treatment). Metal artifacts result in a "black-hole" type appearance, being hypointense rounded to oval to oblong shaped. There is usually a hyperintense rim or edge to abnormalities.

Movement of the animal during the imaging process results in a wavy or "window blind" appearance to the image. Fold-over and wrapping may produce superimposition of structures on one another, the appearance of which may mimic pathologic alterations. Intravenous contrast in vessels external to the intracranial structures may "bleed" this contrast into the intracranial structures. This appears as focal, usually more than one, hyperintense regions within brain parenchyma.

Many apparent abnormalities are also the result of animal position during imaging combined with image slice selection. Even subtle malposition of the head and neck can result in slightly tangential image acquisitions resulting in slightly asymmetrical appearance of intracranial anatomy. As symmetry is one of the important features of the image that leads to diagnosis of disease, slight asymmetry of intracranial structures if often interpreted as abnormal. It is important when evaluating an MR study to keep in mind the effect of animal positioning and slice plane acquisition when interpreting asymmetry within the brain. Evaluation of normal symmetric anatomical structures external to the intracranial structure such as the bulla may help in determining the degree of asymmetry of animal position during image acquisition. Finally, overall poor quality images may preclude subsequent interpretation (Figure 2.105).

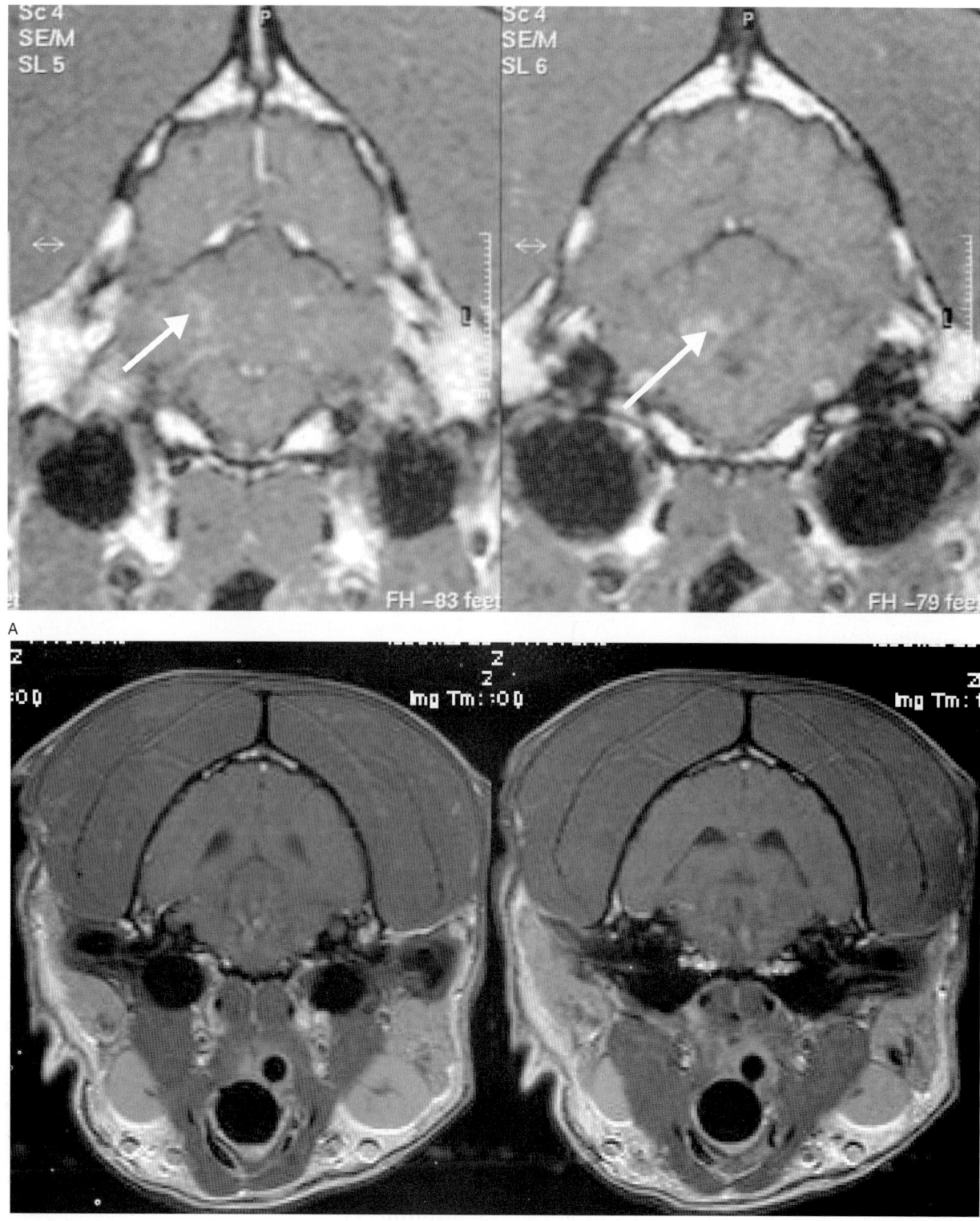

Figure 2.103.   Transverse T1-weighted MR images following intravenous contrast administration from two dogs ((A) and (B)) showing a flow artifact (arrows).

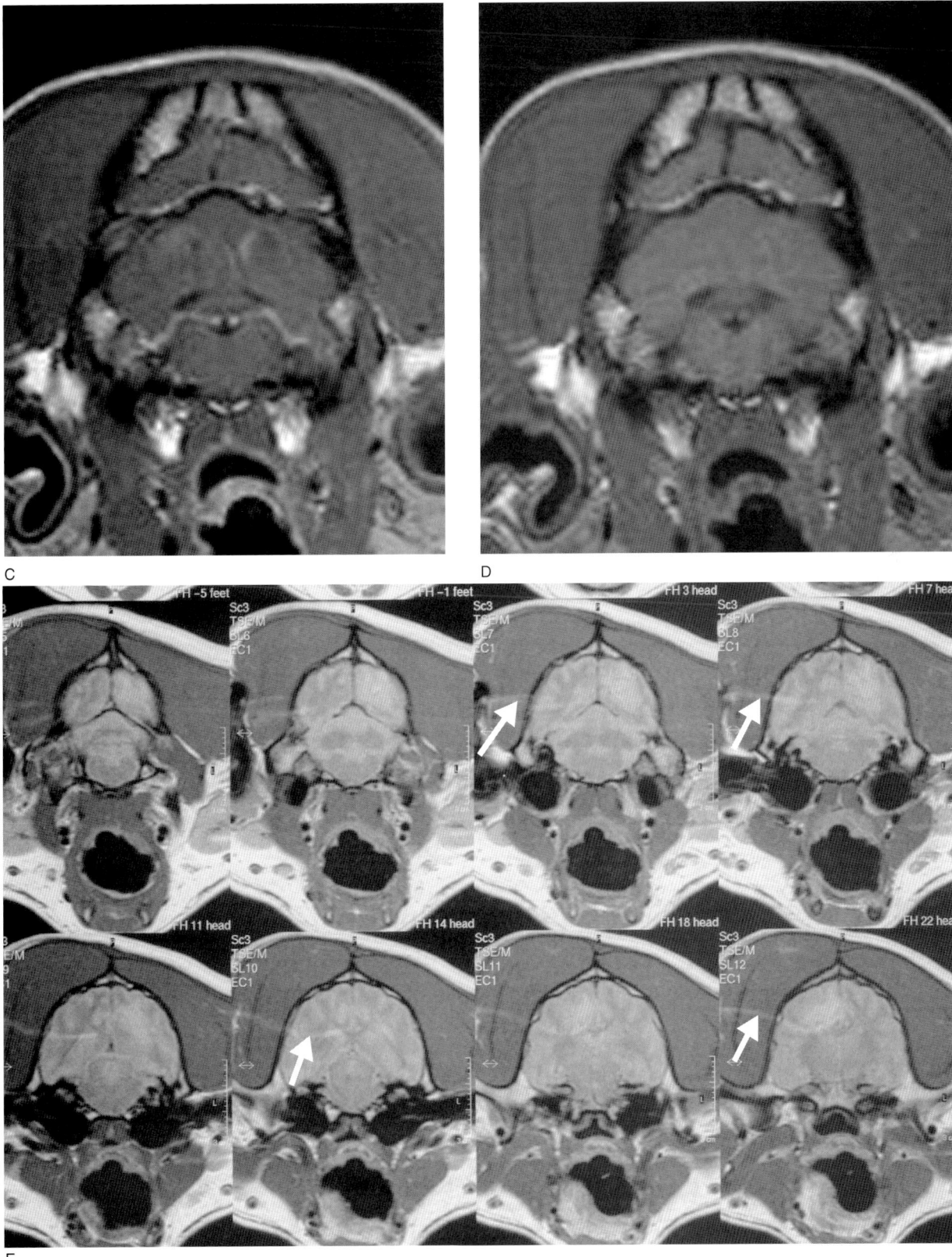

Figure 2.103. (*Continued*) Transverse, T1-weighted image following intravenous contrast administration from a dog showing a flow artifact (C). In part (D), the frequency direction has been changed 90° and the artifact is no longer present. (E) Transverse proton density image from a dog showing fold-over artifact.

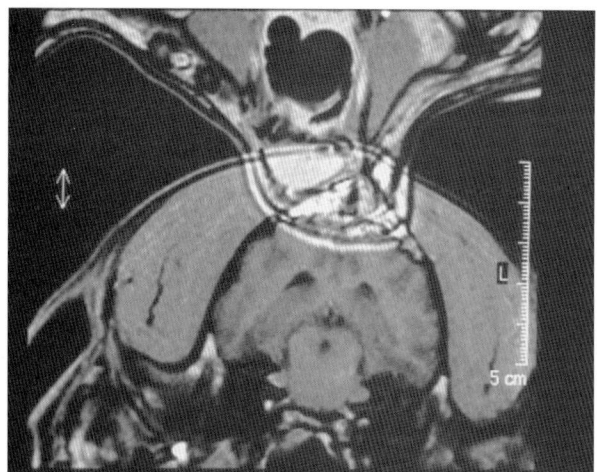

Figure 2.104. Transverse T1-weighted MR image showing a fold-over artifact.

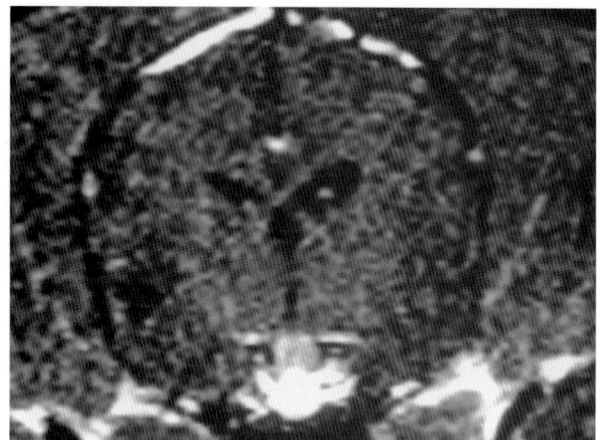

Figure 2.105. Transverse MR image of poor quality making interpretation difficult.

BIBLIOGRAPHY

Neuroanatomy

Beitz AJ and Fletcher TF. 1993. The brain. In: Evans HE (ed), Miller's Anatomy of the Dog, 3rd edn, WB Saunders, Philadelphia, pp. 894–952.

deLahunta A. 1983. Veterinary Neuroanatomy and Clinical Neurology, 2nd edn, WB Saunders, Philadelphia.

Dyce KM, Sack WO, and Wensing CJG. 1996. The nervous system. In: Dyce KM, Sack WO, and Wensing CJG (eds), Textbook of Veterinary Anatomy, 2nd edn, WB Saunders, Philadelphia, pp. 259–324.

Evans HE and Kitchell RL. 1993. Cranial nerves and cutaneous innervation of the head. In: Evans HE (ed), Miller's Anatomy of the Dog, 3rd edn, WB Saunders, Philadelphia, pp. 953–986.

Fletcher TF. 1993. Spinal cord and meninges. In: Evans HE (ed), Miller's Anatomy of the Dog, 3rd edn, WB Saunders, Philadelphia, pp. 800–828.

Hudson LC. 1993. Nervous system. In: Hudson LC and Hamilton WP (eds), Atlas of Feline Anatomy for Veterinarians, WB Saunders, Philadelphia, pp. 190–226.

Jenkins TW. 1978. In: Jenkins TW (ed), Functional Mammalian Neuroanatomy, 2nd edn, Lea & Febiger, Philadelphia, 264 p.

King AS. 1987. Physiological and Clinical Anatomy of the Domestic Mammals, Oxford University Press, Oxford.

Kitchell RL. 1993. Introduction to the nervous system. In: Evans HE (ed), Miller's Anatomy of the Dog, 3rd edn, WB Saunders, Philadelphia, pp. 758–799.

Pathophysiology

Bagley RS. 1996a. Intracranial pressure in dogs and cats. Physiology and treatment. Comp Contin Ed Pract Vet 18:605–621.

Bagley RS. 1996b. Pathophysiologic sequelae of intracranial disease. Vet Clin North Am 26:711–733.

Enevoldsen EM and Jensen FT. 1979. Autoregulation and CO_2 responses of cerebral blood flow in patients with acute severe head injury. J Neurosurg 48:689–703.

Fishman RA. 1975. Brain edema. N Eng J Med 293:706–711.

Kornegay JN. 1993. Pathogenesis of diseases of the central nervous system. In: Slatter D (ed), Textbook of Small Animal Surgery, 2nd edn, WB Saunders, Philadelphia, pp. 1022–1037.

Kornegay JN, Oliver JE, and Gorgacz EJ. 1983. Clinicopathologic features of brain herniation in animals. J Am Vet Med Assoc 182:1111–1116.

March PA. 1998. Seizures: classification, etiology, and pathophysiology. Clin Tech Small Anim Pract 13:119–131.

Olby N and Jeffery N. 2003. Pathogenesis of diseases of the central nervous system. In: Slatter D (ed), Textbook of Small Animal Surgery, WB Saunders, Philadelphia, pp. 1132–1147.

Reulen HJ. 1976. Vasogenic brain oedema. New aspects in its formation, resolution and therapy. Br J Anaesth 48:741–752.

Rosenberg GA, Saland L, and Kyner WT. 1983. Pathophysiology of periventricular tissue changes with raised CSF pressure. J Neurosurg 59:606–611.

Russo ME. 1981. The pathophysiology of epilepsy. Cornell Vet 71:221–247.

Shapiro HM. 1975. Intracranial hypertension: therapeutic and anesthetic considerations. Anesthesiology 43:445–471.

Summers BA, Cummings JF, and deLahunta A. 1995. Veterinary Neuropathology, WB Saunders, Philadelphia.

Intracranial MR Bibliography

Dogs

Abramson C, Garosi L, Platt S, and Penderis J. 2001. Metabolic defect in Staffordshire bull terriers. Vet Rec 149(17):532.

Abramson C, Platt S, Garosi L, and Penderis J. 2003a. L-2-hydroxyglutaric aciduria in Staffordshire bull terriers. Vet Rec 153(3):95–96.

Abramson CJ, Platt SR, Jakobs C, Verhoeven NM, Dennis R, Garosi L, et al. 2003b. L-2-hydroxyglutaric aciduria in Staffordshire bull terriers. J Vet Intern Med 17(4):551–556.

Adamo PF, Crawford JT, and Stepien RL. 2005. Subdural hematoma of the brainstem in a dog: magnetic resonance findings and treatment. J Am Anim Hosp Assoc 41(6):400–405.

Ahmed SH, Shaikh AY, Shaikh Z, and Hsu CY. 2000. What animal models have taught us about the treatment of acute stroke and brain protection. Curr Atheroscler Rep 2(2):167–180.

Allen JW, Horais KA, Tozier NA, Wegner K, Corbeil JA, Mattrey RF, et al. 2006. Time course and role of morphine dose and concentration in intrathecal granuloma formation in dogs: a combined magnetic resonance imaging and histopathology investigation. Anesthesiology 105(3):581–589.

Anderson ML, Smith DS, Nioka S, Subramanian H, Garcia JH, Halsey JH, et al. 1990. Experimental brain ischaemia: assessment of injury by magnetic resonance spectroscopy and histology. Neurol Res 12(4):195–204.

Anor S, Sturges BK, Lafranco L, Jang SS, Higgins RJ, Koblik PD, et al. 2001. Systemic phaeohyphomycosis (Cladophialophora bantiana) in a dog—clinical diagnosis with stereotactic computed tomographic-guided brain biopsy. J Vet Intern Med 15(3):257–261.

Bagley RS. 1997. Common neurologic diseases of older animals. Vet Clin North Am Small Anim Pract 27(6):1451–1486.

Bagley RS and Gavin PR. 1998. Seizures as a complication of brain tumors in dogs. Clin Tech Small Anim Pract 13(3):179–184.

Bagley RS, Harrington ML, and Moore MP. 1996a. Surgical treatments for seizure. Adaptability for dogs. Vet Clin North Am Small Anim Pract 26(4):827–842.

Bagley RS, Harrington ML, Pluhar GE, Gavin PR, and Moore MP. 1997. Acute, unilateral transverse sinus occlusion during craniectomy in seven dogs with space-occupying intracranial disease. Vet Surg 26(3):195–201.

Bagley RS, Kornegay JN, Lane SB, Thrall DL, and Page RL. 1996b. Cystic meningiomas in 2 dogs. J Vet Intern Med 10(2):72–75.

Bagley RS, Silver GM, and Gavin PR. 2000. Cerebellar cystic meningioma in a dog. J Am Anim Hosp Assoc 36(5):413–415.

Bagley RS, Wheeler SJ, Klopp L, Sorjonen DC, Thomas WB, Wilkens BE, et al. 1998. Clinical features of trigeminal nerve-sheath tumor in 10 dogs. J Am Anim Hosp Assoc 34(1):19–25.

Bailey MQ. 1990. Diagnostic imaging of intracranial lesions [Review]. Semin Vet Med Surg (Small Anim) 5(4):232–236.

Barone G, deLahunta A, and Sandler J. 2000. An unusual neurological disorder in the Labrador retriever. J Vet Intern Med 14(3):315–318.

Bayens-Simmonds J, Purcell TP, and Nation NP. 1997. Use of magnetic resonance imaging in the diagnosis of central vestibular disease. Can Vet J 38(1):38.

Behrend EN and Kemppainen RJ. 2001. Diagnosis of canine hyperadrenocorticism. Vet Clin North Am Small Anim Pract 31(5):985–1003.

Behrend EN, Kemppainen RJ, Clark TP, Salman MD, and Peterson ME. 2002. Diagnosis of hyperadrenocorticism in dogs: a survey of internists and dermatologists. J Am Vet Med Assoc 220(11):1643–1649.

Benczik J, Tenhunen M, Snellman M, Joensuu H, Farkkila M, Joensuu R, et al. 2002. Late radiation effects in the dog brain: correlation of MRI and histological changes. Radiother Oncol 63(1):107–120.

Benigni L and Lamb CR. 2005. Comparison of fluid-attenuated inversion recovery and T2-weighted magnetic resonance images in dogs and cats with suspected brain disease. Vet Radiol Ultrasound 46(4):287–292.

Berg JM and Joseph RJ. 2003. Cerebellar infarcts in two dogs diagnosed with magnetic resonance imaging. J Am Anim Hosp Assoc 39(2):203–207.

Bergstrom K, Thuomas KA, Ponten U, Nilsson P, Zwetnow NN, and Vlajkovic S. 1986. Magnetic resonance imaging of brain tissue displacement and brain tissue water contents during progressive brain compression. An experimental study in dogs. Acta Radiol Suppl 369:350–352.

Bertoy EH, Feldman EC, Nelson RW, Dublin AB, Reid MH, and Feldman MS. 1996. One-year follow-up evaluation of magnetic resonance imaging of the brain in dogs with pituitary-dependent hyperadrenocorticism. J Am Vet Med Assoc 208(8):1268–1273.

Bertoy EH, Feldman EC, Nelson RW, Duesberg CA, Kass PH, Reid MH, et al. 1995. Magnetic resonance imaging of the brain in dogs with recently diagnosed but untreated pituitary-dependent hyperadrenocorticism. J Am Vet Med Assoc 206(5):651–656.

Bischoff MG and Kneller SK. 2004. Diagnostic imaging of the canine and feline ear. Vet Clin North Am Small Anim Pract 34(2):437–458.

Bishop TM, Morrison J, Summers BA, deLahunta A, and Schatzberg SJ. 2004. Meningioangiomatosis in young dogs: a case series and literature review. J Vet Intern Med 18(4):522–528.

Bohn AA, Wills TB, West CL, Tucker RL, and Bagley RS. 2006. Cerebrospinal fluid analysis and magnetic resonance imaging in the diagnosis of neurologic disease in dogs: a retrospective study. Vet Clin Pathol 35(3):315–320.

Brady CA, Vite CH, and Drobatz KJ. 1999. Severe neurologic sequelae in a dog after treatment of hypoadrenal crisis. J Am Vet Med Assoc 215(2):222–225, 210.

Brennan KM, Roos MS, Budinger TF, Higgins RJ, Wong ST, and Bristol KS. 1993. A study of radiation necrosis and edema in the canine brain using positron emission tomography and magnetic resonance imaging. Radiat Res 134(1):43–53.

Buback JL, Schulz KS, Walker MA, and Snowden KF. 1996. Magnetic resonance imaging of the brain for diagnosis of neurocysticercosis in a dog. J Am Vet Med Assoc 208(11):1846–1848. Erratum in: 1996 J Am Vet Med Assoc 209(6):1113.

Bush WW, Barr CS, Darrin EW, Shofer FS, Vite CH, and Steinberg SA. 2002. Results of cerebrospinal fluid analysis, neurologic examination findings, and age at the onset of seizures as predictors for results of magnetic resonance imaging of the brain in dogs examined because of seizures: 115 cases (1992–2000). J Am Vet Med Assoc 220(6):781–784.

Bush WW, Throop JL, McManus PM, Kapatkin AS, Vite CII, and Van Winkle TJ. 2003. Intravascular lymphoma involving the central and peripheral nervous systems in a dog. J Am Anim Hosp Assoc 39(1):90–96.

Caruso K, Marrion R, and Silver G. 2002. What is your diagnosis? Retrobulbar mass indenting the inferior aspect of the right globe. J Am Vet Med Assoc 221(11):1553–1554.

Castillo V, Giacomini D, Paez-Pereda M, Stalla J, Labeur M, Theodoropoulou M, et al. 2006. Retinoic acid as a novel medical therapy for Cushing's disease in dogs. Endocrinology 147(9):4438–4444.

Cherubini GB, Mantis P, Martinez TA, Lamb CR, and Cappello R. 2005. Utility of magnetic resonance imaging for distinguishing neoplastic from non-neoplastic brain lesions in dogs and cats. Vet Radiol Ultrasound 46(5):384–387.

Cherubini GB, Platt SR, Anderson TJ, Rusbridge C, Lorenzo V, Mantis P, et al. 2006. Characteristics of magnetic resonance images of granulomatous meningoencephalomyelitis in 11 dogs. Vet Rec 159(4):110–115.

Cizinauskas S, Lang J, Maier R, Fatzer R, and Jaggy A. 2001. Paradoxical vestibular disease with trigeminal nerve-sheath tumor in a dog. Schweiz Arch Tierheilkd 143(8):419–425.

Clifford C, Jennings D, Maslin WR, and Weigand C. 2000. What is your neurologic diagnosis? Unilateral otitis externa or media, cerebellar meningioma, and a solitary mammary adenoma. J Am Vet Med Assoc 216(8):1217–1219.

Coates JR, O'Brien DP, Kline KL, Storts RW, Johnson GC, Shelton GD, et al. 2002. Neonatal cerebellar ataxia in Coton de Tulear dogs. J Vet Intern Med 16(6):680–689.

Coderre JA, Gavin PR, Capala J, Ma R, Morris GM, Button TM, et al. 2000. Tolerance of the normal canine brain to epithermal neutron irradiation in the presence of p-boronophenylalanine. J Neurooncol 48(1):27–40.

Couturier L, Degueurce C, Ruel Y, Dennis R, and Begon D. 2005. Anatomical study of cranial nerve emergence and skull foramina in the dog using magnetic resonance imaging and computed tomography. Vet Radiol Ultrasound 46(5):375–383.

Cozzi F, Vite CH, Wenger DA, Victoria T, and Haskins ME. 1998. MRI and electrophysiological abnormalities in a case of canine globoid cell leucodystrophy. J Small Anim Pract 39(8):401–405.

Dennis R. 2000. Use of magnetic resonance imaging for the investigation of orbital disease in small animals. J Small Anim Pract 41(4):145–155.

Dennis R. 2003. Images in medicine. The haunted brain. Vet Radiol Ultrasound 44(5):593.

Deo-Narine V, Gomez DG, Vullo T, Manzo RP, Zimmerman RD, Deck MD, et al. 1994. Direct in vivo observation of transventricular absorption in the hydrocephalic dog

using magnetic resonance imaging. Invest Radiol 29(3):287–293.

Dewey CW, Berg JM, Barone G, Marino DJ, and Stefanacci JD. 2005. Foramen magnum decompression for treatment of caudal occipital malformation syndrome in dogs. J Am Vet Med Assoc 227(8):1270–1275, 1250–1251.

Di Terlizzi R, Platt SR, and Dennis R. 2004. What is your diagnosis? Cerebrovascular hemorrhage. J Small Anim Pract 45(10):483, 526–528.

Drake JM, Potts DG, and Lemaire C. 1989. Magnetic resonance imaging of silastic-induced canine hydrocephalus. Surg Neurol 31(1):28–40.

Duesberg CA, Feldman EC, Nelson RW, Bertoy EH, Dublin AB, and Reid MH. 1995. Magnetic resonance imaging for diagnosis of pituitary macrotumors in dogs. J Am Vet Med Assoc 206(5):657–662.

Dvir E, Kirberger RM, and Terblanche AG. 2000. Magnetic resonance imaging of otitis media in a dog. Vet Radiol Ultrasound 41(1):46–49.

Ellinwood NM, Wang P, Skeen T, Sharp NJ, Cesta M, Decker S, et al. 2003. A model of mucopolysaccharidosis IIIB (Sanfilippo syndrome type IIIB): N-acetyl-alpha-D-glucosaminidase deficiency in Schipperke dogs. J Inherit Metab Dis 26(5):489–504.

Ellison GW, Donnell RL, and Daniel GB. 1995. Nasopharyngeal epidermal cyst in a dog. J Am Vet Med Assoc 207(12):1590–1592.

Esteve-Ratsch B, Kneissl S, and Gabler C. 2001. Comparative evaluation of the ventricles in the Yorkshire Terrier and the German Shepherd dog using low-field MRI. Vet Radiol Ultrasound 42(5):410–413.

Farrow CS and Tyron K. 2000. Fathoming the mysteries of magnetic resonance imaging. J Am Anim Hosp Assoc 36(3):192–198.

Feldman EC, Nelson RW, and Feldman MS. 1996. Use of low- and high-dose dexamethasone tests for distinguishing pituitary-dependent from adrenal tumor hyperadrenocorticism in dogs. J Am Vet Med Assoc 209(4):772–775.

Fernandez T, Diez-Bru N, Rios A, Gomez L, and Pumarola M. 2001. Intracranial metastases from an ovarian dysgerminoma in a 2-year-old dog. J Am Anim Hosp Assoc 37(6):553–556.

Fisher M. 2002. Disseminated granulomatous meningoencephalomyelitis in a dog. Can Vet J 43(1):49–51.

Fransson B, Kippenes H, Silver GE, and Gavin PR. 2000. Magnetic resonance diagnosis: cavernous sinus syndrome in a dog. Vet Radiol Ultrasound 41(6):536–538.

Frendin J, Funkquist B, Hansson K, Lonnemark M, and Carlsten J. 1999. Diagnostic imaging of foreign body reactions in dogs with diffuse back pain. J Small Anim Pract 40(6):278–285.

Fujisawa I, Asato R, and Kawata M. 1989. Hyperintense signals of the posterior lobe of the pituitary gland on MR images. AJNR Am J Neuroradiol 10(6):1280–1282. No abstract available.

Fukuhara T, Luciano MG, Brant CL, and Klauscie J. 2001. Effects of ventriculoperitoneal shunt removal on cerebral oxygenation and brain compliance in chronic obstructive hydrocephalus. J Neurosurg 94(4):573–581.

Fulton LM and Steinberg HS. 1990. Preliminary study of lomustine in the treatment of intracranial masses in dogs following localization by imaging techniques. Semin Vet Med Surg (Small Anim) 5(4):241–245.

Galloway RL, Jr, Maciunas RJ, and Failinger AL. 1993. Factors affecting perceived tumor volumes in magnetic resonance imaging. Ann Biomed Eng 21(4):367–375.

Galloway RL, Jr, Maciunas RJ, Failinger AL, and Whelan HT. 1990. Volumetric measurement of canine gliomas using MRI. Magn Reson Imaging 8(2):161–165.

Ganz JC, Thuomas KA, Vlajkovic S, Nilsson P, Bergstrom K, Ponten U, et al. 1993. Changes in intracranial morphology, regional cerebral water content and vital physiological variables during epidural bleeding. An experimental MR study in dogs. Acta Radiol 34(3):279–288.

Garosi L, McConnell JE, Platt SR, Barone G, Baron JC, de Lahunta A, et al. 2005a. Results of diagnostic investigations and long-term outcome of 33 dogs with brain infarction (2000–2004). J Vet Intern Med 19(5):725–731.

Garosi L, McConnell JF, Platt SR, Barone G, Baron JC, de Lahunta A, et al. 2006. Clinical and topographic magnetic resonance characteristics of suspected brain infarction in 40 dogs. J Vet Intern Med 20(2):311–321.

Garosi LS, Dennis R, Penderis J, Lamb CR, Targett MP, Cappello R, et al. 2001. Results of magnetic resonance imaging in dogs with vestibular disorders: 85 cases (1996–1999). J Am Vet Med Assoc 218(3):385–391.

Garosi LS, Dennis R, Platt SR, Corletto F, de Lahunta A, and Jakobs C. 2003. Thiamine deficiency in a dog: clinical, clinicopathologic, and magnetic resonance imaging findings. J Vet Intern Med 17(5):719–723.

Garosi LS, Dennis R, and Schwarz T. 2003. Review of diagnostic imaging of ear diseases in the dog and cat. Vet Radiol Ultrasound 44(2):137–146.

Garosi LS, Lamb CR, and Targett MP. 2000. MRI findings in a dog with otitis media and suspected otitis interna. Vet Rec 146(17):501–502.

Garosi LS and McConnell JF. 2005. Ischaemic stroke in dogs and humans: a comparative review. J Small Anim Pract 46(11):521–529.

Garosi LS, McConnell JF, and Lujan A. 2005b. What is your diagnosis? Pneumocephalus. J Am Vet Med Assoc; 226(7):1057–1058.

Garosi LS, Penderis J, Brearley MJ, Brearley JC, Dennis R, and Kirkpatrick PJ. 2002. Intraventricular tension pneumocephalus as a complication of transfrontal craniectomy: a case report. Vet Surg 31(3):226–231.

Garosi LS, Penderis J, McConnell JF, and Jakobs C. 2005c. L-2-hydroxyglutaric aciduria in a West Highland white terrier. Vet Rec 156(5):145–147.

Garosi LS, Platt SR, McConnell JF, Wray JD, and Smith KC. 2005d. Intracranial haemorrhage associated with Angiostrongylus vasorum infection in three dogs. J Small Anim Pract 46(2):93–99.

Gavin PR. 1997. Future of veterinary radiation oncology. Vet Clin North Am Small Anim Pract 27(1):157–165.

Gavin PR, Fike JR, and Hoopes PJ. 1995. Central nervous system tumors. Semin Vet Med Surg (Small Anim) 10(3):180–189.

Gavin PR, Kraft SL, DeHaan CE, Swartz CD, and Griebenow ML. 1994. Large animal normal tissue tolerance with boron neutron capture. Int J Radiat Oncol Biol Phys 28(5):1099–1106.

Gavin PR, Kraft SL, Huiskamp R, and Coderre JA. 1997. A review: CNS effects and normal tissue tolerance in dogs. J Neurooncol 33(1–2):71–80.

George MS, Malloy LC, Slate SO, and Uhde TW. 1994/1995. Pilot MRI study of brain size in nervous pointer dogs. Anxiety 1(3):129–133.

Glass EN, Kapatkin A, Vite C, and Steinberg SA. 2000. A modified bilateral transfrontal sinus approach to the canine frontal lobe and olfactory bulb: surgical technique and five cases. J Am Anim Hosp Assoc 36(1):43–50.

Goossens MM, Feldman EC, Theon AP, and Koblik PD. 1998. Efficacy of cobalt 60 radiotherapy in dogs with pituitary-dependent hyperadrenocorticism. J Am Vet Med Assoc 212(3):374–376.

Gopal MS and Jeffery ND. 2001. Magnetic resonance imaging in the diagnosis and treatment of a canine spinal cord injury. J Small Anim Pract 42(1):29–31.

Graham JP, Newell SM, Voges AK, Roberts GD, and Harrison JM. 1998. The dural tail sign in the diagnosis of meningiomas. Vet Radiol Ultrasound 39(4):297–302.

Graham JP, Roberts GD, and Newell SM. 2000. Dynamic magnetic resonance imaging of the normal canine pituitary gland. Vet Radiol Ultrasound 41(1):35–40.

Gruber A, Leschnik M, Kneissl S, and Schmidt P. 2006. Gliomatosis cerebri in a dog. J Vet Med A Physiol Pathol Clin Med 53(8):435–438.

Hamann F, Kooistra HS, Mol JA, Gottschalk S, Bartels T, and Rijnberk A. 1999. Pituitary function and morphology in two German shepherd dogs with congenital dwarfism. Vet Rec 144(23):644–646.

Harkin KR, Goggin JM, DeBey BM, Kraft SL, and de Lahunta A. 1999. Magnetic resonance imaging of the brain of a dog with hereditary polioencephalomyelopathy. J Am Vet Med Assoc 214(9):1342–1344.

Harrington ML, Bagley RS, and Moore MP. 1996. Hydrocephalus. Vet Clin North Am Small Anim Pract 6(4):843–856.

Hasegawa D, Yayoshi N, Fujita Y, Fujita M, and Orima H. 2005. Measurement of interthalamic adhesion thickness as a criteria for brain atrophy in dogs with and without cognitive dysfunction (dementia). Vet Radiol Ultrasound 46(6):452–457.

Hasegawa T, Taura Y, Kido H, Shibazaki A, and Katamoto H. 2005. Surgical management of combined hydrocephalus, syringohydromyelia, and ventricular cyst in a dog. J Am Anim Hosp Assoc 41(4):267–272.

Higgins RJ, LeCouteur RA, Vernau KM, Sturges BK, Obradovich JE, and Bollen AW. 2001. Granular cell tumor of the canine central nervous system: two cases. Vet Pathol 38(6):620–627.

Itoh T, Nishimura R, Matsunaga S, Kadosawa T, Mochizuki M, and Sasaki N. 1996. Syringomyelia and hydrocephalus in a dog. J Am Vet Med Assoc 209(5):934–936.

Jakobsson KE, Thuomas KA, Bergstrom K, Ponten U, and Zwetnow NN. 1990. Rebound of ICP after brain compression. An MRI study in dogs. Acta Neurochir (Wien) 104(3–4):126–135.

Jeffery N. 2005. Ethmoidal encephalocoele associated with seizures in a puppy. J Small Anim Pract 46(2):89–92.

Jeffery ND, Lakatos A, and Franklin RJ. 2005. Autologous olfactory glial cell transplantation is reliable and safe in naturally occurring canine spinal cord injury. J Neurotrauma 22(11):1282–1293.

Jeffery ND, Watson PJ, Abramson C, and Notenboom A. 2003. Brain malformations associated with primary adipsia identified using magnetic resonance imaging. Vet Rec 152(14):436–438.

Johnson RP, Neer TM, Partington BP, Cho DY, and Partington CR. 2001. Familial cerebellar ataxia with hydrocephalus in bull mastiffs. Vet Radiol Ultrasound 42(3):246–249.

Jull BA, Merryman JI, Thomas WB, and McArthur A. 1997. Necrotizing encephalitis in a Yorkshire Terrier. J Am Vet Med Assoc 211(8):1005–1007.

Kacher DF, Frerichs K, Pettit J, Campbell PK, Meunch T, and Norbash AM. 2006. DuraSeal magnetic resonance and computed tomography imaging: evaluation in a canine craniotomy model. Neurosurgery 58(Suppl. 1):ONS140–ONS147.

Kaneda T, Minami M, Curtin HD, Utsunomiya T, Shirouzu I, Yamashiro M, et al. 1998. Dental bur fragments causing metal artifacts on MR images. AJNR Am J Neuroradiol 19(2):317–319.

Katayama KI, Kuroki K, Uchida K, Nakayama H, Sakai M, Mochizuki M, et al. 2001. A case of canine primitive neuroectodermal tumor (PNET). J Vet Med Sci 63(1):103–105.

Kaye EM, Alroy J, Raghavan SS, Schwarting GA, Adelman LS, Runge V, et al. 1992. Dysmyelinogenesis in animal model of GM1 gangliosidosis. Pediatr Neurol 8(4):255–261.

Kent M, Delahunta A, and Tidwell AS. 2001. MR imaging findings in a dog with intravascular lymphoma in the brain. Vet Radiol Ultrasound 42(6):504–510.

Kii S, Uzuka Y, Taura Y, Nakaichi M, Inokuma H, and Onishi T. 1998. Developmental change of lateral ventricular volume and ratio in Beagle-type dogs up to 7 months of age. Vet Radiol Ultrasound 39(3):185–189.

Kii S, Uzuka Y, Taura Y, Nakaichi M, Takeuchi A, Inokuma H, et al. 1997. Magnetic resonance imaging of the lateral ventricles in beagle-type dogs. Vet Radiol Ultrasound 38(6):430–433.

Kim H, Itamoto K, Watanabe M, Nakaichi M, and Taura Y. 2006. Application of ventriculoperitoneal shunt as a treatment for hydrocephalus in a dog with syringomyelia and Chiari I malformation. J Vet Sci 7(2):203–206.

Kimotsuki T, Nagaoka T, Yasuda M, Tamahara S, Matsuki N, and Ono K. 2005. Changes of magnetic resonance imag-ing on the brain in beagle dogs with aging. J Vet Med Sci 67(10):961–967.

Kippenes H, Gavin PR, Kraft SL, Sande RD, and Tucker RL. 2001. Mensuration of the normal pituitary gland from magnetic resonance images in 96 dogs. Vet Radiol Ultrasound 42(2):130–133.

Kipperman BS, Feldman EC, Dybdal NO, and Nelson RW. 1992. Pituitary tumor size, neurologic signs, and relation to endocrine test results in dogs with pituitary-dependent hyperadrenocorticism: 43 cases (1980–1990). J Am Vet Med Assoc 201(5):762–767.

Kitagawa M, Kanayama K, and Sakai T. 2002. Cystic meningioma in a dog. J Small Anim Pract 43(6):272–274.

Kitagawa M, Kanayama K, and Sakai T. 2003. Quadrigeminal cisterna arachnoid cyst diagnosed by MRI in five dogs. Aust Vet J 81(6):340–343.

Kitagawa M, Kanayama K, and Sakai T. 2004a. Cerebellopontine angle meningioma expanding into the sella turcica in a dog. J Vet Med Sci 66(1):91–93.

Kitagawa M, Kanayama K, Satoh T, and Sakai T. 2004b. Cerebellar focal granulomatous meningoencephalitis in a dog: clinical findings and MR imaging. J Vet Med A Physiol Pathol Clin Med 51(6):277–279.

Kitagawa M, Kanayama K, and Sakai T. 2005a. Subdural accumulation of fluid in a dog after the insertion of a ventriculoperitoneal shunt. Vet Rec 156(7):206–208.

Kitagawa M, Kanayama K, and Sakai T. 2005b. Subtotal agenesis of the cerebellum in a dog. Aust Vet J 83(11):680–681.

Kitagawa M, Okada M, Kanayama K, and Sakai T. 2005c. Traumatic intracerebral hematoma in a dog: MR images and clinical findings. J Vet Med Sci 67(8):843–846.

Kitagawa M, Okada M, Oogushi N, Dei H, Yamamura H, Kanayama K, et al. 2002. A canine case of gliosis with cyst formation in the posterior fossa. J Vet Med Sci 64(7):611–614.

Kitagawa M, Okada M, Yamamura H, Kanayama K, and Sakai T. 2006. Diagnosis of olfactory neuroblastoma in a dog by magnetic resonance imaging. Vet Rec 159(9):288–289.

Kneissl S, Probst A, and Konar M. 2004. Low-field magnetic resonance imaging of the canine middle and inner ear. Vet Radiol Ultrasound 45(6):520–522.

Knutzon RK, Poirier VC, Gerscovich EO, Brock JM, and Buonocore M. 1991. The effect of intravenous gadolinium on the magnetic resonance appearance of cerebrospinal fluid. Invest Radiol 26(7):671–673.

Koie H, Shibuya H, Sato T, Sato A, Nawa K, Nawa Y, et al. 2004. Magnetic resonance imaging of neuronal ceroid lipofuscinosis in a border collie. J Vet Med Sci 66(11):1453–1456.

Kraft SL and Gavin PR. 1999. Intracranial neoplasia. Clin Tech Small Anim Pract 14(2):112–123.

Kraft SL, Gavin PR, DeHaan C, Moore M, Wendling LR, and Leathers CW. 1997. Retrospective review of 50 canine intracranial tumors evaluated by magnetic resonance imaging. J Vet Intern Med 11(4):218–225.

Kraft SL, Gavin PR, Leathers CW, Wendling LR, Frenier S, and Dorn RV, III. 1990. Diffuse cerebral and leptomeningeal astrocytoma in dogs: MR features. J Comput Assist Tomogr 14(4):555–560.

Kraus KH and McDonnell J. 1996. Identification and management of brain tumors. Semin Vet Med Surg (Small Anim) 11(4):218–224.

Krisht AF, Yoo K, Arnautovic KI, and Al-Mefty O. 2005. Cavernous sinus tumor model in the canine: a simulation model for cavernous sinus tumor surgery. Neurosurgery 56(6):1361–1365; discussion 1365–1366.

Kube SA, Bruyette DS, and Hanson SM. 2003. Astrocytomas in young dogs. J Am Anim Hosp Assoc 39(3):288–293.

Kucharczyk J, Kucharczyk W, Berry I, de Groot J, Kelly W, Norman D, et al. 1989. Histochemical characterization and functional significance of the hyperintense signal on MR images of the posterior pituitary. AJR Am J Roentgenol 152(1):153–157.

Kuwabara M, Tanaka S, and Fujiwara K. 1998. Magnetic resonance imaging and histopathology of encephalitis in a Pug. J Vet Med Sci 60(12):1353–1355.

Kuwamura M, Adachi T, Yamate J, Kotani T, Ohashi F, and Summers BA. 2002. Necrotising encephalitis in the Yorkshire Terrier: a case report and literature review. J Small Anim Pract 43(10):459–463.

Lamb CR, Croson PJ, Cappello R, and Cherubini GB. 2005. Magnetic resonance imaging findings in 25 dogs with inflammatory cerebrospinal fluid. Vet Radiol Ultrasound 46(1):17–22.

Lamb CR and Garosi L. 2000. Two little ducks went swimming one day. Vet Radiol Ultrasound 41(3):292.

Larocca RD. 2000. Unilateral external and internal ophthalmoplegia caused by intracranial meningioma in a dog. Vet Ophthalmol 3(1):3–9.

Lavely J and Lipsitz D. 2005. Fungal infections of the central nervous system in the dog and cat. Clin Tech Small Anim Pract 20(4):212–219.

LeCouteur RA. 1999. Current concepts in the diagnosis and treatment of brain tumours in dogs and cats. J Small Anim Pract 40(9):411–416.

Lester NV, Hopkins AL, Bova FJ, Friedman WA, Buatti JM, Meeks SL, et al. 2001. Radiosurgery using a stereotactic headframe system for irradiation of brain tumors in dogs. J Am Vet Med Assoc 219(11):1562–1567, 1550.

Lipsitz D, Higgins RJ, Kortz GD, Dickinson PJ, Bollen AW, Naydan DK, et al. 2003. Glioblastoma multiforme: clinical findings, magnetic resonance imaging, and pathology in five dogs. Vet Pathol 40(6):659–669.

Lipsitz D, Levitski RE, and Berry WL. 2001. Magnetic resonance imaging features of multilobular osteochondrosarcoma in 3 dogs. Vet Radiol Ultrasound 42(1):14–19.

Lipsitz D, Levitski RE, and Chauvet AE. 1999. Magnetic resonance imaging of a choroid plexus carcinoma and meningeal carcinomatosis in a dog. Vet Radiol Ultrasound 40(3):246–250.

Liu CH, Liu CI, Liang SL, Cheng CH, Huang SC, Lee CC, et al. 2004. Intracranial granular cell tumor in a dog. J Vet Med Sci 66(1):77–79.

Lorenzo V, Pumarola M, and Munoz A. 1998. Meningioangiomatosis in a dog: magnetic resonance imaging and neuropathological studies. J Small Anim Pract 39(10):486–489.

Lotti D, Capucchio MT, Gaidolfi E, and Merlo M. 1999. Necrotizing encephalitis in a Yorkshire Terrier: clinical, imaging, and pathologic findings. Vet Radiol Ultrasound 40(6):622–626.

Lu D, Lamb CR, Pfeiffer DU, and Targett MP. 2003. Neurological signs and results of magnetic resonance imaging in 40 Cavalier King Charles spaniels with Chiari type 1-like malformations. Vet Rec 153(9):260–263.

Lynch GL, Broome MR, and Scagliotti RH. 2006. What is your diagnosis? Mass originating from the pituitary fossa. J Am Vet Med Assoc 228(11):1681–1682.

Mariani CL, Clemmons RM, Graham JP, Phillips LA, and Chrisman CL. 2001. Magnetic resonance imaging of spongy degeneration of the central nervous system in a Labrador Retriever. Vet Radiol Ultrasound 42(4):285–290.

Mariani CL, Platt SR, Newell SM, Terrell SP, Chrisman CL, and Clemmons RM. 2001. Magnetic resonance imaging of cerebral cortical necrosis (polioencephalomalacia) in a dog. Vet Radiol Ultrasound 42(6):524–531.

Matsuki N, Yamato O, Kusuda M, Maede Y, Tsujimoto H, and Ono K. 2005. Magnetic resonance imaging of GM2-gangliosidosis in a golden retriever. Can Vet J 46(3):275–278.

Mattoon JS and Walker MA. 1998. MRI case presented as part of the 1997 A.C.V.R. oral certification examination: computed tomography/magnetic resonance imaging elective. Vet Radiol Ultrasound 39(2):154–155. No abstract available.

Mazur WJ and Lazar T. 2005. What is your diagnosis? Chondrosarcoma. J Am Vet Med Assoc 226(8):1301–1302.

McConnell JF, Garosi L, and Platt SR. 2005. Magnetic resonance imaging findings of presumed cerebellar cerebrovascular accident in twelve dogs. Vet Radiol Ultrasound 46(1):1–10.

McConnell JF, Hayes A, Platt SR, and Smith KC. 2006. Calvarial hyperostosis syndrome in two bullmastiffs. Vet Radiol Ultrasound 47(1):72–77.

McConnell JF, Platt S, and Smith KC. 2004. Magnetic resonance imaging findings of an intracranial medulloblastoma in a Polish Lowland Sheepdog. Vet Radiol Ultrasound 45(1):17–22.

McConnell JF, Platt SR, and Feliu-Pascual AL. 2005. What is your diagnosis? Intracranial meningiomas. J Small Anim Pract 46(11):555–557.

McGowan JC, Haskins M, Wenger DA, and Vite C. 2000. Investigating demyelination in the brain in a canine model of globoid cell leukodystrophy (Krabbe disease) using magnetization transfer contrast: preliminary results. J Comput Assist Tomogr 24(2):316–321.

Meij B, Voorhout G, and Rijnberk A. 2002. Progress in transsphenoidal hypophysectomy for treatment of pituitary-dependent hyperadrenocorticism in dogs and cats. Mol Cell Endocrinol 197(1–2):89–96.

Mellema LM, Koblik PD, Kortz GD, LeCouteur RA, Chechowitz MA, and Dickinson PJ. 1999. Reversible magnetic resonance imaging abnormalities in dogs following seizures. Vet Radiol Ultrasound 40(6):588–595.

Mellema LM, Samii VF, Vernau KM, and LeCouteur RA. 2002. Meningeal enhancement on magnetic resonance imaging in 15 dogs and 3 cats. Vet Radiol Ultrasound 43(1): 10–15.

Miyabayashi T, Smith M, and Tsuruno Y. 2000. Comparison of fast spin-echo and conventional spin-echo magnetic resonance spinal imaging techniques in four normal dogs. Vet Radiol Ultrasound 41(4):308–312.

Moore MP, Bagley RS, Harrington ML, and Gavin PR. 1996. Intracranial tumors. Vet Clin North Am Small Anim Pract 26(4):759–777.

Morozumi M, Miyahara K, Sato M, and Hirose T. 1997. Computed tomography and magnetic resonance findings in two dogs and a cat with intracranial lesions. J Vet Med Sci 59(9):807–810.

Muhle AC, Kircher P, Fazer R, Scheidegger J, Lang J, and Jaggy A. 2004. Intracranial haemorrhage in an eight-week-old puppy. Vet Rec 154(11):338–339.

Nakaichi M, Taura Y, Nakama S, Takeuchi A, Matsunaga N, Ebe K, et al. 1996. Primary brain tumors in two dogs treated by surgical resection in combination with postoperative radiation therapy. J Vet Med Sci 58(8):773–775.

O'Brien DP, Kroll RA, Johnson GC, Covert SJ, and Nelson MJ. 1994. Myelinolysis after correction of hyponatremia in two dogs. J Vet Intern Med 8(1):40–48.

Ohashi F, Kotani T, Onishi T, Katamoto H, Nakata E, and Fritz-Zieroth B. 1993. Magnetic resonance imaging in a dog with choroid plexus carcinoma. J Vet Med Sci 55(5):875–876.

Olby N, Munana K, De Risio L, Sebestyen P, and Hansen B. 2002. Cervical injury following a horse kick to the head in two dogs. J Am Anim Hosp Assoc 38(4):321–326.

Ota S, Komiyama A, Johkura K, Hasegawa O, and Kondo K. 1994. Eosinophilic meningo-encephalo-myelitis due to Toxocara canis [Japanese]. Rinsho Shinkeigaku 34(11):1148–1152.

O'Toole TE, Sato AF, and Rozanski EA. 2003. Cryptococcosis of the central nervous system in a dog. J Am Vet Med Assoc 222(12):1722–1725, 1706. Erratum in: 2003 J Am Vet Med Assoc 223(5):653.

Owen MC, Lamb CR, Lu D, and Targett MP. 2004. Material in the middle ear of dogs having magnetic resonance imaging for investigation of neurologic signs. Vet Radiol Ultrasound 45(2):149–155.

Patterson EE, Mickelson JR, Da Y, Roberts MC, McVey AS, O'Brien DP, et al. 2003. Clinical characteristics and inheritance of idiopathic epilepsy in Vizslas. J Vet Intern Med 17(3):319–325.

Pease A, Sullivan S, Olby N, Galano H, Cerda-Gonzalez S, Robertson ID, et al. 2006. Value of a single-shot turbo spin-echo pulse sequence for assessing the architecture of the subarachnoid space and the constitutive nature of cerebrospinal fluid. Vet Radiol Ultrasound 47(3):254–259.

Pellegrino FC and Sica RE. 2004. Canine electroencephalographic recording technique: findings in normal and epileptic dogs. Clin Neurophysiol 115(2):477–487.

Platt SR, Alleman AR, Lanz OI, and Chrisman CL. 2002. Comparison of fine-needle aspiration and surgical-tissue biopsy in the diagnosis of canine brain tumors. Vet Surg 31(1):65–69.

Platt SR, Chrisman CL, Graham J, and Clemmons RM. 1999. Secondary hypoadrenocorticism associated with craniocerebral trauma in a dog. J Am Anim Hosp Assoc 35(2):117–122.

Platt SR and Garosi L. 2003. Canine cerebrovascular disease: do dogs have strokes? J Am Anim Hosp Assoc 39(4):337–342.

Platt SR, Graham J, Chrisman CL, Adjiri-Awere A, and Clemmons RM. 1999. Canine intracranial epidermoid cyst. Vet Radiol Ultrasound 40(5):454–458.

Platt SR, Scase TJ, Adams V, Wieczorek L, Miller J, Adamo F, et al. 2006. Vascular endothelial growth factor expression in canine intracranial meningiomas and association with patient survival. J Vet Intern Med 20(3):663–668.

Polizopoulou ZS, Koutinas AF, Souftas VD, Kaldrymidou E, Kazakos G, and Papadopoulos G. 2004. Diagnostic correlation of CT-MRI and histopathology in 10 dogs with brain neoplasms. J Vet Med A Physiol Pathol Clin Med 51(5):226–231.

Ponten U, Thuomas KA, Bergstrom K, Nilsson P, Zwetnow NN, Vlajkovic S, et al. 1986. Evaluation of intracranial pressure rebound after evacuation of intracranial expanding lesions. An experimental study in dogs. Acta Radiol Suppl 369:360–364.

Ramsey IK, Dennis R, and Herrtage ME. 1999. Concurrent central diabetes insipidus and panhypopituitarism in a German shepherd dog. J Small Anim Pract 40(6):271–274.

Rusbridge C, Greitz D, and Iskandar BJ. 2006. Syringomyelia: current concepts in pathogenesis, diagnosis, and treatment. J Vet Intern Med 20(3):469–479.

Rusbridge C and Knowler SP. 2003. Hereditary aspects of occipital bone hypoplasia and syringomyelia (Chiari type I malformation) in Cavalier King Charles spaniels. Vet Rec 153(4):107–112.

Rusbridge C, MacSweeny JE, Davies JV, Chandler K, Fitzmaurice SN, Dennis R, et al. 2000. Syringohydromyelia in Cavalier King Charles spaniels. J Am Anim Hosp Assoc 36(1):34–41.

Sage JE, Samii VF, Abramson CJ, Green EM, Smith M, and Dingus C. 2006. Comparison of conventional spin-echo and fast spin-echo magnetic resonance imaging in the canine brain. Vet Radiol Ultrasound 47(3):249–253.

Saito M, Sharp NJ, Kortz GD, de Lahunta A, Leventer RJ, Tokuriki M, et al. 2002. Magnetic resonance imaging features of lissencephaly in 2 Lhasa Apsos [Review]. Vet Radiol Ultrasound 43(4):331–337..

Sarwar M, Virapongse C, and Carbo P. 1985. Experimental production of superior sagittal sinus thrombosis in the dog. AJNR Am J Neuroradiol 6(1):19–22.

Saunders JH, Clercx C, Snaps FR, Sullivan M, Duchateau L, van Bree HJ, et al. 2004. Radiographic, magnetic resonance imaging, computed tomographic, and rhinoscopic features of nasal aspergillosis in dogs. J Am Vet Med Assoc 225(11):1703–1712.

Saunders JH, Poncelet L, Clercx C, Snaps FR, Flandroy P, Capasso P, et al. 1998. Probable trigeminal nerve schwannoma in a dog. Vet Radiol Ultrasound 39(6):539–542.

Sawashima Y, Sawashima K, Taura Y, Shimada A, and Umemura T. 1996. Clinical and pathological findings of a Yorkshire terrier affected with necrotizing encephalitis. J Vet Med Sci 58(7):659–661.

Schoeman JP, Stidworthy MF, Penderis J, and Kafka U. 2002. Magnetic resonance imaging of a cerebral cavernous haemangioma in a dog. J S Afr Vet Assoc 73(4):207–210.

Seiler G, Cizinauskas S, Scheidegger J, and Lang J. 2001. Low-field magnetic resonance imaging of a pyocephalus and a suspected brain abscess in a German Shepherd dog. Vet Radiol Ultrasound 42(5):417–422.

Sharkey LC, McDonnell JJ, and Alroy J. 2004. Cytology of a mass on the meningeal surface of the left brain in a dog. Vet Clin Pathol 33(2):111–114

Sheppard BJ, Chrisman CL, Newell SM, Raskin RE, and Homer BL. 1997. Primary encephalic plasma cell tumor in a dog. Vet Pathol 34(6):621–627.

Shores A. 1993a. Magnetic resonance imaging. Vet Clin North Am Small Anim Pract 23(2):437–459..

Shores A. 1993b. New and future advanced imaging techniques. Vet Clin North Am Small Anim Pract 23(2):461–469.

Shubitz LF and Dial SM. 2005. Coccidioidomycosis: a diagnostic challenge [Review]. Clin Tech Small Anim Pract 20(4):220–226.

Singh M, Thompson M, Sullivan N, and Child G. 2005. Thiamine deficiency in dogs due to the feeding of sulphite preserved meat. Aust Vet J 83(7):412–417.

Snellman M, Benczik J, Joensuu R, Ramadan UA, Tanttu J, and Savolainen S. 1999. Low-field magnetic resonance imaging of beagle brain with a dedicated receiver coil. Vet Radiol Ultrasound 40(1):36–39.

Snyder JM, Shofer FS, Van Winkle TJ, and Massicotte C. 2006. Canine intracranial primary neoplasia: 173 cases (1986–2003). J Vet Intern Med 20(3):669–675.

Steiss JE, Cox NR, and Hathcock JT. 1994. Brain stem auditory-evoked response abnormalities in 14 dogs with confirmed central nervous system lesions. J Vet Intern Med 8(4):293–298.

Straszek SP, Taagehoj F, Graff S, and Pedersen OF. 2003. Acoustic rhinometry in dog and cat compared with a fluid-displacement method and magnetic resonance imaging. J Appl Physiol 95(2):635–642.

Strother CM, Unal O, Frayne R, Turk A, Omary R, Korosec FR, et al. 2000. Endovascular treatment of experimental canine aneurysms: feasibility with MR imaging guidance. Radiology 215(2):516–519.

Stubbs JB, Frankel RH, Schultz K, Crocker I, Dillehay D, and Olson JJ. 2002. Preclinical evaluation of a novel device for delivering brachytherapy to the margins of resected brain tumor cavities. J Neurosurg 96(2):335–343.

Sturges BK, Dickinson PJ, Kortz GD, Berry WL, Vernau KM, Wisner ER, et al. 2006. Clinical signs, magnetic resonance imaging features, and outcome after surgical and medical

treatment of otogenic intracranial infection in 11 cats and 4 dogs. J Vet Intern Med 20(3):648–656.

Su MY, Head E, Brooks WM, Wang Z, Muggenburg BA, Adam GE, et al. 1998. Magnetic resonance imaging of anatomic and vascular characteristics in a canine model of human aging. Neurobiol Aging 19(5):479–485.

Su MY, Tapp PD, Vu L, Chen YF, Chu Y, Muggenburg B, et al. 2005. A longitudinal study of brain morphometrics using serial magnetic resonance imaging analysis in a canine model of aging. Prog Neuropsychopharmacol Biol Psychiatry 29(3):389–397.

Suzuki M, Nakayama H, Ohtsuka R, Yasoshima A, Katayama K, Uetsuka K, et al. 2002. Cerebellar myxoid type meningioma in a Shih Tzu dog. J Vet Med Sci 64(2):155–157.

Swensen SJ, Keller PL, Berquist TH, McLeod RA, and Stephens DH. 1985. Magnetic resonance imaging of hemorrhage. AJR Am J Roentgenol 145(5):921–927.

Takagi S, Kadosawa T, Ohsaki T, Hoshino Y, Okumura M, and Fujinaga T. 2005. Hindbrain decompression in a dog with scoliosis associated with syringomyelia. J Am Vet Med Assoc 226(8):1359–1363, 1347.

Tamura S, Tamura Y, Tsuka T, and Uchida K. 2006. Sequential magnetic resonance imaging of an intracranial hematoma in a dog. Vet Radiol Ultrasound 47(2):142–144.

Taoda T, Hara Y, Takekoshi S, Itoh J, Teramoto A, Osamura RY, et al. 2006. Effect of mitotane on pituitary corticotrophs in clinically normal dogs. Am J Vet Res 67(8):1385–1394.

Tapp PD, Head K, Head E, Milgram NW, Muggenburg BA, and Su MY. 2006. Application of an automated voxel-based morphometry technique to assess regional gray and white matter brain atrophy in a canine model of aging. Neuroimage 29(1):234–244.

Tapp PD, Siwak CT, Gao FQ, Chiou JY, Black SE, Head E, et al. 2004. Frontal lobe volume, function, and beta-amyloid pathology in a canine model of aging. J Neurosci 24(38):8205–8213.

Targett MP, McInnes E, and Dennis R. 1999. Magnetic resonance imaging of a medullary dermoid cyst with secondary hydrocephalus in a dog. Vet Radiol Ultrasound 40(1):23–26.

Theisen SK, Podell M, Schneider T, Wilkie DA, and Fenner WR. 1996. A retrospective study of cavernous sinus syndrome in 4 dogs and 8 cats. J Vet Intern Med 10(2):65–71. Erratum in: 1996 J Vet Intern Med 10(3):197.

Thomas WB. 1996. Cerebrovascular disease. Vet Clin North Am Small Anim Pract 26(4):925–943.

Thomas WB. 1998. Inflammatory diseases of the central nervous system in dogs. Clin Tech Small Anim Pract 13(3):167–178.

Thomas WB. 1999. Nonneoplastic disorders of the brain. Clin Tech Small Anim Pract 14(3):125–147.

Thomas WB, Adams WH, McGavin MD, and Gompf RE. 1997. Magnetic resonance imaging appearance of intracranial hemorrhage secondary to cerebral vascular malformation in a dog. Vet Radiol Ultrasound 38(5):371–375.

Thomas WB, Sorjonen DC, Hudson JA, and Cox NR. 1993. Ultrasound-guided brain biopsy in dogs. Am J Vet Res 54(11):1942–1947.

Thuomas KA, Vlajkovic S, Ganz JC, Nilsson P, Bergstrom K, Ponten U, et al. 1993. Progressive brain compression. Changes in vital physiological variables, correlated with brain tissue water content and brain tissue displacement. Experimental MR imaging in dogs. Acta Radiol 34(3):289–295.

Tiches D, Vite CH, Dayrell-Hart B, Steinberg SA, Gross S, and Lexa F. 1998. A case of canine central nervous system cryptococcosis: management with fluconazole. J Am Anim Hosp Assoc 34(2):145–151.

Tidwell AS and Jones JC. 1999. Advanced imaging concepts: a pictorial glossary of CT and MRI technology. Clin Tech Small Anim Pract 14(2):65–111.

Tidwell AS, Ross LA, and Kleine LJ. 1997. Computed tomography and magnetic resonance imaging of cavernous sinus enlargement in a dog with unilateral exophthalmos. Vet Radiol Ultrasound 38(5):363–370.

Tidwell AS, Solano M, and Schelling SH. 1994. Pediatric neuroimaging. Semin Vet Med Surg (Small Anim) 9(2):68–85.

Tieber LM, Axlund TW, Simpson ST, and Hathcock JT. 2006. Survival of a suspected case of central nervous system cuterebrosis in a dog: clinical and magnetic resonance imaging findings. J Am Anim Hosp Assoc 42(3):238–242.

Torisu S, Washizu M, Hasegawa D, and Orima H. 2005. Brain magnetic resonance imaging characteristics in dogs and cats with congenital portosystemic shunts. Vet Radiol Ultrasound 46(6):447–451.

Triolo AJ, Howard MO, and Miles KG. 1994. Oligodendroglioma in a 15-month-old dog. J Am Vet Med Assoc 205(7):986–988.

Troxel MT, Drobatz KJ, and Vite CH. 2005. Signs of neurologic dysfunction in dogs with central versus peripheral vestibular disease. J Am Vet Med Assoc 227(4):570–574.

Tucker RL and Gavin PR. 1996. Brain imaging. Vet Clin North Am Small Anim Pract 26(4):735–758.

Van Der Merwe LL and Lane E. 2001. Diagnosis of cerebellar cortical degeneration in a Scottish terrier using magnetic resonance imaging. J Small Anim Pract 42(8):409–412.

Van Der Vlugt-Meijer RH, Voorhout G, and Meij BP. 2002. Imaging of the pituitary gland in dogs with pituitary-dependent hyperadrenocorticism. Mol Cell Endocrinol 197(1–2):81–87.

Varejao AS, Munoz A, and Lorenzo V. 2006. Magnetic resonance imaging of the intratemporal facial nerve in idiopathic facial paralysis in the dog. Vet Radiol Ultrasound 47(4):328–333.

Vermeersch K, Van Ham L, Caemaert J, Tshamala M, Taeymans O, Bhatti S, et al. 2004. Suboccipital craniectomy, dorsal laminectomy of C1, durotomy and dural graft placement as a treatment for syringohydromyelia with cerebellar tonsil herniation in Cavalier King Charles spaniels. Vet Surg 33(4):355–360.

Vernau KM, Kortz GD, Koblik PD, LeCouteur RA, Bailey CS, and Pedroia V. 1997. Magnetic resonance imaging and computed tomography characteristics of intracranial intra arachnoid cysts in 6 dogs. Vet Radiol Ultrasound 38(3):171–176.

Vernau KM, LeCouteur RA, Sturges BK, Samii V, Higgins RJ, Koblik PD, et al. 2002. Intracranial intra-arachnoid cyst with intracystic hemorrhage in two dogs. Vet Radiol Ultrasound 43(5):449–454.

Viitmaa R, Cizinauskas S, Bergamasco LA, Kuusela E, Pascoe P, Teppo AM, et al. 2006. Magnetic resonance imaging findings in Finnish Spitz dogs with focal epilepsy. J Vet Intern Med 20(2):305–310.

Vite CH, Insko EK, Schotland HM, Panckeri K, and Hendricks JC. 1997. Quantification of cerebral ventricular volume in English bulldogs. Vet Radiol Ultrasound 38(6):437–443.

Vite CH and McGowan JC. 2001. Magnetization transfer imaging of the canine brain: a review [Review]. Vet Radiol Ultrasound 42(1):5–8.

Vlajkovic S, Zwetnow NN, Thuomas KA, Bergstrom K, Ponten U, and Nilsson P. 1986. Magnetic resonance imaging of water intoxication. An experimental study in dogs. Acta Radiol Suppl 369:353–355.

von Praun F, Matiasek K, Grevel V, Alef M, and Flegel T. 2006. Magnetic resonance imaging and pathologic findings associated with necrotizing encephalitis in two Yorkshire terriers. Vet Radiol Ultrasound 47(3):260–264.

Vullo T, Korenman E, Manzo RP, Gomez DG, Deck MD, and Cahill PT. 1997. Diagnosis of cerebral ventriculomegaly in normal adult beagles using quantitative MRI. Vet Radiol Ultrasound 38(4):277–281.

Vullo T, Manzo R, Gomez DG, Deck MD, and Cahill PT. 1998. A canine model of acute hydrocephalus with MR correlation. AJNR Am J Neuroradiol 19(6):1123–1125.

Vural SA, Besalti O, Ilhan F, Ozak A, and Haligur M. 2006. Ventricular ependymoma in a German Shepherd dog. Vet J 172(1):185–187.

Wakshlag JJ, de Lahunta A, Robinson T, Cooper BJ, Brenner O, O'Toole TD, et al. 1999. Subacute necrotising encephalopathy in an Alaskan husky. J Small Anim Pract 40(12):585–589.

Walmsley GL, Herrtage ME, Dennis R, Platt SR, and Jeffery ND. 2006. The relationship between clinical signs and brain herniation associated with rostrotentorial mass lesions in the dog. Vet J 172(2):258–264.

Webb AA, Cullen CL, Rose P, Eisenbart D, Gabor L, and Martinson S. 2005. Intracranial meningioma causing internal ophthalmoparesis in a dog. Vet Ophthalmol 8(6):421–425.

Weingarten K, Zimmerman RD, Deo-Narine V, Markisz J, Cahill PT, and Deck MD. 1991. MR imaging of acute intracranial hemorrhage: findings on sequential spin-echo and gradient-echo images in a dog model. AJNR Am J Neuroradiol 12(3):457–467.

Weiss KL, Schroeder CE, Kastin SJ, Gibson JP, Yarrington JT, Heydorn WE, et al. 1994. MRI monitoring of vigabatrin-induced intramyelinic edema in dogs. Neurology 44(10):1944–1949.

Wenger DA, Victoria T, Rafi MA, Luzi P, Vanier MT, Vite C, et al. 1999. Globoid cell leukodystrophy in cairn and West Highland white terriers. J Hered 90(1):138–142.

Whelan HT, Clanton JA, Wilson RE, and Tulipan NB. 1988. Comparison of CT and MRI brain tumor imaging using a canine glioma model. Pediatr Neurol 4(5):279–283.

Whelan HT, Schmidt MH, Segura AD, McAuliffe TL, Bajic DM, Murray KJ, et al. 1993. The role of photodynamic therapy in posterior fossa brain tumors. A preclinical study in a canine glioma model. J Neurosurg 79(4):562–568.

Widmer WR and Kneller SK. 1997. Artifacts and technical errors presented as part of the 1996 ACVR oral certification examination. Vet Radiol Ultrasound 38(2):156–158.

Wilson J. 2001. Solving the neurological dilemma. J Small Anim Pract 42(2):98.

Wood AK, Kundel HL, McGrath JT, and Wortman JA. 1987. Computed tomography, magnetic resonance imaging, and pathologic observations of the effects of intrathecal metrizamide and iohexol on the canine central nervous system. Invest Radiol 22(8):672–677.

Yamada K, Miyahara K, Nakagawa M, Kobayashi Y, Furuoka H, Matsui T, et al. 1999. A case of a dog with thickened calvaria with neurologic symptoms: magnetic resonance imaging (MRI) findings. J Vet Med Sci 61(9):1055–1057.

Yamaya Y, Iwakami E, Goto M, Koie H, Watari T, Tanaka S, et al. 2004. A case of shaker dog disease in a miniature dachshund. J Vet Med Sci 66(9):1159–1160.

Zwetnow NN, Vlajkovic S, Thuomas KA, Bergstrom K, Ponten U, and Nilsson P. 1986. Magnetic resonance imaging of cerebral compression and local brain tissue water content during continuous extradural bleeding. An experimental study in dogs. Acta Radiol Suppl 369:356–359.

Cats

Allgoewer I, Grevel V, Philipp K, Schmidt P, and Brunnberg L. 1998. Somatotropic pituitary adenoma with lesions of the oculomotor nerve in a cat [German]. Tierarztl Prax Ausg K Klientiere Heimtiere 26(4):267–272.

Allgoewer I, Lucas S, and Schmitz SA. 2000. Magnetic resonance imaging of the normal and diseased feline middle ear. Vet Radiol Ultrasound 41(5):413–418.

Bagley RS. 1997. Common neurologic diseases of older animals. Vet Clin North Am Small Anim Pract 27(6):1451–1486.

Bagley RS and Gavin PR. 1998. Seizures as a complication of brain tumors in dogs. Clin Tech Small Anim Pract 13(3):179–184.

Bailey MQ. 1990. Diagnostic imaging of intracranial lesions. Semin Vet Med Surg (Small Anim) 5(4):232–236.

Baratti C, Barnett AS, and Pierpaoli C. 1999. Comparative MR imaging study of brain maturation in kittens with T1, T2, and the trace of the diffusion tensor. Radiology 210(1):133–142.

Barnes D, Harvey I, McDonald WI, Ron MA, and Moore S. 1991. The effect of chlorpromazine and methylprednisolone on NMR relaxation times in the normal cat brain. Magn Reson Med 18(1):232–236.

Bayens-Simmonds J, Boisvert DP, Castro ME, and Johnson ES. 1988. A feline model for experimental studies of peritumor brain edema. J Neurooncol 6(4):371–378.

Benigni L and Lamb CR. 2005. Comparison of fluid-attenuated inversion recovery and T2-weighted magnetic resonance images in dogs and cats with suspected brain disease. Vet Radiol Ultrasound 46(4):287–292.

Berry I, Brant-Zawadzki M, and Manelfe C. 1988. MRI study of a feline model of acute cerebral ischaemia. Contribution of paramagnetic contrast media to the diagnosis. J Neuroradiol 15(2):95–107.

Bischoff MG and Kneller SK. 2004. Diagnostic imaging of the canine and feline ear. Vet Clin North Am Small Anim Pract 34(2):437–458.

Bockhorst KH, Smith JM, Smith MI, Bradley DP, Houston GC, Carpenter TA, et al. 2000. A quantitative analysis of cortical spreading depression events in the feline brain characterized with diffusion-weighted MRI. J Magn Reson Imaging 12(5):722–733.

Boisvert DP, Lazareff JA, and Allen PS. 1990. Quantitative magnetic resonance imaging assessment of mannitol's effect on peritumoral brain edema. Adv Neurol 52:560.

Bose B, Jones SC, Lorig R, Friel HT, Weinstein M, and Little JR. 1988. Evolving focal cerebral ischemia in cats: spatial correlation of nuclear magnetic resonance imaging, cerebral blood flow, tetrazolium staining, and histopathology. Stroke 19(1):28–37.

Bottcher P, Maierl J, Hecht S, Matis U, and Liebich HG. 2004. Automatic image registration of three-dimensional images of the head of cats and dogs by use of maximization of mutual information. Am J Vet Res 65(12):1680–1687.

Bradley DP, Smith JM, Smith MI, Bockhorst KH, Papadakis NG, Hall LD, et al. 2002. Cortical spreading depression in the feline brain following sustained and transient stimuli studied using diffusion-weighted imaging. J Physiol 544 (Pt 1):39–56.

Branch CA, Ewing JR, Helpern JA, Ordidge RJ, Butt S, and Welch KM. 1992. Atraumatic quantitation of cerebral perfusion in cats by 19 F magnetic resonance imaging. Magn Reson Med 28(1):39–53.

Buonanno FS, Pykett IL, Kistler JP, Vielma J, Brady TJ, Hinshaw WS, et al. 1982. Cranial anatomy and detection of ischemic stroke in the cat by nuclear magnetic resonance imaging. Radiology 143(1):187–193.

Chan KH, Swarts JD, Hashida Y, Doyle WJ, Kardatzke D, and Wolf GL. 1992. Experimental otitis media evaluated by magnetic resonance imaging: an in vivo model. Ann Otol Rhinol Laryngol 101(3):248–254.

Cherubini GB, Mantis P, Martinez TA, Lamb CR, and Cappello R. 2005. Utility of magnetic resonance imaging for distinguishing neoplastic from non-neoplastic brain lesions in dogs and cats. Vet Radiol Ultrasound 46(5):384–387.

Chew W, Kucharczyk J, Moseley M, Derugin N, and Norman D. 1991. Hyperglycemia augments ischemic brain injury: in vivo MR imaging/spectroscopic study with nicardipine in cats with occluded middle cerebral arteries. AJNR Am J Neuroradiol 12(4):603–609.

De Crespigny AJ, Wendland MF, Derugin N, Kozniewska E, and Moseley ME. 1992. Real-time observation of transient focal ischemia and hyperemia in cat brain. Magn Reson Med 27(2):391–397.

de Crespigny AJ, Wendland MF, Derugin N, Vexler ZS, and Moseley ME. 1993. Rapid MR imaging of a vascular challenge to focal ischemia in cat brain. J Magn Reson Imaging 3(3):475–481.

Dennis R. 2000. Use of magnetic resonance imaging for the investigation of orbital disease in small animals. J Small Anim Pract 41(4):145–155.

Detre JA, Subramanian VH, Mitchell MD, Smith DS, Kobayashi A, Zaman A, et al. 1990. Measurement of regional cerebral blood flow in cat brain using intracarotid ^2H_2O and ^2H NMR imaging. Magn Reson Med 14(2):389–395.

Dewey CW, Coates JR, Ducote JM, Stefanacci JD, Walker MA, and Marino DJ. 2003. External hydrocephalus in two cats. J Am Anim Hosp Assoc 39(6):567–572.

Dickinson PJ, Keel MK, Higgins RJ, Koblik PD, LeCouteur RA, Naydan DK, et al. 2000. Clinical and pathologic features of oligodendrogliomas in two cats. Vet Pathol 37(2):160–167.

Elliott DA, Feldman EC, Koblik PD, Samii VF, and Nelson RW. 2000. Prevalence of pituitary tumors among diabetic cats with insulin resistance. J Am Vet Med Assoc 216(11):1765–1768.

Foley JE, Lapointe JM, Koblik P, Poland A, and Pedersen NC. 1998. Diagnostic features of clinical neurologic feline infectious peritonitis. J Vet Intern Med 12(6):415–423.

Forterre F, Tomek A, Konar M, Vandevelde M, Howard J, and Jaggy A. 2006. Multiple meningiomas: clinical, radiological, surgical, and pathological findings with outcome in four cats. J Feline Med Surg 9(1):36–43.

Foster SF, Charles JA, Parker G, Krockenberger M, Churcher RM, and Malik R. 2001. Cerebral cryptococcal granuloma in a cat. J Feline Med Surg 3(1):39–44.

Garosi LS, Dennis R, and Schwarz T. 2003. Review of diagnostic imaging of ear diseases in the dog and cat. Vet Radiol Ultrasound 44(2):137–146.

Gavin PR, Fike JR, and Hoopes PJ. 1995. Central nervous system tumors. Semin Vet Med Surg (Small Anim) 10(3):180–189.

Graham JP, Newell SM, Voges AK, Roberts GD, and Harrison JM. 1998. The dural tail sign in the diagnosis of meningiomas. Vet Radiol Ultrasound 39(4):297–302.

Hayman LA, McArdle CB, Taber KH, Saleem A, Baskin D, Lee HS, et al. 1989. MR imaging of hyperacute intracranial hemorrhage in the cat. AJNR Am J Neuroradiol 10(4):681–686.

Henderson LA, Frysinger RC, Yu PL, Bandler R, and Harper RM. 2001. A device for feline head positioning and stabilization during magnetic resonance imaging. Magn Reson Imaging 19(7):1031–1036.

Holland M. 1993. Contrast agents. Vet Clin North Am Small Anim Pract 23(2):269–279.

Hossmann KA, Szymas J, Seo K, Assheuer J, and Krajewski S. 1989. Experimental transplantation gliomas in the adult cat brain. 2. Pathophysiology and magnetic resonance imaging. Acta Neurochir (Wien) 98(3–4):189–200.

Ide H, Kobayashi H, Handa Y, Kubota T, Maeda M, Itoh S, et al. 1993. Correlation between somatosensory-evoked potentials and magnetic resonance imaging of focal cerebral ischemia in cats. Surg Neurol 40(3):216–223.

Inada S, Mochizuki M, Izumo S, Kuriyama M, Sakamoto H, Kawasaki Y, et al. 1996. Study of hereditary cerebellar degeneration in cats. Am J Vet Res 57(3):296–301.

Kaser-Hotz B, Rohrer CR, Stankeova S, Wergin M, Fidel J, and Reusch C. 2002. Radiotherapy of pituitary tumours in five cats. J Small Anim Pract 43(7):303–307.

Kim HJ, Lee CH, Kim HG, Lee SD, Son SM, Kim YW, et al. 2004. Reversible MR changes in the cat brain after cerebral fat embolism induced by triolein emulsion. AJNR Am J Neuroradiol 25(6):958–963. Erratum in: 2004 AJNR Am J Neuroradiol. 25(7):1301.

Kitagawa M, Koie H, Kanayamat K, and Sakai T. 2003. Medulloblastoma in a cat: clinical and MRI findings. J Small Anim Pract 44(3):139–142.

Kline RA, Negendank WG, McCoy LE, Lester M, and Berguer R. 1990. MRI quantitation of edema in focal cerebral ischemia in cats: correlation with cytochrome aa3 oxidation state. Magn Reson Med 13(2):319–323.

Klopp LS, Hathcock JT, and Sorjonen DC. 2000. Magnetic resonance imaging features of brain stem abscessation in two cats. Vet Radiol Ultrasound 41(4):300–307.

Kobayashi H, Ide H, Kabuto M, Handa Y, Kubota T, and Ishii Y. 1995. Effect of mannitol on focal cerebral ischemia evaluated by somatosensory-evoked potentials and magnetic resonance imaging. Surg Neurol 44(1):55–61; discussion 61–62.

Kobayashi H, Ide H, Kodera T, Handa Y, Kabuto M, Kubota T, et al. 1994. Effect of mannitol on focal cerebral ischemia evaluated by magnetic resonance imaging. Acta Neurochir Suppl (Wien) 60:228–230.

Kraft SL and Gavin PR. 1999. Intracranial neoplasia. Clin Tech Small Anim Pract 14(2):112–123.

Kraus KH and McDonnell J. 1996. Identification and management of brain tumors. Semin Vet Med Surg (Small Anim) 11(4):218–224.

Kroll RA, Pagel MA, Roman-Goldstein S, Barkovich AJ, D'Agostino AN, and Neuwelt EA. 1995. White matter changes associated with feline GM2 gangliosidosis (Sandhoff disease): correlation of MR findings with pathologic and ultrastructural abnormalities. AJNR Am J Neuroradiol 16(6):1219–1226.

Kucharczyk J, Vexler ZS, Roberts TP, Asgari HS, Mintorovitch J, Derugin N, et al. 1993. Echo-planar perfusion-sensitive MR imaging of acute cerebral ischemia. Radiology 188(3):711–717.

Kudnig ST. 2002. Nasopharyngeal polyps in cats. Clin Tech Small Anim Pract 17(4):174–177.

Kuwabara M, Kitagawa M, Sato T, Ohba S, and Tsubokawa T. 2002. Early diagnosis of feline medulloblastoma in the vermis. Vet Rec 150(15):488–489. No abstract available.

Lavely J and Lipsitz D. 2005. Fungal infections of the central nervous system in the dog and cat. Clin Tech Small Anim Pract 20(4):212–219.

LeCouteur RA. 1999. Current concepts in the diagnosis and treatment of brain tumours in dogs and cats. J Small Anim Pract 40(9):411–416.

LeCouteur RA. 2003. Advanced diagnostic techniques in feline brain disease. J Feline Med Surg 5(2):117–119.

Lu D, Pocknell A, Lamb CR, and Targett MP. 2003. Concurrent benign and malignant multiple meningiomas in a cat: clinical, MRI and pathological findings. Vet Rec 152(25):780–782. No abstract available.

Lujan A, Philbey AW, and Anderson TJ. 2003. Intradural epithelial cyst in a cat. Vet Rec 153(12):363–364.

Maeda M, Itoh S, Ide H, Matsuda T, Kobayashi H, Kubota T, et al. 1993. Acute stroke in cats: comparison of dynamic susceptibility-contrast MR imaging with T2- and diffusion-weighted MR imaging. Radiology 189(1):227–232.

Mattoon JS and Wisner ER. 2004. What's under the cat's hat: feline intracranial neoplasia and magnetic resonance imaging. J Vet Intern Med 18(2):139–140.

McKay JS, Targett MP, and Jeffery ND. 1999. Histological characterization of an ependymoma in the fourth ventricle of a cat. J Comp Pathol 120(1):105–113.

Meij B, Voorhout G, and Rijnberk A. 2002. Progress in transsphenoidal hypophysectomy for treatment of pituitary-dependent hyperadrenocorticism in dogs and cats. Mol Cell Endocrinol 197(1–2):89–96.

Mellanby RJ, Jeffery ND, Gopal MS, and Herrtage ME. 2005. Secondary hypothyroidism following head trauma in a cat. J Feline Med Surg 7(2):135–139.

Mellema LM, Samii VF, Vernau KM, and LeCouteur RA. 2002. Meningeal enhancement on magnetic resonance imaging in 15 dogs and 3 cats. Vet Radiol Ultrasound 43(1):10–15.

Moore MP, Bagley RS, Harrington ML, and Gavin PR. 1996. Intracranial tumors. Vet Clin North Am Small Anim Pract 26(4):759–777.

Morozumi M, Miyahara K, Sato M, and Hirose T. 1997. Computed tomography and magnetic resonance findings in two dogs and a cat with intracranial lesions. J Vet Med Sci 59(9):807–810.

Morozumi M, Sasaki N, Oyama Y, Uetsuka K, Nakayama H, and Goto N. 1993. Computed tomography and magnetic resonance findings of meningeal syndrome in a leukemic cat. J Vet Med Sci 55(6):1035–1037.

Okada Y, Hoehn-Berlage M, Bockhorst K, Tolxdorff T, and Hossmann KA. 1990. Magnetic resonance imaging and regional biochemical analysis of experimental brain tumours in cats. Acta Neurochir Suppl (Wien) 51:128–130.

Parent JM and Quesnel AD. 1996. Seizures in cats. Vet Clin North Am Small Anim Pract 26(4):811–825.

Pease A, Sullivan S, Olby N, Galano H, Cerda-Gonzalez S, Robertson ID, et al. 2006. Value of a single-shot turbo spin-echo pulse sequence for assessing the architecture of the subarachnoid space and the constitutive nature of cerebrospinal fluid. Vet Radiol Ultrasound 47(3):254–259.

Pfohl JC and Dewey CW. 2005. Intracranial Toxoplasma gondii granuloma in a cat. J Feline Med Surg 7(6):369–374.

Podell M, Hadjiconstantinou M, Smith MA, and Neff NH. 2003. Proton magnetic resonance imaging and spectroscopy identify metabolic changes in the striatum in the MPTP feline model of Parkinsonism. Exp Neurol 179(2):159–166.

Podell M, Maruyama K, Smith M, Hayes KA, Buck WR, Ruehlmann DS, et al. 1999. Frontal lobe neuronal injury correlates to altered function in FIV-infected cats. J Acquir Immune Defic Syndr 22(1):10–18.

Podell M, Oglesbee M, Mathes L, Krakowka S, Olmstead R, and Lafrado L. 1993. AIDS-associated encephalopathy with experimental feline immunodeficiency virus infection. J Acquir Immune Defic Syndr 6(7):758–771.

Quesnel AD and Parent JM. 1995. Paradoxical vestibular syndrome in a cat with a cerebellar meningioma. Can Vet J 36(4):230–232. No abstract available.

Quesnel AD, Parent JM, McDonell W, Percy D, and Lumsden JH. 1997. Diagnostic evaluation of cats with seizure disorders: 30 cases (1991–1993). J Am Vet Med Assoc 210(1):65–71.

Runge VM, Kirsch JE, Wells JW, Dunworth JN, and Woolfolk CE. 1994. Visualization of blood-brain barrier disruption on MR images of cats with acute cerebral infarction: value of administering a high dose of contrast material. AJR Am J Roentgenol 162(2):431–435.

Sato T, Ikebata Y, Koie H, Shibuya H, Shirai W, and Nogami S. 2003. Magnetic resonance imaging and pathological findings in a cat with brain contusions. J Vet Med A Physiol Pathol Clin Med 50(4):222–224.

Sharp NJ, Davis BJ, Guy JS, Cullen JM, Steingold SF, and Kornegay JN. 1999. Hydranencephaly and cerebellar hypoplasia in two kittens attributed to intrauterine parvovirus infection. J Comp Pathol 121(1):39–53.

Shirakuni T, Nagashima T, Tamaki N, and Matsumoto S. 1985. Magnetic resonance imaging of experimental brain edema in cats. Neurosurgery 17(4):557–563.

Sturges BK, Dickinson PJ, Kortz GD, Berry WL, Vernau KM, Wisner ER, et al. 2006. Clinical signs, magnetic resonance imaging features, and outcome after surgical and medical treatment of otogenic intracranial infection in 11 cats and 4 dogs. J Vet Intern Med 20(3):648–656.

Tanaka S, Tanaka T, Kondo S, Hori T, Fukuda H, Yonemasu Y, et al. 1993. Magnetic resonance imaging in kainic acid-induced limbic seizure status in cats. Neurol Med Chir (Tokyo) 33(5):285–289.

Tani K, Taga A, Itamoto K, Iwanaga T, Une S, Nakaichi M, et al. 2001. Hydrocephalus and syringomyelia in a cat. J Vet Med Sci 63(12):1331–1334.

Theisen SK, Podell M, Schneider T, Wilkie DA, and Fenner WR. 1996. A retrospective study of cavernous sinus syndrome in 4 dogs and 8 cats. J Vet Intern Med 10(2):65–71. Erratum in: 1996 J Vet Intern Med 10(3):197.

Torisu S, Washizu M, Hasegawa D, and Orima H. 2005. Brain magnetic resonance imaging characteristics in dogs and cats with congenital portosystemic shunts. Vet Radiol Ultrasound 46(6):447–451.

Troxel MT, Vite CH, Massicotte C, McLear RC, Van Winkle TJ, Glass EN, et al. 2004. Magnetic resonance imaging features of feline intracranial neoplasia: retrospective analysis of 46 cats. J Vet Intern Med 18(2):176–189.

Vexler ZS, Ayus JC, Roberts TP, Fraser CL, Kucharczyk J, and Arieff AI. 1994. Hypoxic and ischemic hypoxia exacerbate brain injury associated with metabolic encephalopathy in laboratory animals. J Clin Invest 93(1):256–264.

Vexler ZS, Roberts TP, Kucharczyk J, and Arieff AI. 1994. Severe brain edema associated with cumulative effects of hyponatremic encephalopathy and ischemic hypoxia. Acta Neurochir Suppl (Wien) 60:246–249.

Vite CH, McGowan JC, Braund KG, Drobatz KJ, Glickson JD, Wolfe JH, et al. 2001. Histopathology, electrodiagnostic testing, and magnetic resonance imaging show significant peripheral and central nervous system myelin abnormalities in the cat model of alpha-mannosidosis. J Neuropathol Exp Neurol 60(8):817–828.

Vite CH, McGowan JC, Niogi SN, Passini MA, Drobatz KJ, Haskins ME, et al. 2005. Effective gene therapy for an inherited CNS disease in a large animal model. Ann Neurol 57(3):355–364.

Wallack ST, Wisner ER, and Feldman EC. 2003. Mensuration of the pituitary gland from magnetic resonance images in 17 cats. Vet Radiol Ultrasound 44(3):278–282.

Widmer WR and Kneller SK. 1997. Artifacts and technical errors presented as part of the 1996 ACVR oral certification examination. Vet Radiol Ultrasound 38(2):156–158.

Yamada K, Miyahara K, Sato M, Hirose T, Yasugi Y, Matsuda Y, et al. 1995. Magnetic resonance imaging of the central nervous system in the kitten. J Vet Med Sci 57(1):155–156.

Yamada K, Miyahara K, Sato M, Miyabayashi T, and Hirose T. 1998. The contrecoup injury in a cat case of traffic accident: MRI findings. J Vet Med Sci 60(5):647–649.

Diagnosis of Spinal Disease

Rodney S. Bagley, Patrick R. Gavin, and Shannon P. Holmes

Similar to intracranial disease processes, spinal diseases may result in anatomical alterations of spinal tissues or affect spinal cord elements at a microscopic, physiologic, or functional level. Magnetic resonance (MR) imaging yields the most complete anatomical information and is currently the "gold standard" for evaluation of the spine and spinal cord. MR imaging yields superior images of the soft tissue such as the spinal cord, intervertebral disks, nerve roots, or peripheral nerves in close proximity to the spinal cord, as well as other paraspinal anatomical structures.

ANATOMY

Normal Neuroanatomy

At the level of the foramen magnum, the brain stem becomes contiguous with the spinal cord (Figure 2.106). The spinal cord serves as a conduit for transmission of information to and from the intracranial structures. Also, the spinal cord contains, primarily in the gray matter, the neuronal cell bodies that are responsible for motor functions in the limbs and trunk.

Both the spinal cord and the overlying vertebral structures are divided into segments (Figure 2.107). The vertebral segments are defined by the individual vertebral structures. The spinal segments, comparatively, are not as anatomically discretely identifiable, but are often within proximity to the overlying vertebral segments. In some regions of the spinal cord, notably in the caudal cervical and lumbar regions, the individual spinal cord segments may not lie within the associated vertebral segments of the same number. The relationship between spinal segments and the vertebral segments may also vary between differing species such as cats and dogs.

There are approximately 36 spinal segments with some variability in this absolute number occurring between individual animals. The cervical spinal cord normally contains 8 of these spinal segments, the thoracic area has 13 segments, and the lumbar region has 7 segment structures. The sacral segments are generally divided into three segments, with the caudal segments being somewhat variable, but often five segments. The spinal cord segmental arrangement is variable, both between species and even among individuals within the species. Spinal segments are encased within the vertebrae from the foramen magnum to approximately the caudal aspect of the lumbar 6 (L6) vertebrae in dogs. In relatively smaller dogs, the spinal cord may terminate more caudally; in larger dogs, the spinal cord may terminate more cranially. In cats, spinal cord segments may be found more caudally extending into the sacral vertebrae.

In the cervical area, there are 7 cervical vertebrae (vertebral segments) and 8 associated spinal cord segment structures. Therefore, there is a slight discontinuity between the location of the cervical spinal cord segments and the cervical vertebral segments, with the spinal cord segments lying within or slightly cranial to the vertebrae. A single spinal cord segment will give rise to a paired set of associated spinal nerves numbered similarly as the spinal segment. For example, the first cervical, or C1, spinal cord segment will produce the first cervical, or C1, nerve. There is also a first cervical vertebrae, the C1 vertebrae. To reiterate, it is important not to confuse the spinal cord segments, associated spinal nerves, and cervical vertebrae during clinical communication even though each of these structures is commonly referred to as "C1." Obviously there is an extra cervical spinal segment and associated nerves (C8 segment and nerves) compared to only seven cervical vertebrae. Spinal nerves that arise from a spinal segment must traverse the vertebral canal to terminate peripherally on a muscle or organ or to provide afferent information from the periphery into the spinal cord. Spinal nerves traverse between vertebrae in the intervertebral foramen just ventral to the articular facets of the adjacent

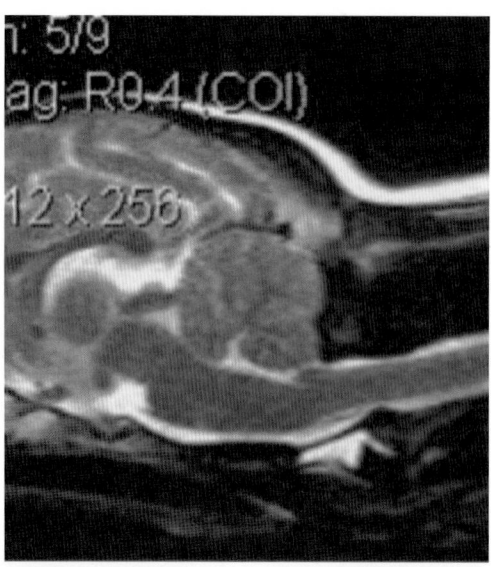

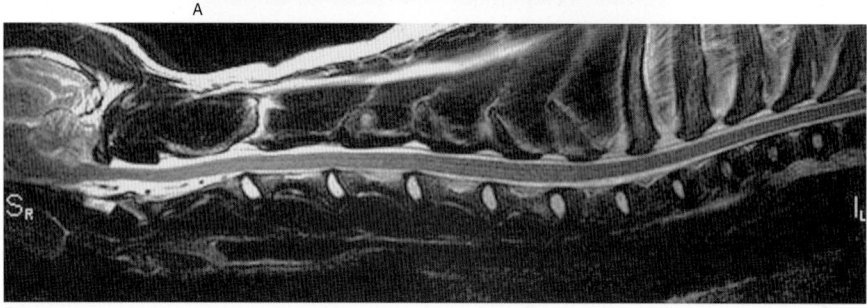

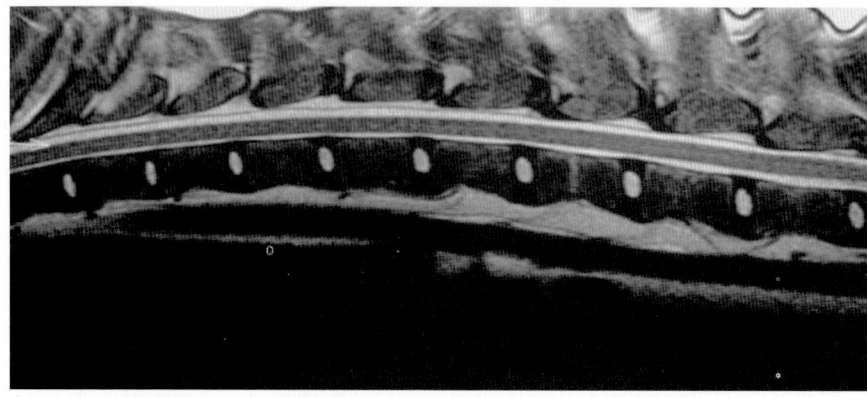

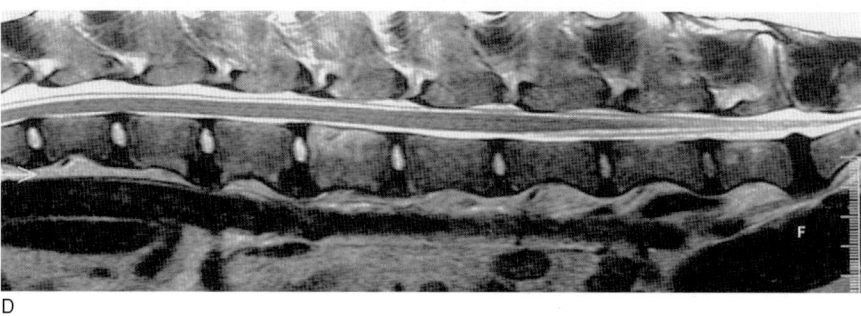

Figure 2.106. (A) Sagittal T2-weighted MR image of a dog at the level of caudal brain stem and cranial cervical spinal cord. (B) Sagittal T2-weighted MR image of a dog at the cervical spinal cord. (C) Sagittal T2-weighted MR image of a dog at the level of thoracolumbar spinal cord. (D) Sagittal T2-weighted MR image of a dog at the level of lumbar spinal cord.

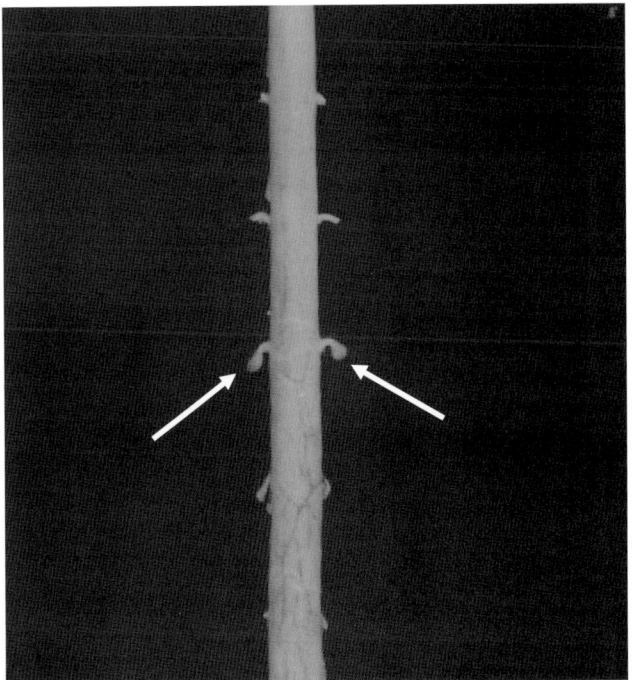

A

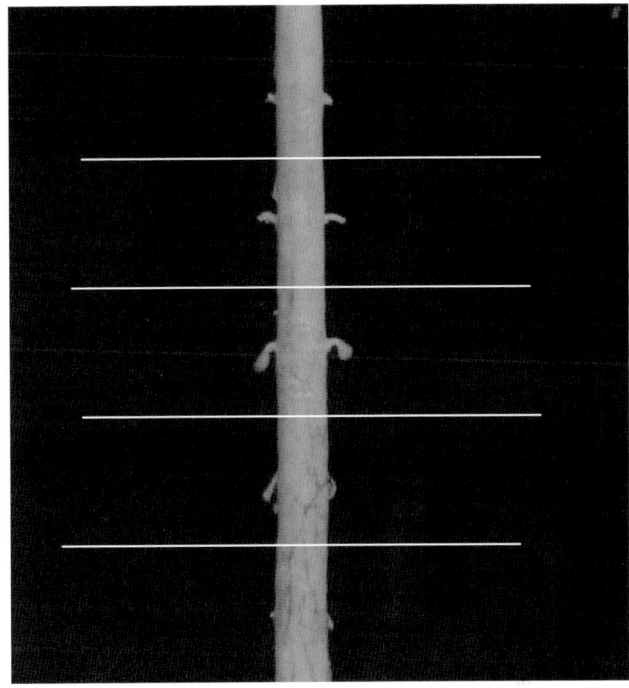

B

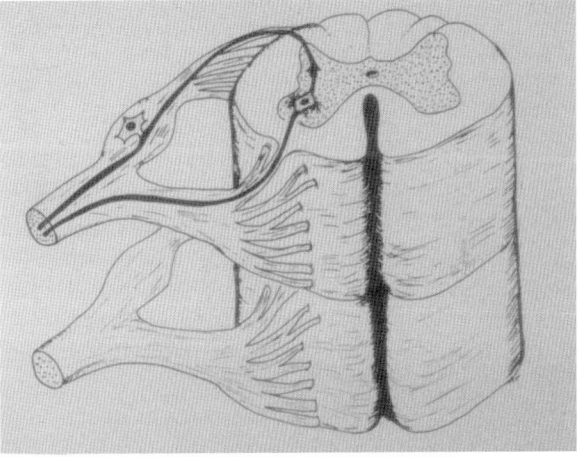

C   D

Figure 2.107.   Gross section of the spinal cord (A) showing the associated dorsal nerve roots (arrows). The spinal cord (B) is anatomically divided into adjacent spinal segments (lines). Schematic drawing of an individual spinal cord segment with associated peripheral connections to a muscle (C). Schematic drawing of adjacent spinal cord segments (D).

vertebrae. In the cervical area, the first cervical nerve will traverse from the vertebral canal peripherally through the lateral vertebral foramen located within the dorsal arch of C1 vertebrae. The C2 spinal nerve will traverse between C1 and C2 vertebrae. The additional cervical spinal nerves will traverse the vertebral foramen cranial to the vertebrae of the same number. For example, the C7 spinal nerve will traverse the foramen between the C6 and C7 vertebrae and the C8 spinal nerve will traverse the foramen between the C8 and T1 vertebrae. The T1 spinal nerve will exit the spinal canal through the foramen between T1 and T2.

The thoracic spinal cord contains 13 thoracic spinal cord segments and 13 associated pairs of spinal nerves. Generally, the spinal segments overlie the vertebrae of the same number. The spinal nerves traverse the foramen caudal to the vertebrae of the same spinal cord segment. For example, the T6 spinal nerve will traverse the foramen between the T6 and T7 vertebrae.

The discontinuity between spinal segment location and associated vertebral segment is more pronounced in the lumbar and sacral areas of the spine. In the mid to caudal lumbar area, the spinal cord segments lie cranial to the corresponding vertebral segments, even though there are the same number of vertebral segments and spinal segments (i.e., 7). In dogs, the sacral segments generally are found within the lumbar (L) 5 vertebrae. Remembering that an S for sacral segments looks like a 5 for lumbar vertebra 5 may help in remembering the relationship between these segments and the lumbar vertebrae. Generally, the L1 and L2 spinal segments lie approximately over the L1 and L2 vertebrae, respectively. Spinal segments L3 to L7 lie between L3 and L5 vertebrae.

The spinal cord terminates in the caudal half of the L6 vertebrae to the cranial half of L7 in dog structures (Figure 2.106D). In larger breeds, the spinal cord may terminate more cranially. In smaller breeds, the spinal cord may terminate more caudally. In cats, the spinal cord ends at the L7 vertebrae or the sacrum.

Spinal nerves that arise from a spinal segment must traverse the vertebral canal to terminate peripherally on a muscle or organ or to provide afferent information from the periphery into the spinal cord structures. Spinal nerves traverse between vertebrae in the intervertebral foramen just ventral to the articular facets of the adjacent vertebrae. In the lumbar area, as in the thoracic area, the first lumbar nerve will traverse from the vertebral canal peripherally through the foramen between L1 and L2 vertebrae or caudal to the vertebrae of the same number. The additional lumbar spinal nerves will traverse the vertebral foramen caudal to the vertebrae of the same number. The L7 spinal nerve will traverse between L7 and the cranial aspect of the sacrum. The sacral spinal nerves will traverse through foramen within the sacrum.

As the spinal cord proper terminates at approximately the L6 vertebrae and the spinal nerves traverse foramen progressively farther away from their spinal segment origin, the nervous system overlying the L6, L7, and sacral vertebrae is more a collection of spinal nerves than spinal cord proper. This collection of nerves viewed grossly gives off the appearance of hairs within a horse's tail, and thus is often referred to as the cauda equina.

Peripheral nerves are formed usually by the combination of extensions of axonal processes from nerve cell bodies (ventral nerve) and the entering afferent fibers from sensory fibers (dorsal nerve) (Figures 2.107A, B). These fibers form the paired dorsal and ventral nerves or roots associated with each spinal cord segment. The dorsal root consists primarily of axons projecting into the spinal cord from the periphery. The cell bodies of these axons primarily reside with an enlargement of the dorsal root referred to as the dorsal root ganglion. Prior to their entrance into the spinal cord proper, the nerve roots form multiple rootlets. The ventral root is formed primarily from axons of efferent or exiting nerves to the periphery. At the origin of these nerve roots are nerve rootlets, which coalesce to form the nerve root and, ultimately, the peripheral nerve. While the dorsal root usually contains sensory axons and the ventral root contains motor axons, these are not exclusive relationships.

A cross-section of a spinal segment reveals the relationship between the central gray matter and the more peripheral white matter structures (Figures 2.107C, D). Spinal cord white matter contains groups of axons or tracts traversing through the spinal cord from peripheral sensory receptors and their projections to the intracranial structures. In addition, within the white matter, there are tracts descending from the intracranial structures that traverse through the spinal cord to synapse on the neuronal cells that form nerves that exit the spinal cord and project to the peripheral axial or appendicular structures.

The central gray matter of the spinal cord tends to have the appearance of an H, but has also been described as a butterfly or animal horns. The dorsal and ventral arms of the H are contiguous with the nerve rootlets either entering (dorsal) or exiting (ventral). The white matter is isolated more peripherally by the H-shaped gray matter and associated nerve rootlets into discrete regions. These regions of white matter are referred to as funiculi. Between the parallel sides of the H and the cross bar dorsally is the dorsal funiculus (or bilateral funiculi). Lateral to the parallel sides of the H is the lateral funiculus (funiculi). Ventral to the parallel sides of the H and the cross bar is the ventral funiculus (funiculi).

The peripheral nerves often coalesce distal to their traversing the intervertebral foramen. This coalescence of nerves is commonly referred to as a plexus. In the thoracic limb axillary area, these nerves are referred to as the brachial plexus. In the medial pelvic limb area, these peripheral nerves form the pelvic plexus.

The innervation of regional nerves, as well as the corresponding origin of these nerves from spinal segments forming the plexus, may vary between animals.

When regional nerves are formed by more cranial spinal rootlets than is usually seen, the plexus is said to be prefixed. When the nerves originate from more caudal spinal cord segments than normal, the plexus is said to be post-fixed. Allam studied the nerves that form the brachial plexus in dogs and found the following percentages of dogs had the brachial plexus derived from the associated spinal segments: 58.6% were formed by C6, C7, C8, and T1; 20.7% were formed by C5, C6, C7, C8, and T1; 17.24% were formed by C6, C7, C8, T1, and T2; and 3.4% were formed by C5, C6, C7, C8, T1, and T2 (Allam et al. 1952). The ratio of dogs with prefixed, median, and post-fixed plexus types is approximately 1:3:1.

The Vertebral Structures

The spinal cord is contained within the vertebral canal formed by adjacent vertebral structures (Figure 2.108). The vertebrae are relatively complex bony structures, which vary in configuration and size throughout the spinal column. In the cervical region, essentially all of the vertebral structures have a unique shape; however, C3 through C5 are more similarly shaped (Figure 2.109). The first (C1) and second (C2) vertebrae have distinct appearances (Figure 2.109). The prominent dorsal spinous process of C2 affords a commonly used landmark for establishing this vertebral segment in the sagittal MR image of this area (Figure 2.110). The more prominent transverse processes of C6 often serve as an anatomical landmark and are more obvious in the transverse image (Figure 2.111).

The thoracic vertebrae also have relatively unique shapes. The cranial most vertebrae have prominent dorsal spinous processes. The dorsal spinous process of T1 being comparatively larger and directly more upright compared to the relatively smaller and directed more cranial dorsal spinous process of C7 can be used as an anatomical landmark to distinguish this vertebral level. In general, the cranial thoracic vertebrae have "heart or V-shaped" vertebral bodies, prominent dorsal spinouses, and articulations with the associated ribs. At the anticlinal region, the cranial/caudal direction of the dorsal spinous processes changes from being relatively more caudally directed to a more cranially directed process. From this point to the last thoracic vertebrae, the articular facets become independent structures compared to the ribs. At the first lumbar vertebrae, the transverse process becomes apparent, and the vertebral shape becomes more similar to the level of the last lumbar vertebrae. The unique shape of the sacrum is another useful anatomical landmark for determining the location of the associated vertebral segments.

While many animals have these more standard vertebral features, not all individual animals will have this "normal" vertebral column components. Abnormalities of formation of vertebral structures are important to identify to avoid misinterpretation of spinal segment location. For example, some animals will have one less lumbar vertebrae structures. The interpreter of any MR image should be aware of these types of anatomical diversity to avoid mislabeling of a vertebral level. Other vertebral defects such as block vertebrae or hemivertebrae may result in abnormal anatomical orientation of the spinal column (see congenital spinal cord defects within this chapter).

The Meninges

As within the intracranial region, the neural tissue of the spinal cord and proximal nerve roots are covered by the meninges (Figure 2.112). The normal meninges, however, are usually not apparent on standard T1- and T2 sequences. Normal meningeal tissue does not enhance following contrast administration as a general rule.

Spinal Cord Blood Flow

The spinal cord receives blood flow segmentally at multiple levels along the vertebral axis. In the cervical area, blood flows to the spinal cord from the heart, brachiocephalic trunk, and left subclavian arteries. From these arteries, blood flows into the vertebral arteries, as well as the dorsal scapular artery, deep cervical artery, and thoracic vertebral artery. The vertebral arteries will primarily supply the C1 to C7 spinal segments. The dorsal scapular artery gives rise to the C8 cervical spinal branch. The deep cervical artery gives rise to the first thoracic spinal branch. The thoracic vertebral artery gives rise to the spinal branches between T2 and T4. Primarily in the lumbar vertebrae, the arterial vascular canals that enter the center of the vertebral body are often apparent on MR sequences (Figure 2.113).

Within the spinal canal, the spinal branch arteries divide into a dorsal and ventral branch. The dorsal branch is smaller than the ventral branch. The ventral branches become contiguous and form the ventral spinal artery. This artery is unpaired and is present in the ventral median fissure. The ventral spinal artery extends longitudinally along the ventral aspect of the spinal cord. This artery is usually not apparent on standard MR sequences unless it is enlarged. The ventral spinal artery will give rise to numerous dorsally directed branches

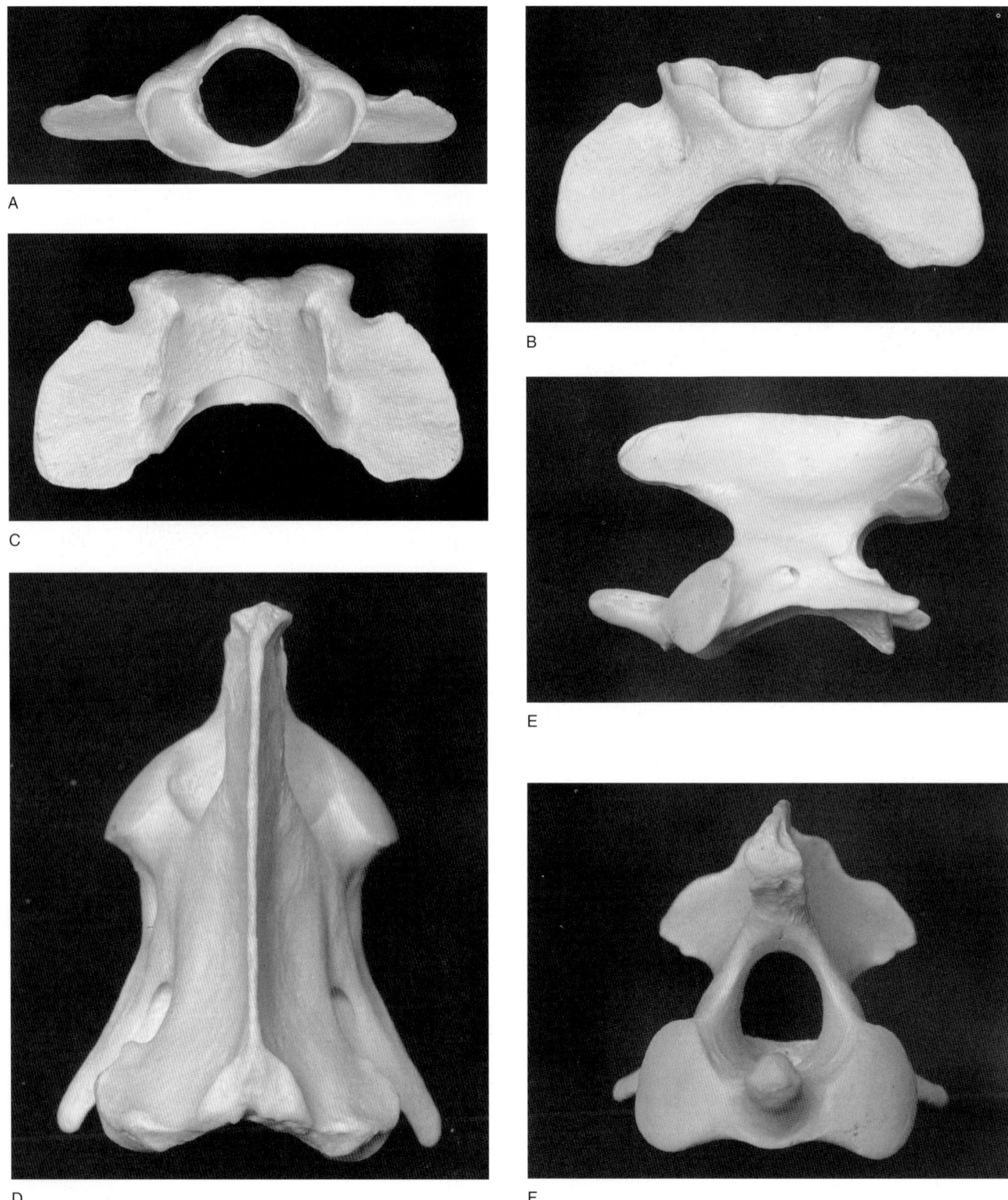

Figure 2.108. Transverse gross appearance of the cranial (A), ventral (B), and dorsal (C) aspect of the C1 vertebrae. Dorsal (D), lateral (E), and transverse (cranial aspect) (F) of the C2 vertebrae.

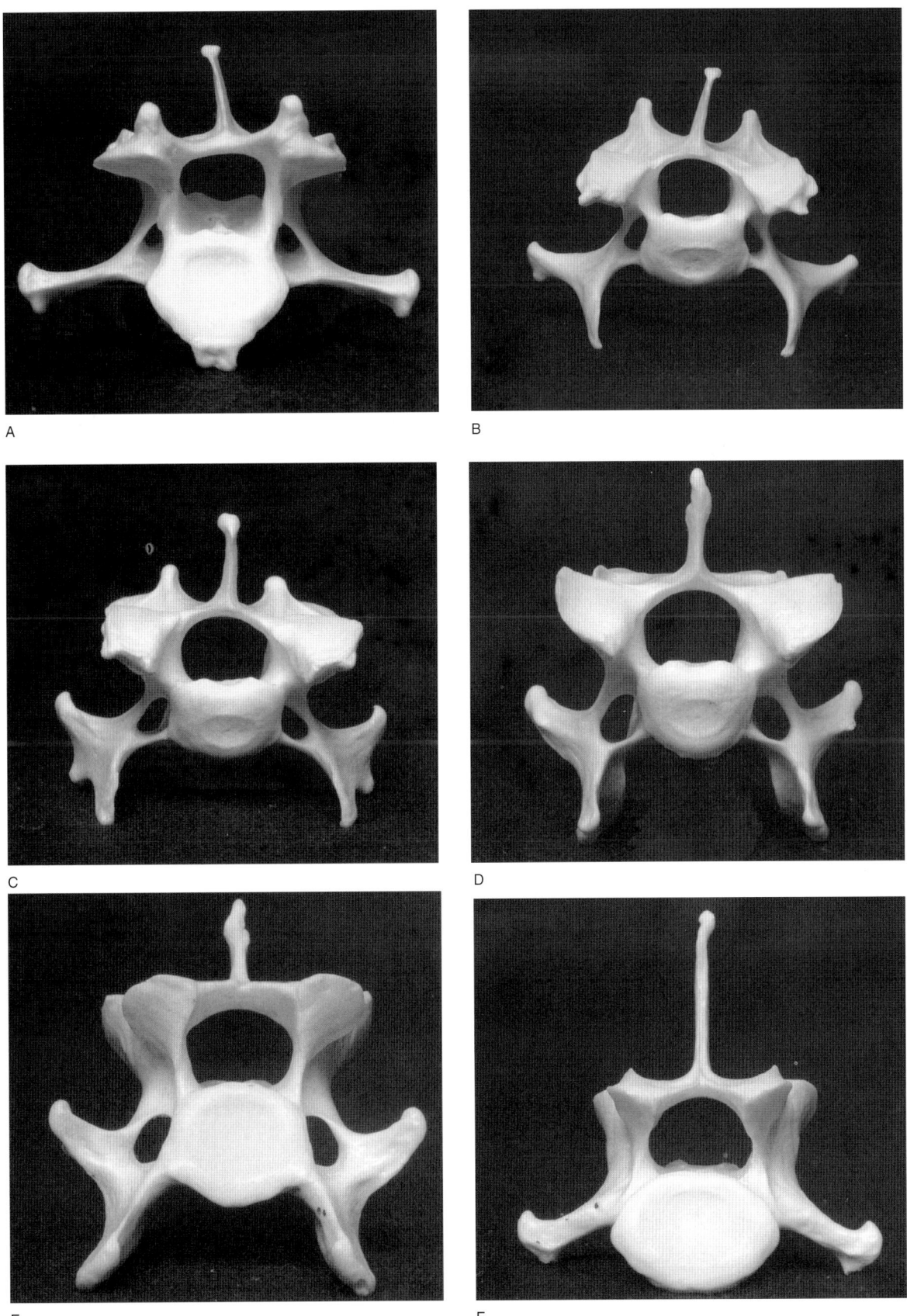

Figure 2.109. Transverse gross appearance of the vertebrae of C3 (A), C 4 (B), C5 (C), C6 (cranial aspect) (D), C6 (caudal aspect) (E), and C7 (F).

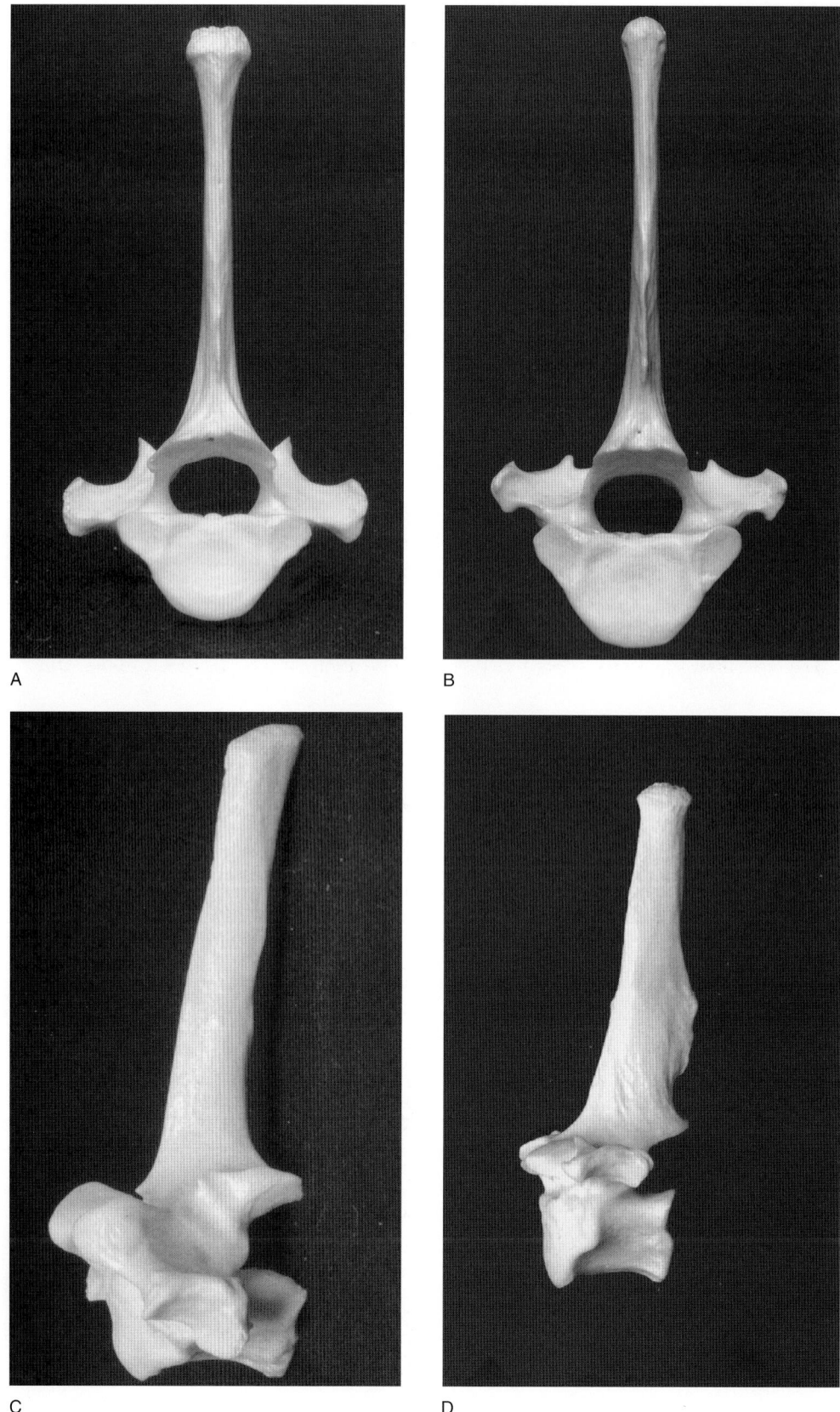

A

B

C

D

Figure 2.110.   Transverse gross appearance of two thoracic vertebrae ((A)—T2; (B)—T3). Lateral gross appearance of the thoracic vertebrae ((C)—T1; (D)—T3;

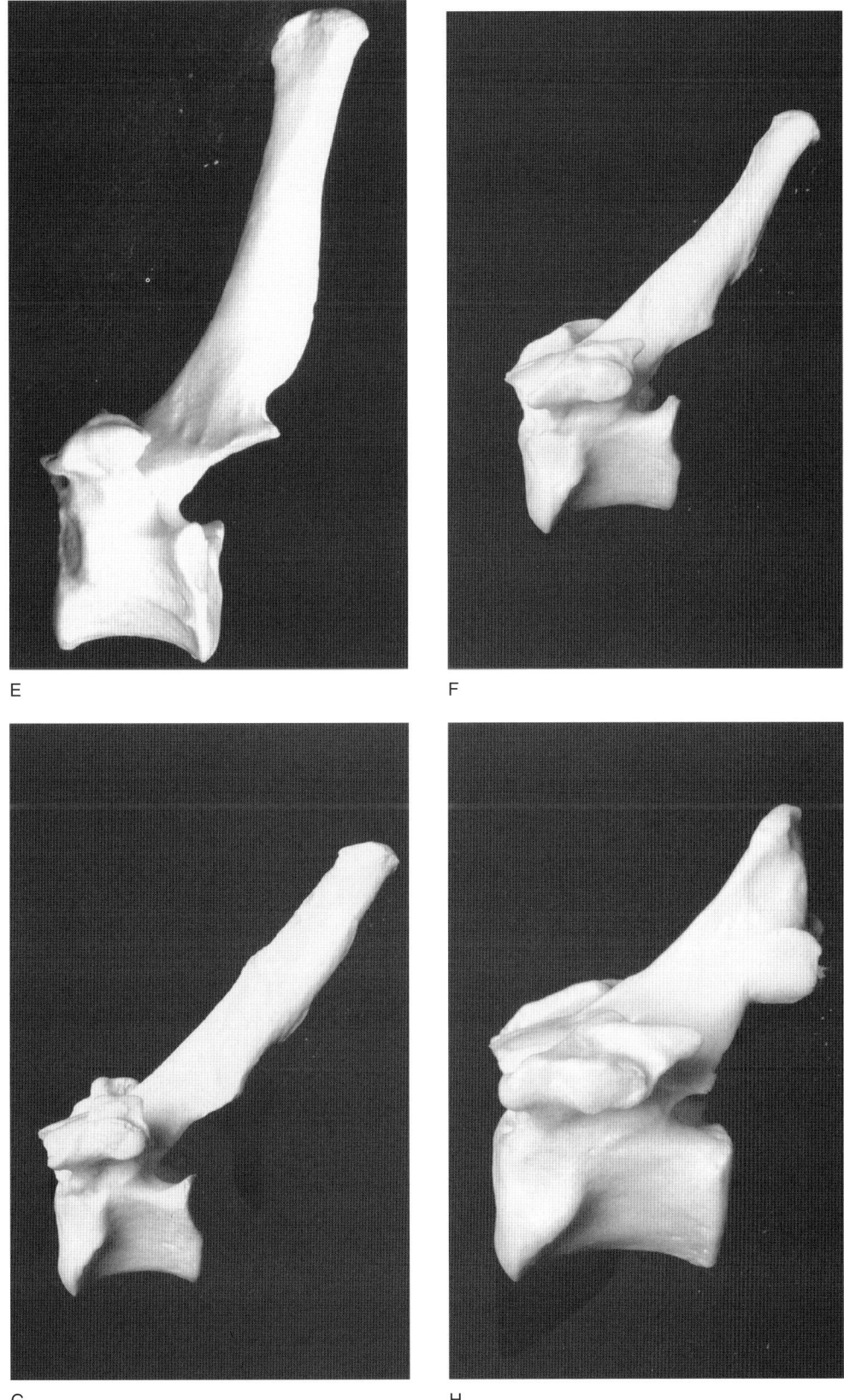

Figure 2.110. (*Continued*) (E)—T5; (F)—T7; (G)—T8; (H)—T10;

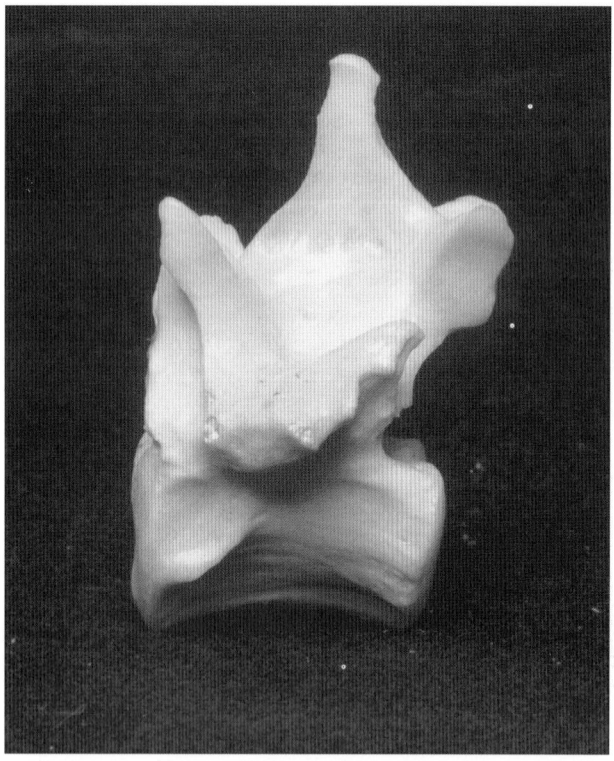

that enter the spinal cord ventrally to supply the ventral gray matter and ventral funiculi.

The dorsal branches enter the spinal cord around the dorsal nerve roots to primarily supply the dorsal lateral gray and white matter. On the surface of the cord in the pia there are incomplete anastomotic connects which may encircle the spinal cord. In some instances, the dorsal lateral arteries can also travel longitudinally along the length of the spinal cord in a dorsal lateral direction. While this basic pattern occurs in the arterial blood supply to the spinal cord, there is often significant individual variation among these arterial channels. The ventral spinal artery system is more consistent in location and anatomy.

Within a spinal cord segment, the arteries that penetrate into the parenchyma tend to be relatively small and thin-walled. While some region of a spinal segment is supplied by one primary arterial system (ventral or dorsal), some regions of the spinal cord are in an overlapping zone, being supplied partially by both arterial systems. These areas of arterial overlap may be more susceptible to ischemic changes and subsequent spinal damage.

The venous drainage from within and around the spinal cord occurs through the associated vertebral venous plexus (venous sinuses) and associated branches. The venous vascular system exits the intervertebral

Figure 2.110. *(Continued)* (I)—T11).

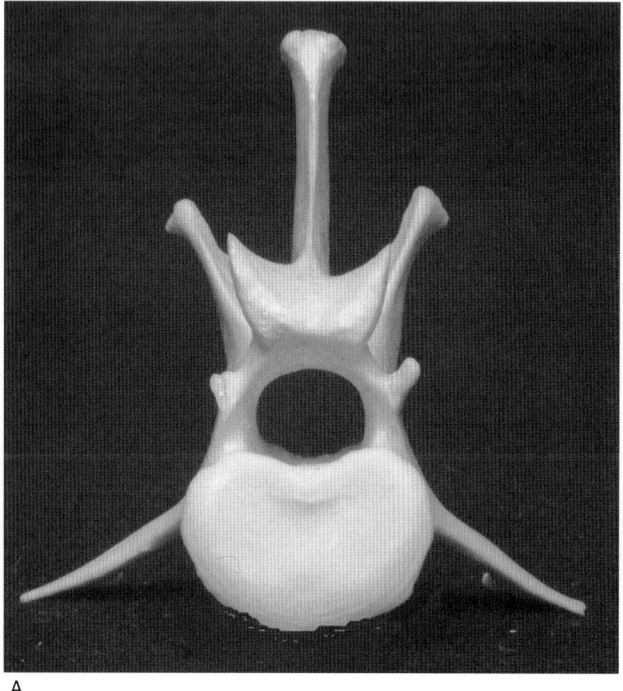

A

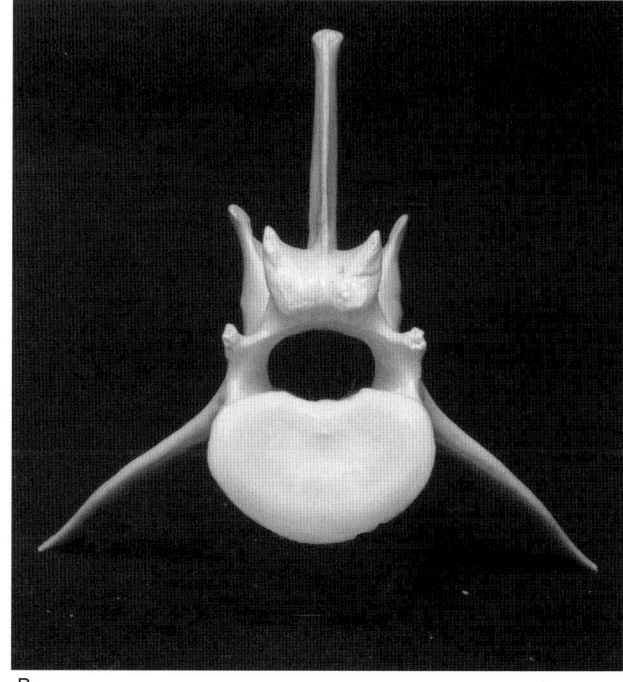

B

Figure 2.111. Transverse gross appearance of three lumbar vertebrae ((A)—L4 (caudal aspect); (B)—L5 caudal aspect;

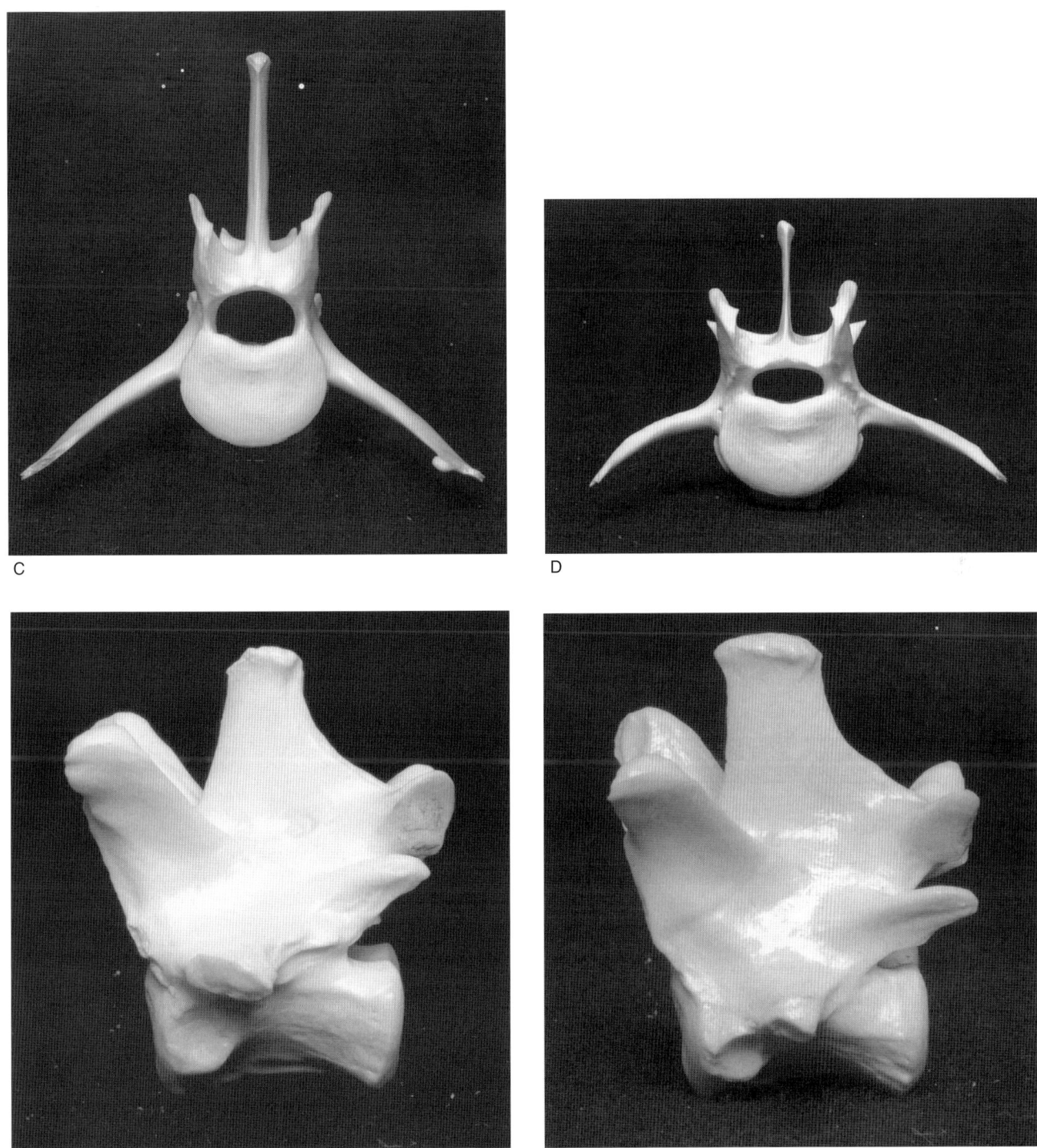

Figure 2.111. (*Continued*) (C)—L5 cranial aspect; (D)—L7). Lateral gross appearance of the thoracic ((E)—T12; (F)—T13) and lumbar vertebrae

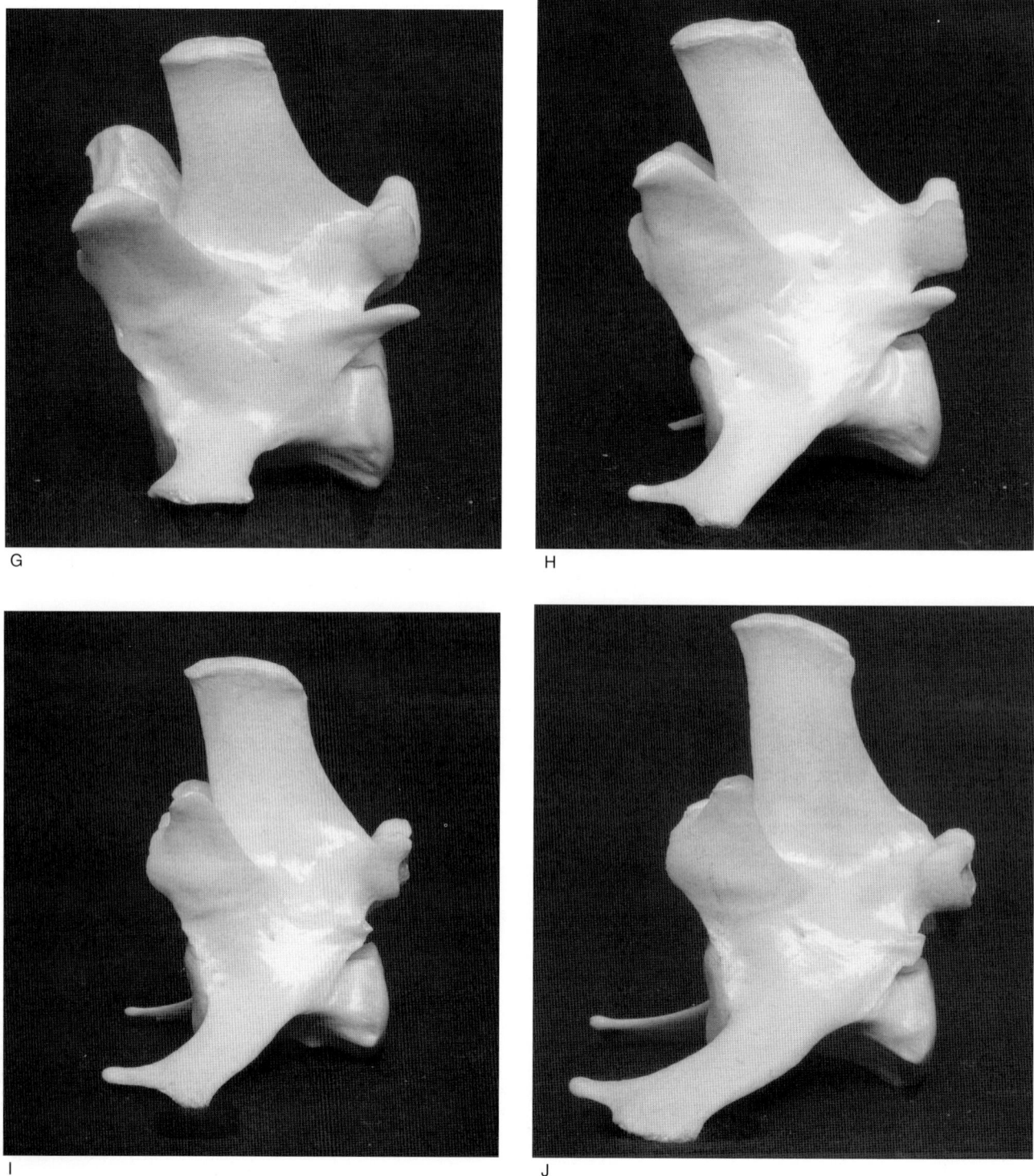

Figure 2.111.   (*Continued*) ((G)—L1; (H)—L2; (I)—L3; (J)—L5;

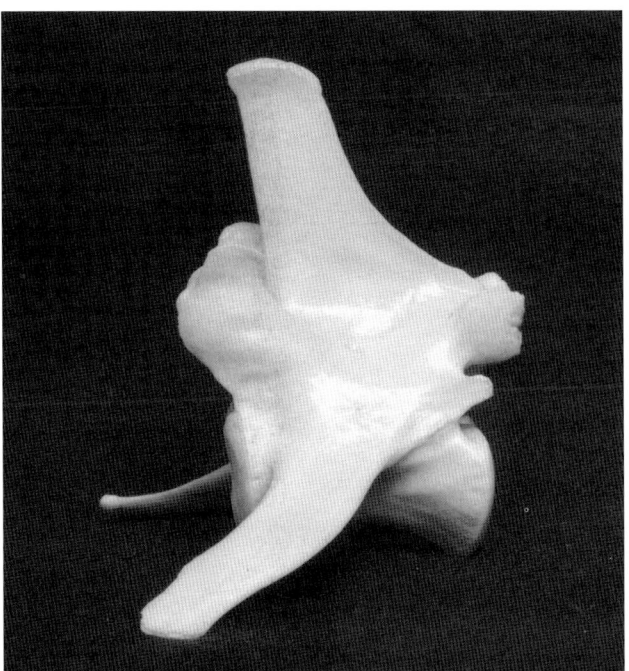

K

Figure 2.111. (*Continued*) (K)—L6). (See Color Plate 2.111H.)

foramen ventral to exiting nerves, and is contiguous with the venous sinus. These vascular structures may be apparent primarily in MR images of the spinal canal and vertebral column (Figures 2.114–2.116).

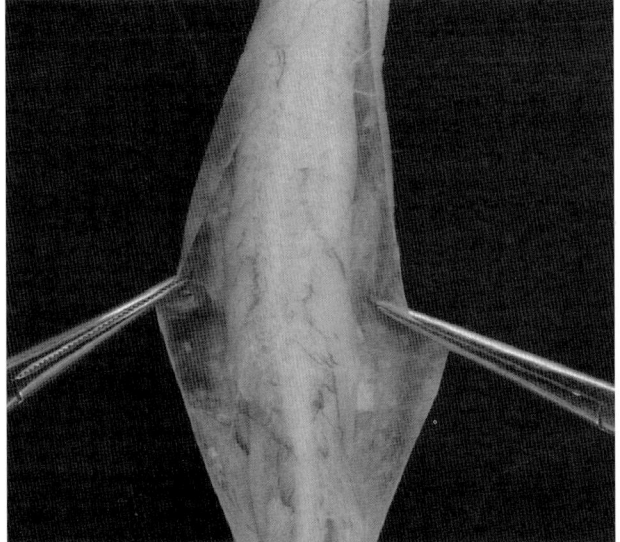

Figure 2.112. Dorsal view of the formaldehyde-fixed meninges and spinal cord from a normal dog. The outer meninges have been incised to reveal the underlying spinal cord.

GENERAL TYPES OF SPINAL CORD PATHOPHYSIOLOGY

There are a number of pathophysiologic changes that occur in association with spinal cord diseases. These include, but are not limited to, ischemia, edema, demyelination, obstruction to cerebrospinal fluid (CSF) flow, hemorrhage, syringo- and hydromyelia, and malacia. These nonspecific pathophysiologic events often occur in the presence of a specific disease entity. The MR signal changes associated with the various spinal cord diseases reflect the combination of these primary disease entities and associated secondary pathophysiologic events.

DIAGNOSIS OF SPINAL CORD DISEASE PROCESSES

In the following section, MR features of differing spinal cord diseases are discussed. Diseases are presented following major categories of disease using a DAMNNIITTV scheme (Degenerative, Anomalous, Metabolic, Neoplastic, Nutritional, Inflammatory, Idiopathic, Traumatic, Toxic, Vascular).

Degenerative Disease

Early-onset degenerative spinal cord disease usually occurs in specific breeds of animals and younger animals are more often affected. Examples of primary degenerative spinal cord diseases of younger animals include Afghan myelomalacia, hereditary ataxia of smooth-haired fox terriers and Jack Russell terriers, Labrador retriever axonopathy, encephalomyelopathy of young cats, leukoencephalomyelopathy of Rottweilers, and miniature poodle demyelination. An etiology for the neural element degeneration in many of these diseases has not been established.

Antemortem diagnostics either have not been consistently performed or are invariably normal in animals with primary degenerative spinal cord disease. MR imaging features of many of these primary degenerative diseases either have not been identified or have not been evaluated for. In many of the degenerative

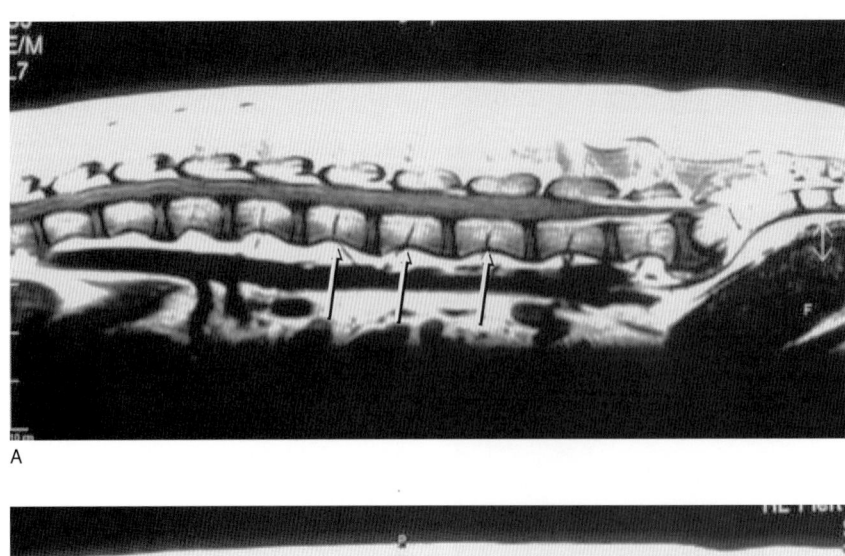

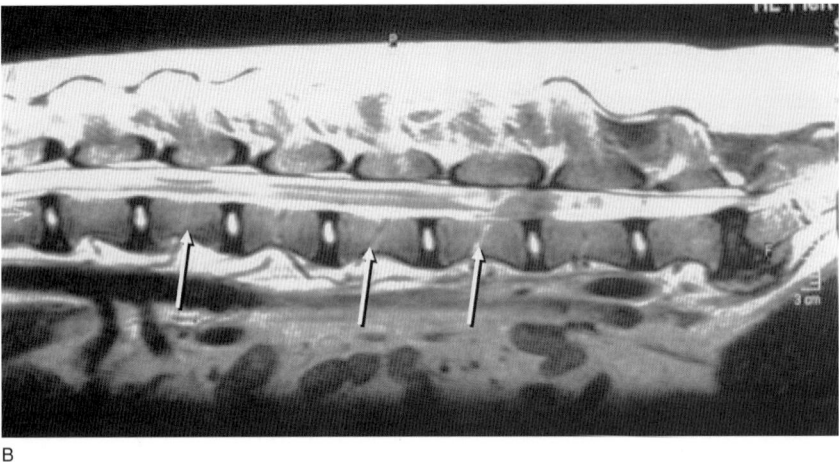

Figure 2.113. Sagittal T1-weighted (A) and T2-weighted (B) MR images of the lumbar spinal cord. The arterial vascular channels are apparent at approximately the middle of the vertebral body (arrows).

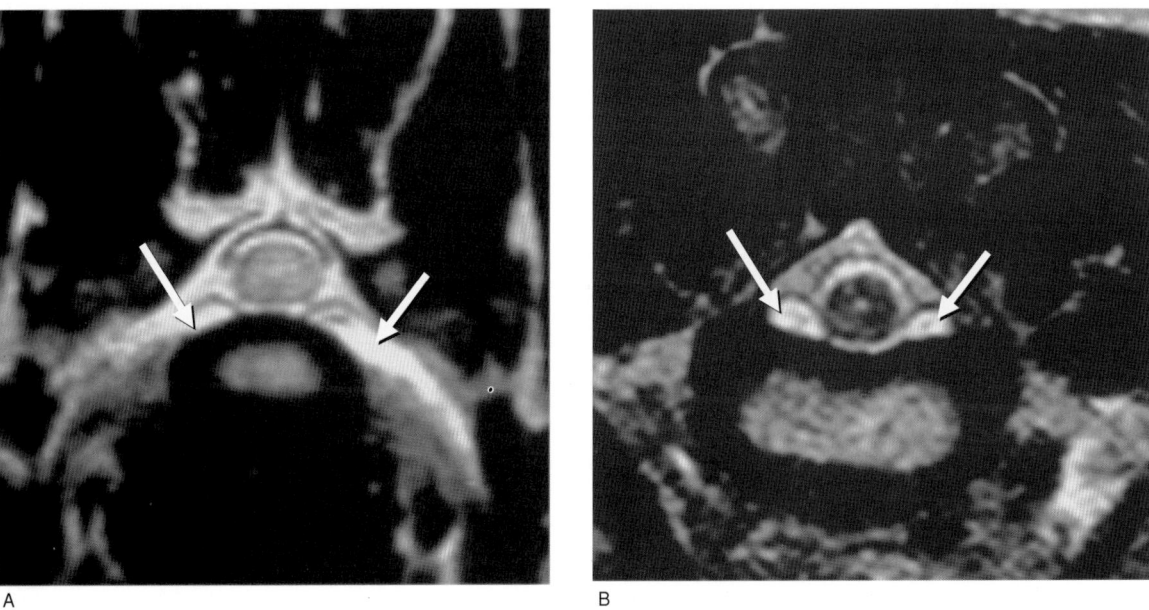

Figure 2.114. Transverse T2-weighted MR images from two separate dogs ((A) and (B)) showing the appearance and location of the vertebral venous sinuses and veins (arrows).

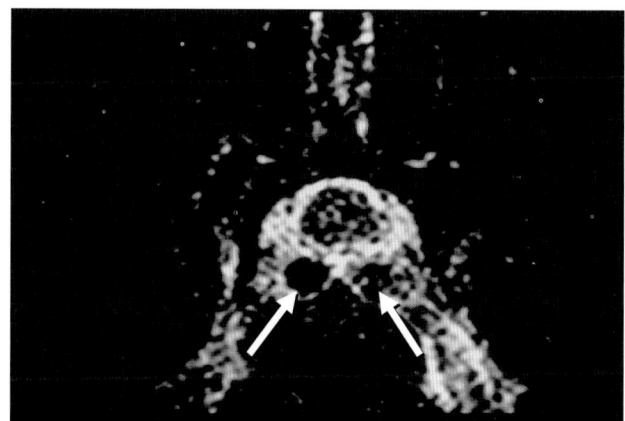

Figure 2.115. Transverse T2-weighted MR image from a dog showing different signal characteristics due to differing flow characteristics in the venous sinuses (arrows).

spinal cord diseases where MR evaluations have been performed, no definitive changes have been identified.

Degenerative Myelopathy

Degenerative myelopathy is the name commonly used to describe a specific degenerative spinal cord disease of mature dogs and cats that results in paraparesis, eventually evolving to tetraparesis and possibly, CN signs. Dogs most often become paralyzed in the pelvic limbs prior to clinically detectable thoracic limbs abnormalities. This disease most commonly is reported in middle-aged to older German shepherds, but also affects other breeds of dogs and has been occasionally reported in cats. Similar disease processes have been described in young (<2 years of age) dogs including German shepherds and Siberian huskies. Clinical signs are usually more gradual in onset, chronic in duration, and progressively worsen. Clinical features most notably reflect an abnormality of the T3-L3 spinal cord segments; however, the actual histopathological lesions may be more severe in the caudal cervical area.

Conventional MR images from affected dogs are also normal. In many dogs with clinical features suggestive of "degenerative myelopathy" evaluated in the modern era with MR spinal imaging there is evidence of disk protrusion affecting various regions of the spinal cord. In some instances this disk protrusion occurs at a single site. In other instances compression is present at multiple intervertebral disk spaces (Figure 2.117). The relationship between the presence of intervertebral disk

protrusion and degenerative myelopathy is currently unknown. Most likely, these are separate disease entities with, unfortunately, similar clinical features. Concurrent disease processes such as spinal cord compression (i.e., with intervertebral disk disease (IVDD)) may occur in association with degenerative myelopathy in the same animal. This creates a diagnostic dilemma as there are no currently established pathognomonic MR imaging features that will indicate the presence of degenerative disease. Definitive diagnosis of a true degenerative myelopathic condition is made only at necropsy.

Intervertebral Disk Disease

IVDD is one of the most common abnormalities seen in clinical practice in animals with spinal disease. Selected breeds of dogs such as dachshunds have a greater incidence of IVDD, however, this problem can be found in almost all breeds. Clinical features such as spinal pain, paresis, or paralysis are suggestive of IVDD but are also associated with other spinal cord conditions. Importantly, there is no pathognomonic clinical feature of IVDD.

MR images can be collected in multiple planes to allow for viewing of IVDD in various dimensions (Figures 2.118–2.135). Degeneration of the nucleus pulposus and the anatomical structure of the disk itself is readily seen in the T2-weighted sagittal and transverse (axial) images of the spinal column (Figures 2.122–2.124). Normal hydrated nucleus pulposus has a hyperintense signal compared to the annulus fibrosis (Figure 2.118). As the nucleus pulposus loses hydration (seen in chondroid metaplasia or Hansen's type I disk disease), the signal becomes less intense and may appear iso- or hypointense relative to the annulus fibrosis. Most acute disk extrusions of this type of degenerated disk material appear primarily as a hypointense lesion surrounding the spinal cord in the T2-weighted sagittal image (Figures 2.118–2.132). Traumatic rupture of previously healthy nucleus pulposus results in a high signal intensity (hyperintense) material in or around the spinal cord as this material is usually (at least initially) normally hydrated (Figures 2.128C, D). The axial MR view provides important information regarding the location of any compressive material surrounding the spinal cord in a cross-sectional dimension (Figures 2.120, 2.121, 2.126, 2.127, 2.130–2.132). If one area (side) of the spinal cord is exclusively or more compressed than others, this can readily be determined with spinal MR imaging.

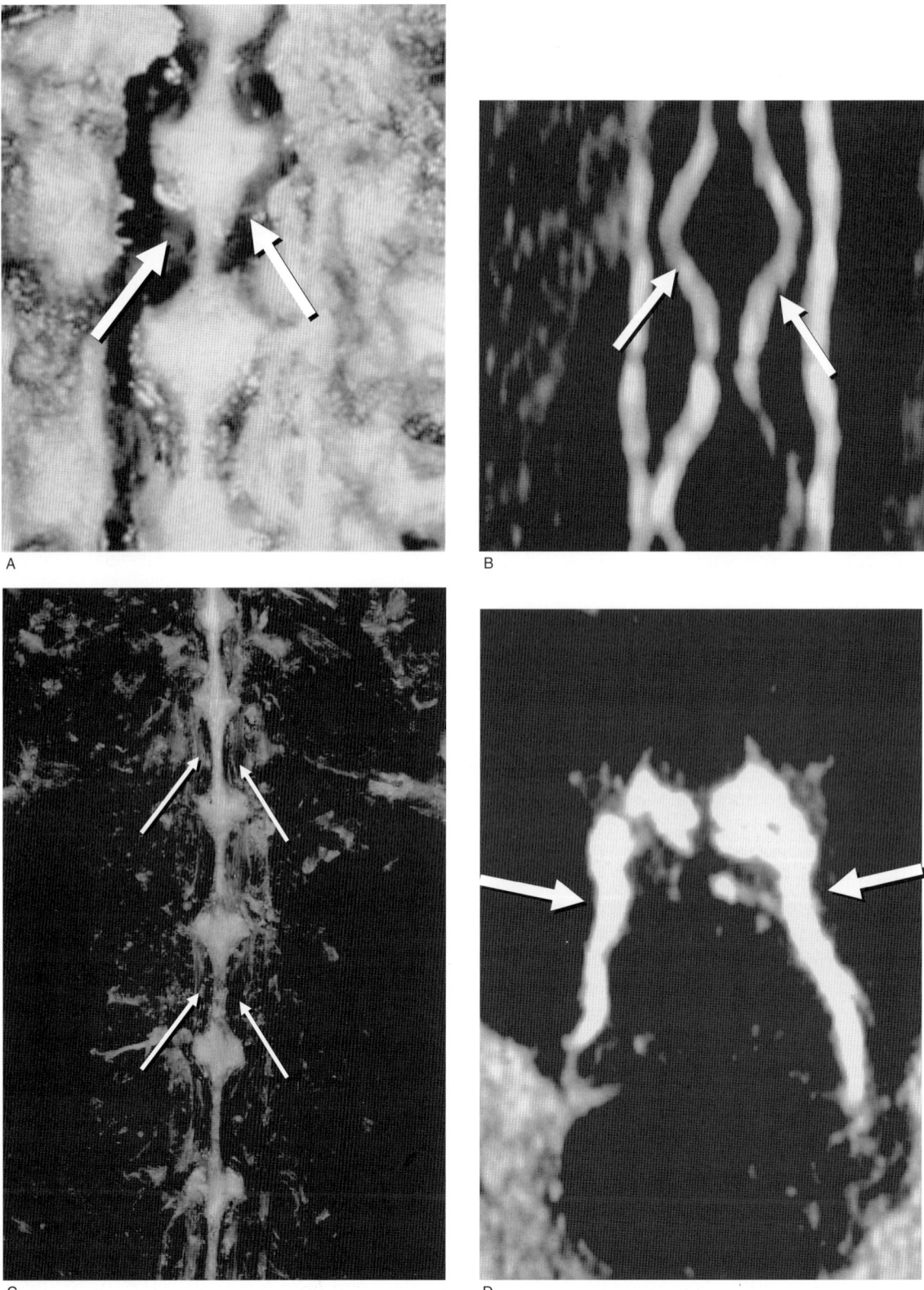

Figure 2.116.   Gross anatomical view (A) following removal of the dorsal vertebral elements showing the location and course of the vertebral sinuses in the cervical region (arrows). MR angiographic appearance (dorsal plane reconstruction) (B) of the venous structures of the cervical region (arrows). Gross anatomical view (C) following removal of the dorsal vertebral elements showing the location and course of the vertebral sinuses in the lumbar region (arrows). Transverse MR angiographic appearance (D) of the vertebral veins (arrows) exiting through the intervertebral foramen ventral to the associated exiting peripheral nerve.

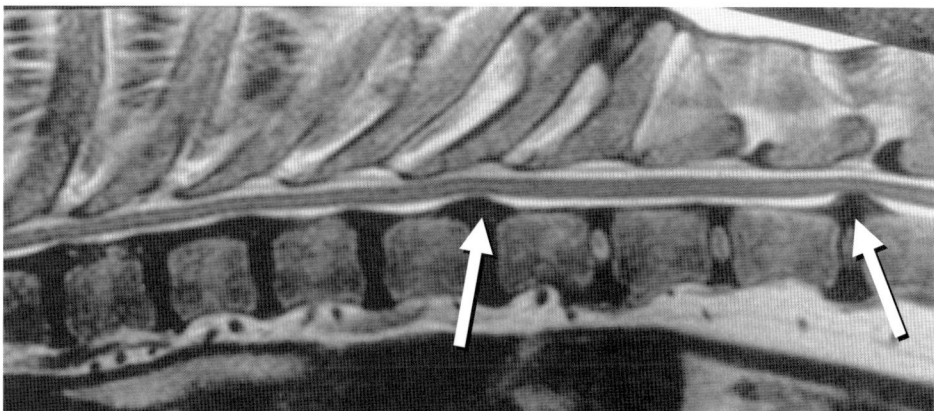

Figure 2.117. Sagittal T2-weighted MR image from a dog presumptively diagnosed with degenerative myelopathy which had multiple chronic protrusions of the intervertebral disk components (arrows).

Oftentimes and especially with acute IVD extrusions, there is associated hemorrhage and inflammation in the region of the IVD rupture. Hemorrhage usually is the result of damage or rupture of the ventral vertebral venous sinus (venous blood). In some instances, epidural hematomas may form as a result of this hemorrhage. This hemorrhage or hematoma formation can extend for multiple disk space levels in or around the regions of the acute disk rupture. Hemorrhage associated with IVD extrusion may be present in the ventral, lateral, or even dorsal aspects of the spinal canal. Also commonly, the acutely extruded IVD material will become admixed with hemorrhage to result in spinal cord compression. The combination of varying consistencies of extruded intervertebral disk material and/or stages of hemorrhage mixed with disk material may create a spectrum of MR imaging characteristics of disk material herniation. Most often, the combination of herniated intervertebral disk material and hemorrhage often results in a heterogeneous signal intensity in T2-weighted MR images.

Intervertebral disk extrusion or protrusion can occur at multiple levels of the spinal column. Historically, thoracolumbar and cervical IVDD has been recognized commonly. In some dogs, however, cranial to mid thoracic verterbral level IVDD have been found with MR imaging (Figure 2.133). These types of IVDD are more often protrusions with hypertrophy of the dorsal longitudinal ligament. In rarer instances, acute extrusions may occur.

In addition to the variety of levels of spinal column that may be affected with IVDD, IVD elements may extrude or protrude dorsally, laterally, ventrally, or some combination of these directions at the affected IVD space. Dorsally extruded or protruded disk elements enter the spinal canal as described previously within this section. Ventrally extruded or protruded IVD elements have been suggested to contribute or result in spondylosis deformans.

Laterally extruded or protruded elements may not affect the spinal cord, but can result in compression and impingement of the peripheral nerves as these nerves

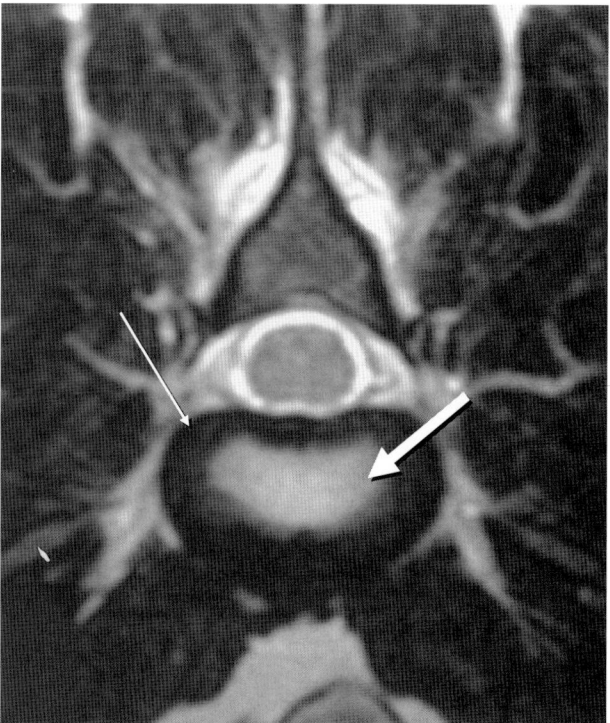

Figure 2.118. Transverse T2-weighted MR image at the level a lumbar IVD from a healthy dog. Note the hyperintense signal from the healthy nucleus pulposus (larger arrow) compared to the hypointense signal from the annulus fibrosis (smaller arrow).

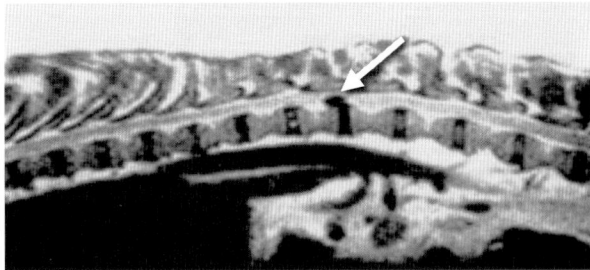

A

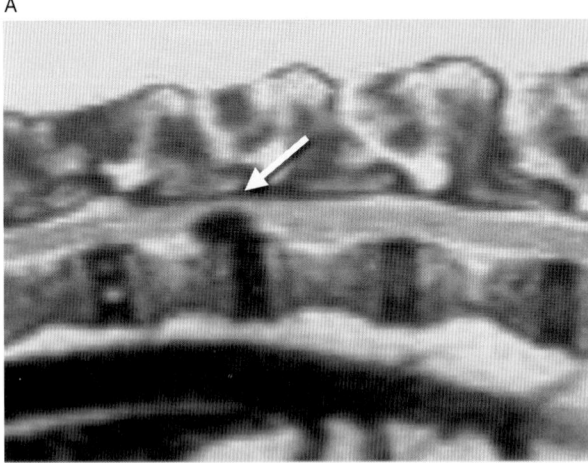

B

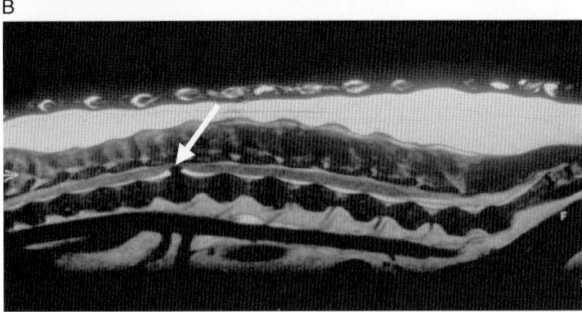

C

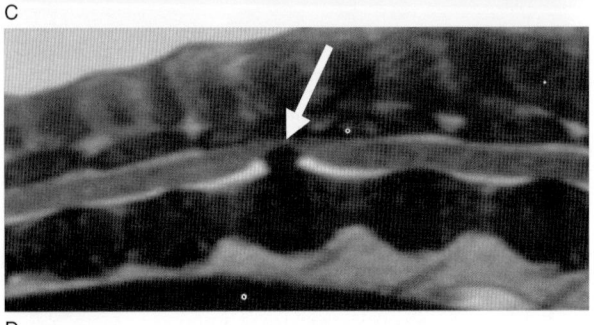

D

Figure 2.119. Sagittal T2-weighted MR images from two dogs ((A) and (C)) with intervertebral disk extrusions (arrows). Parts (B) and (D) show enlarged views of (A) and (C), respectively.

exit the spinal column through the intervertebral foramen (Figure 2.134). In instances of lateral disk extrusion, the location of the lesion may not be identified with myelography, especially if the extruded disk material is either within or lateral to the intervertebral

foramen. In these situations, however, the degenerative disk is generally identifiable in the T2-sagittal MR image as decreased signal intensity and an abnormally shaped (smaller) nucleus pulposus. The transverse (axial) image often confirms the laterally extruded disk impinging on a nerve root.

Occasionally, and especially with more chronic IVD extrusion or protrusion, IVD material within or around the spinal canal may show contrast enhancement following intravenous administration of contrast media (Figure 2.135). Contrast enhancement is most likely due to increased vascularization within the extruded or protruded disk material and/or associated inflammation. In some instances, the contrast enhancement will occur at the peripheral edges of the IVD material ("ring enhancement"). It is important to recognize this feature of IVDD to avoid misdiagnosis of other disease processes showing contrast enhancement such as spinal tumors.

As with all imaging studies, knowledge of the location of the lesion in a sagittal as well as axial plane is imperative, especially if surgical correction is to occur. Localization can be slightly more difficult using MR imaging as body landmarks such as ribs are not always present within the plane of section. Additional views, such as a dorsal plane image, may be helpful in establishing lesion location and normal anatomical variations (Figure 2.136).

Imaging Following Spinal Surgery

While currently used as a pre-surgical diagnostic tool, MR imaging may also provide information regarding the status of the spinal cord following spinal surgical decompressive surgeries such as laminectomies and ventral slots (Figures 2.137–2.141). MR imaging in the immediate time (within hours) following spinal surgery may show the degree of decompression, ongoing hemorrhage, and other information that may help in assessing potential complications following surgery. In some instances, MR imaging is performed days, weeks, or months following spinal surgery because of persistence or recurrence of clinical signs. In some instances where animals have recovered poorly or even worsened following surgery, persistent spinal cord compression can be identified. In most instances of IVD, this persistent compression from IVD elements is not the result of "new" extrusion or protrusion of IVD material, but rather the result of unsuccessful IVD element removal at the time of surgery. In other instances, even animals that have recovered well following surgery may have persistent compression at the surgery site. Therefore, it may be difficult, based on evaluation of MR

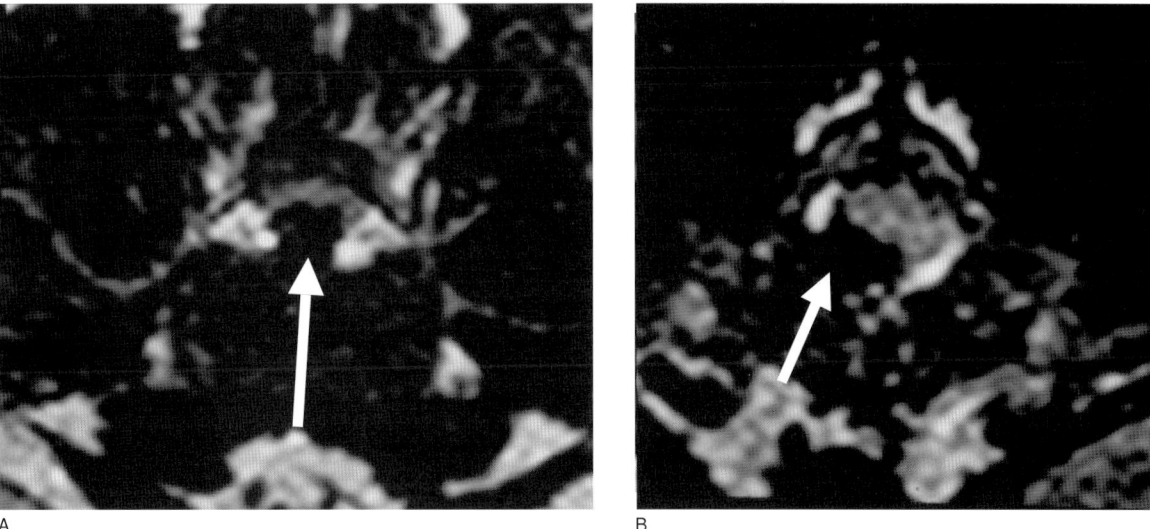

A

B

Figure 2.120. Transverse T2-weighted MR images from two dogs ((A) and (B)) with intervertebral disk extrusions (arrows).

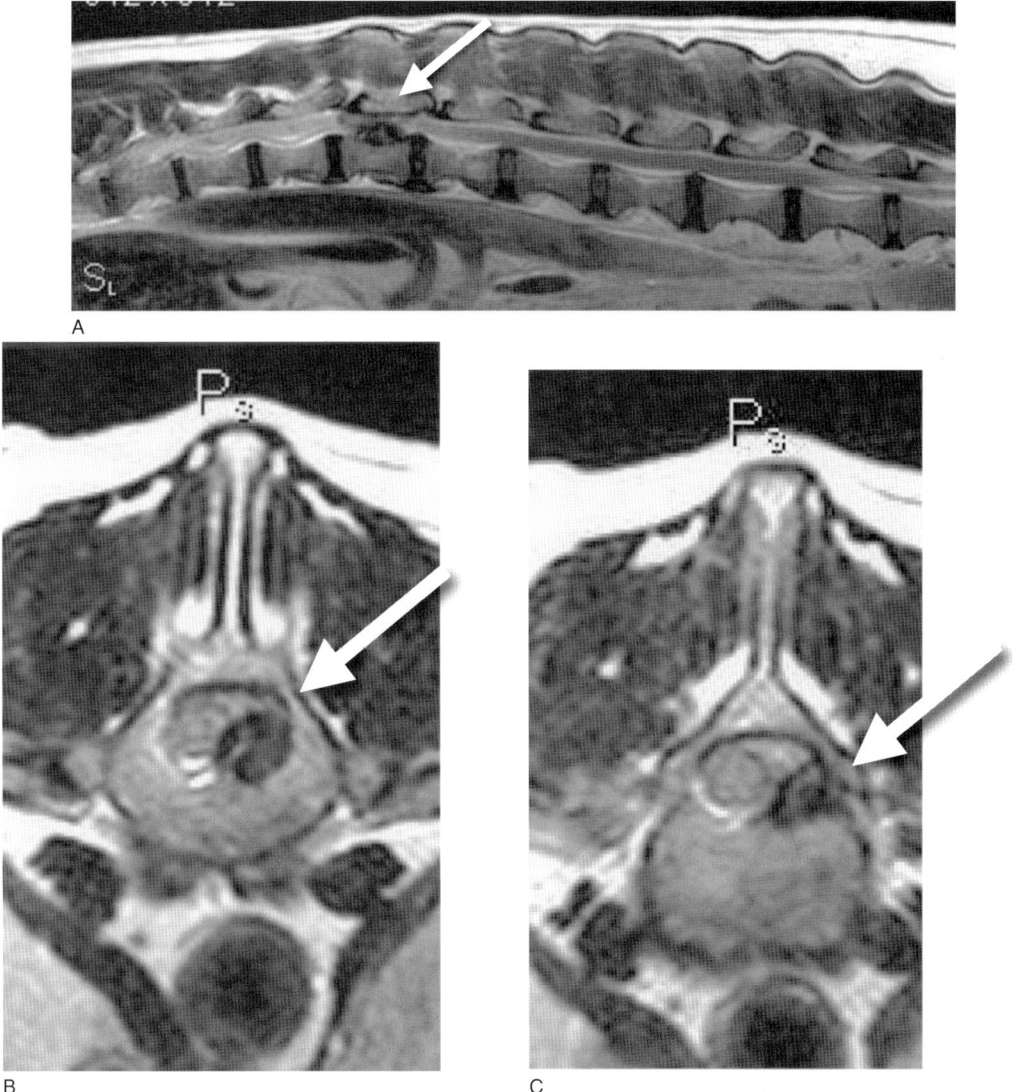

A

B

C

Figure 2.121. Sagittal T2-weighted MR images from a dog (A) with an intervertebral disk extrusion (arrow). Adjacent transverse T2-weighted images ((B) and (C)) from the same dog at the level of the intervertebral disk extrusion (arrows).

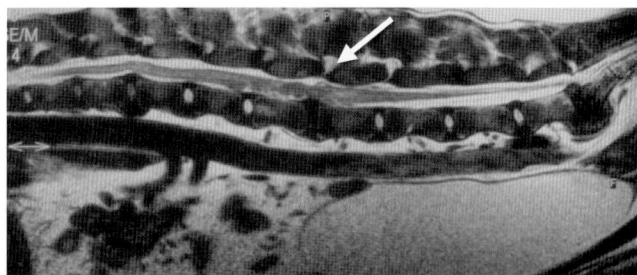

Figure 2.122. Sagittal T2-weighted MR image from a dog with an acute lumbar intervertebral disk extrusion (arrow).

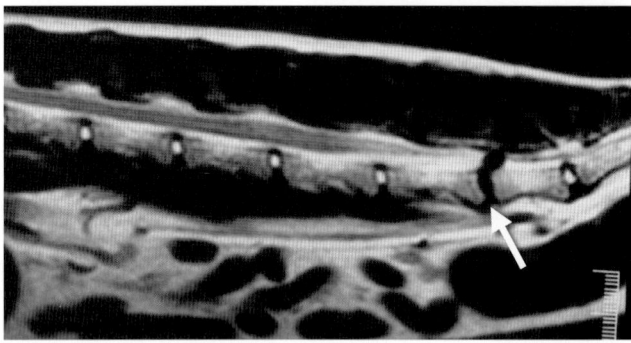

Figure 2.123. Sagittal T2-weighted MR image from a cat with an acute lumbar intervertebral disk extrusion (arrow).

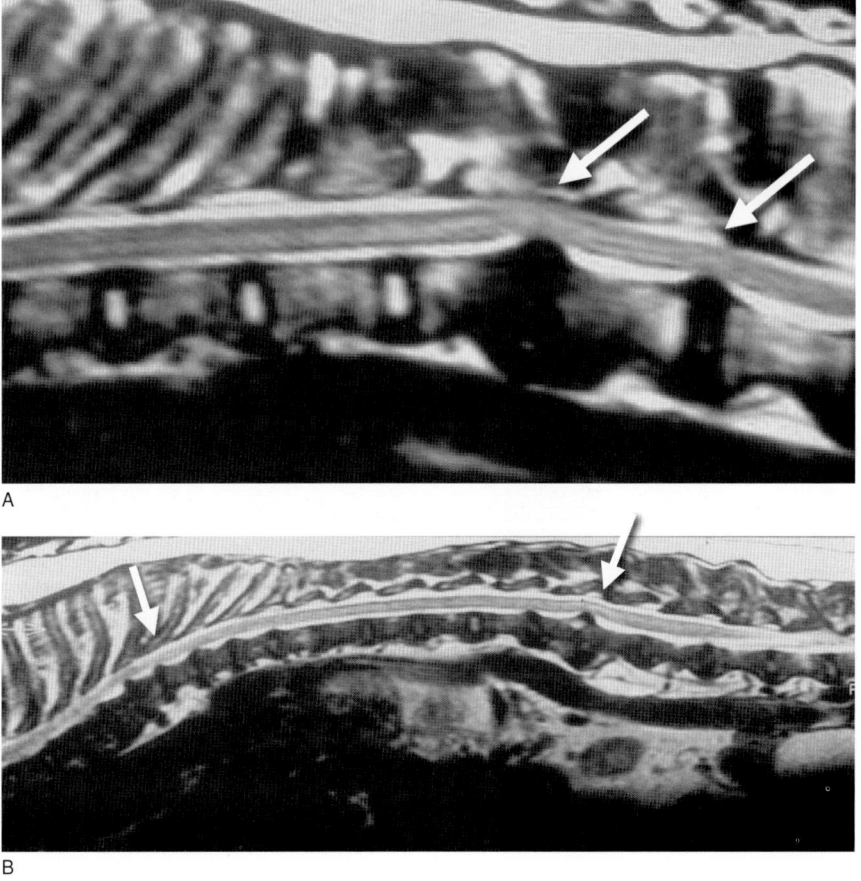

A

B

Figure 2.124. Sagittal T2-weighted MR images from two dogs ((A) and (B)) with intervertebral disk protrusions (arrows).

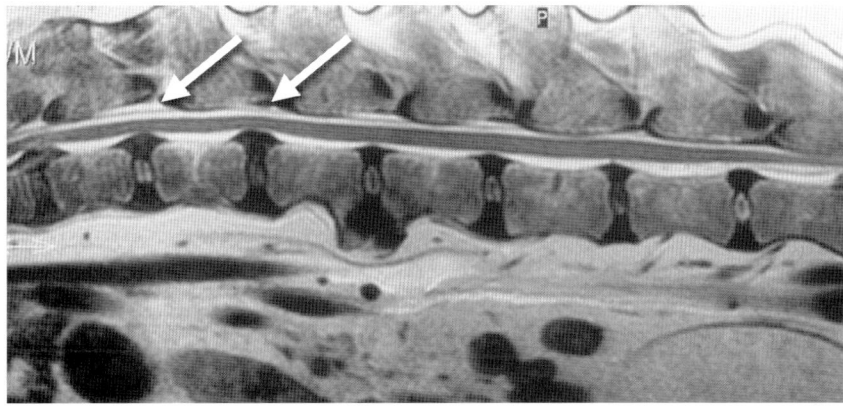

A

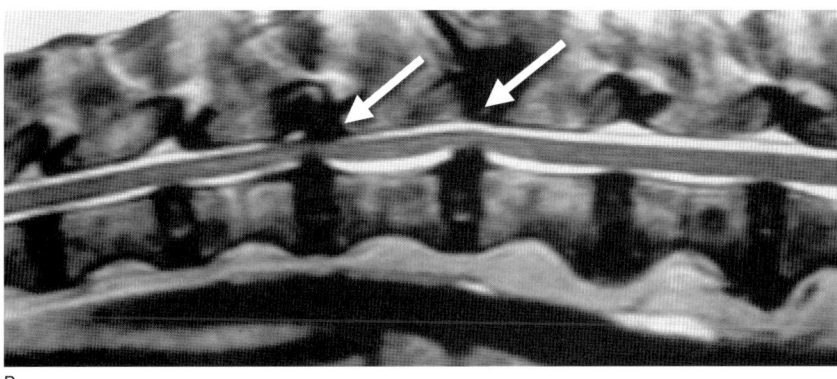

B

Figure 2.125. Sagittal T2-weighted MR images from two large-breed dogs ((A) and (B)) with intervertebral disk protrusions (arrows).

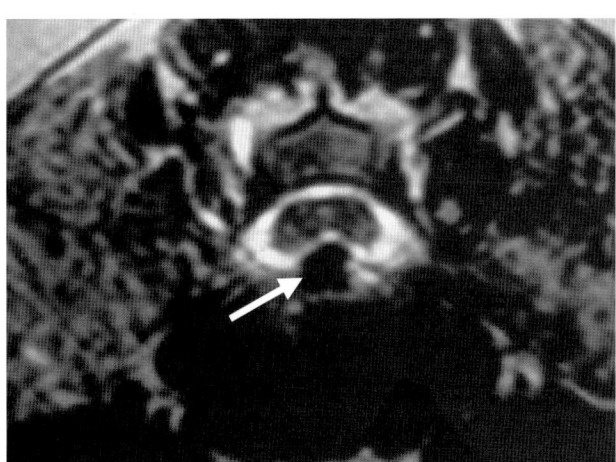

Figure 2.126. Transverse T2-weighted MR image from a dog with an intervertebral disk protrusion (arrow).

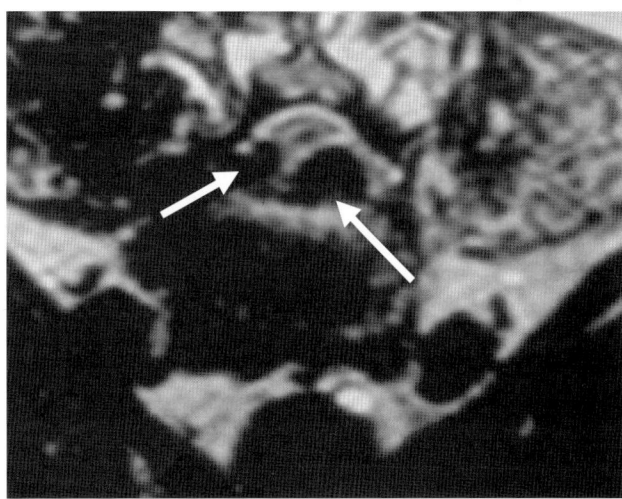

Figure 2.127. Transverse T2-weighted MR image from a dog with two separate intervertebral disk protrusions/extrusions (arrows) at the same intervertebral level.

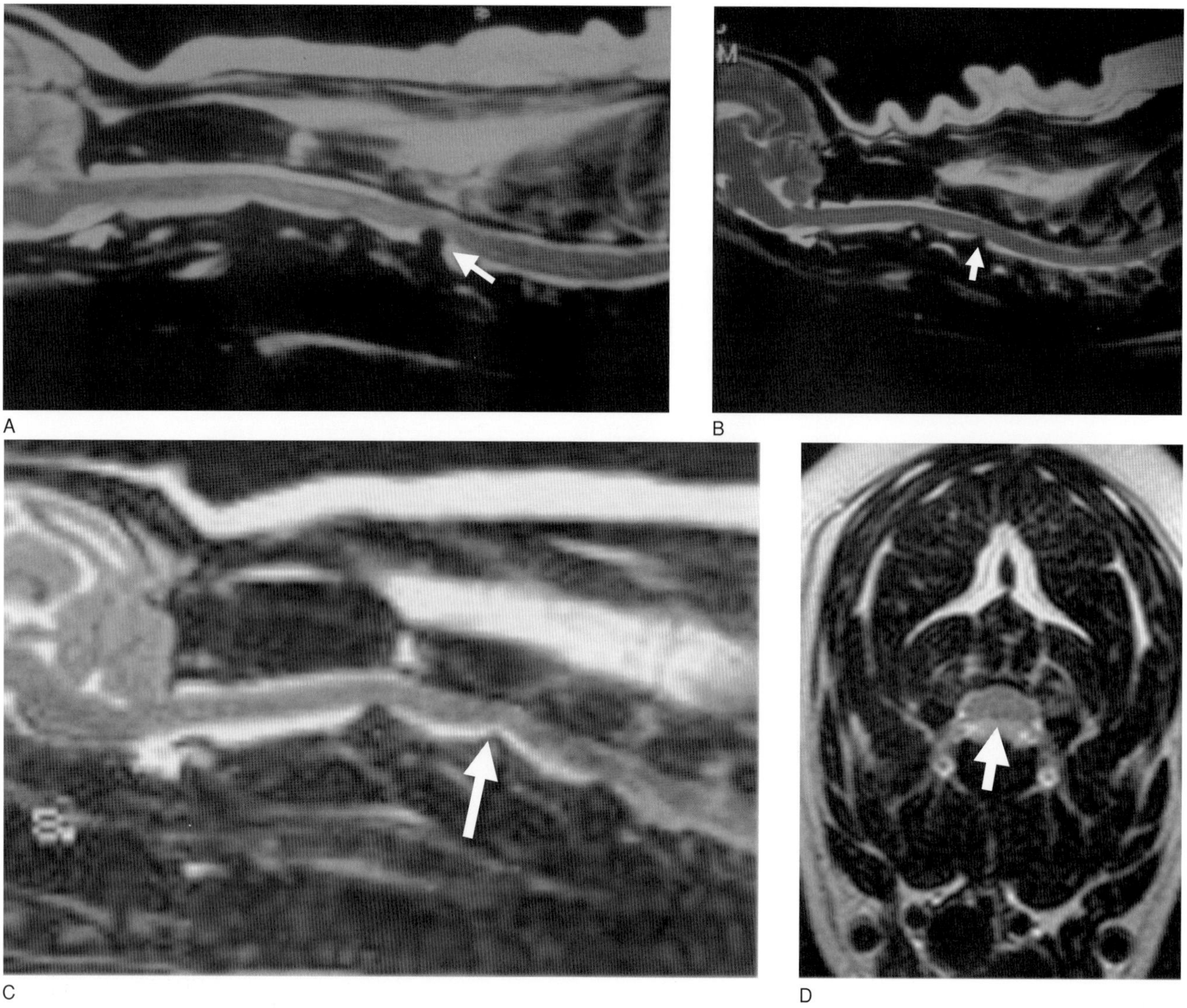

Figure 2.128.   Sagittal T2-weighted MR images from three dogs (A)–(C) with cervical intervertebral disk extrusions (arrows). (D) Transverse T2-weighted MR image from dog in part (C). In this dog the extrusion was of acute normal nucleus pulposus, hence the hyperintense signal (arrow) rather than the hypointense signal.

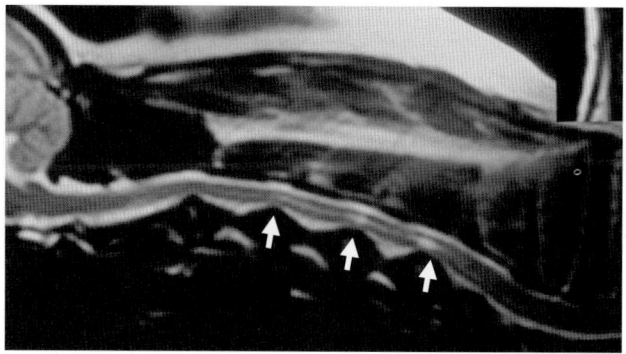

Figure 2.129.   Sagittal T2-weighted MR image from a dog with multiple cervical intervertebral disk protrusions (arrows).

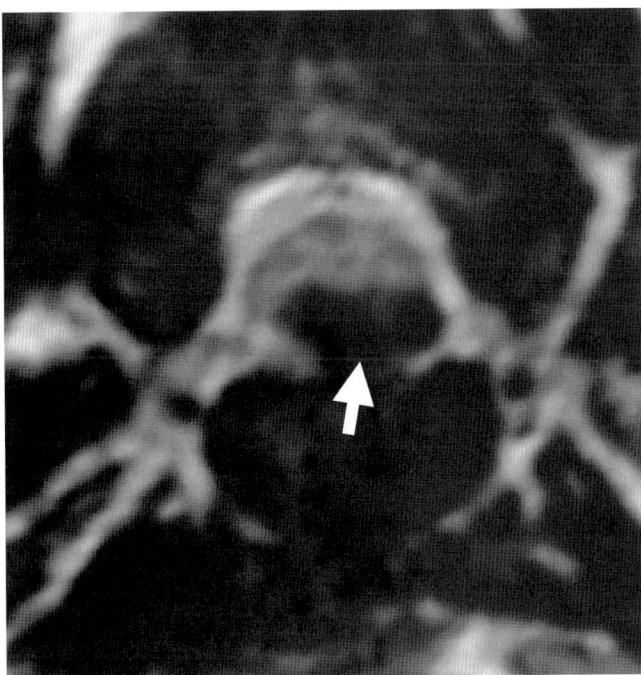

Figure 2.130. Transverse T2-weighted MR image from a dog with a midline cervical intervertebral disk extrusion (arrow).

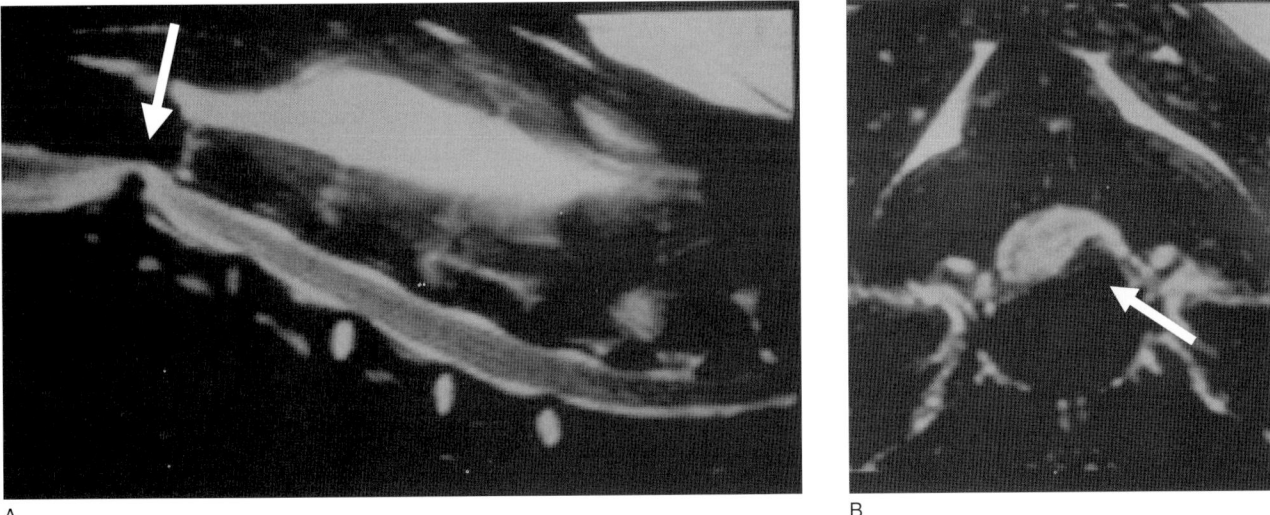

A   B

Figure 2.131. Sagittal (A) and transverse (B) T2-weighted MR images from a dog with a more lateralized cervical intervertebral disk extrusion (arrows).

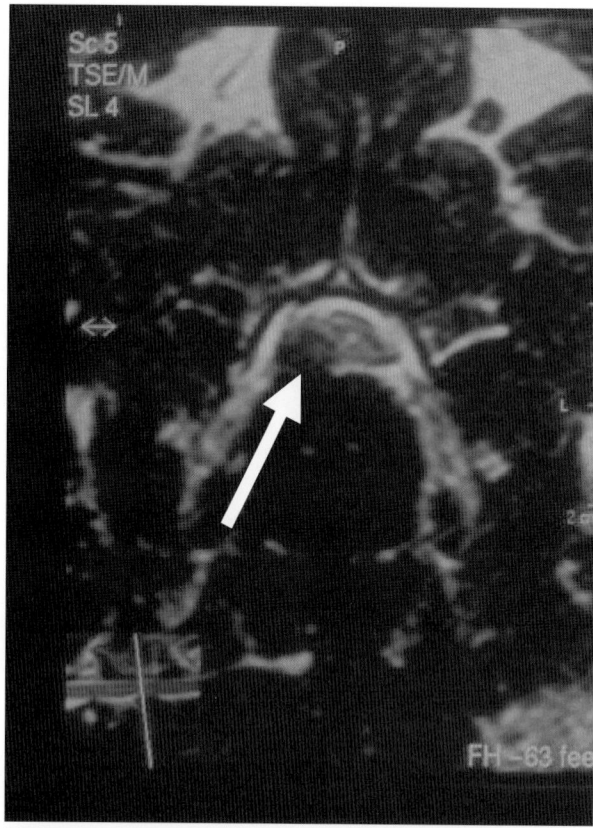

A

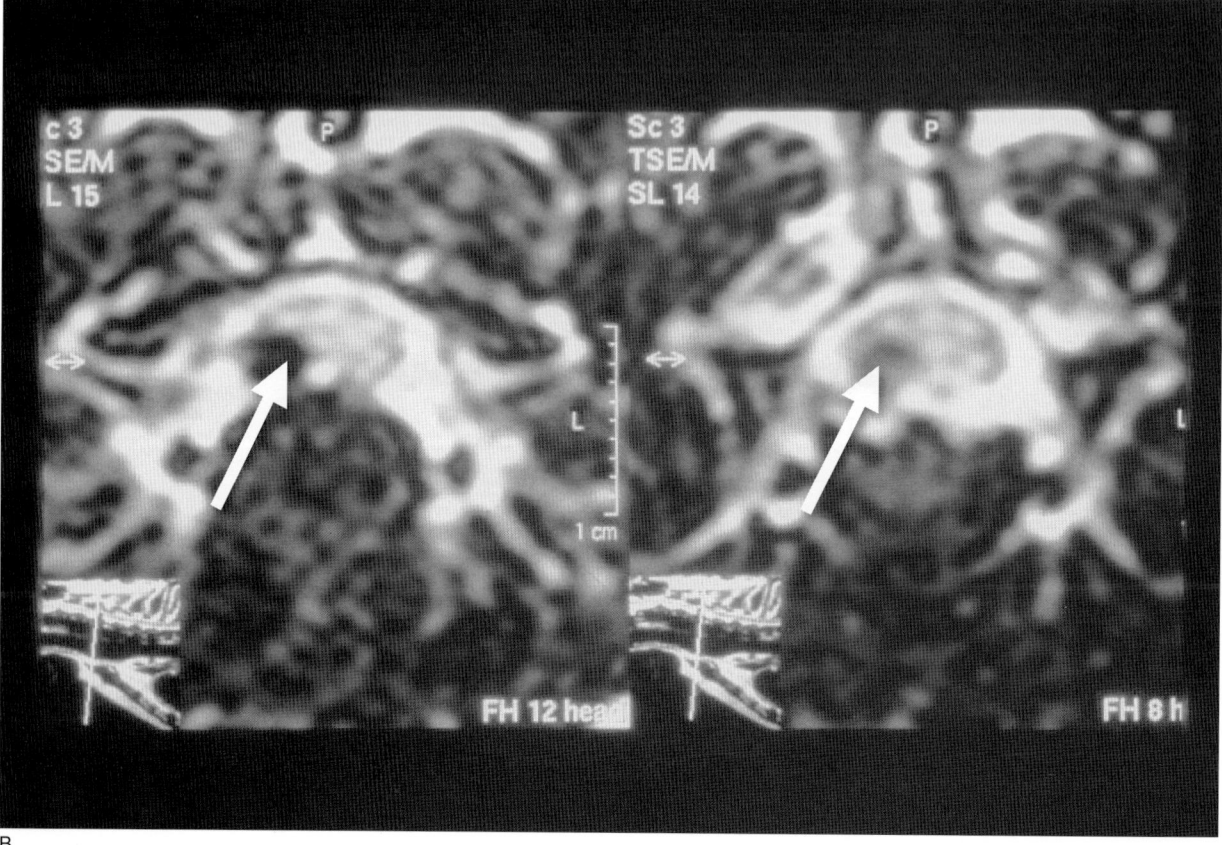

B

Figure 2.132. Transverse T2-weighted MR images from two dogs ((A) and (B)) with more laterally displaced cervical intervertebral disk extrusions (arrows).

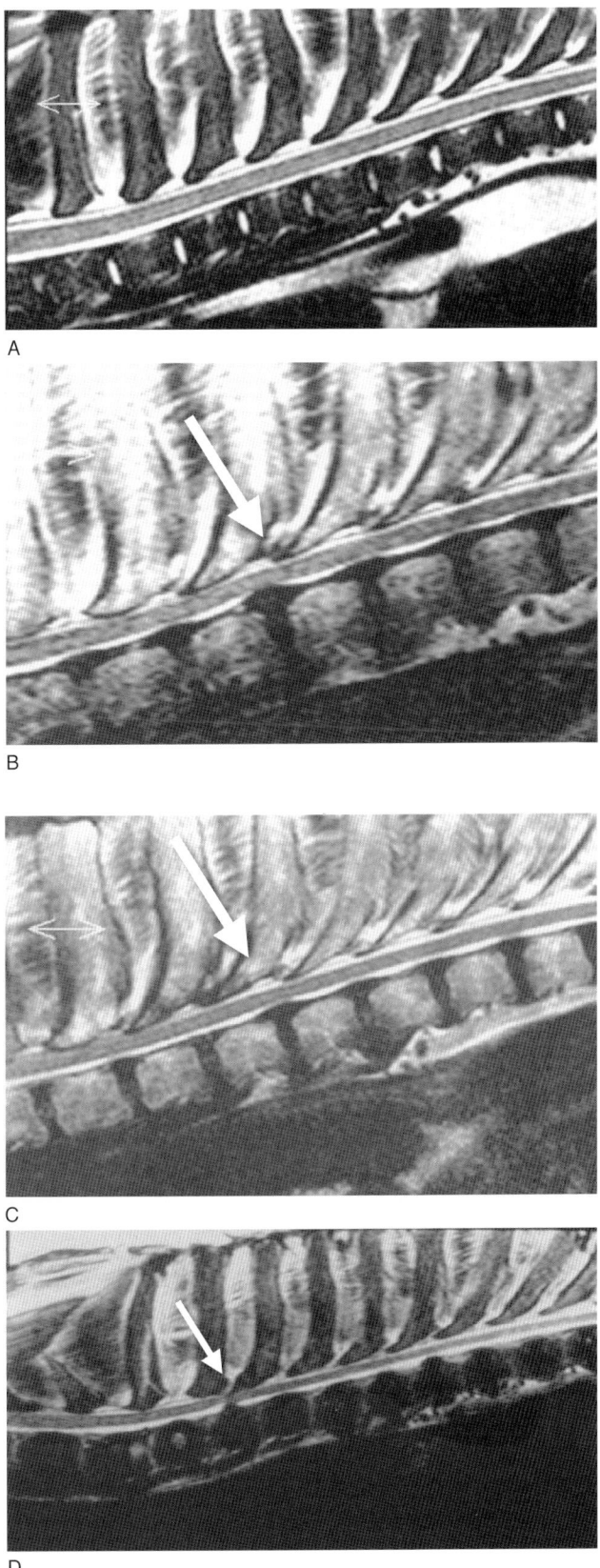

Figure 2.133. Sagittal T2-weighted MR images through the cranial thoracic region from a healthy dog (A) and from three dogs (B)–(D) with thoracic intervertebral disk protrusion (arrows).

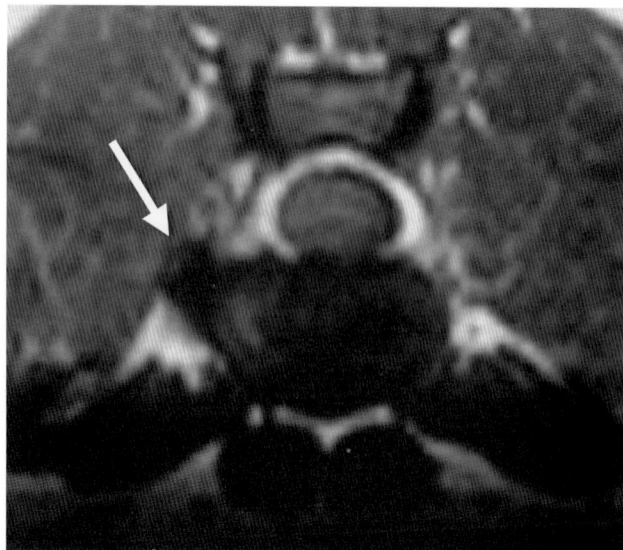

Figure 2.134.   Transverse T2-weighted MR images from a dog with a far lateral lumbar intervertebral disk extrusion (arrow).

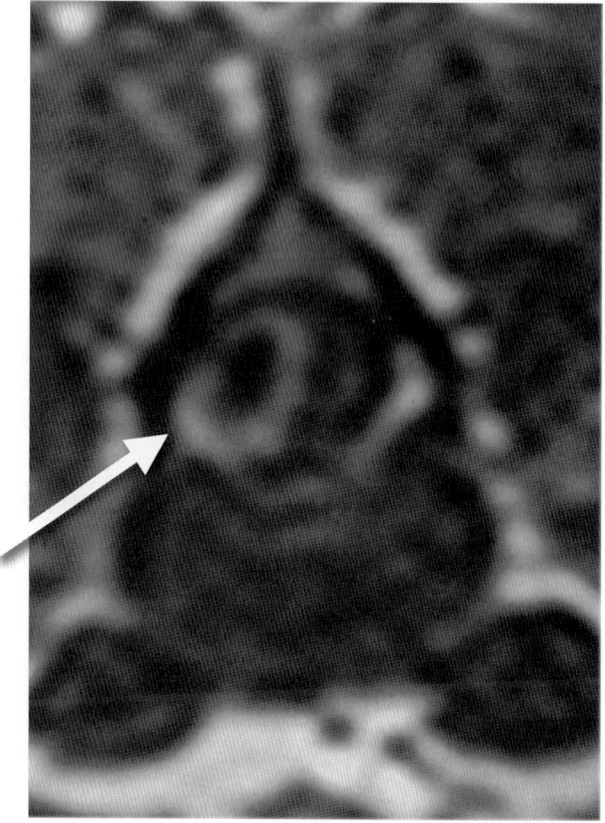

Figure 2.135.   Transverse T1-weighted MR image following intravenous contrast (gadolinium) from a dog with intervertebral disk extrusion (arrow). There was peripheral contrast enhancement of the extruded intervertebral disk material.

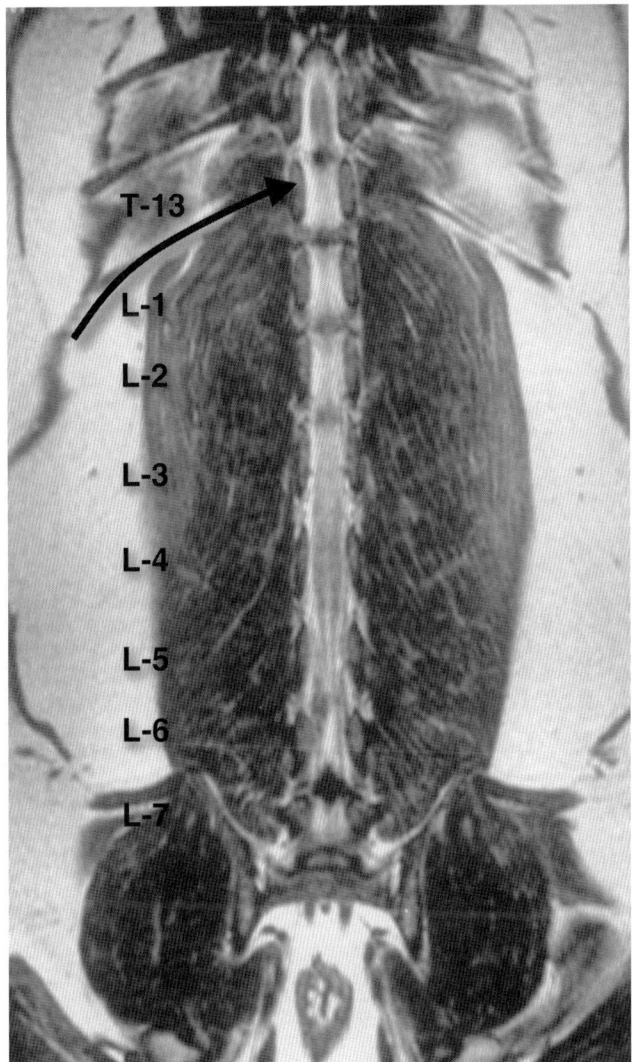

Figure 2.136. Dorsal plane, T2-weighted MR image through the lumbar and caudal thoracic region from a healthy dog showing the relationship of the last rib and the sacrum.

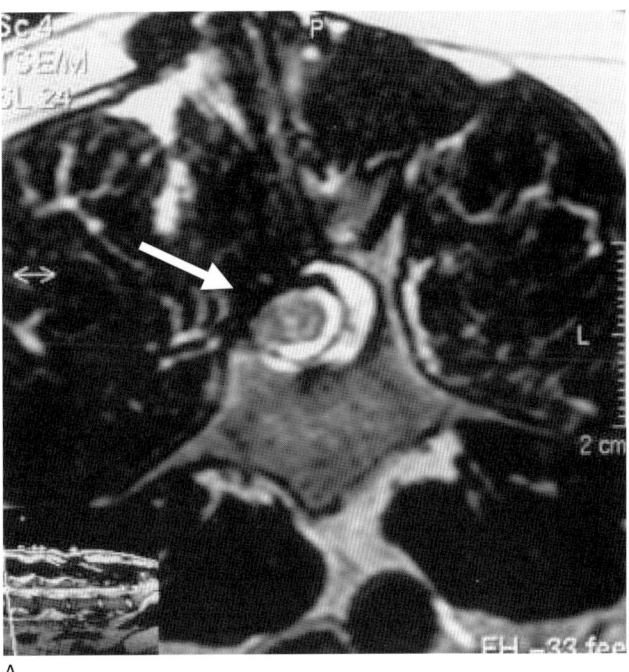

A

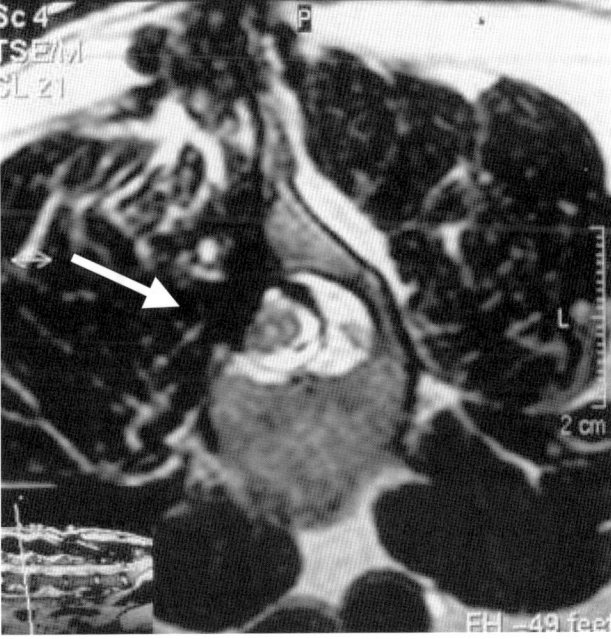

B

Figure 2.137. Transverse T2-weighted MR images from a dog ((A) and (B)) immediately following a hemilaminectomy (arrow).

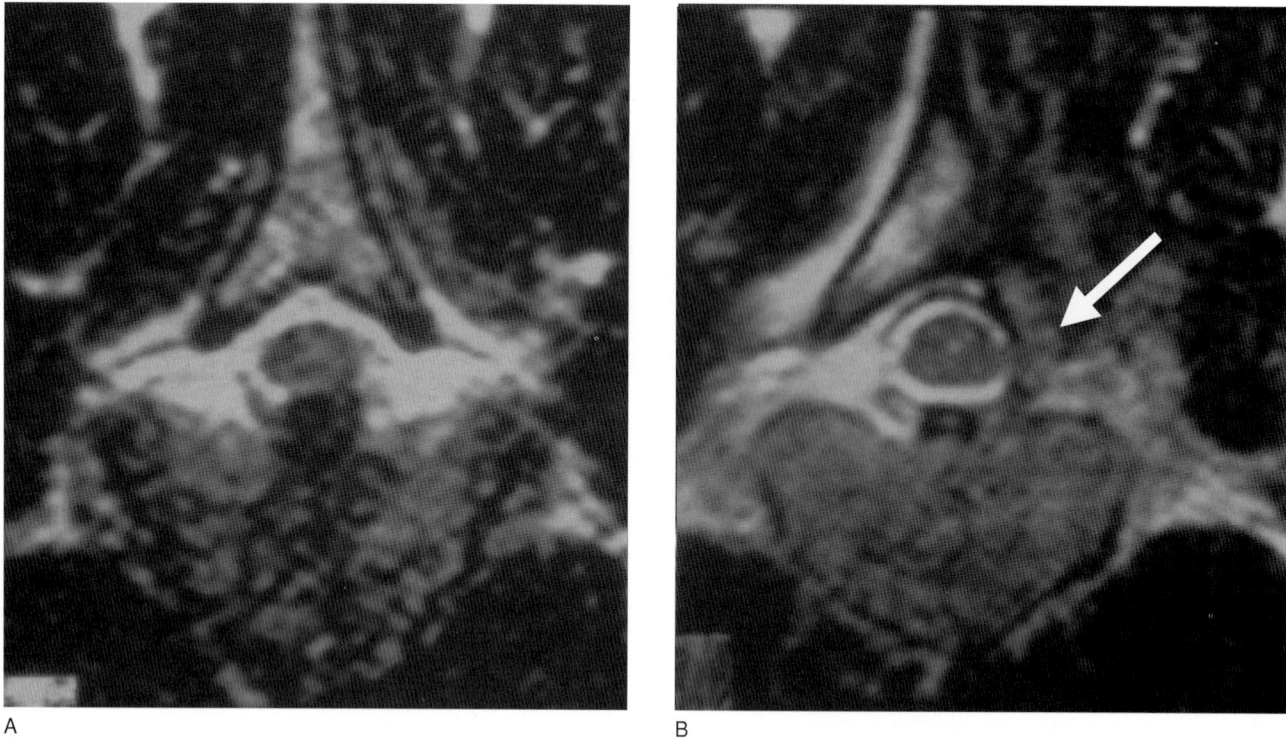

Figure 2.138. Transverse T2-weighted MR images from a dog before (A) and immediately following (B) a hemilaminectomy (arrow).

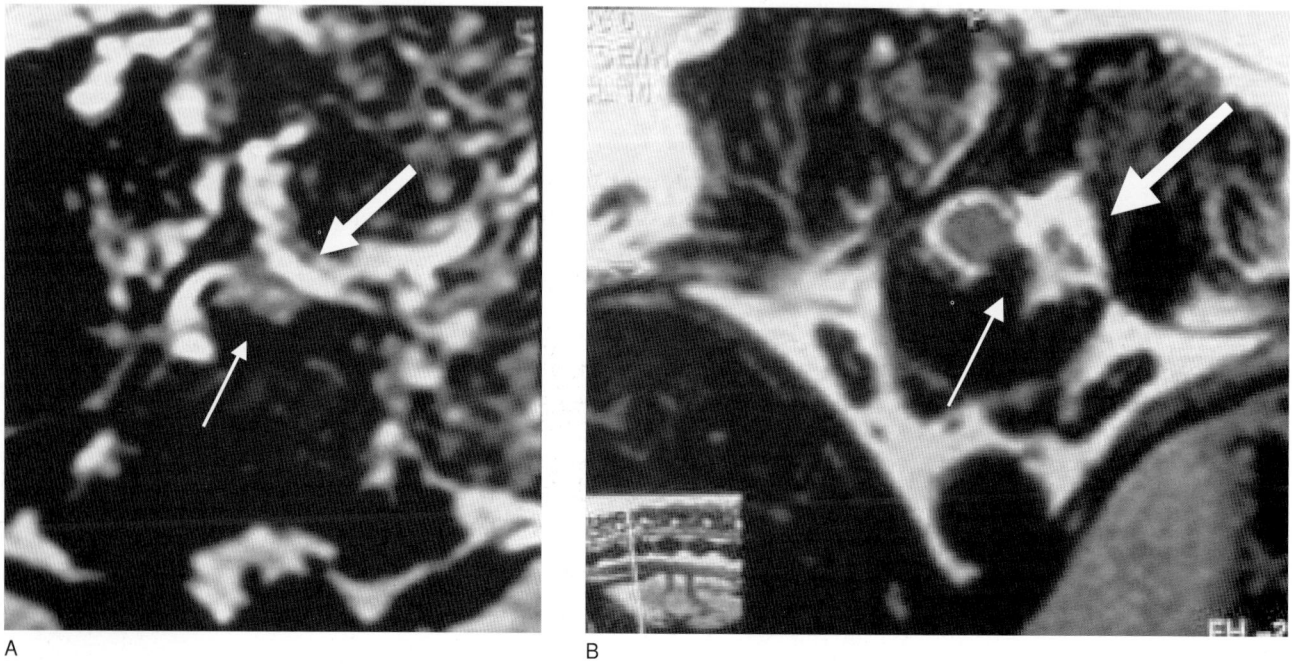

Figure 2.139. Transverse T2-weighted MR images from two dogs ((A) and (B)) following a hemilaminectomy (larger arrow) where intervertebral disk material (smaller arrow) has been incompletely removed.

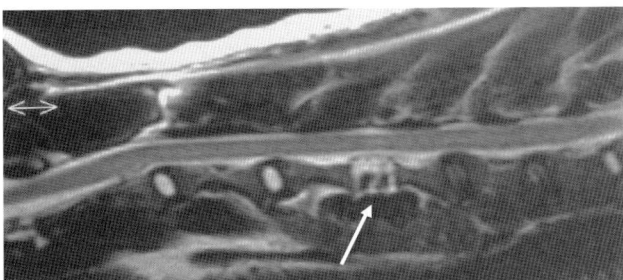

Figure 2.140.   Sagittal T2-weighted MR image from a dog following a ventral slot procedure (arrow).

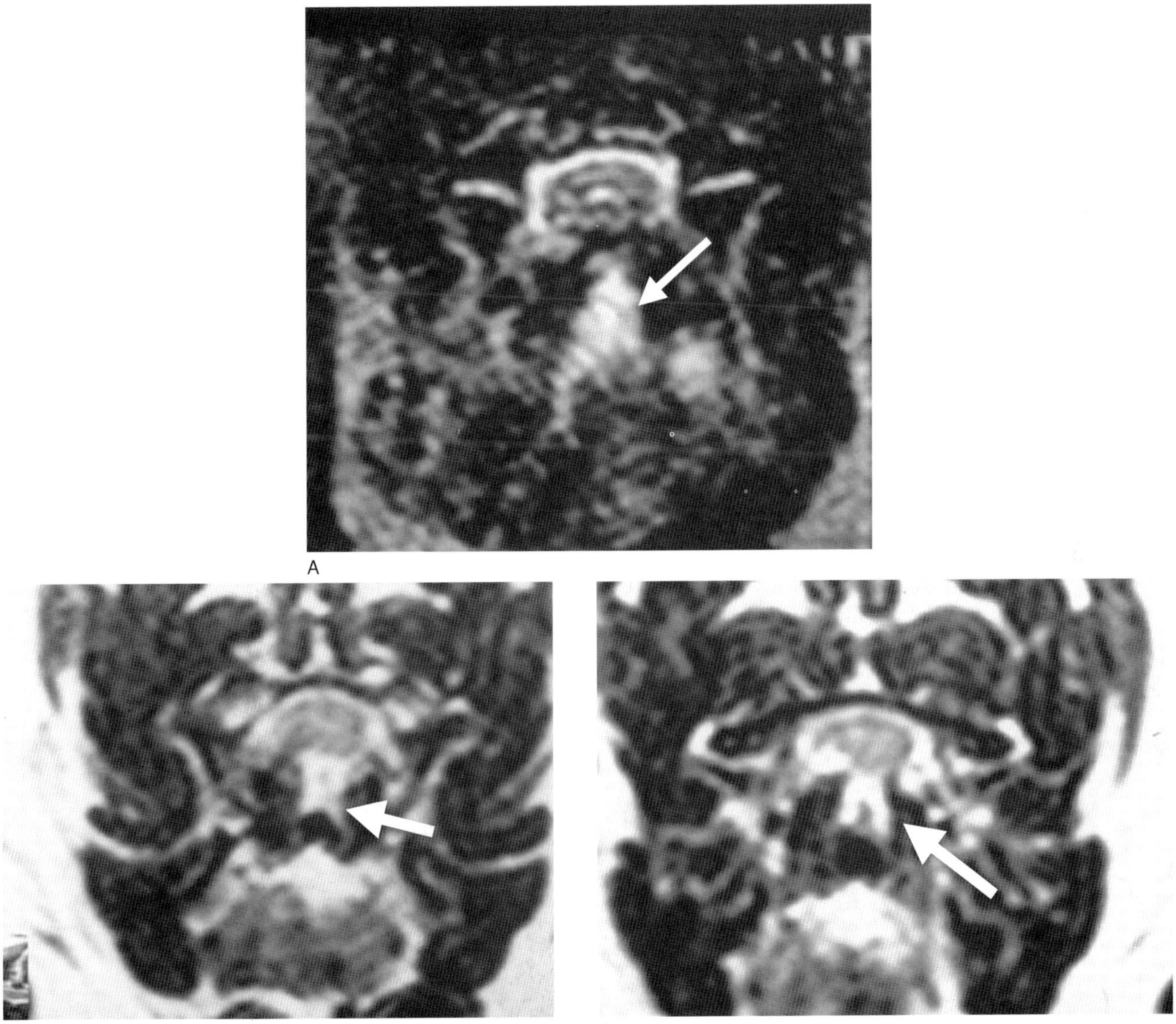

A

B   C

Figure 2.141.   Transverse T2-weighted MR images from three dogs (A)–(C) immediately following a ventral slot procedure (arrows).

images alone, to predict outcome following surgery. MR imaging performed weeks to months following spinal surgery may also reveal intraspinal cord abnormalities such as syringomyelia or focal gray matter malacia, usually at the level of the previous spinal injury or IVD compression. Obviously, if metal surgical implants have been placed for spinal stabilization, metal artifacts in the local spinal region will distort the MR signal and prevent adequate MR imaging interpretation (Figure 2.142).

Wobbler's Syndrome

The term "Wobbler's syndrome" encompasses a number of cervical vertebral abnormalities. These include vertebral malarticulation/malformation, intervertebral disk extrusion and protrusion, articular facet hypertrophy, and spinal ligament hypertrophy. Two general clinical presentations, however, are usually included under the "Wobbler's syndrome" heading. One of these clinical presentations is classically seen in middle-aged to older Doberman pinschers. Other breeds, however, including both large and small body types can also be affected. The disease in these animals is characterized primarily by ventral compressive lesions of the caudal cervical area resulting from ligamentous hypertrophy and intervertebral disk (usually annulus fibrosis) protrusion (Figures 2.143 and 2.144). While the pathophysiology of this disease is not fully understood, some caudal cervical instability coupled with increased flexion force due to the pull of gravity in a comparatively large head size may predispose one to damage to the intervertebral disk space and the associated articulations. Damage to the intervertebral disk elements may contribute to vertebral unit instability. Hypertrophy of the associated ligamentous supporting structures (dorsal longitudinal ligament, dorsal intervertebral ligament, or ligamentum flavum) is most likely an attempt by the body to decrease this instability and to naturally fuse these articulations. This hypertrophied tissue, in combination with protruded intervertebral disk elements (annulus) however, encroaches into the vertebral canal leading eventually to spinal cord compression (Figures 2.143–2.145). This compression may be static or dynamic (Figures 2.145–2.149). In addition to compressive damage to axons and neurons, impingement of spinal cord vessels can result in ischemic damage to the spinal cord. In some instances, there are acute extrusions of IVD nucleus pulposus (Figure 2.145).

MR imaging is often helpful in determining the exact location of any spinal cord compressed segments (Figures 2.143–2.145). MR imaging may be helpful in assessing vertebral changes, spinal cord atrophy, and the degree of spinal cord compression. The transverse imaging view afforded by these imaging modalities provides for the most accurate visualization of spinal cord compression in a 360° orientation surrounding the spinal cord. With ventral compression from annulus fibrosis or hypertrophied spinal ligaments, a ventral extradural compressive lesion is more apparent. This tissue is usually hypointense on T2-weighted sequences. It is common to have focal hyperintense abnormalities within the central spinal cord (gray matter) in T2-weighted images directly dorsal to the ventral spinal compression (Figures 2.148 and 2.149). As both dynamic and static spinal cord compression may be present with these diseases, flexed and extended (positional) imaging views may be needed to reveal the dynamic nature of the compressive lesion if the disease is suspected but not obvious in neutral position images. Commonly in dogs with lesions such as those classically seen in Doberman pinschers ventral compression is worse when the head (and neck) is extended dorsally.

Younger, large-breed dogs, such as Great Danes, mastiffs, and Saint Bernards, have a similarly named disease, but with a differing pathophysiology. In these younger and larger dogs, the disease involves the dorsal articular facets with secondary hypertrophy of the associated joint capsules and ligaments (Figures 2.150–2.155). This hypertrophy results in a more dorsal and lateral anatomical location of spinal compression. If the compressive tissue is fibrous connective (ligamentous) tissue or cortical bone, the compressive lesion will appear hypointense in T2-weighted images (Figures 2.151, 2.153, and 2.154). Some animals may have congenital bony malformations of the articular facets predisposing to a stenotic vertebral canal. The articular facet joints may inherently degenerate, or may be damaged due to ineffectual ability to support the weight of the head. This will result in hyperintense (on T2 sequences) alterations in these joints. In still other instances, small portions of synovial tissue may become entrapped and "pinched off" containing synovial fluid (Figures 2.156–2.158). These sacs of inspissated synovial fluid are known as synovial cysts and are usually hyperintense in T2-weighted images. These cysts may also compress the spinal cord, either statically or with vertebral movement (dynamic compression). A similar-type spinal compression from hypertrophied dorsal ligaments and abnormal articular facet joints is possible (Figure 2.154).

As some animals with this category of disease are treated surgically, MR imaging may be performed following surgery (Figures 2.161 and 2.162). Assessments made are similar to those as described under treatment of IVDD.

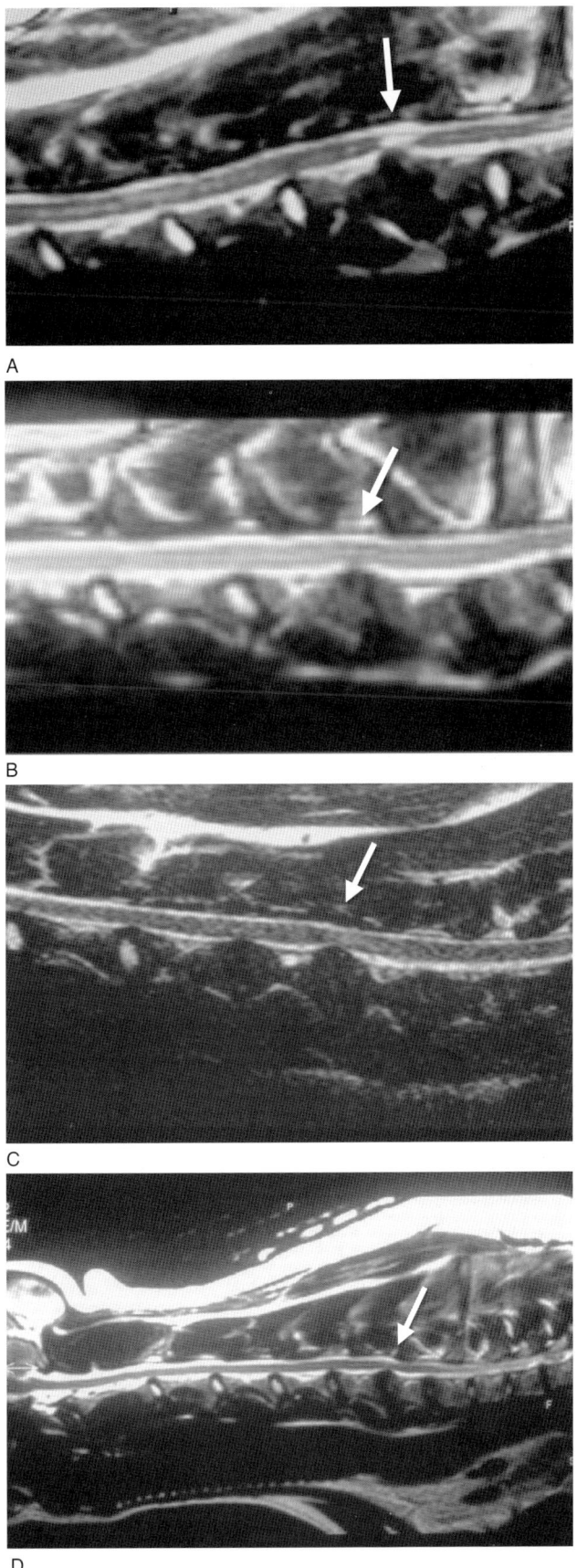

Figure 2.142. Sagittal T2-weighted MR images from four dogs (A)–(D) with ventral cervical spinal cord compression (arrows) associated with cervical vertebral malformation/malarticulation or "Wobbler's syndrome."

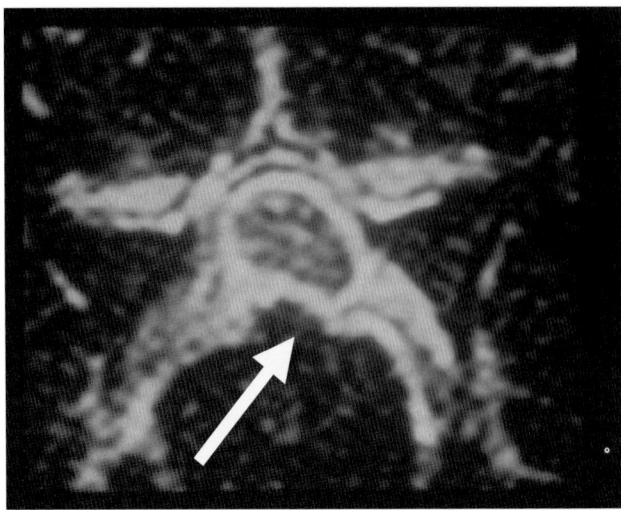

Figure 2.143. Transverse T2-weighted MR image from a dog with ventral cervical spinal cord compression (arrow) associated with cervical vertebral malformation/malarticulation or "Wobbler's syndrome."

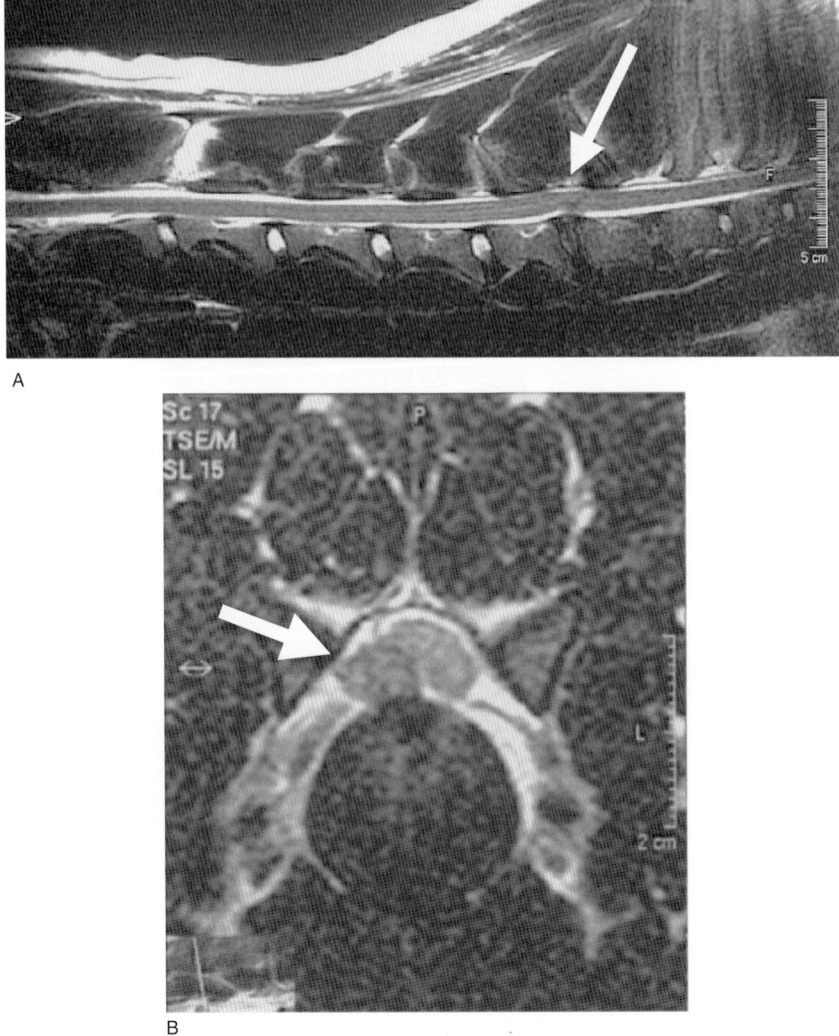

Figure 2.144. Sagittal (A) and transverse (B) T2-weighted MR images from a large dog with a ventral cervical spinal cord compression (arrow) associated with an acute IVD extrusion.

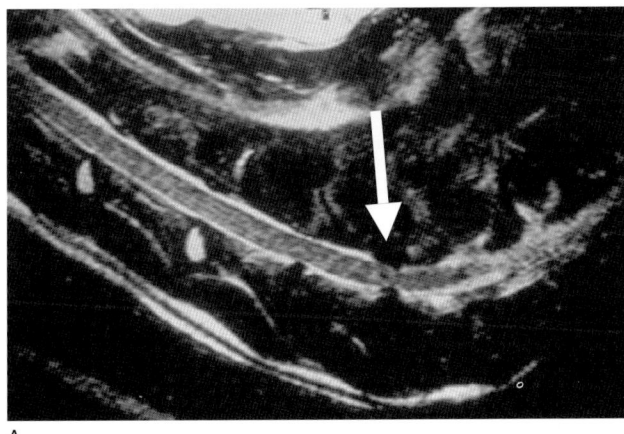

A

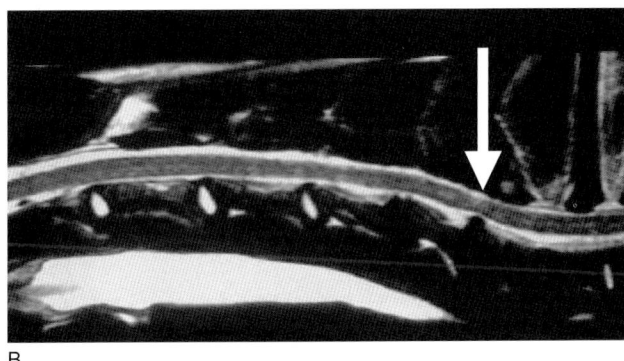

B

Figure 2.145. Sagittal T2-weighted MR images from a dog with ventral cervical spinal cord compression (arrow) associated with cervical vertebral malformation/malarticulation or "Wobbler's syndrome" when the head and neck is placed in an extended (A) compared to a flexed (B) position.

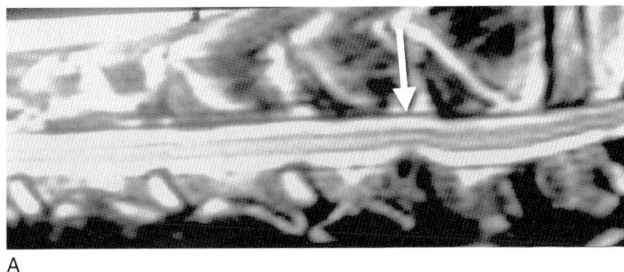

A

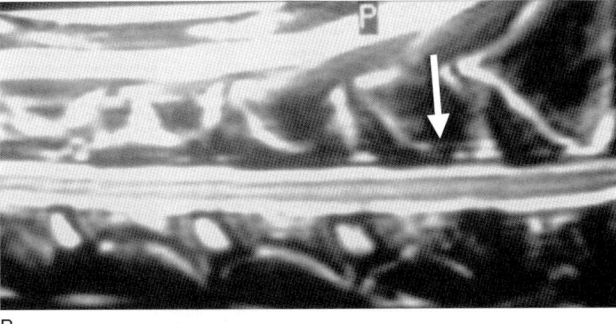

B

Figure 2.146. Sagittal T2-weighted MR images from a dog with ventral cervical spinal cord compression (arrow) associated with cervical vertebral malformation/malarticulation or "Wobbler's syndrome" when the head and neck is in a neutral position (A) compared to when a traction force is placed on the head and neck (B).

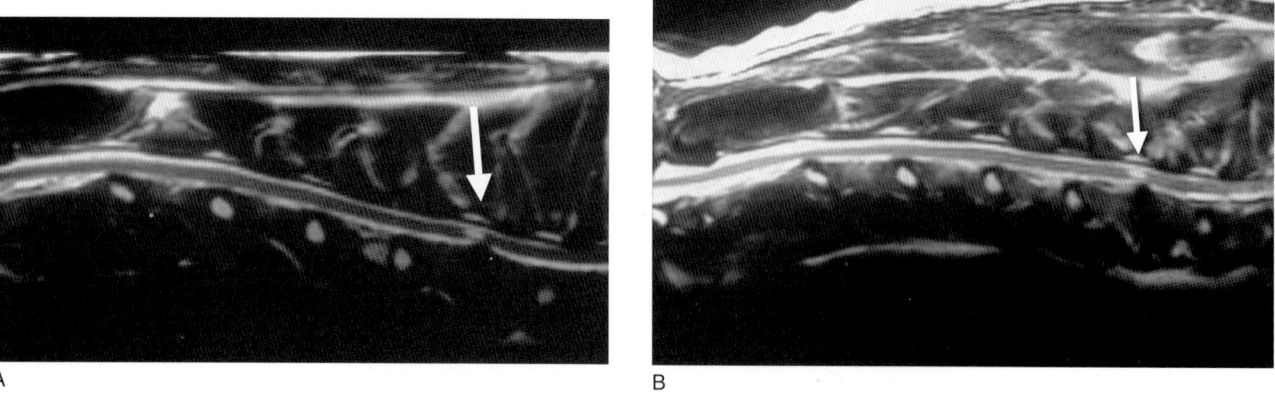

A

B

Figure 2.147.   Sagittal T2-weighted MR images from two dogs (A)–(B) with intramedullary increased signal intensity (arrows) associated with cervical vertebral malformation/malarticulation or "Wobbler's syndrome."

A

B

C

D

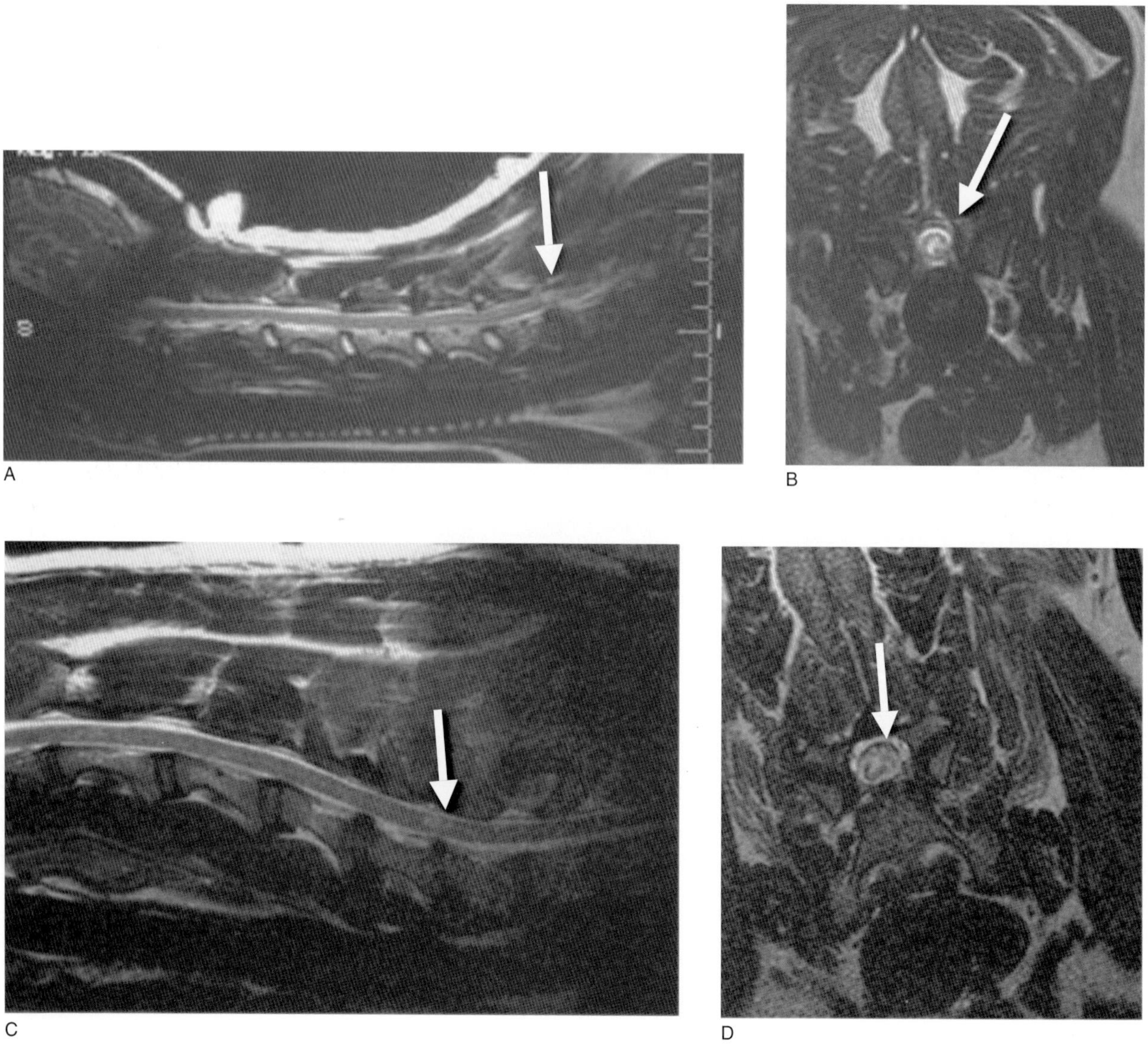

Figure 2.148.   Sagittal ((A) and (C)) and transverse ((B) and (D)) T2-weighted MR images from two large dogs ((A), (B) and (C), (D)) with intramedullary increased signal intensity (arrows) associated with cervical vertebral malformation/malarticulation or "Wobbler's syndrome."

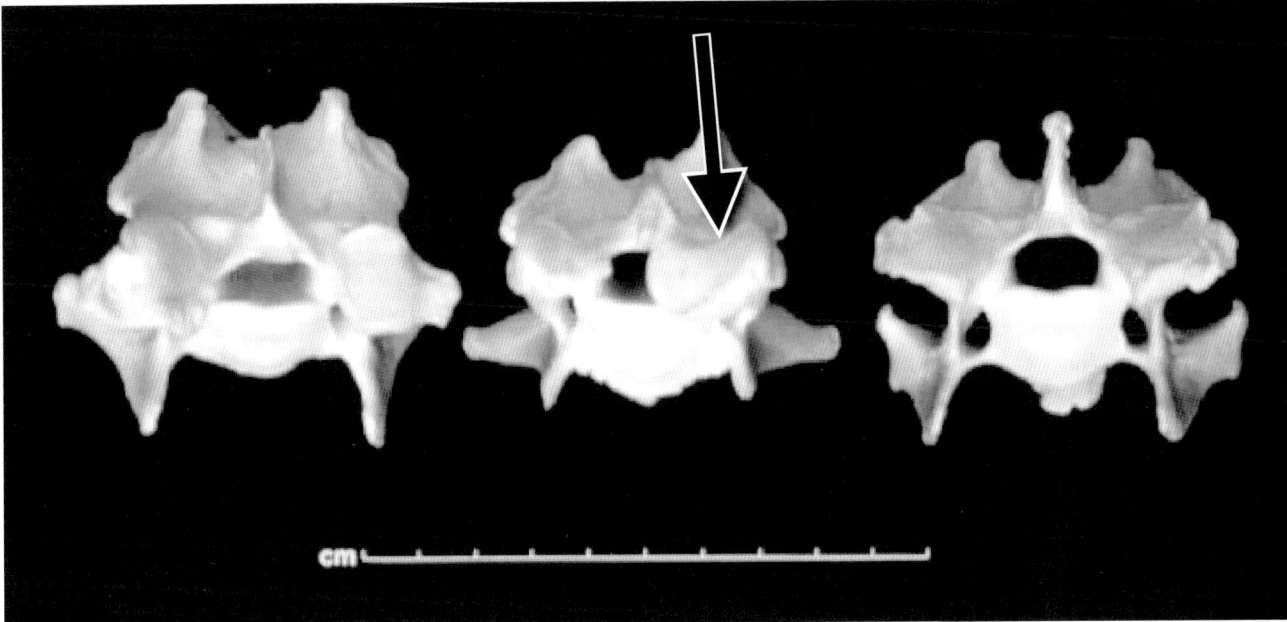

Figure 2.149. Pathologic vertebral specimen from a young dog with "Wobbler's syndrome" showing the malformation of the dorsal articular facets (arrow).

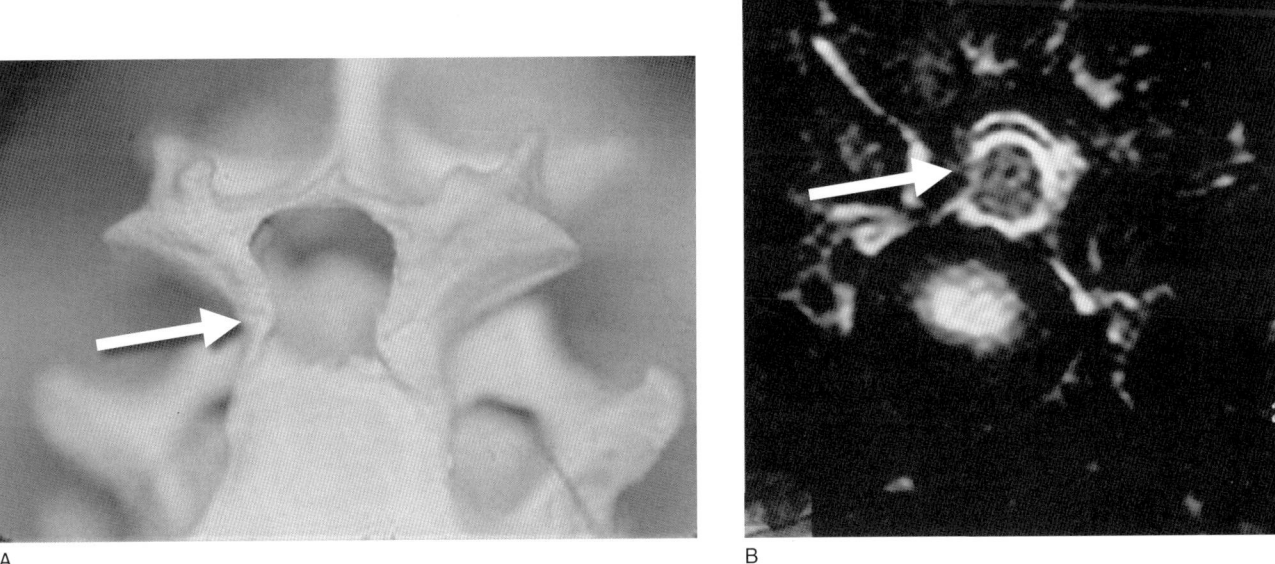

A

B

Figure 2.150. Pathologic vertebral specimen (A) from a young dog with "Wobbler's syndrome" showing the malformation of the dorsal articular facets (arrow). Transverse T2-weighted MR image (B) from a similarly affected dog showing bony impingement on the spinal canal (arrow).

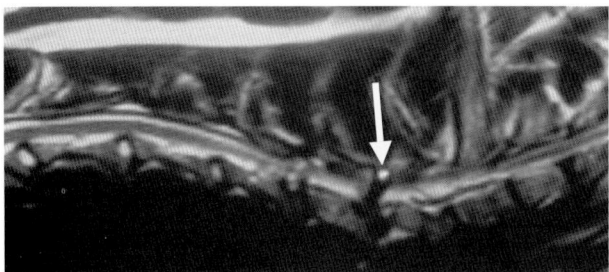

Figure 2.151. Parasagittal T2-weighted MR image from a young dog with "Wobbler's syndrome" due to hypertrophy of the dorsal articular facets (arrow). The focal, round, hyperintense signal at this level was the result of an associated synovial cyst.

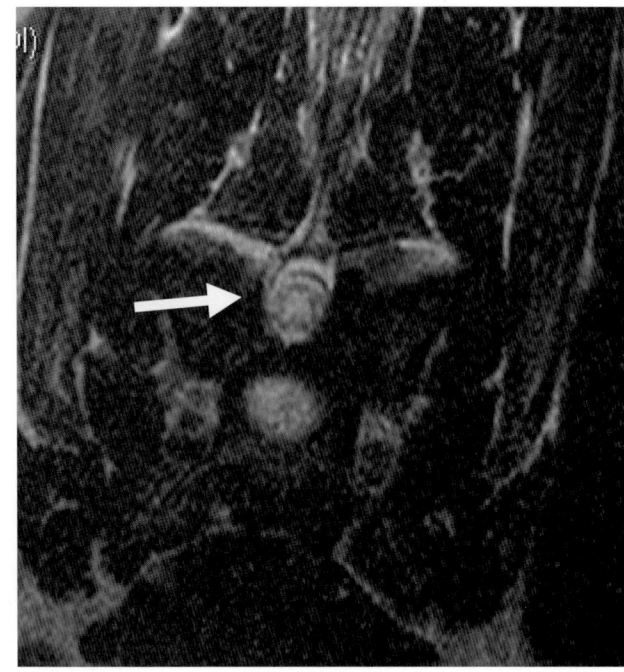

Figure 2.153. Transverse T2-weighted MR image from a young dog with "Wobbler's syndrome" due to bony spinal canal stenosis (arrow) with associated intramedullary gray matter hyperintense signal.

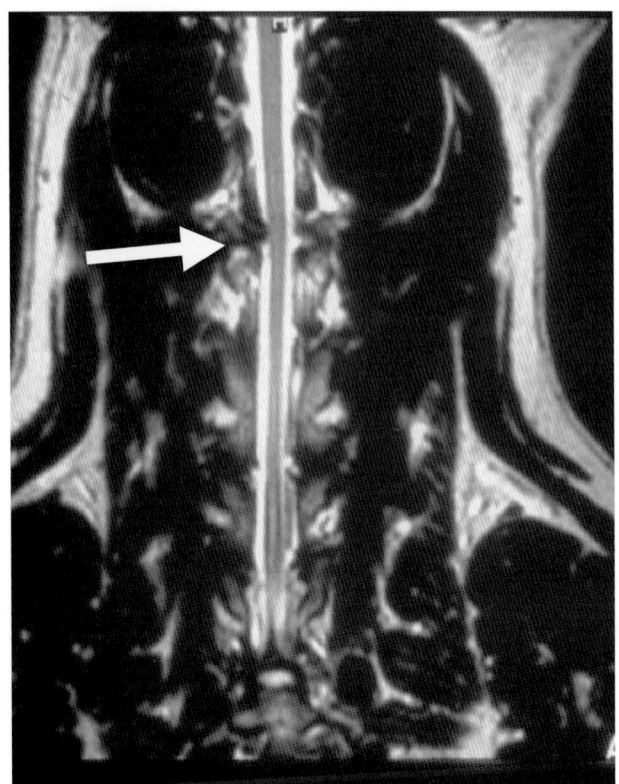

Figure 2.152. Dorsal plane, T2-weighted MR image from a young dog with "Wobbler's syndrome" due to hypertrophy of the dorsal articular facets (arrow).

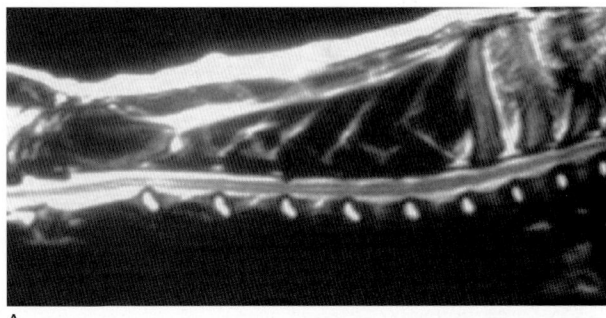

A

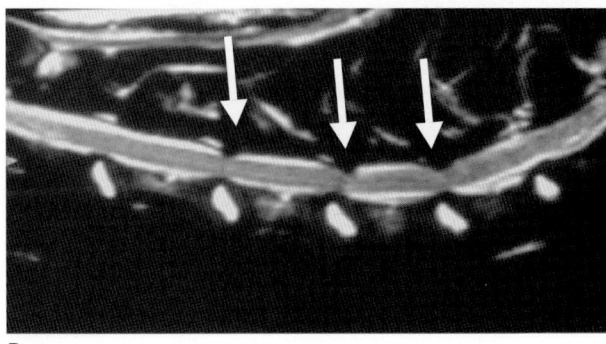

B

Figure 2.154. Sagittal T2-weighted MR images from a young large dog with the head and neck in a neutral position (A) compared to a dorsally extended position (B). Note the dorsal spinal cord compression which is more evident in the extended head position (arrows).

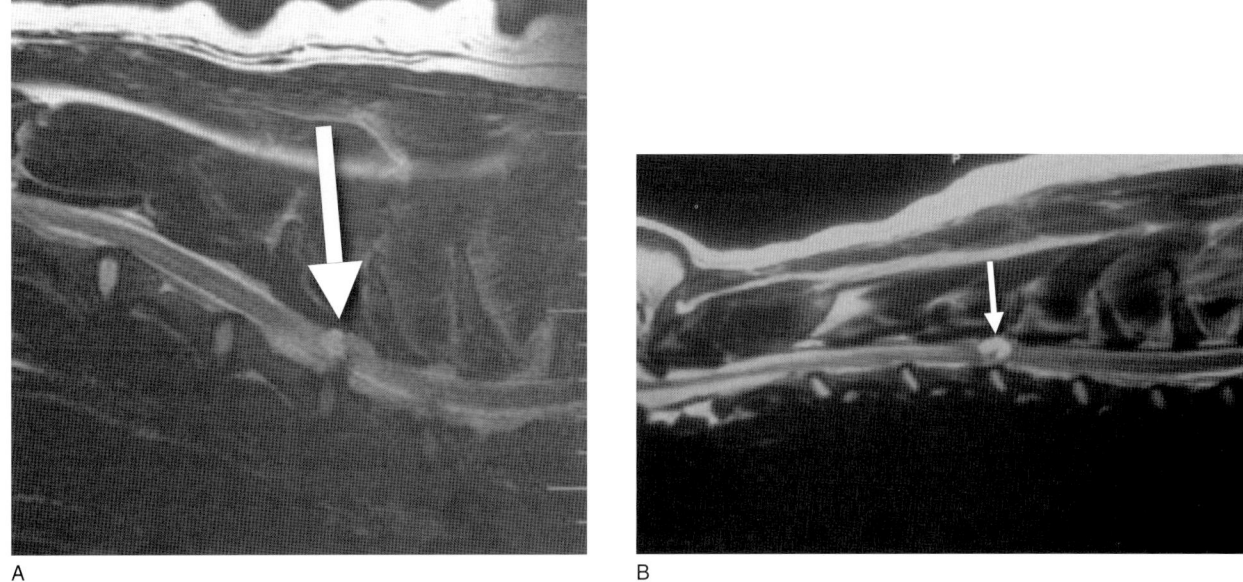

Figure 2.155.   Sagittal T2-weighted MR images from two young large dogs ((A) and (B)) with synovial cysts (arrows).

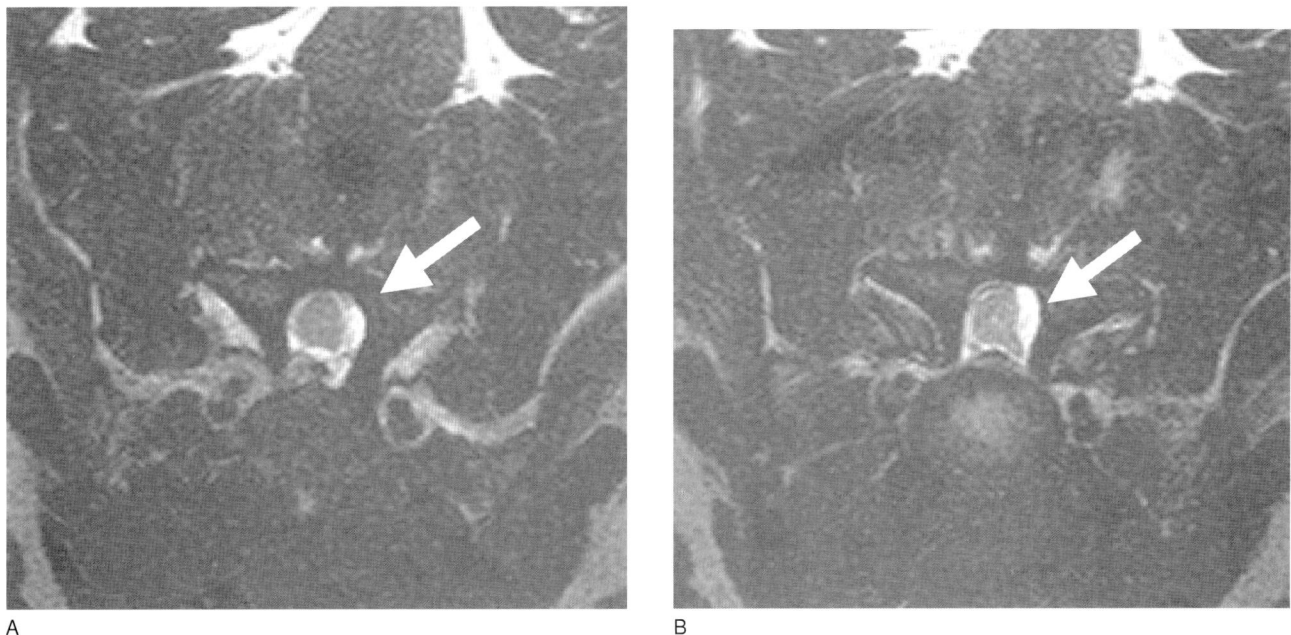

Figure 2.156.   Transverse T2-weighted MR images from a young large dog ((A) and (B)) with a synovial cyst (arrows).

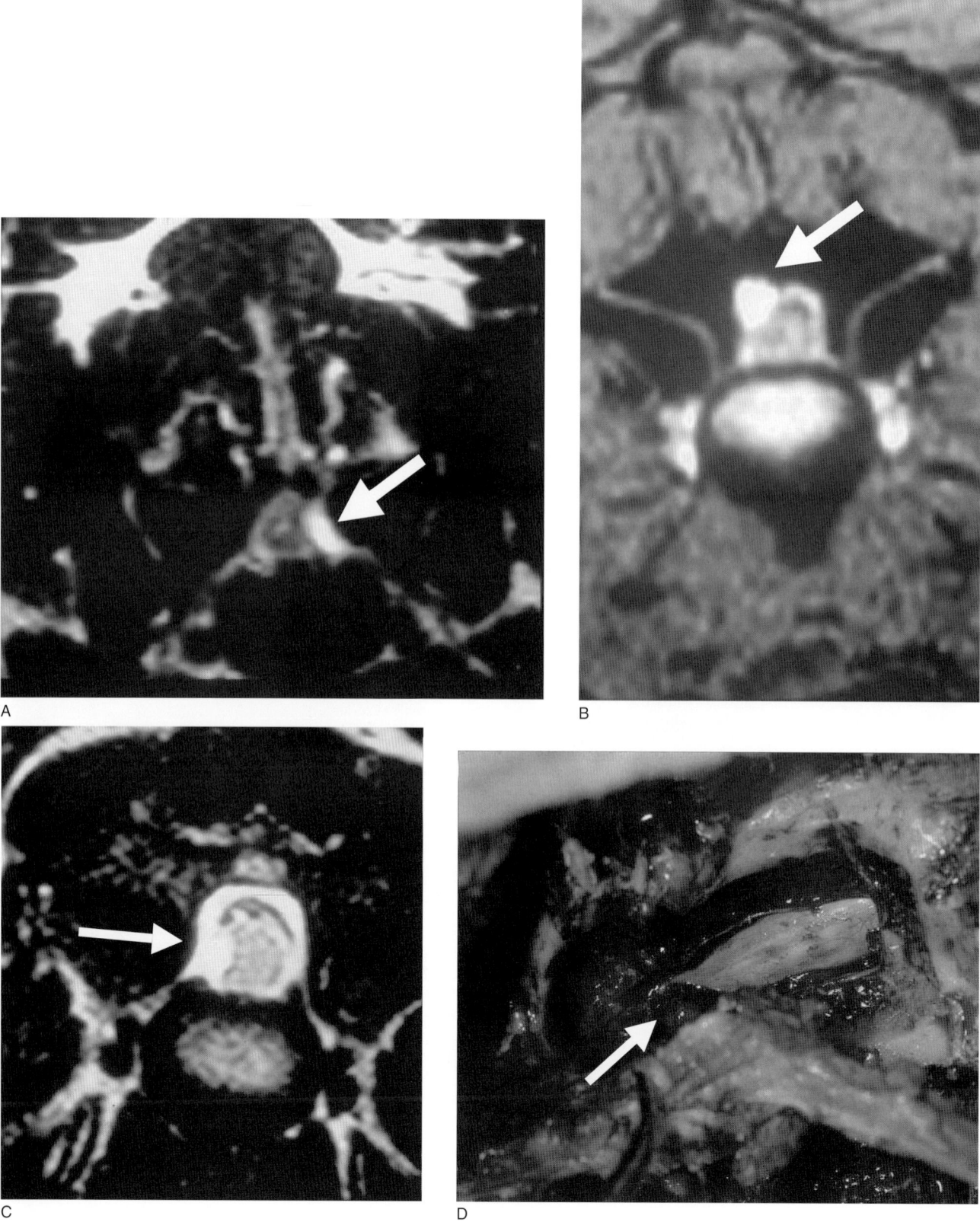

Figure 2.157.   Transverse T2-weighted MR images from two young large dogs ((A) and (B)) with a synovial cyst (arrows). Transverse T2-weighted MR images from a young large dog (C) with a synovial cyst (arrow). Appearance of the cyst (arrow) at surgery (D).

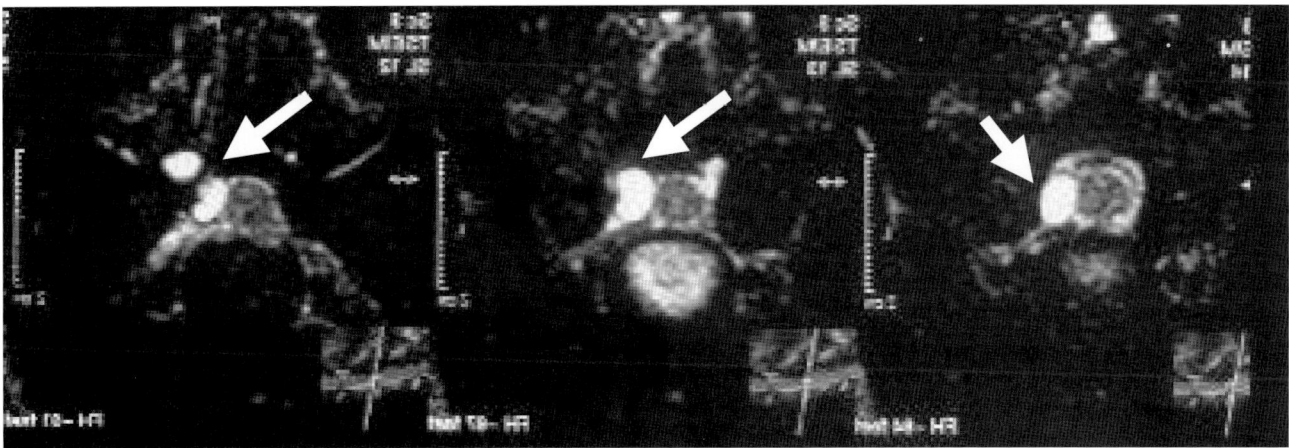

Figure 2.158.   Transverse T2-weighted MR images from a young large dog with multiple synovial cysts (arrows).

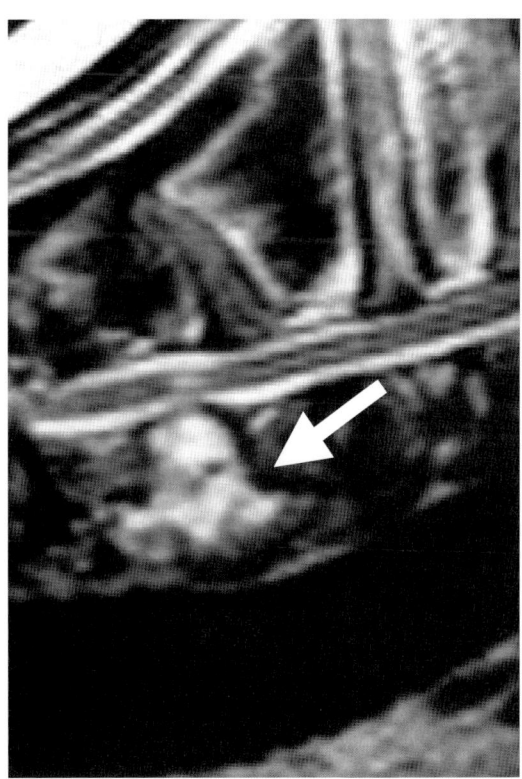

Figure 2.159.   Sagittal T2-weighted MR image from a large dog following a ventral slot (arrow).

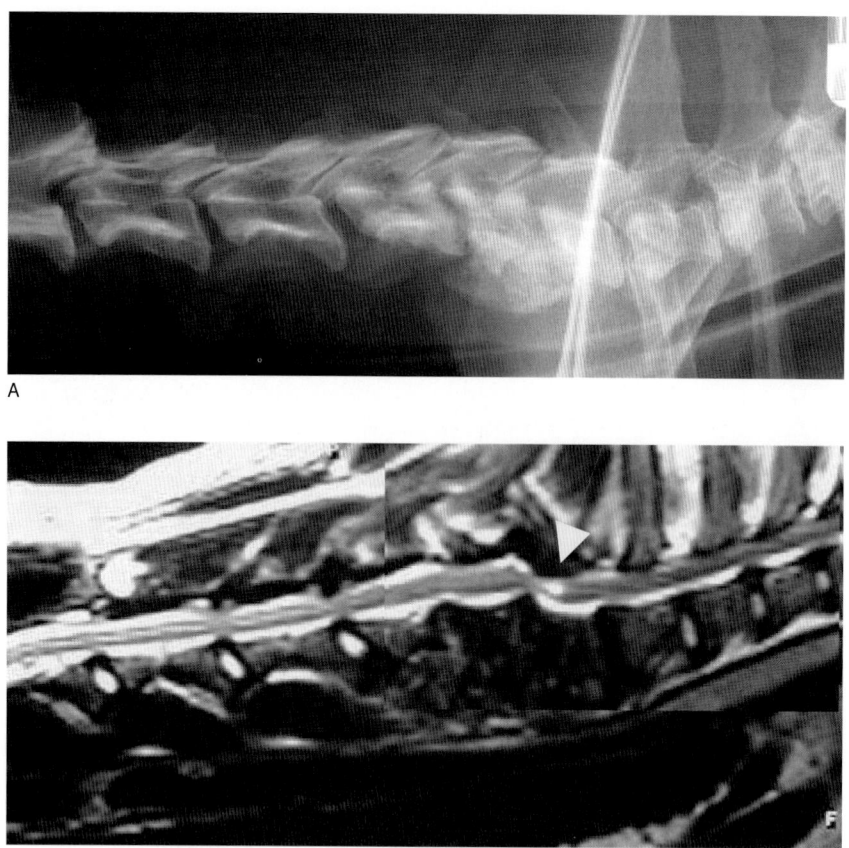

Figure 2.160. Lateral radiograph (A) and sagittal T2-weighted MR image (B) from a large dog following a failed ventral slot (arrow).

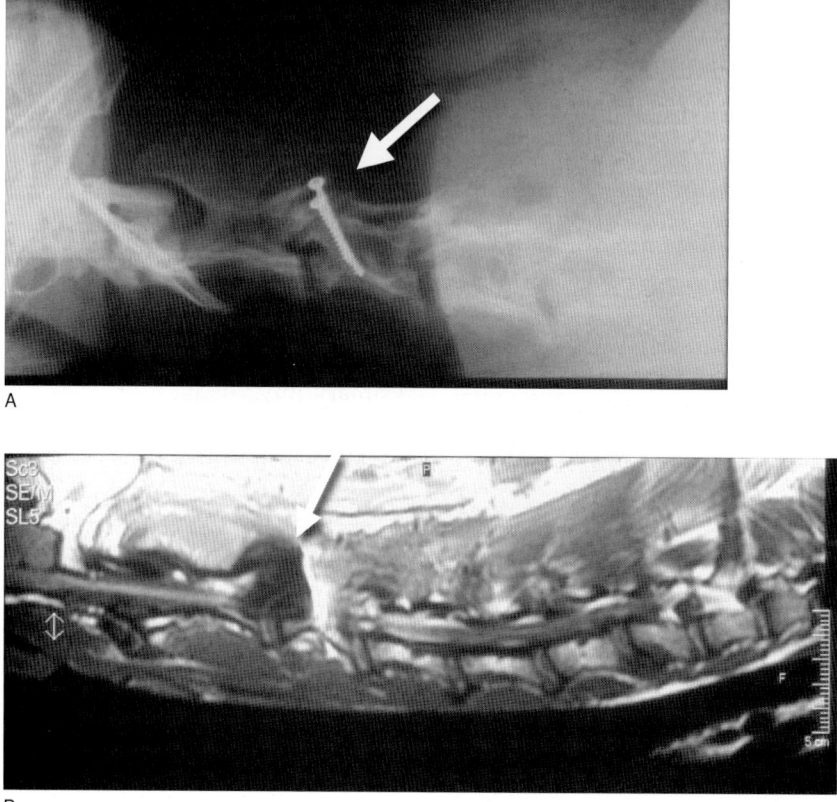

Figure 2.161. (A) Lateral radiographic view of a dog with metal surgical implants (cortical bone screws) through the C2-3 dorsal articular facets (arrow). (B) Sagittal T1-weighted MR image from the same dog showing metal artifact (arrow).

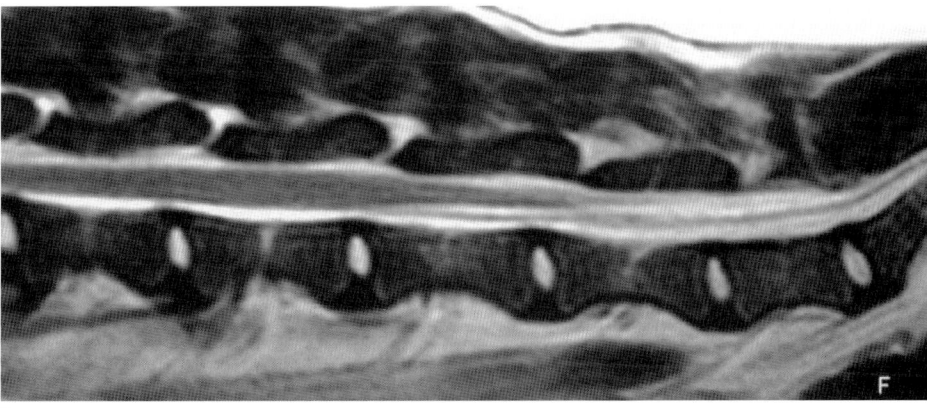

A

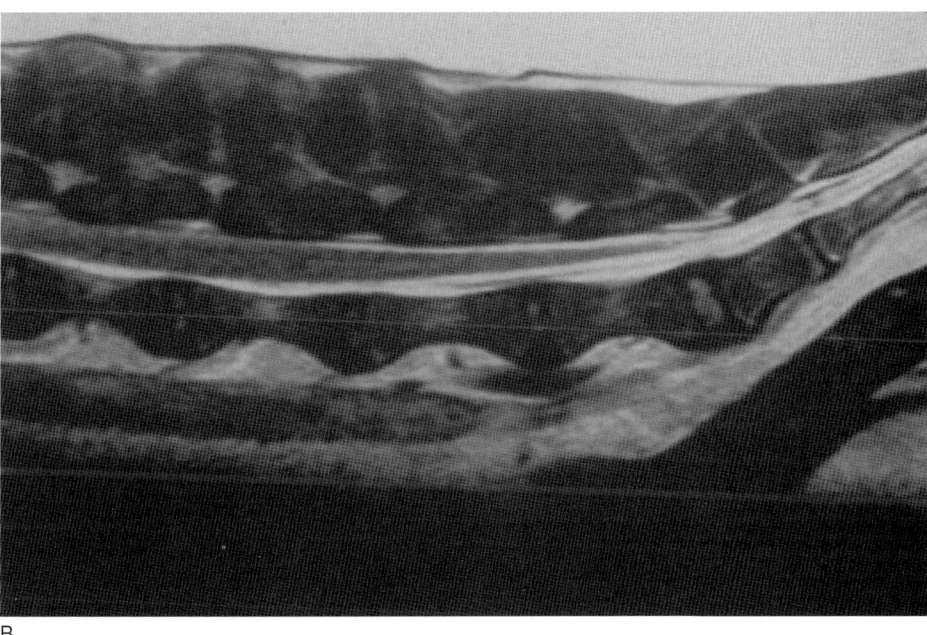

B

Figure 2.162. Sagittal T2-weighted MR images from two healthy dogs ((A) and (B)) with normal appearing LS articulations.

Lumbosacral Disease

Lumbosacral (LS) disease can occur as a congenital stenosis of the LS region or be acquired due to malarticulation, malformation, occult osteochondritis dessicans lesions, or, most commonly, IVD degeneration and protrusion. The associated spinal nerve compression usually affects the L7, sacral, and caudal nerve roots as these traverse through the LS area. Compression can result dorsally from the interarcuate ligament, or ventrally from the bulging or tearing of the annulus fibrosis. The L7 nerves are often also compressed from a ventral and lateral direction as they exit the vertebral canal at the intervertebral foramen from collapse of the foraminal area or secondary osteophyte production. Occasionally, other diseases such as neoplasia, fracture, or

diskospondylitis can result in LS nerve compression. Primary inflammation of these nerves (cauda equina neuritis) is rare.

MR imaging is often helpful in establishing disease of the LS region, especially as myelography is generally poor in establishing nerve compression in this region. Sagittal, parasagittal, and transverse plane images may be needed to determine the spectrum of compression present (Figures 2.162–2.167). Both parasagittal and transverse images allow for an assessment of the foraminal areas where exiting nerves are often compressed as well as the spinal cord and associated paraspinal vertebral, ligament, and joint structure. However, interpretation of these advanced imaging studies may be associated with both over- and underrepresentation of

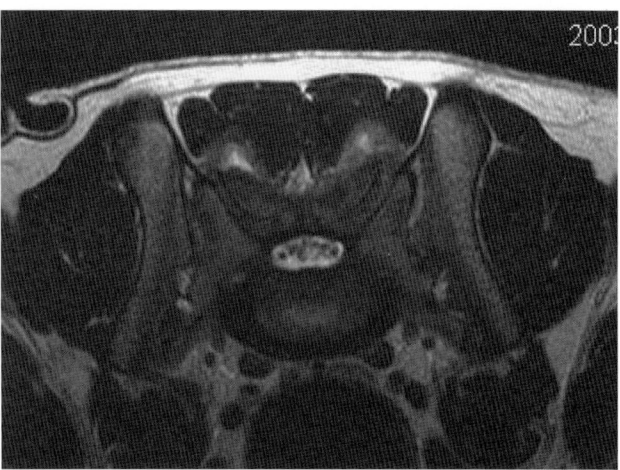

Figure 2.163. Transverse T2-weighted MR image from a healthy dog through the LS intervertebral articulation.

spinal and nerve compression. It is important in the diagnosis of LS disease, as with any disease, to correlate any imaging abnormality with the appropriate clinical signs.

With degenerative LS diseases, pathophysiologic alterations in vertebral units are similar to those described with "Wobbler's syndrome." Protruded LS IVD elements and hypertrophied ligamentous structures are usually hypointense in T2-weighted images. Alterations in the dorsal articular facet joints may show abnormal hyperintense alterations in T2-weighted images. It is more difficult, however, to determine foraminal alterations due to inconsistencies in slice plane angulation and level.

There is both clinical and radiological evidence that instability may exist in many instances of LS disease. Dynamic imaging studies of the LS joint tend to show that the LS joint is movable and that LS compression is worse in most instances when the joint is in a neutral or extended position as compared to a flexed position (Figure 2.168). We have had similar experiences when using MR imaging to image the LS articulation in various positions. Compression of the spinal cord is worsened when the animal's lower spine is dorsally extended, and improved when the spine is in a ventrally flexed position. Because of this dynamic compression, the position that the animal is placed in at the time of imaging study may influence the detection of any LS compression. Synovial cysts may be found associated with the dorsal LS articular joints (Figure 2.169). In some

instances, parasagittal as well as transverse flexed and extended MR views may show alterations in foraminal size in various positions (Figures 2.170 and 2.171).

Spondylosis Deformans/Ventral Bridging Spondylosis

Spondylosis deformans or ventral bridging spondylosis is commonly encountered on survey radiographic spinal evaluation in dogs. This bony proliferation is thought to be the result of an age-related, degenerative vertebral and paravertebral abnormality and most likely initiated by ventral extrusions or protrusions of IVD components. Spondylosis can be found at all vertebral levels. While it can be acquired in younger animals (disseminated skeletal hyperostosis), it is most often found in middle-aged to older dogs and cats. In cats, hypervitaminosis A results in severe spondylitic change in the vertebrae, usually affecting the cervical region.

In many older animals, spondylosis deformans is found incidentally on spinal MR evaluations (Figures 2.172 and 2.173). Spondylosis deformans may have either a hypointense or hyperintense signal in T2-weighted images. If spondylosis results secondarily to intervertebral disk disease, alterations in vertebral articulation resulting in pain may also occur. Additionally, spondylosis may extend into or around the intervertebral foramen and compress the exiting spinal nerves. In these instances, transverse spinal imaging with MR may reveal bony proliferation into or around exiting spinal nerve.

Dural Ossification

Ossification of the dura can occur in older animals, more commonly in the cervical area. A radiopaque, usually relatively thin, linear density is noted on radiographs in the area where the dura would normally be found. The pathologic significance of this radiographic finding is unknown, however, most feel that this abnormality is not associated with clinical signs of spinal or peripheral nerve disease. Occasionally, mineralized dura plaques will be adherent to the underlying spinal cord, which could result in a spinal cord abnormality. These focal dura mineralizations are rarely evident on survey spinal radiographs. Dural ossification has been difficult to determine with MR imaging if the lesion does not increase the size of the dura.

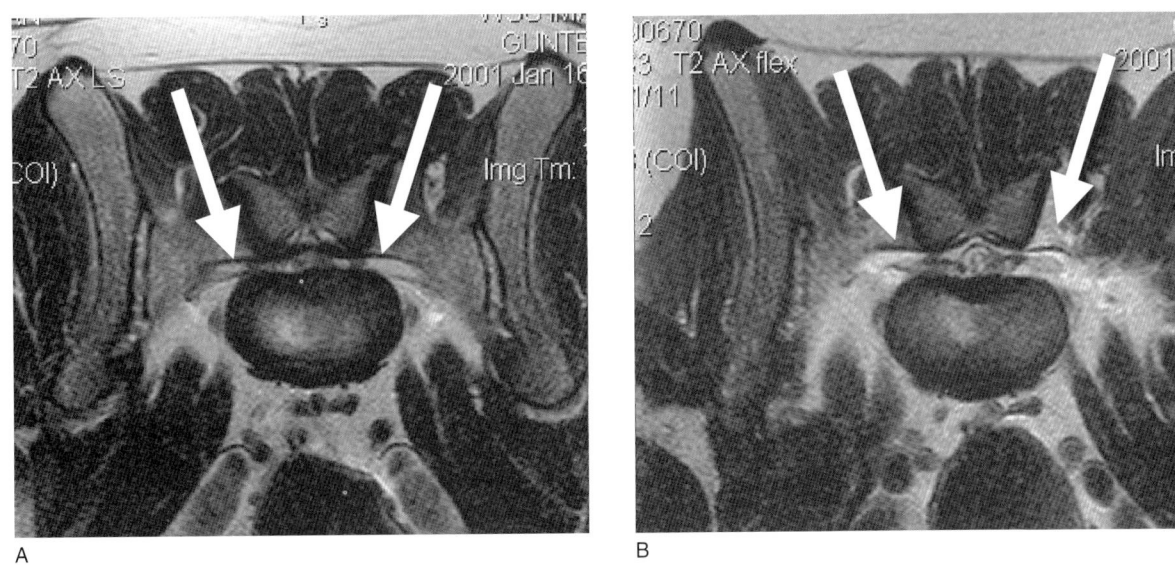

Figure 2.164. Transverse T2-weighted MR images from a healthy dog at immediately adjacent levels through the LS intervertebral foraminal region (arrows).

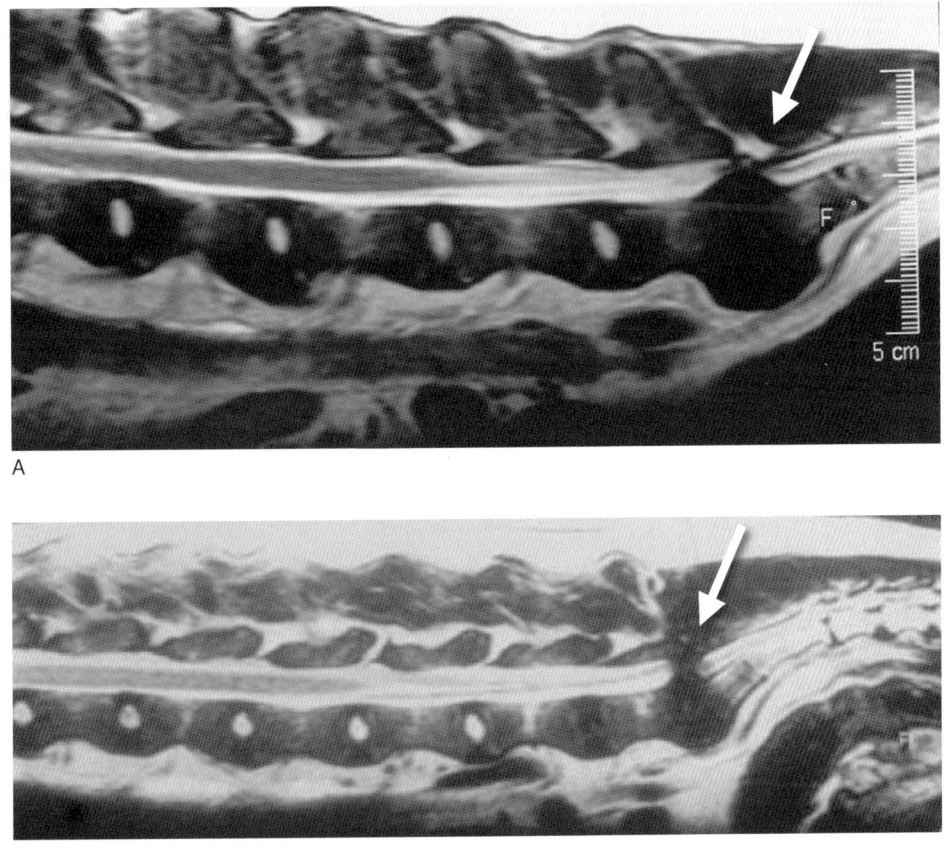

Figure 2.165. Sagittal T2-weighted MR images from six dogs (A)–(F) with LS disease showing a spectrum of MR abnormalities.

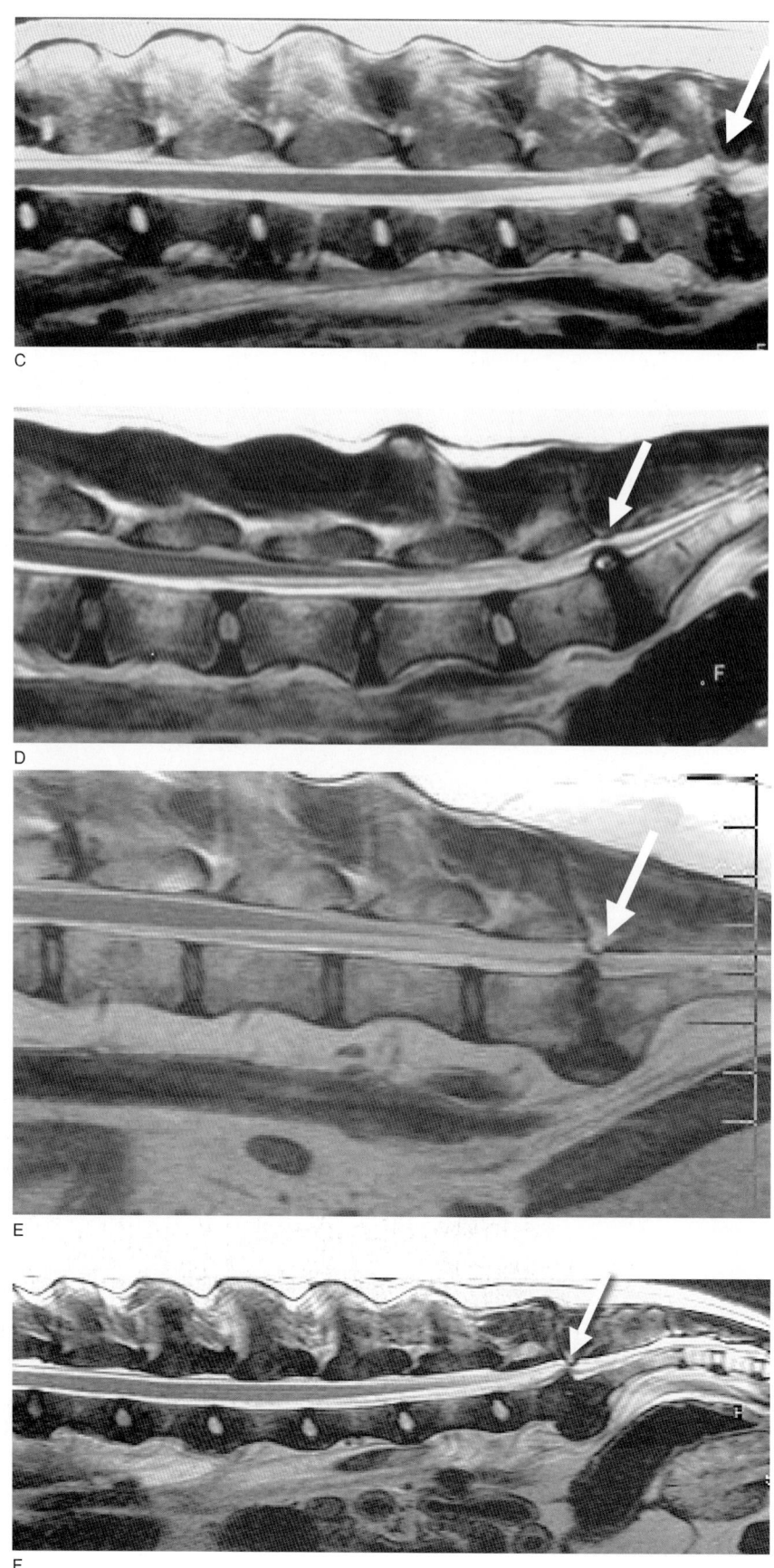

Figure 2.165. (*Continued*)

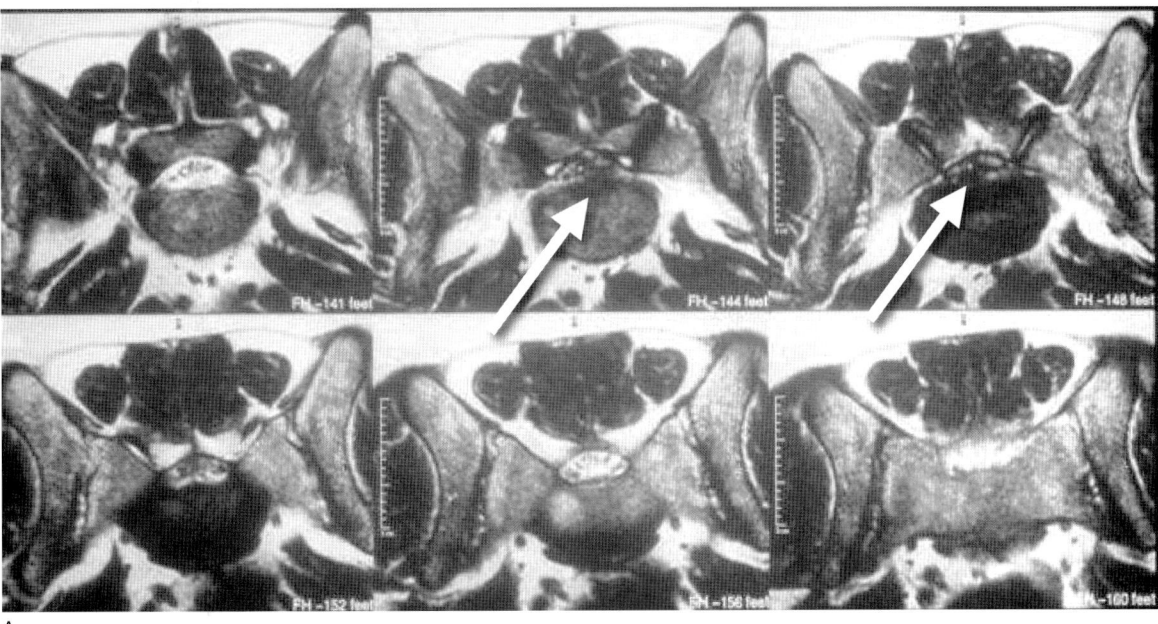

A

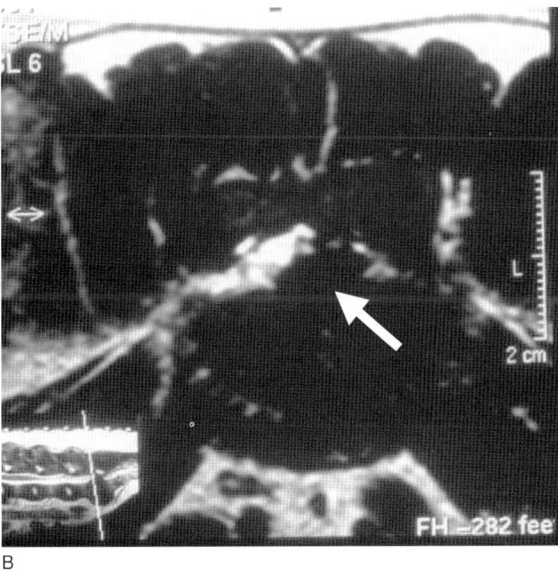

B

Figure 2.166. Transverse T2-weighted MR images from two dogs ((A) and (B)) with LS disease due to protrusion into the spinal canal of the intervertebral disk elements (arrows).

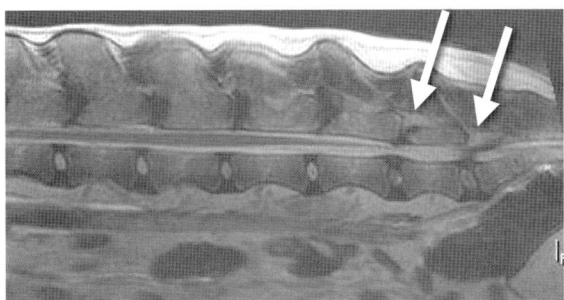

Figure 2.167. Sagittal T2-weighted MR image from a dog with spinal and nerve compression at both L6-7 and at the LS intervertebral disk levels.

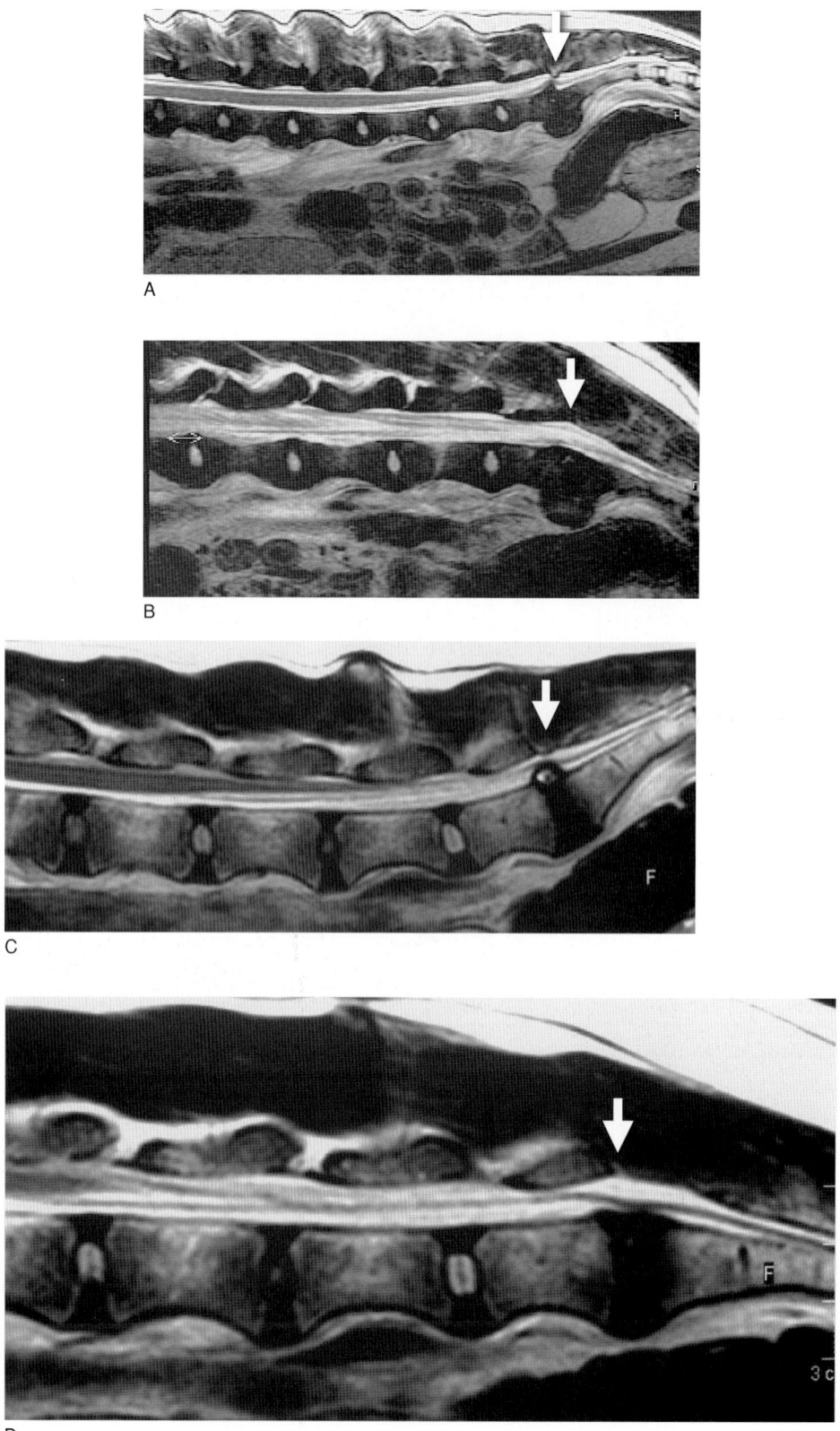

Figure 2.168. Sagittal T2-weighted MR images from four dogs ((A), (B); (C), (D);

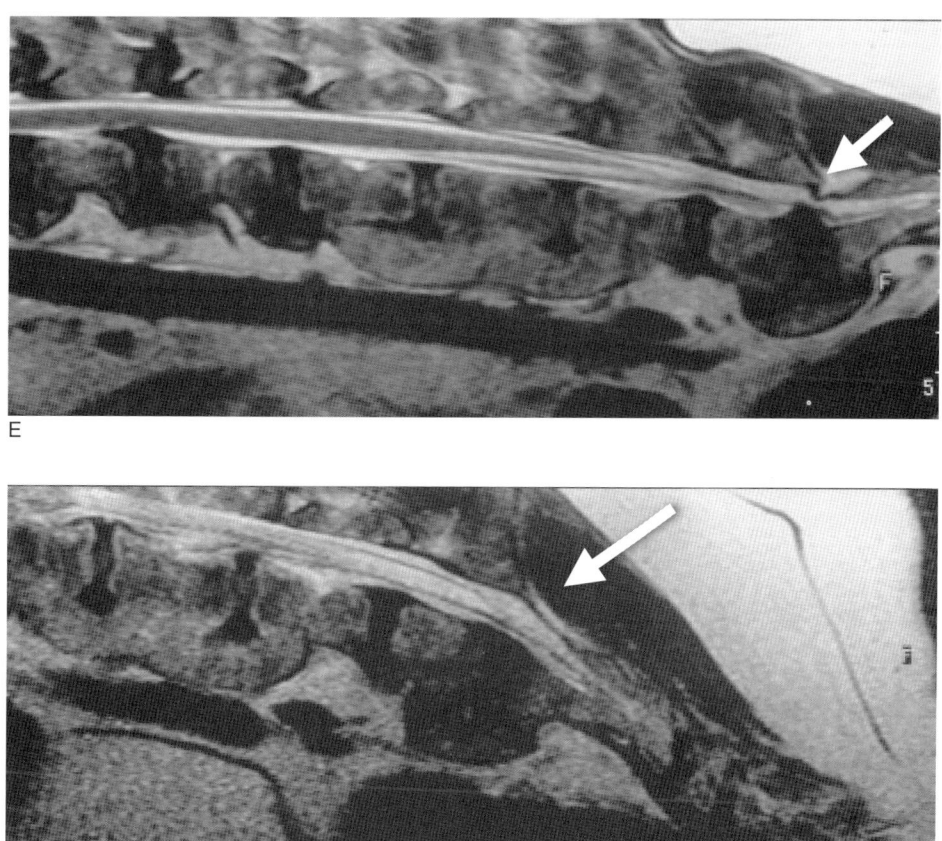

E

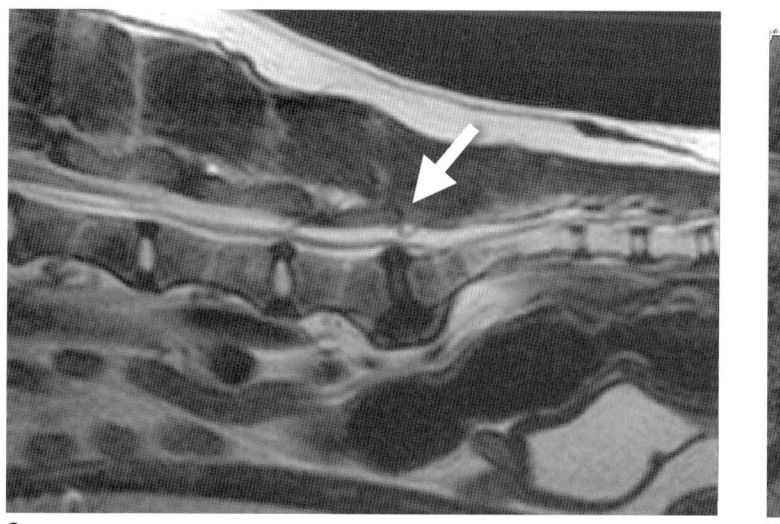

G

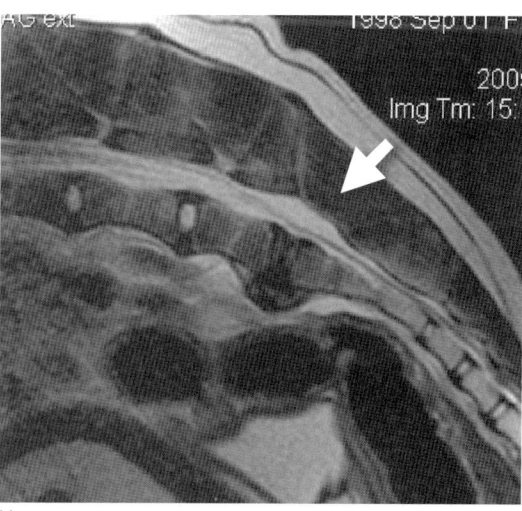

H

Figure 2.168. (*Continued*) (E), (F); and (G), (H)) with LS disease showing the degree of compression in a neutral ((A), (C), (E), and (G)) compared to a flexed ((B), (D), (F), and (H)) spine position (arrows).

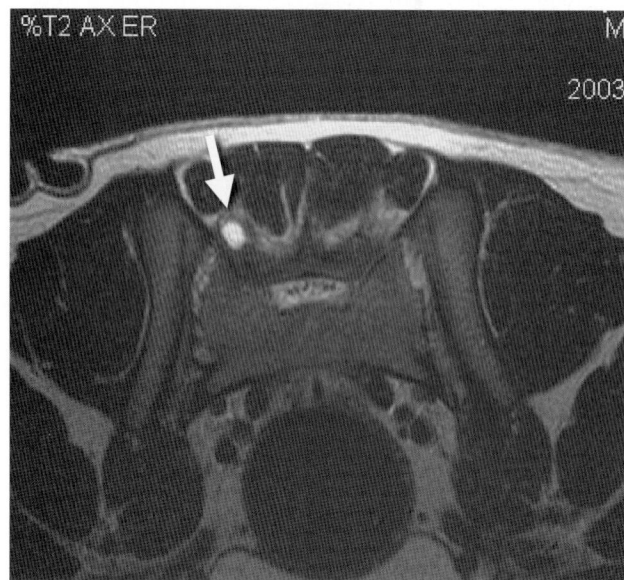

Figure 2.169. Transverse T2-weighted MR image from a dog with a synovial cyst of the dorsal L7-sacrum articulation (arrow).

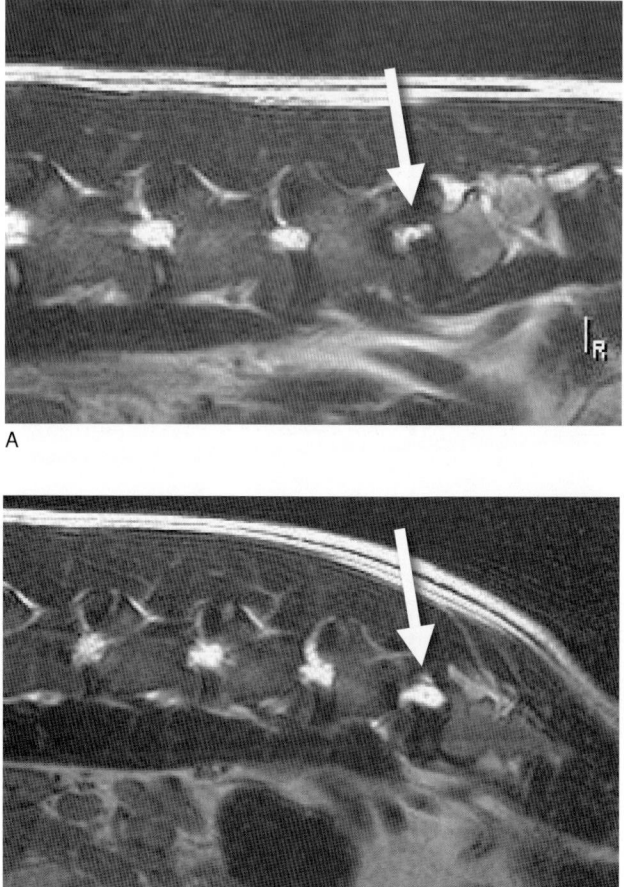

Figure 2.170. Parasagittal T2-weighted MR images from a dog with LS disease showing the intervertebral foramen in a neutral (A) compared to a flexed (B) spine position (arrows).

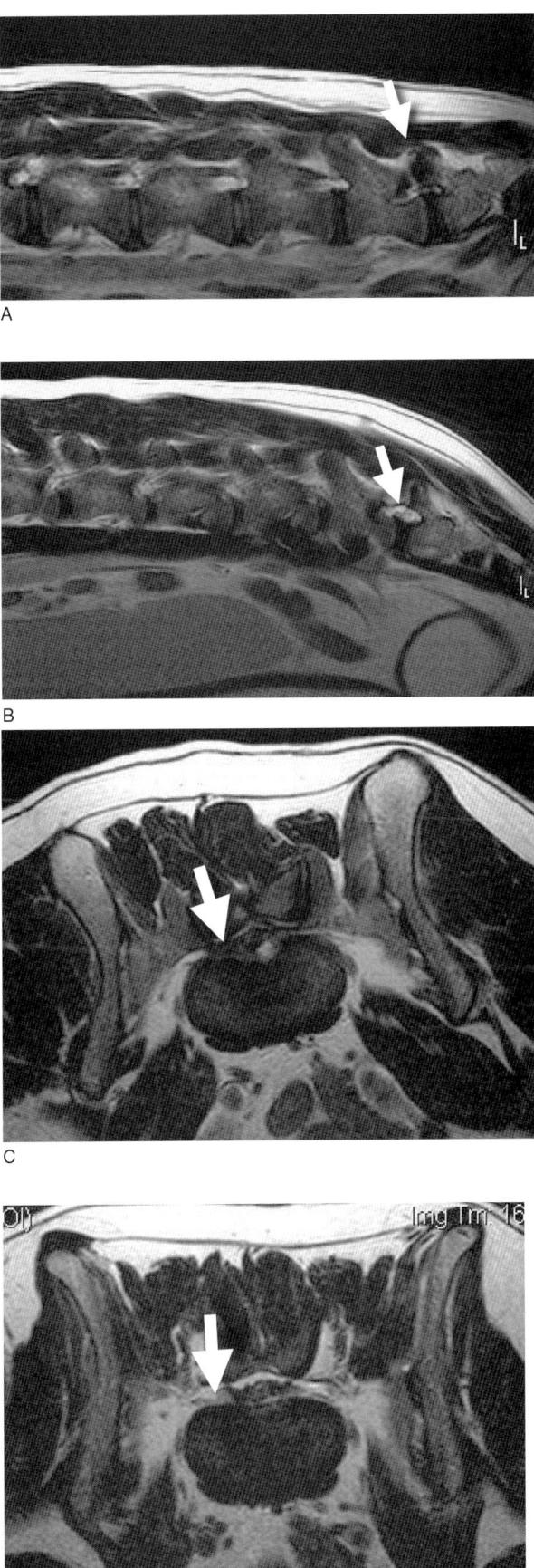

Figure 2.171. Parasagittal T2-weighted MR images from a dog with LS disease showing the intervertebral foramen in a neutral (A) compared to a flexed (B) spine position (arrows). Transverse T2-weighted MR images from the same dog in a neutral (C) compared to a flexed (D) spine position (arrows).

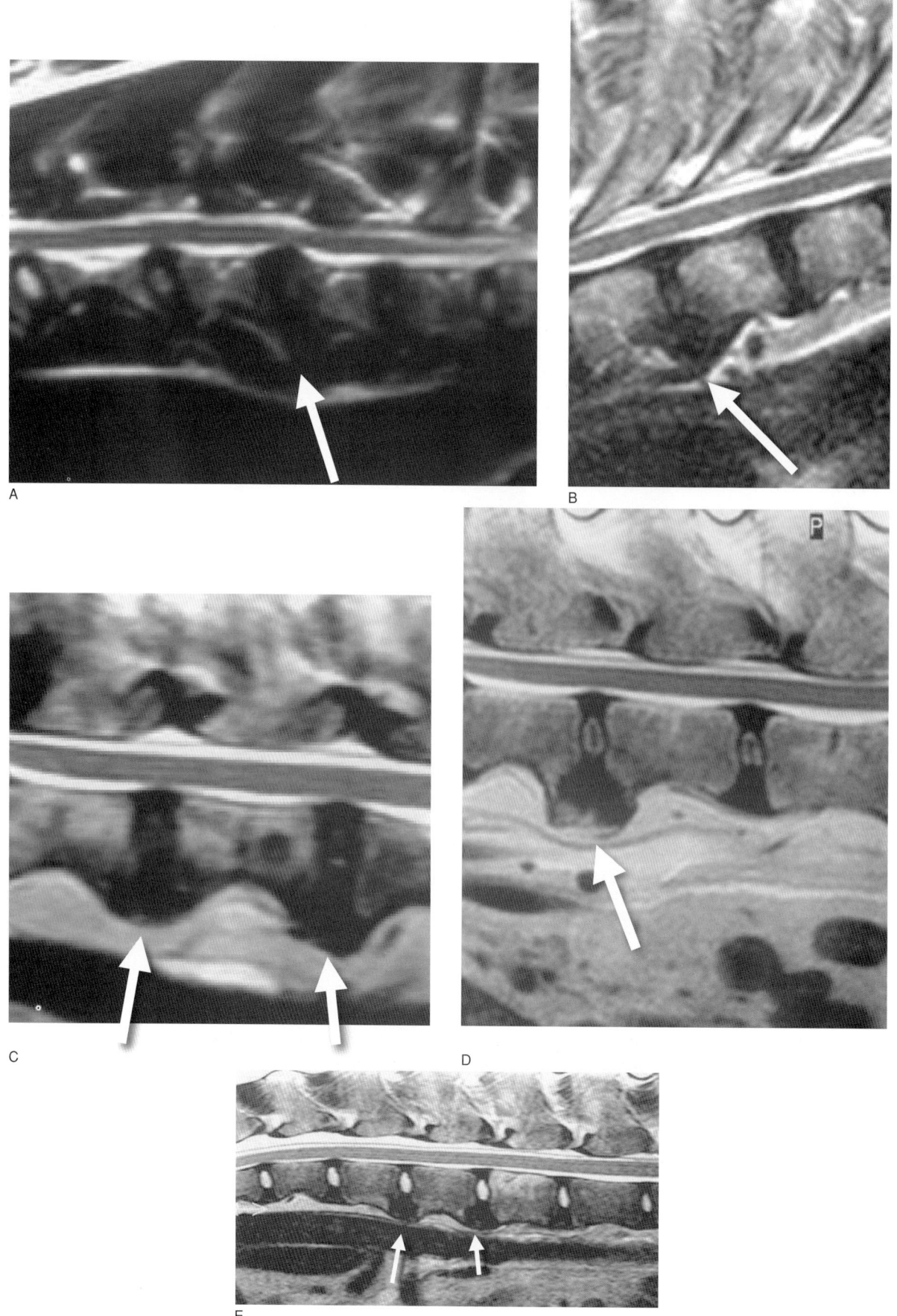

Figure 2.172. Sagittal T2-weighted MR images from five dogs with varying degrees of spondylosis deformans (arrows) in the cervical (A), thoracic (B), and lumbar (C)–(E) regions.

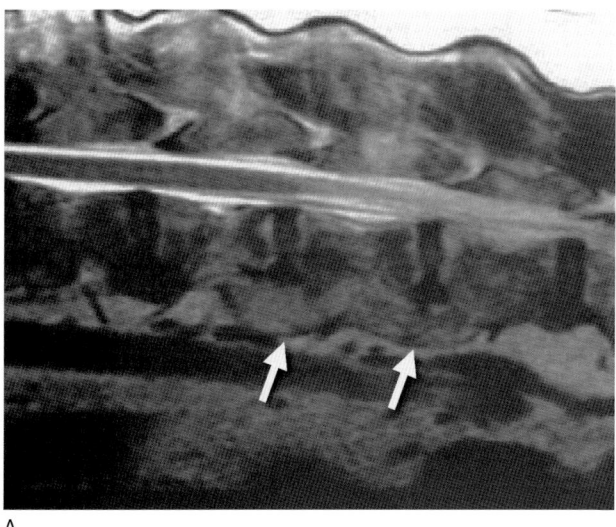
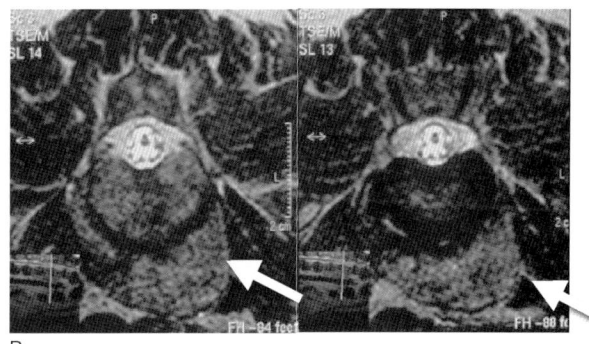

Figure 2.173. Sagittal (A) and transverse (B) T2-weighted MR images from a dog with spondylosis deformans (arrows).

Anomalous Diseases

A variety of spinal cord congenital abnormalities may involve the vertebrae, the meninges, or the spinal cord proper. Spina bifida is a failure of the dorsal aspect of the vertebrae to fuse during development. This may be seen on a dorsal ventral survey spinal radiograph as an ununited dorsal lamina and spinous process. A dorsal spinous process may also not be apparent on a survey radiograph in affected animals. Protrusion or adhesion of the meninges (meningocele), or meninges and spinal cord (meningomyelocele) through an associated vertebral defect may be seen with myelography but is best clarified with MR imaging. Myelography may show communication of these meningeal structures with the spinal cord. Myelodysplasia or abnormal spinal cord development is best evaluated with MR imaging. Abnormalities of the normal spinal architecture usually result in a distortion of the anatomical appearance of the spinal cord. Often, on T2-weighted imaging sequences, the spinal cord contains abnormal hyperintense regions suggesting increases in fluid, malacia, or possibly, hemorrhage (Figures 2.174–2.176).

Vertebral abnormalities such as hemivertebrae, block vertebrae, or transitional vertebrae are often evident on survey radiographs. These abnormalities result in abnormally shaped vertebrae. Vertebral defects may result in malalignment of the vertebral segments with associated scoliosis, kyphosis, or lordosis. Spinal cord compression is only determined with myelography, CT, or MR imaging. Associated spinal cord defects such as myelodysplasia or syringomyelia are most obviously evident on spinal MR imaging as distortions of normal

spinal cord architecture. In instances where the spine is permanently deviated, proper alignment of the patient for MR imaging may be difficult and subsequently affect image quality by creating positional artifacts. CSF may be normal or contain nonspecific increases in protein, nucleated cell counts, or both.

Rhodesian ridgeback dogs, and occasionally other breeds of dogs such as Shih tzus, Yorkshire terriers, and boxers, have a congenital connection from the spinal cord to the skin referred to as a dermoid sinus. This is with the result of failure of separation of the skin from underlying tissues during closure of the neural tube. The characteristic unusual hair pattern on the dorsal neck and back of Rhodesian ridgeback dogs is a reflection of the defect, however, this abnormality does not always connect to the spinal cord. Dermoid sinus may appear as small indentations or openings in the skin. In some instances, fluid will be present from the abnormal skin area with an associated dermatitis. Dermoid sinuses usually occur on midline in the cervical, thoracic, or sacrococcygeal regions. MR imaging is used for diagnosis of spinal cord involvement with this disease (Figure 2.177).

Scoliosis

Scoliosis is usually evident on physical evaluation. Survey radiographs of the affected spinal areas confirm the lateral deviation of the vertebral column. This deviation is often associated with abnormalities of the vertebral structures. The vertebrae may be misshapen and

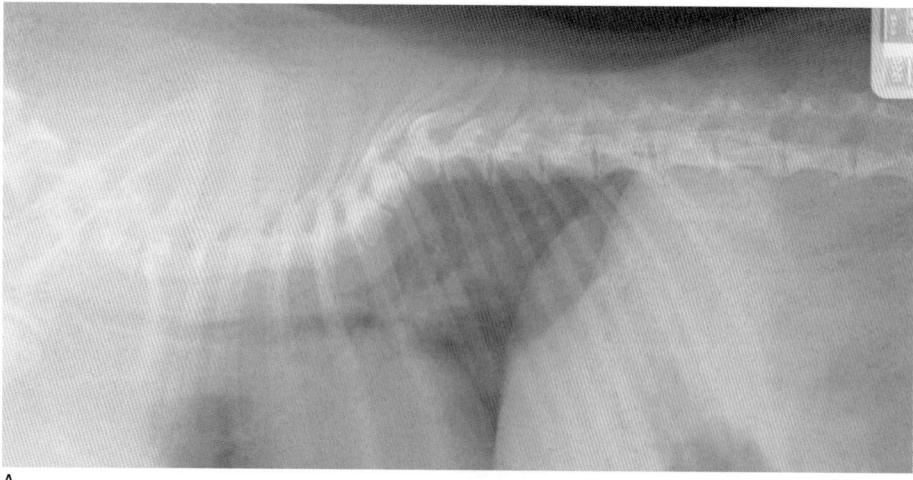

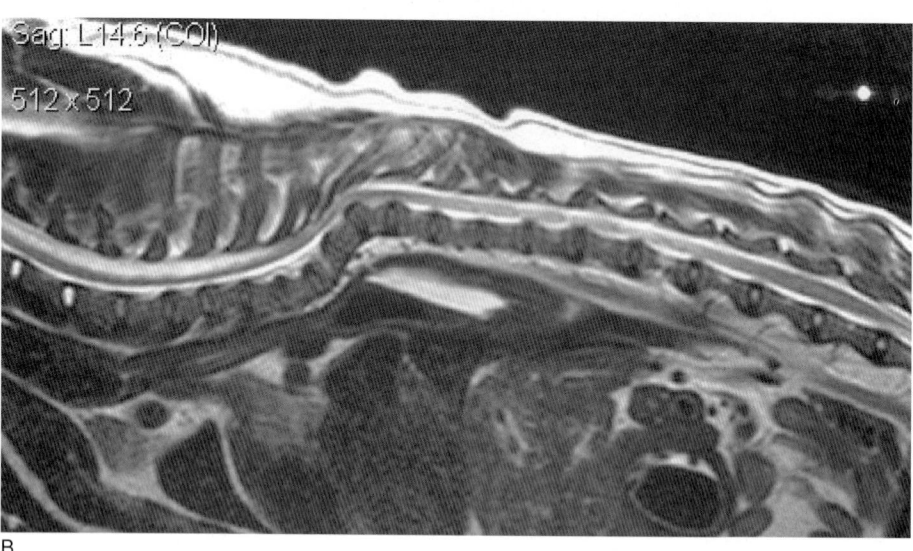

Figure 2.174. Lateral radiograph (A) and sagittal, T2-weighted MR image (B) from a dog with hemivertebrae and kyphosis.

irregular in appearance and contour. In animals that are still growing, abnormalities of the growth plates may be present. However, these vertebrae may not be inherently misshapen, but may develop abnormally due to abnormal forces being placed on the vertebral unit from the pressures associated with spinal bending.

Scoliosis has most commonly been associated with intramedullary cystic spinal lesions such as syringomyelia and hydromyelia in dogs. Evaluation for underlying spinal cord defects in association with scoliosis is most accurately performed with MR spinal evaluations. With MR imaging, the lateral deviation of the vertebral column may make it difficult to achieve acceptable positioning for sagittal imaging. This may create positional artifacts in the images produced. Electromyography of the paraspinal muscles may show abnormal spontaneous activity suggesting denervation of these muscles. CSF may be normal or reveal nonspecific

alterations such as increases in protein concentration, nucleated cells, or both.

Atlantoaxial Subluxation

Atlantoaxial (AA) instability occurs in numerous, usually small, but occasionally large, dog breeds. Yorkshire terriers, Chihuahuas, Lhasa Apsos, and Pomeranians are most often affected. Other breeds affected include the Japanese Chin, toy poodle, Pekingese, Rottweiler, and Doberman pinscher. This disease is occasionally reported in cats.

This disease is most often the result of some degree of abnormal articulation between the C1 and C2 vertebrae. This abnormal articulation may be the result of exogenous trauma with either fracture of the occiput, axis, or atlas, or disruption of the atlantooccipital ligaments. There may also be a congenital abnormality

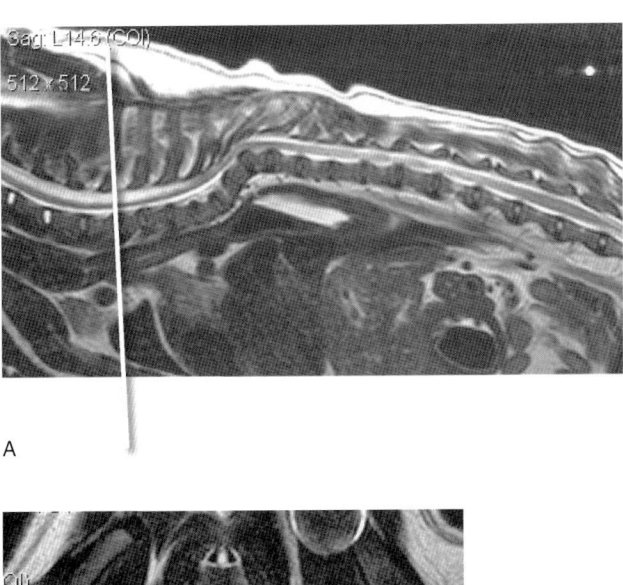

A

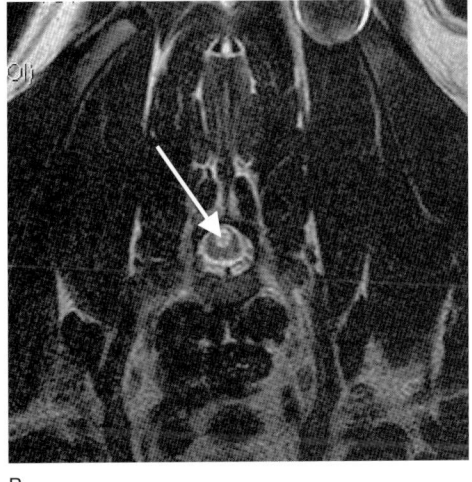

B

Figure 2.175. Sagittal (A) and transverse (B) T2-weighted MR images from the same dog as in Figure 2.174. The line shows the level of the transverse section. The transverse image shows the associated cystic abnormality of the spinal cord (arrow).

of the ligamentous or bony structures associated with this articulation. Various degrees of ligamentous and joint capsule abnormalities may be present. The ventral, cranial aspect of C2 forming the caudal articulation of

this joint is also commonly malformed. Many of these ligamentous abnormalities are assumed to affect the stability of the odontoid process or dens. AA instability may also be associated with an abnormally shaped or

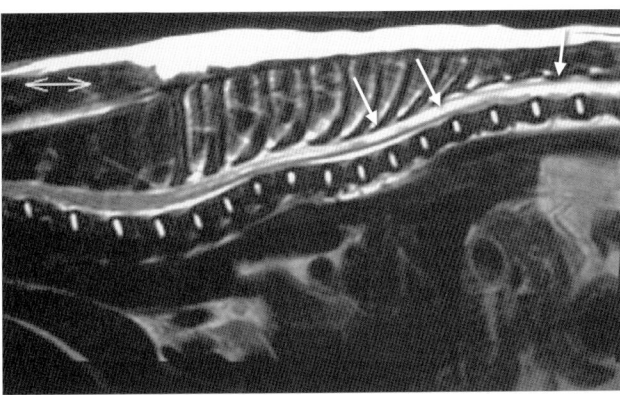

Figure 2.176. Sagittal T2-weighted MR image from a dog with kyphosis and syringomyelia (arrows).

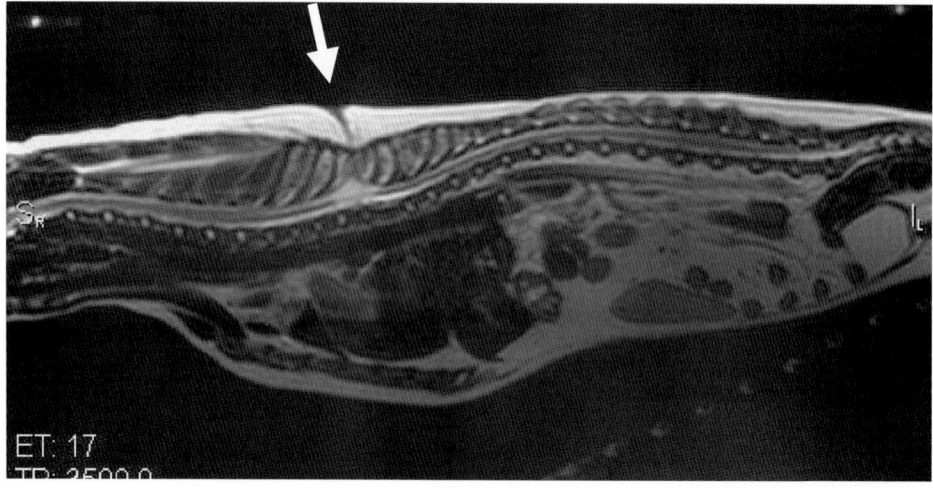

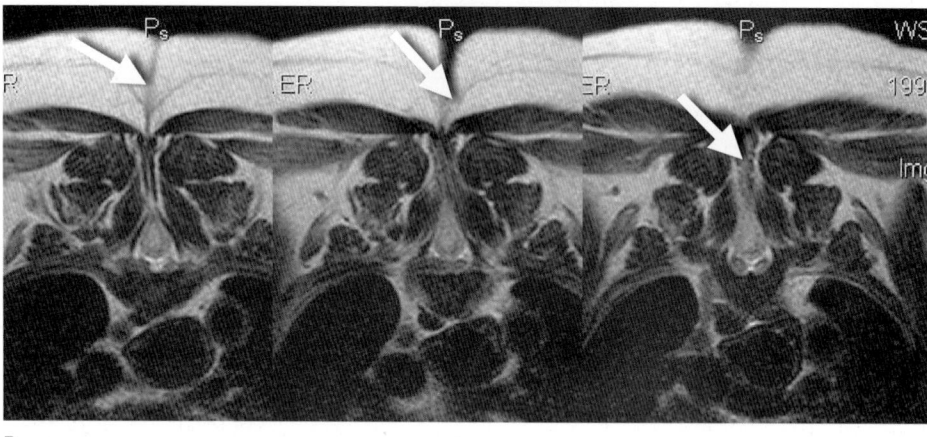

Figure 2.177. Sagittal (A) and transverse (B) T2-weighted MR images from a dog with a dermoid sinus (arrows).

absent dens. In some instances, there is a fracture of the dens. In still other cases, the dens is present but abnormally angulated in a dorsal direction to compress the spinal cord. Clinical signs result from spinal cord compression or alterations in spinal cord blood flow. As this abnormality results in vertebral instability, spinal cord compression may be dynamic depending on the position of the head.

The diagnosis of AA instability is supported by demonstrating an increased distance (greater than a few millimeters) between the dorsal aspects of C1 and C2 when viewed on a lateral survey radiograph. Flexion of the neck may exacerbate the radiographic features, but may also exacerbate clinical signs so should be performed cautiously if not minimally. AA instability may also be associated with an abnormal or absent odontoid process, which also may be evident on survey radiographs. Assessment for associated spinal cord compression or spinal cord parenchymal abnormalities

is most accurately determined with MR imaging (Figure 2.178). Syringomyelia is surprisingly common in association with AA instability and may contribute to any associated clinical signs of spinal cord dysfunction. Imaging of the spinal cord with MR is the most accurate way to determine the presence of syringomyelia (Figure 2.179).

Syringomyelia and Hydromyelia

With the increased utilization of MR imaging for evaluation of animals with CNS disease, syringomyelia and hydromyelia are relatively common encountered spinal cord disease processes. Syringomyelia refers to abnormal cavities filled with fluid in the substance of the spinal cord. A syrinx refers to one of these cavities. Hydromyelia refers to a pathologic condition characterized by accumulation of fluid within an enlarged central canal of the spinal cord. In both of these instances, the

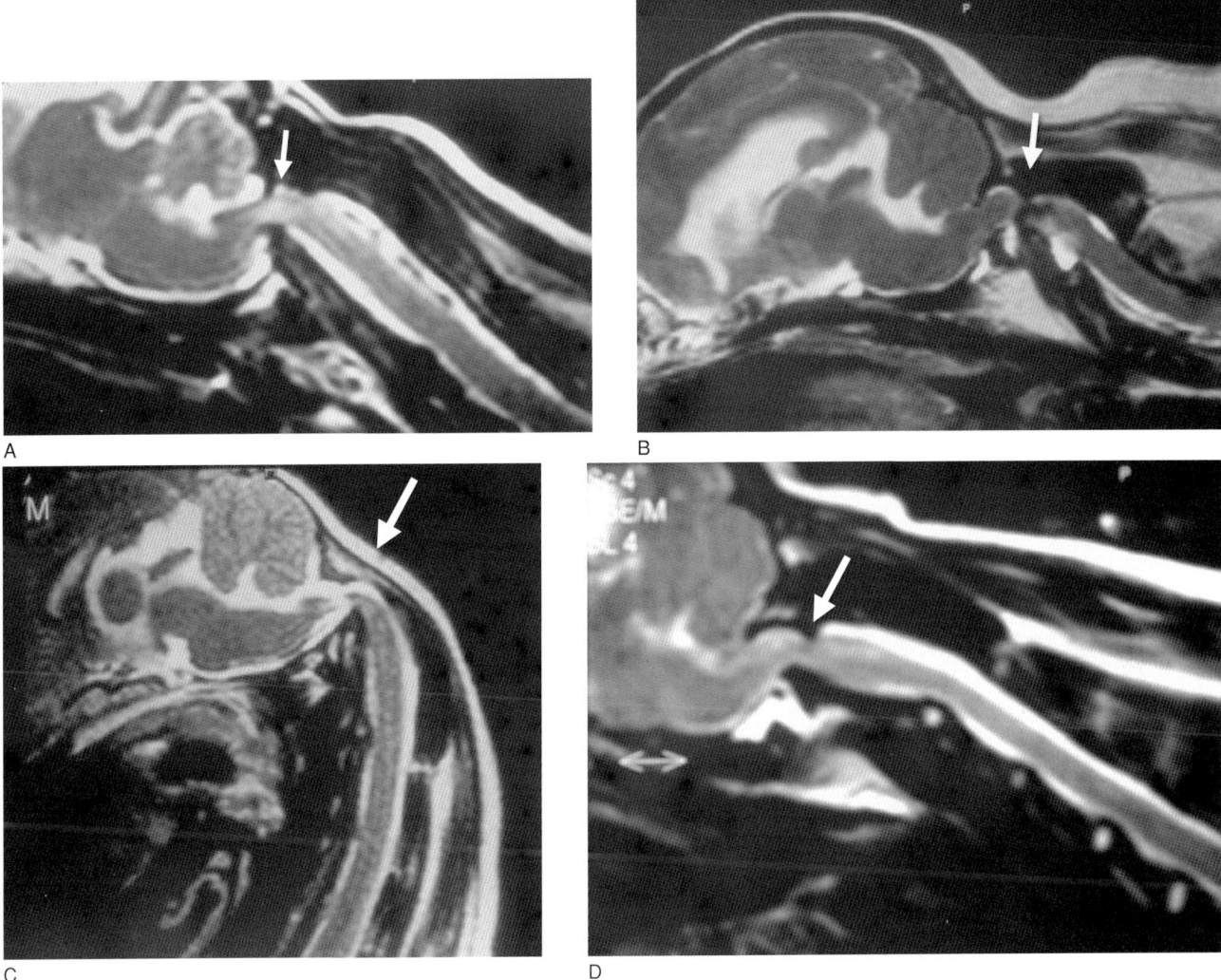

Figure 2.178. Sagittal T2-weighted MR images from four dogs (A)–(D) with varying degrees of AA instability/subluxation (arrows).

fluid that accumulates is similar, if not identical, to CSF. Some authors refer to hydromyelia as a communicating syringomyelia and use the term "syringomyelia" to describe all intraspinal abnormal fluid accumulations.

Clinically and diagnostically, it is often difficult to differentiate between syringomyelia and hydromyelia. Therefore, the term "syringo-/hydromyelia" is used. Ultimately, the diagnosis is made at a histologic evaluation. The fluid cavity within the spinal cord in hydromyelia is lined by ependymal cells characteristic of the central canal. A syringomyelic cavity, on the other hand, is located within the spinal cord external to the central canal and is lined by glial cells. Again, in many instances, these pathologic processes occur concurrently.

Malformations of the foramen magnum and infratentorial anatomical relationships (Chiari malformations) are frequently associated with both hydrocephalus and syringo-/hydromyelia in dogs. Obstruction of CSF flow at the foramen magnum and alterations in CSF pressure seem to be the primary mechanisms of these pathologic changes. Similar abnormalities may occur in dogs and other animals. Intracranial abnormalities resulting in hydrocephalus and a dilated fourth ventricle may also be associated with syringomyelia. The Dandy–Walker syndrome is one such example. With this disease there is a malformation of the cerebellum resulting in a cyst-like abnormality in the cerebellum. The lateral and third ventricles are commonly concurrently dilated. This is a congenital problem assumed to be associated with abnormal embryogenesis. Examples of a similar syndrome have been described in dogs and other animals. Spinal cord abnormalities have not been historically described. However, the spinal cords of affected

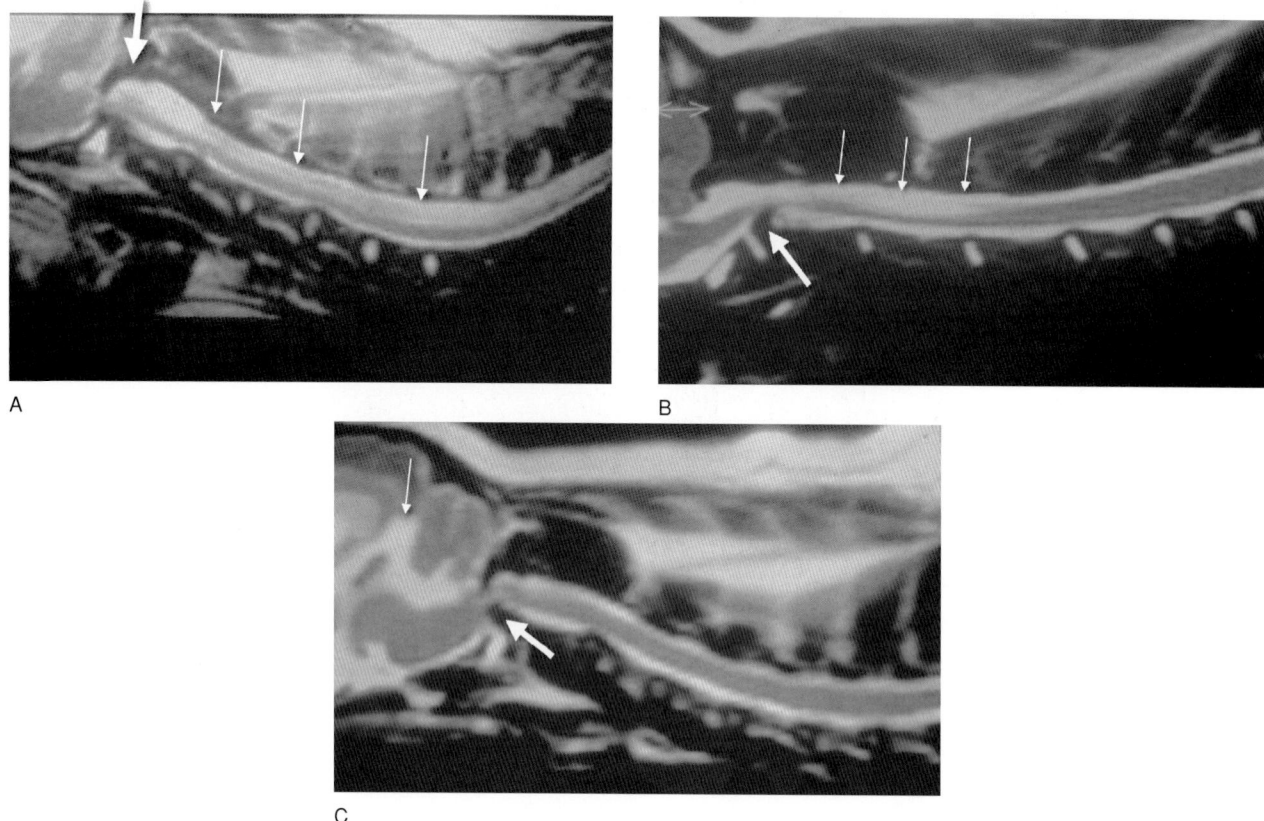

Figure 2.179. Sagittal T2-weighted MR images from three dogs with varying degrees of AA instability/subluxation (larger arrows) and associated syringomyelia ((A) and (B)) (larger arrows) and excessive CSF in the corpora quadgeminal region (C) (smaller arrow).

animals may not have been examined pathologically. Interestingly, a number of dogs and humans with syringomyelia have associated scoliosis (see above under scoliosis).

Syringomyelia is not apparent on survey spinal radiographic evaluation and usually also not apparent on myelography. If during myelography, contrast enters or is injected into the central canal of the spinal cord, hydromyelia may be evident. While this is sometimes attributed to the force of the injection, the enlarged central canal is usually present prior to the injection. That is, the injection is not the cause of the central canal dilation. If syringomyelia is associated with scoliosis, vertebral deviation may be evident on survey spinal radiographs.

MR imaging is the "gold standard" diagnostic test for detection of these spinal intramedullary processes (Figures 2.179–2.183). These cavities are hyperintense or whiter regions compared to the spinal cord in T2-weighted MR images shown, while in T1-weighted MR images these cavities are hypointense or blacker compared to the spinal cord. Often these cavities are more conspicuous with T2-weighted images, but the actual borders of the cavity with the associated spinal cord

parenchyma may be indistinct. MR images of the caudal brain stem and cerebellum (infratentorial area) should be performed in any animal with syringomyelia as associated abnormalities of this portion of the nervous system and foramen magnum region are commonly associated with this disease process (Figures 2.184–2.193).

CSF may be normal or reveal nonspecific alterations such as increases in protein concentration, nucleated cells, or both. If syringomyelia results secondary to myelitis, more obvious evidence of inflammatory CNS disease may be found. CSF should be collected with caution or not at all from the cisterna magna region of animals with syringomyelia as the associated anatomical abnormalities may result in an increased potential for iatrogenic nervous system injury from misplaced needle penetration.

Arachnoid Cysts

Spinal arachnoid cysts have been reported with increasing frequency in dogs. The term "arachnoid cyst" is misleading as there are extramedullary expansion and cord cavitation rather than cyst formation. Additionally,

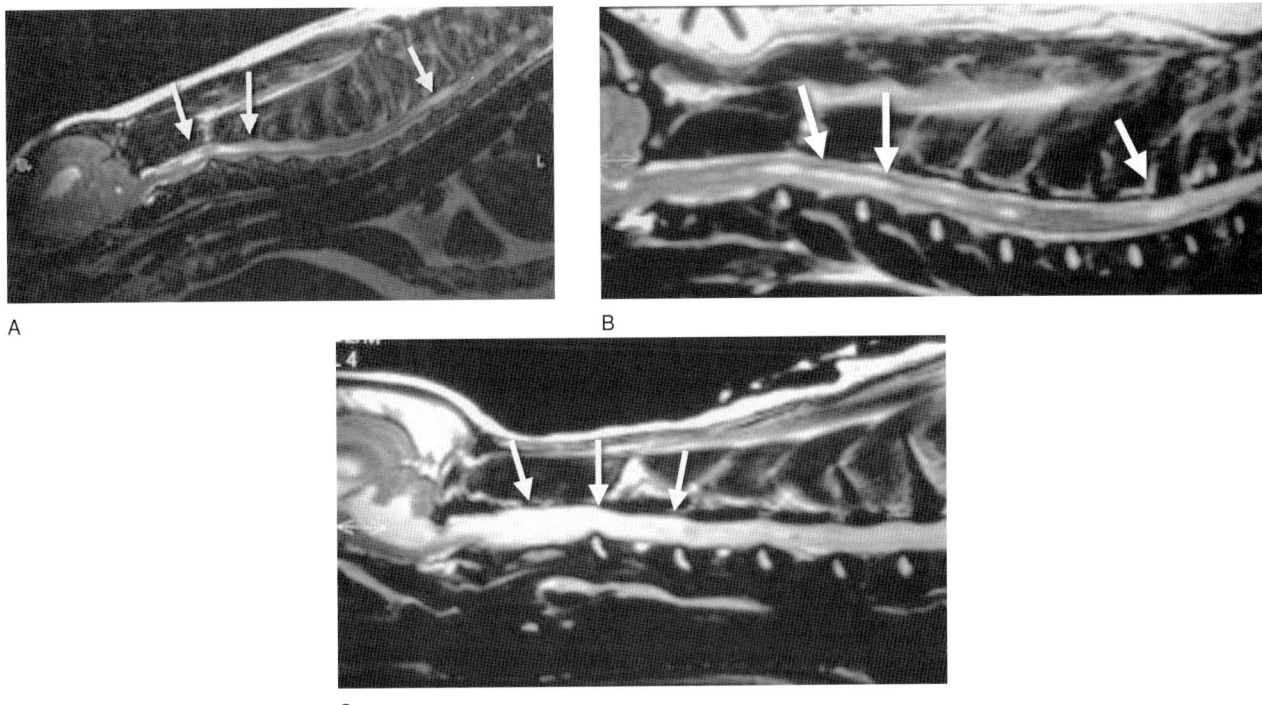

Figure 2.180. Sagittal T2-weighted MR images from three dogs (A)–(C) with syringomyelia (arrows). In dog (C), the spinal cord contains diffuse edema, an early stage of syringomyelia.

there is no epithelial lining to the cyst. A congenital etiology for lesion is most likely, although trauma has been implicated as a potential cause in both human beings and dogs. Scarring and local inflammation of the pia or other meninges may result in the creation of pockets of CSF accumulation. These cystic cavities may expand with each heartbeat and with respirations due to alteration in intracystic pressures. It is also possible that abnormal subarachnoid CSF dynamics contribute to cyst formation.

Arachnoid cysts are not apparent on survey spinal radiographs. Classically, an arachnoid cyst appears as a teardrop-shaped expansile abnormality of the dorsal, or occasionally ventral or lateral, subarachnoid space on myelography. With CT or MR, a similar expansile, fluid-filled structure with a teardrop shape (on a sagittal view) is seen (Figures 2.194–2.199). With MR, this cystic structure is hypointense (darker) and hyperintense (whiter) relative to the spinal cord parenchyma on T1- and T2-weighted MR sequences, respectively. CSF may be normal or reveal nonspecific alterations associated with increases in protein concentration, nucleated cells, or both. Surgical biopsy confirms the type of abnormality present.

We have seen a number of Pug dogs with focal cystic abnormalities of the dorsal and lateral subarachnoid space. Lesions are usually in the thoracolumbar area of the spinal cord, and may be in a location dorsal to an area of chronic disk protrusion. Clinical signs are reflective of a thoracolumbar myelopathy with progressive paraparesis. Interestingly, a number of affected animals with spinal cord scarring, arachnoid cysts, or other focally cystic spinal cord abnormalities have fecal incontinence as a predominant presenting complaint. In many of these dogs, the gross appearance of the lesion is that of a focal cicatrix or scarring involving the pia mater and subarachnoid structures. Fibrous adhesion to the spinal cord is common. In some instances, these abnormalities resemble arachnoid cysts and may, in fact, be a variant of this disease. It is also possible that some arachnoid cysts are actually the result of arachnoid and pial scarring, adhesion, and fibrosis from an inflammatory or chronic irritation etiology. Diagnosis has been made with MR imaging to reveal the location and characteristics of these lesions and surgical biopsy of the offending tissue.

Neoplasia

Spinal neoplasms are often categorized initially by the anatomical area, in relation to the dura and spinal cord, of spinal involvement. Tumors are grouped into those primarily arising from an extradural location (extradural), within the dura but outside the spinal cord

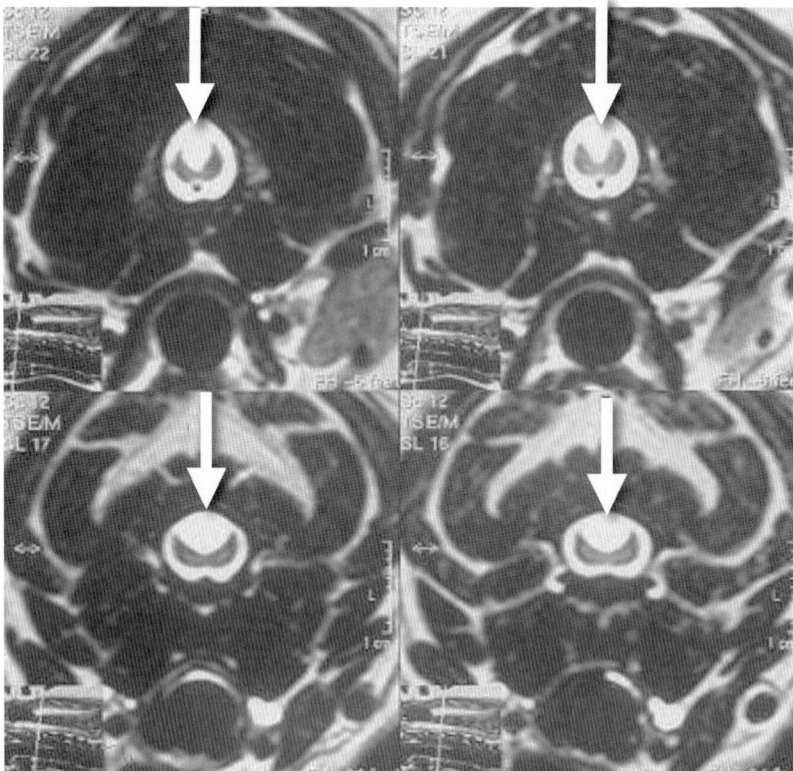

Figure 2.181. Transverse T2-weighted MR images from immediately adjacent cervical spinal cord levels from a dog with syringomyelia (arrows).

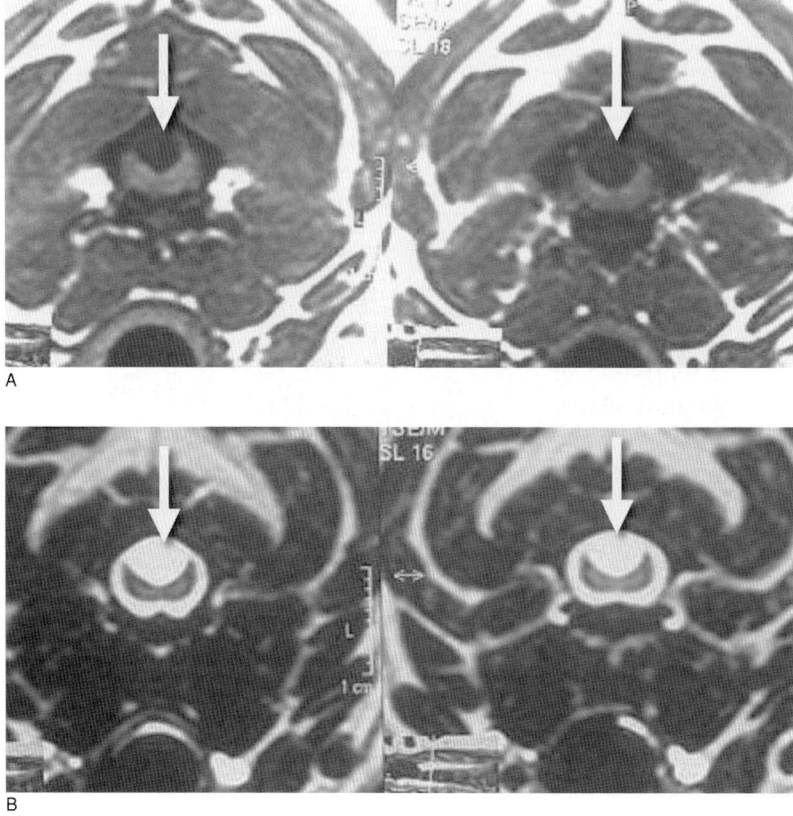

Figure 2.182. (A) Transverse T1-weighted and (B) T2-weighted MR images from immediately adjacent cervical spinal cord levels from a dog with syringomyelia (arrows) showing the differing appearance of the cavity on each sequence.

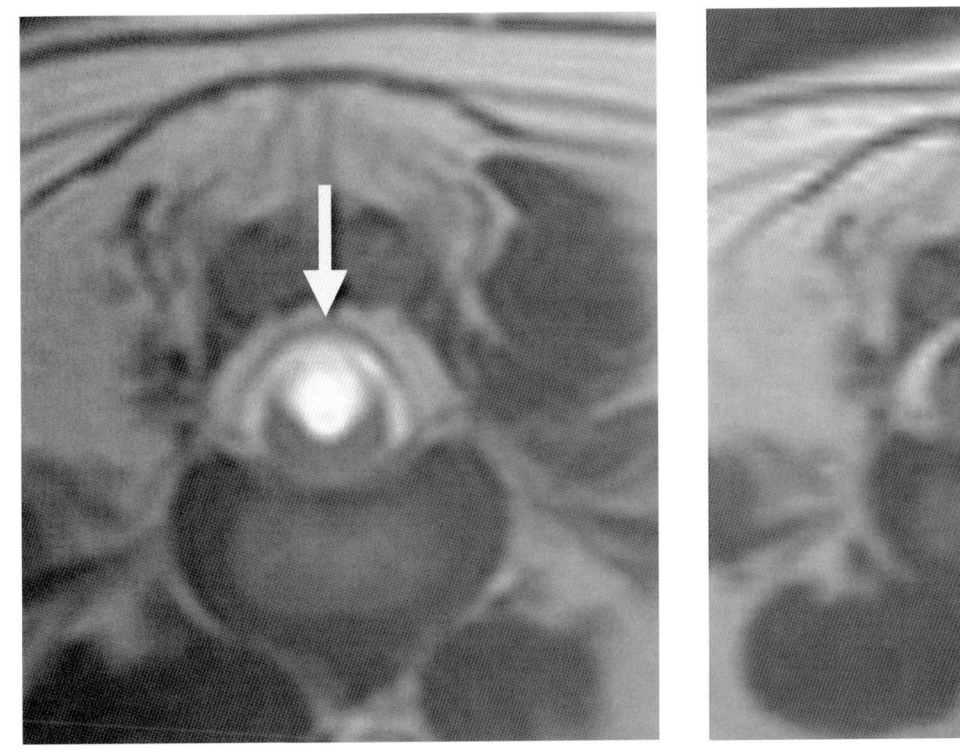
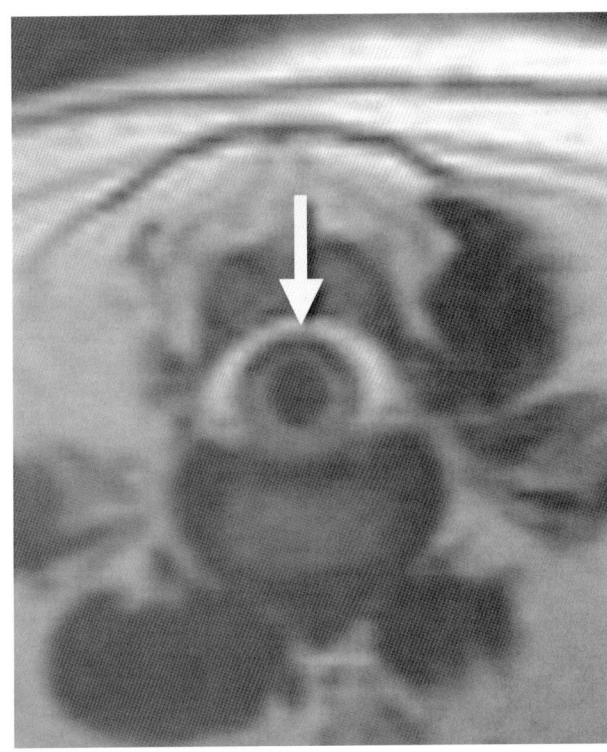

A

B

Figure 2.183. Transverse T2-weighted (A) and T1-weighted (B) MR images from the same spinal cord levels from a dog with syringomyelia (arrows) showing the differing appearance of the cavity on each sequence.

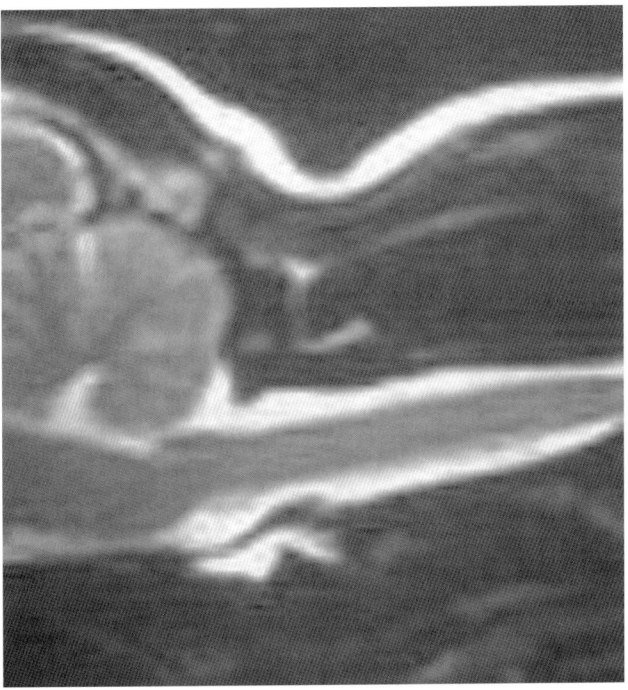

Figure 2.184. Sagittal T2-weighted MR image from a healthy dog at the foramen magnum level.

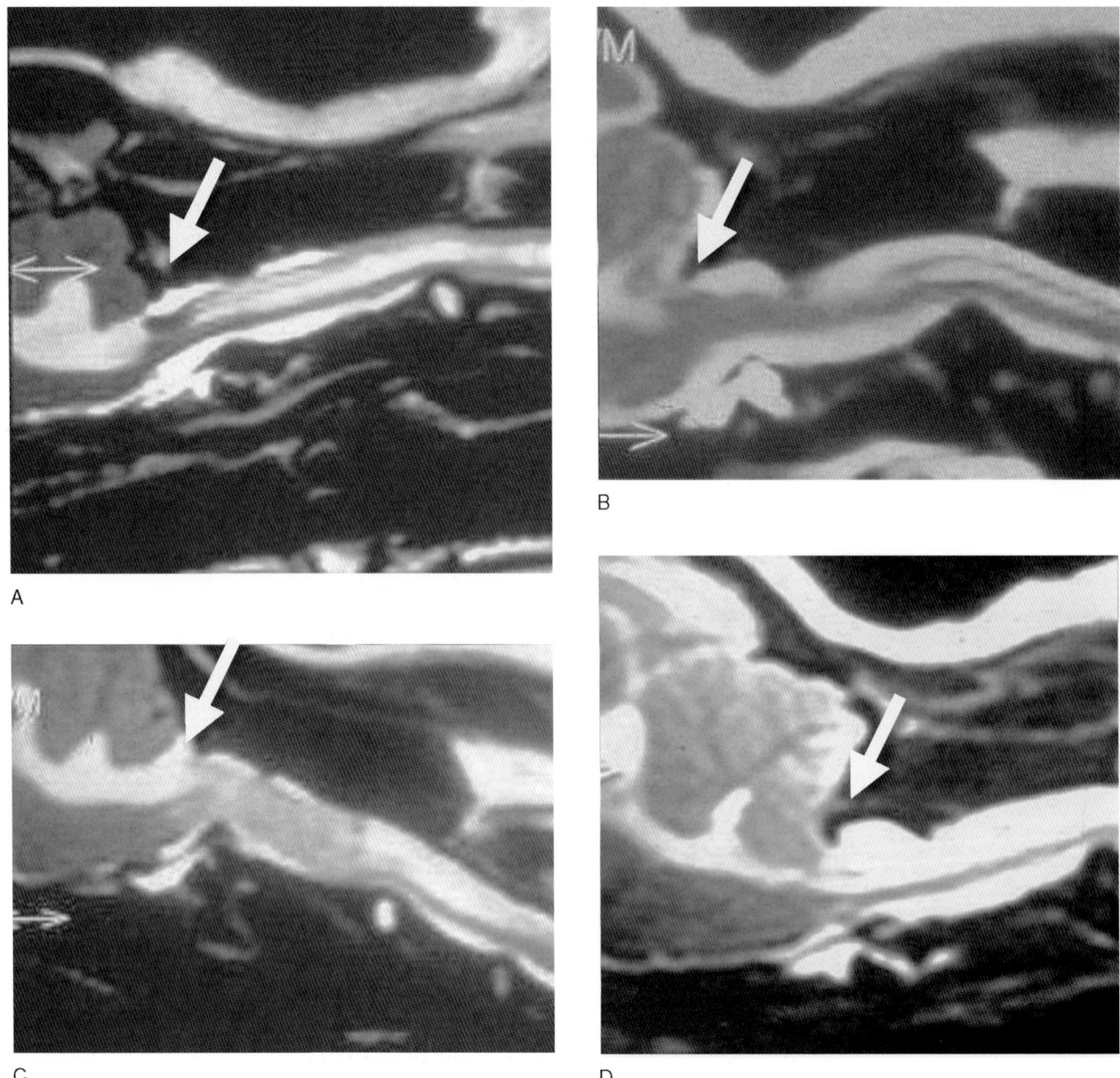

Figure 2.185. Sagittal T2-weighted MR images from four dogs with syringomyelia and abnormalities of the caudal fossa/foramen magnum region.

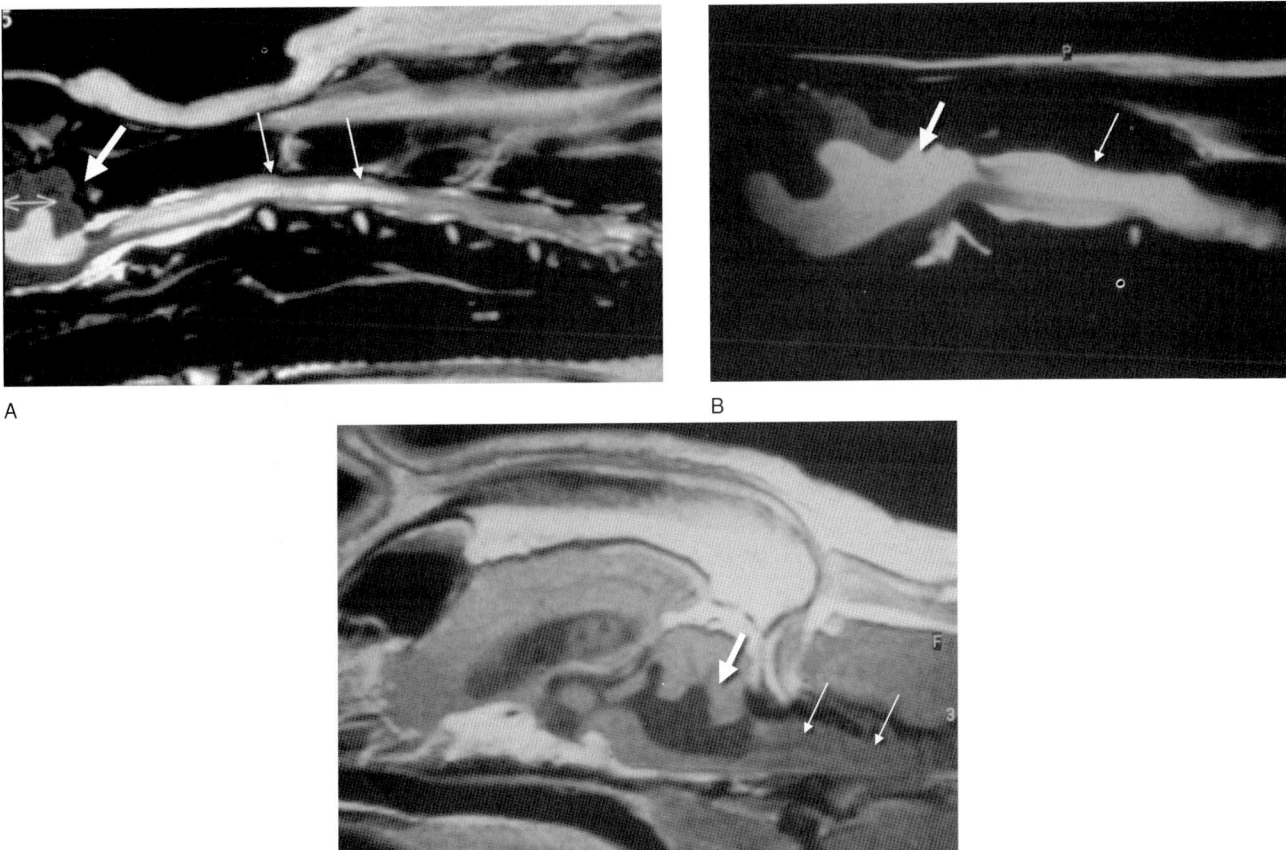

Figure 2.186.   Sagittal T2-weighted MR images ((A) and (B)) and sagittal T1-weighted image (C) from three dogs with syringomyelia (small arrows) and abnormalities of the fourth ventricle (larger arrows).

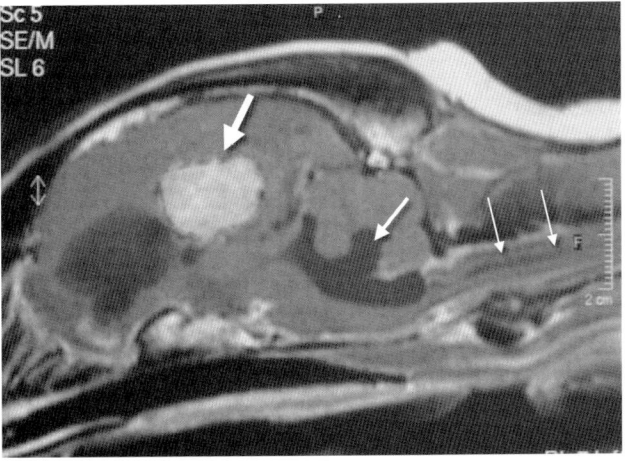

Figure 2.187.   Sagittal T1-weighted MR image following contrast administration in a dog with a third ventricle mass (largest arrow), syringomyelia (smaller arrows) and abnormalities of the fourth ventricle (medium arrow).

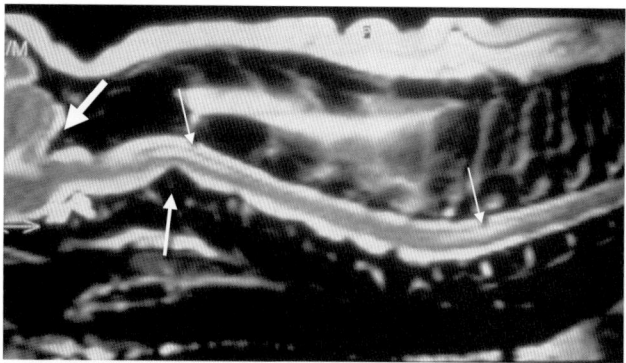

Figure 2.188.   Sagittal T2-weighted MR image from a dog with a caudal displacement of the cerebellum (largest arrow), syringomyelia (smaller arrows), and a protrusion of the C2-3 intervertebral disk (medium arrow).

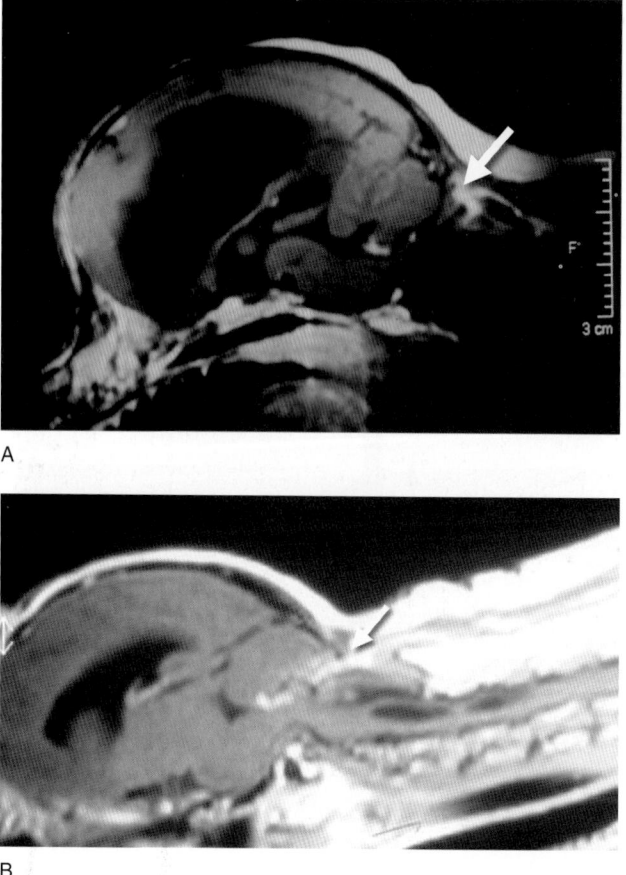

Figure 2.189.   Sagittal T1-weighted MR images from two dogs ((A) and (B)) with crowding and malformation of the foramen magnum region (arrows). (See Color Plate 2.189A.)

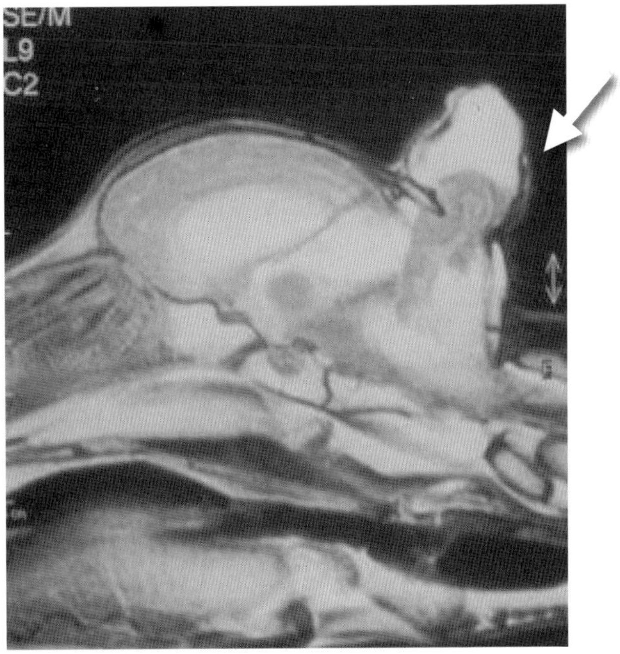

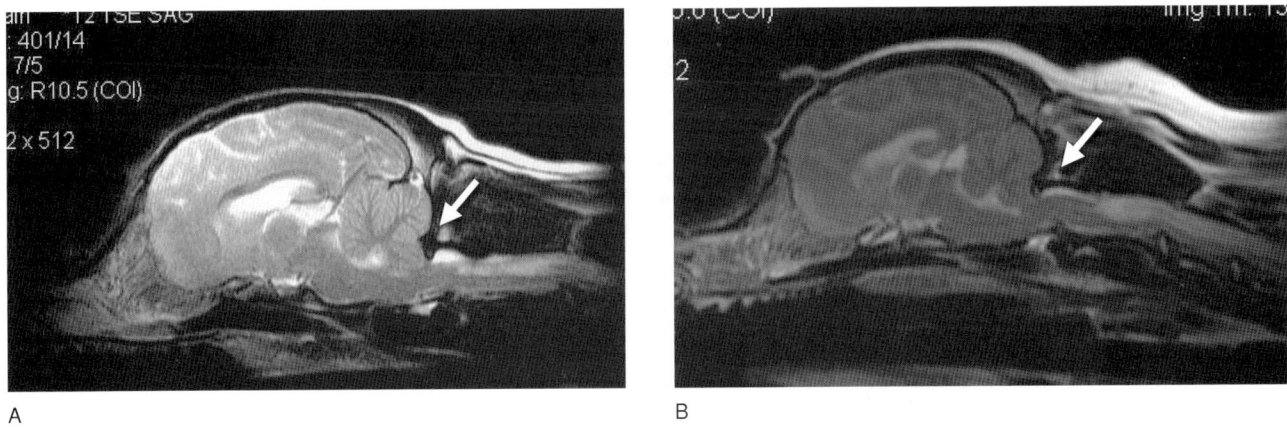

Figure 2.190.   Sagittal T2-weighted MR image from a sheep with a meningoencephalocele (arrow).

A

B

Figure 2.191.   Sagittal T2-weighted MR images from two Cavalier King Charles spaniels ((A) and (B)) with malformations of the foramen magnum region.

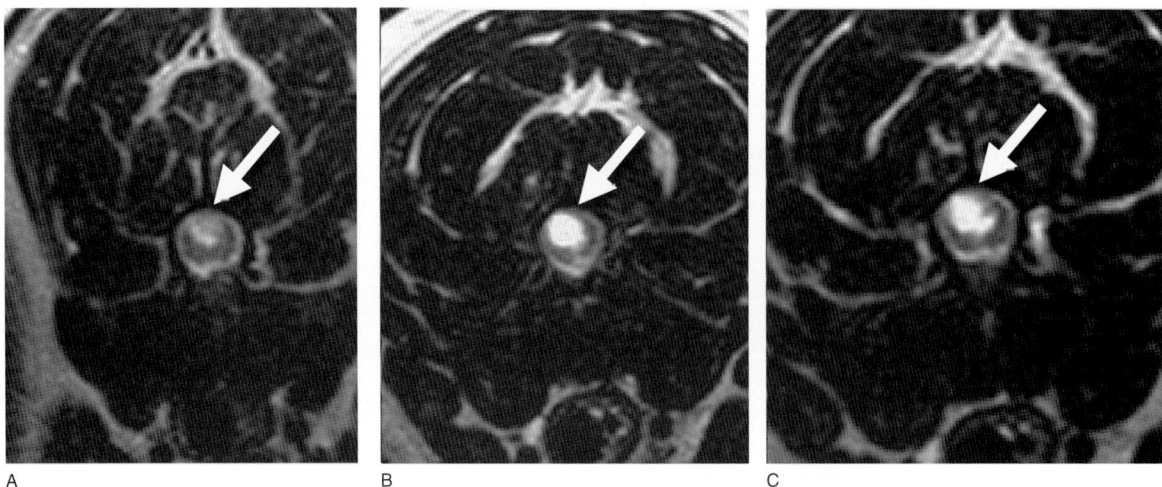

Figure 2.192.   Transverse T2-weighted MR images from a Cavalier King Charles spaniel with syringomyelia (arrows).

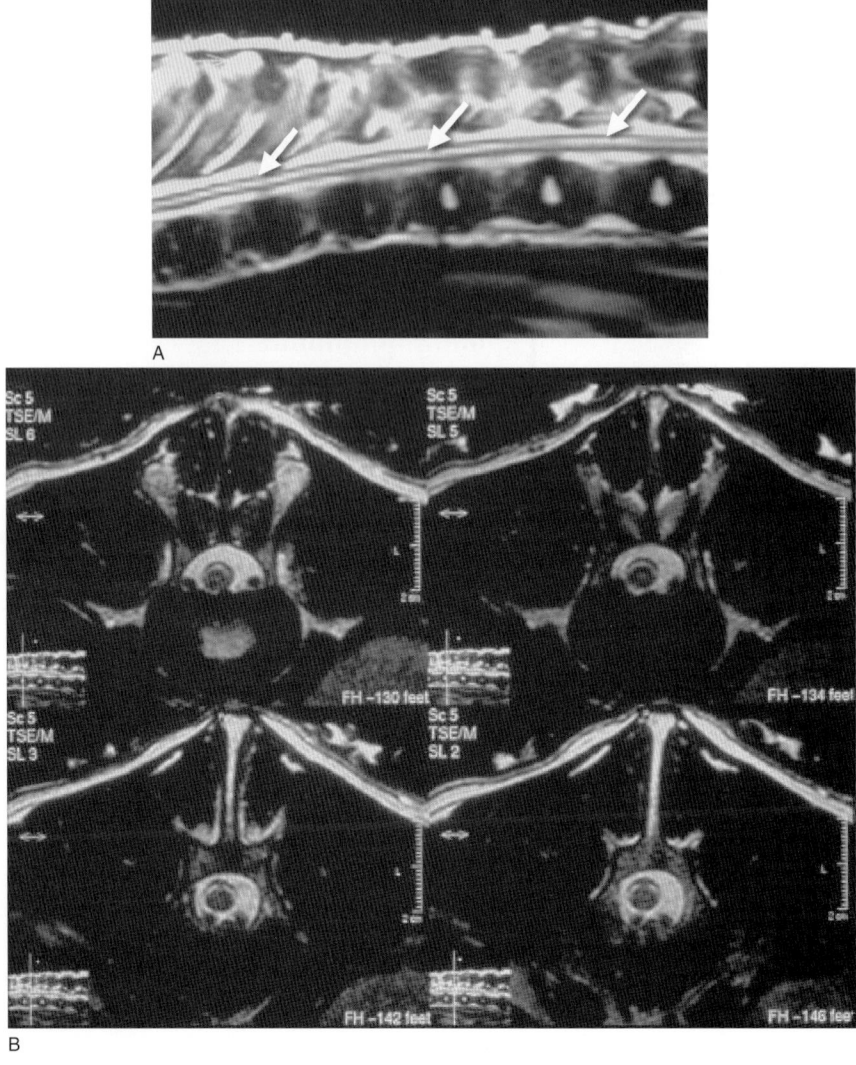

Figure 2.193.   Sagittal T2-weighted MR image (A) from a normal dog showing truncation artifact (arrows). Transverse T2-weighted images (B) showing no abnormalities.

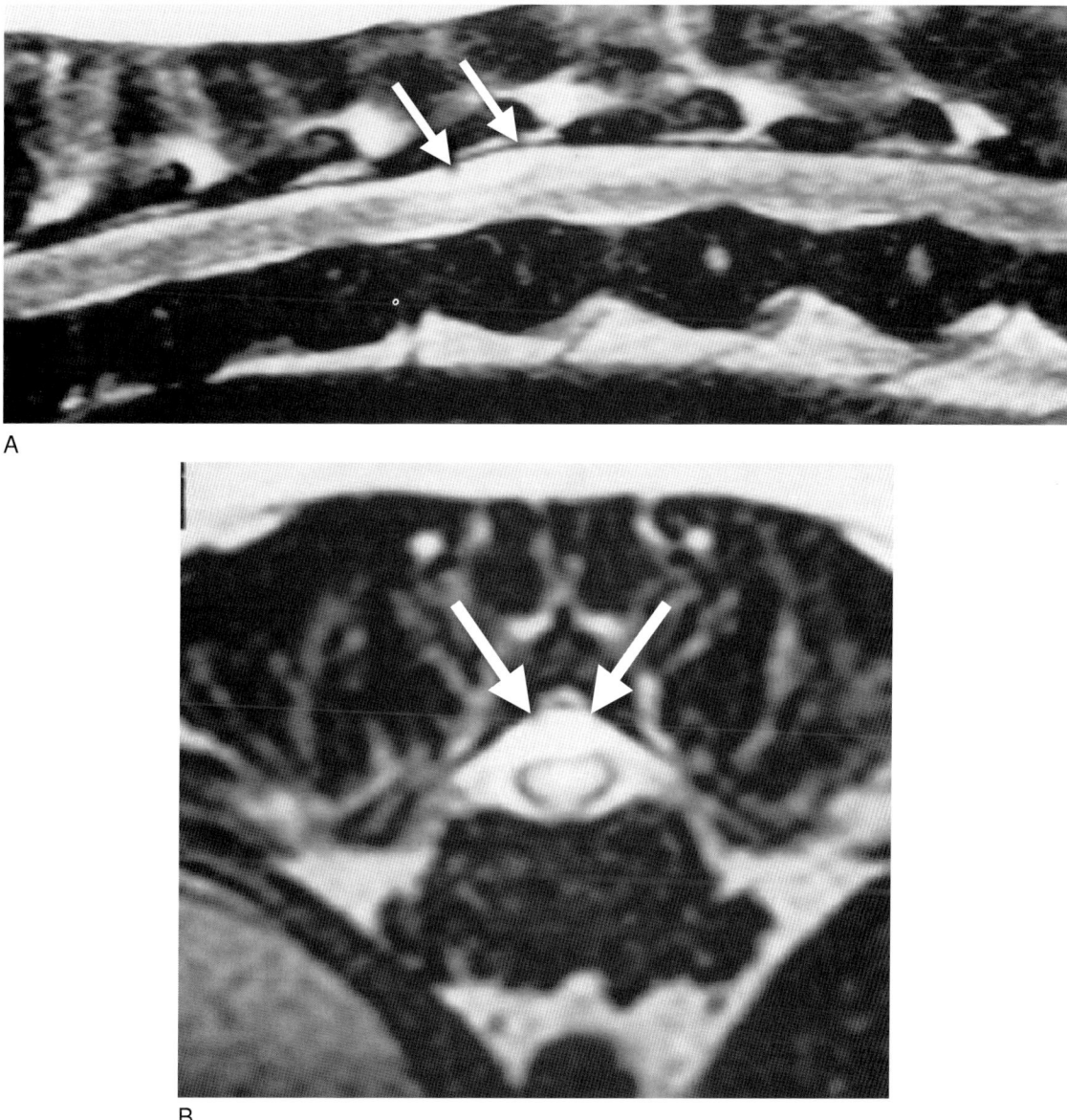

A

B

Figure 2.194.   Sagittal (A) and transverse (B) T2-weighted MR images from a dog with an arachnoid cyst (arrows).

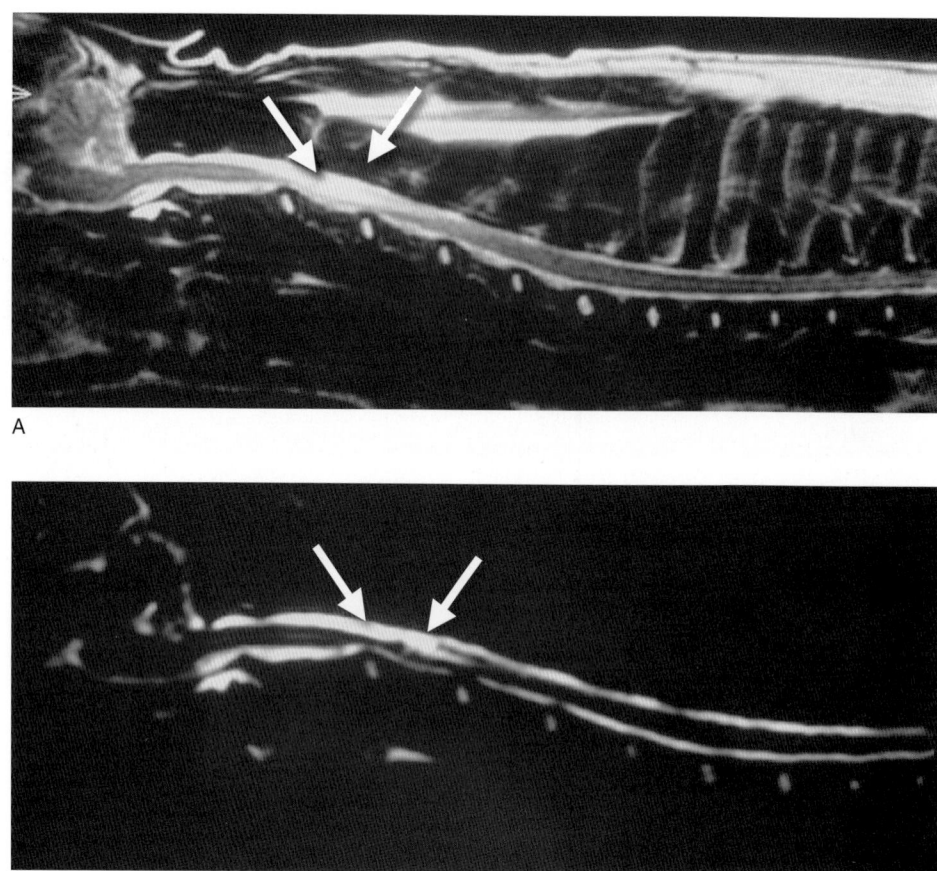

Figure 2.195. Sagittal (A) T2-weighted and myelogram effect (B) MR images from a dog with a cervical arachnoid cyst (arrows).

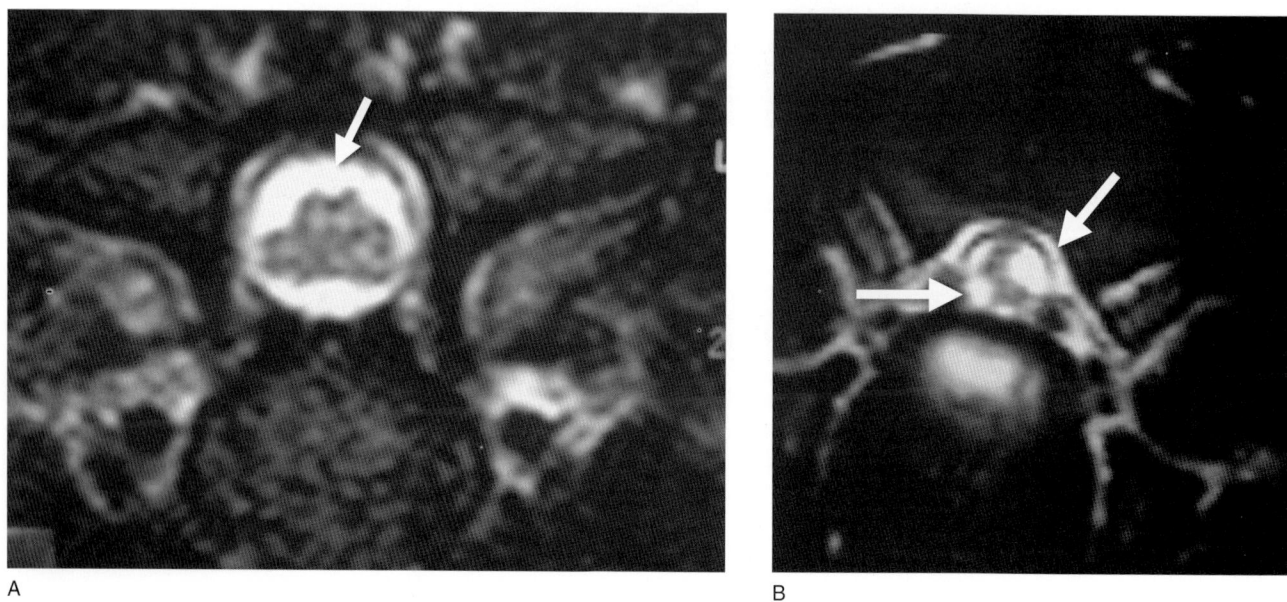

Figure 2.196. Transverse T2-weighted MR images from two dogs ((A) and (B)) with complex or multiple arachnoid cysts (arrows).

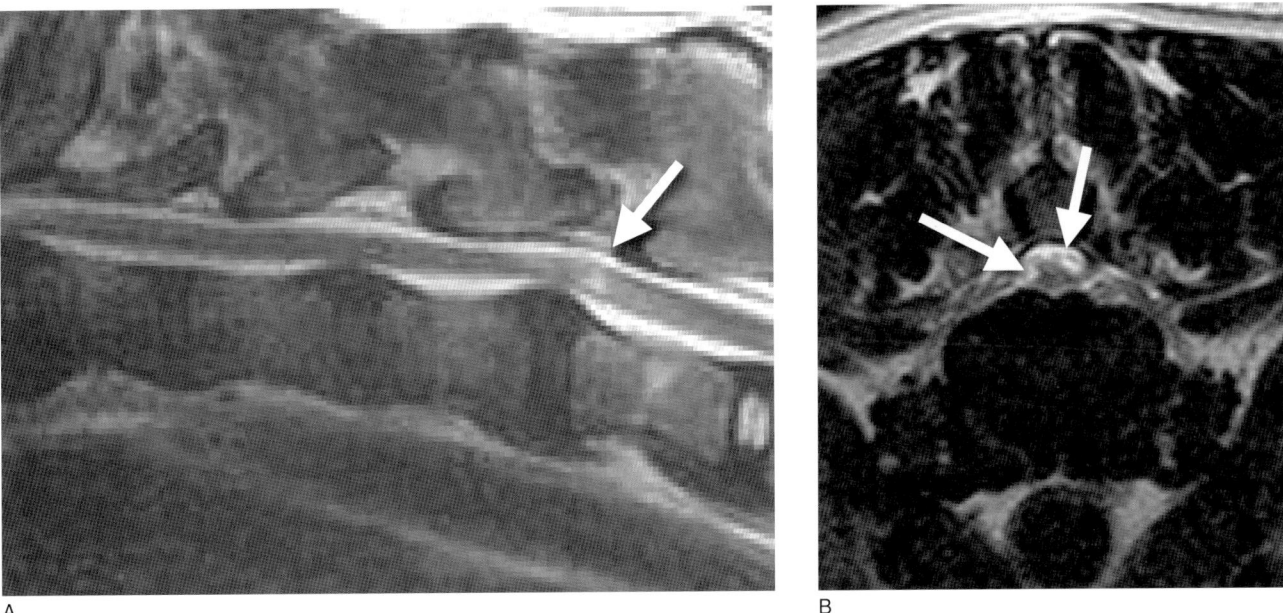

A   B

Figure 2.197. Sagittal (A) and transverse (B) T2-weighted MR images from a dog with multiple arachnoid cysts (arrows) associated with a chronic intervertebral disk protrusion.

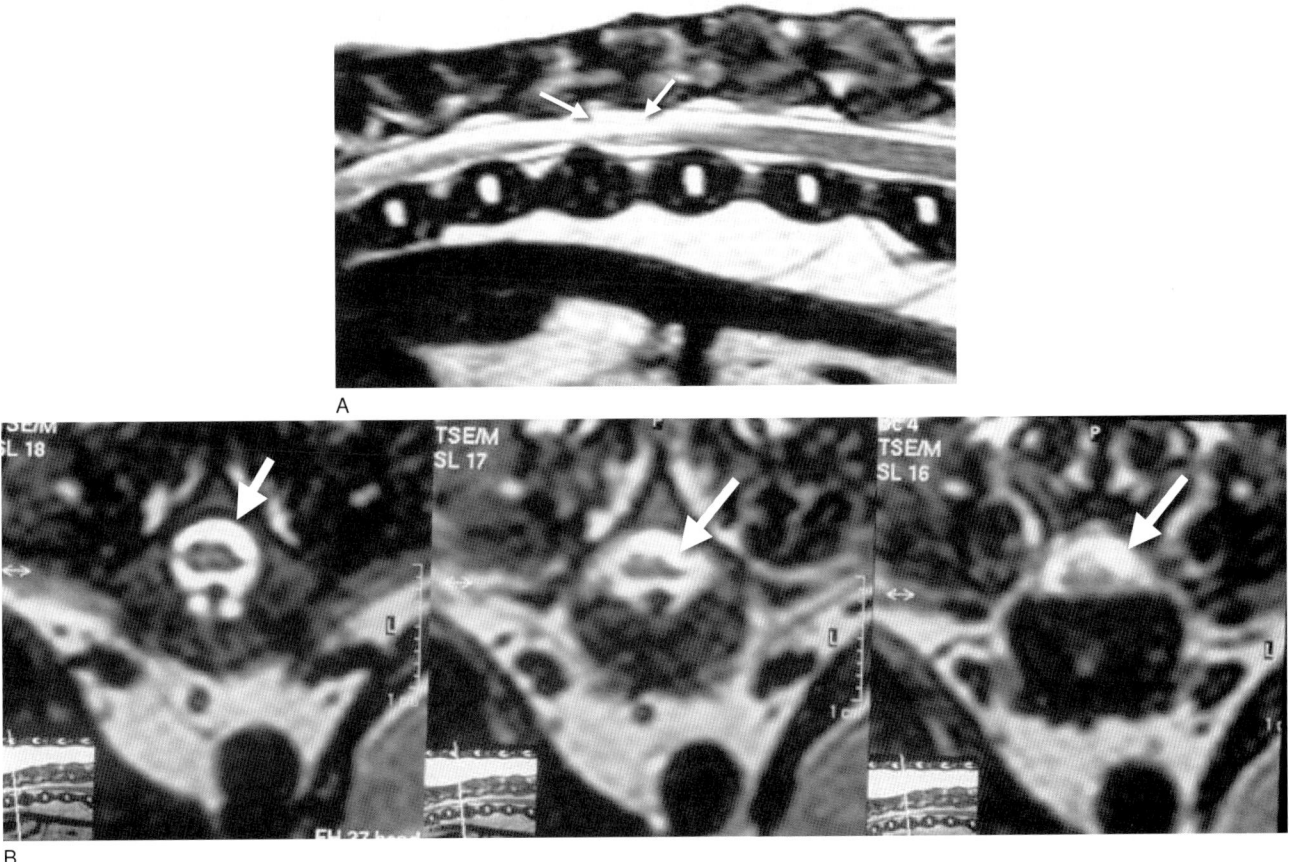

A

B

Figure 2.198. Sagittal (A) and transverse (B) T2-weighted MR images from a Pug dog with an arachnoid cyst (arrows) associated with a chronic intervertebral disk protrusion.

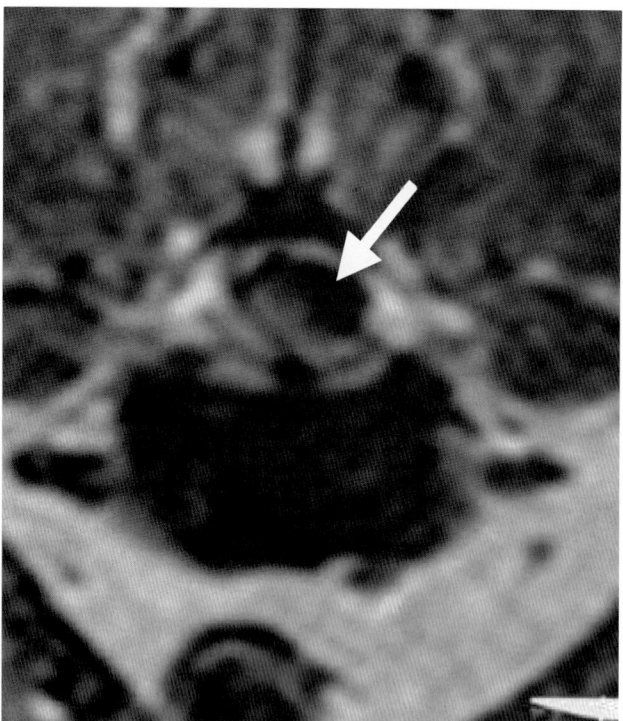

Figure 2.199. Transverse FLAIR MR image from the same Pug dog as in Figure 2.198 showing the hypointense arachnoid cyst (arrow).

proper (intradural/extramedullary), or arising within the spinal cord parenchyma proper (intramedullary). Depending upon growth characteristics and tumor aggressiveness, a tumor can expand and extend from one of these strict anatomical areas to involve another. This is most often seen with peripheral nerve sheath tumors that may begin in an extradural location but may traverse the dura into the intradural/extramedullary space, and eventually, into the spinal cord gray matter.

Diagnosis of a spinal tumor is often presumptively made using survey spinal radiographs, myelography, or advanced imaging (CT, MR). Tumors involving the vertebral bone may be evident on survey radiographs as osteolytic and/or osteoproliferative processes. These bony changes need to be differentiated from diskospondylitis and vertebral body osteomyelitis. Classically, vertebral tumors do not traverse the joint space (intervertebral disk) from one vertebra into an adjacent one. Vertebral tumors are found, however, to invade adjacent vertebral bodies in some instances. Extradural compression of the spinal cord overlying the vertebral body rather than the intervertebral disk space is suspicious for, but not pathognomonic of neoplastic disease.

Soft tissue tumors of the spinal cord or peripheral nerve tumors are usually not apparent on survey radio-

graphs. Nerve sheath tumors, however, may involve exiting peripheral nerves within the intervertebral foramina. The foramen where the abnormal nerve is exiting may be enlarged due to associated bone atrophy and visible on survey radiographs.

Myelography is used to outline the subarachnoid space and determine if spinal cord compression or expansion is present. With extradural tumors, one or both of the contrast columns may be deviated axially (toward the center of the spinal canal). Clues to the presence of an extradural tumor on myelography include compression of the spinal cord primarily overlying a vertebral body rather than the intervertebral disk space and annular compressive lesions of the dura. These same myelographic features may also be seen with IVDD and other spinal cord compressive diseases, and therefore should not be considered pathognomonic for extradural spinal tumor.

With intradural but extramedullary tumor, myelographic spinal imaging will often result in a characteristic pattern of expansion of the subarachnoid space and outlining of the tumor in negative shadow referred to as a "golf tee." Nerve sheath tumors may also expand on either side of where the nerve traverses the dura, giving these tumors a "dumbbell-shaped" appearance. Conversely, expansion of the dural tube in 90° opposed radiographic views is most indicative of an intramedullary or intradural lesion.

Advanced imaging studies such as computed CT and MR imaging have greatly improved the ability to determine the location and extent of any spinal tumor. With CT, a myelogram is often performed initially to outline the subarachnoid space. In some instances, a series of scans are performed before and after intravenous injection of an iodinated contrast material. Abnormalities disrupting the blood-spinal cord or blood-nerve barrier may become more apparent with this technique. Loss of integrity of these barriers or increased vascularity may result in an area of increased uptake (whiteness) after intravenous contrast enhancement. Contrast enhancement is most often seen with tumors, vascular abnormalities, and inflammatory foci; however, it may also be seen with intervertebral disk disease.

MR imaging affords superior anatomical evaluation of soft tissue structures, and therefore is usually excellent in providing detail as to the extent and location of spinal tumors (Figures 2.200–2.214). Tumors may have a variety of appearances with MR imaging, and need to be differentiated from other spinal disease processes such as intervertebral disk herniation. Many epidural tumors invade the surrounding vertebral body before impinging on the spinal cord. Thus, bony destruction of the vertebrae may be a clue to an underlying neoplastic

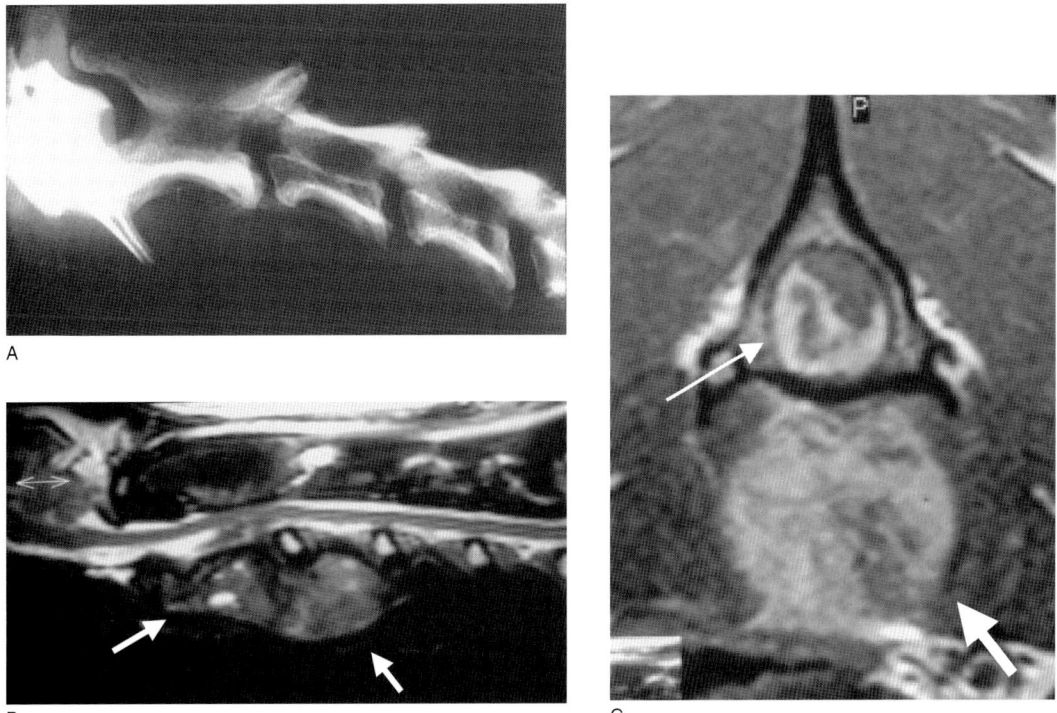

Figure 2.200.   Lateral cervical radiograph (A) and sagittal, T2-weighted MR image (B) from a dog with an extradural tumor. (C) Transverse T1-weighted MR image following intravenous contrast administration from the same dog showing contrast enhancement of the vertebrae (larger arrow) and within the spinal canal (smaller arrow).

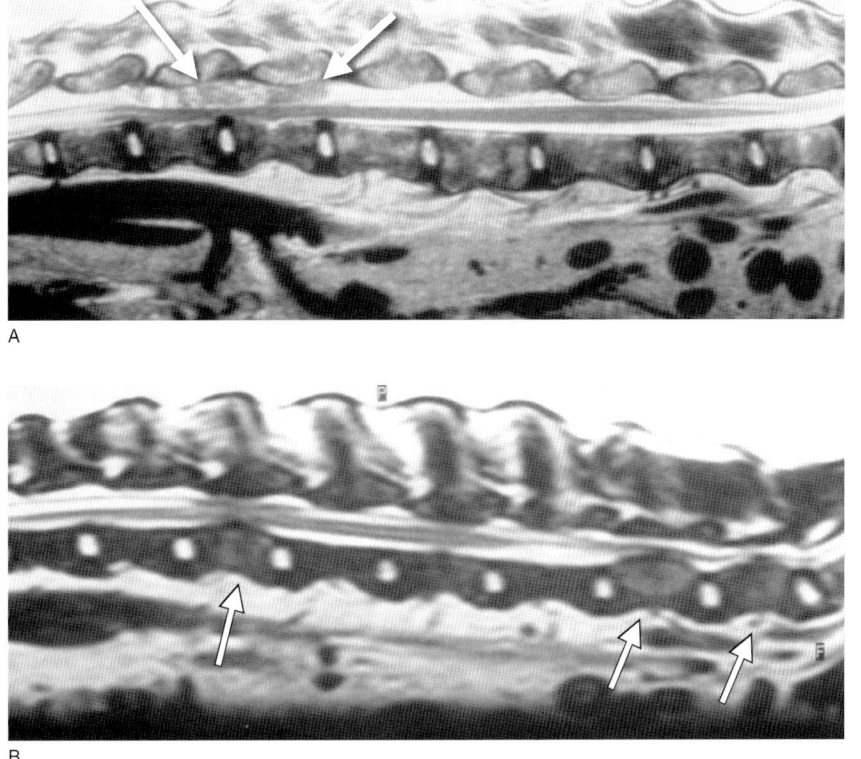

Figure 2.201.   Sagittal T2-weighted MR image (A) from a dog with a dorsally located extradural tumor (arrows). Sagittal T2-weighted MR image (B) from a dog with multiple vertebral masses (arrows).

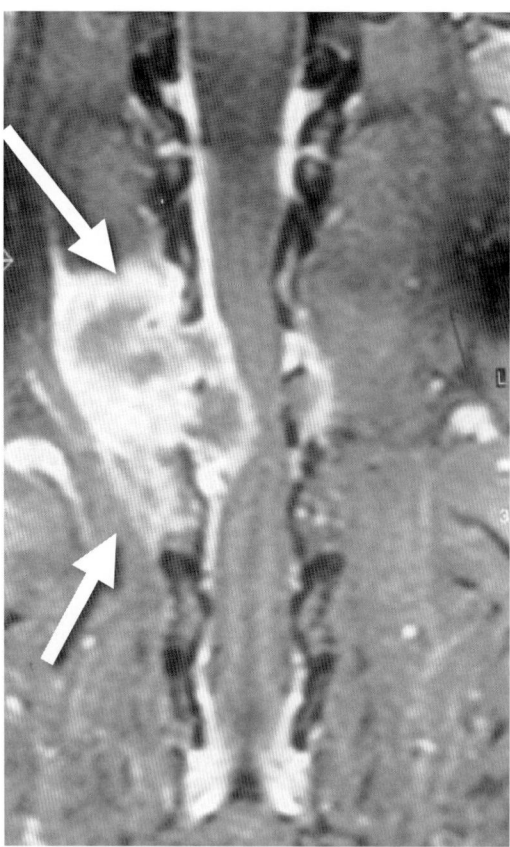

Figure 2.202. Dorsal plane, T1-weighted MR image following intravenous contrast administration from a dog with an extradural tumor showing contrast enhancement of the mass (arrows).

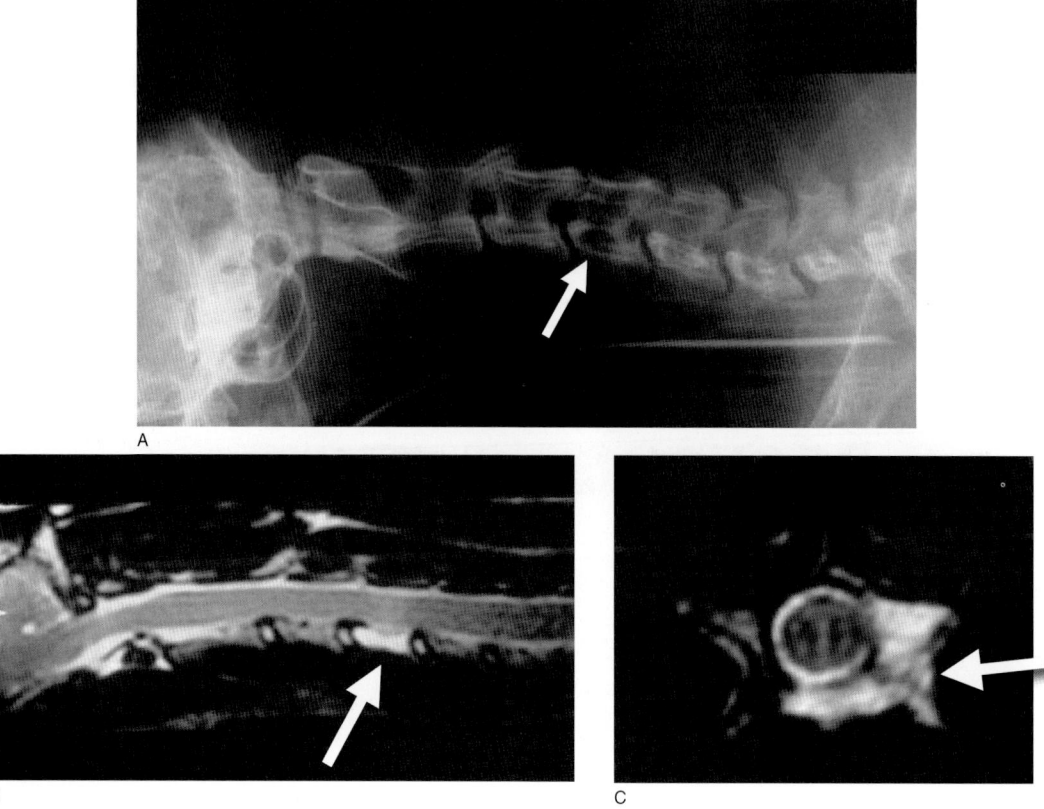

Figure 2.203. Lateral cervical radiograph (A), sagittal (B), and transverse (C) T2-weighted MR images from a cat with a vertebral tumor (arrows).

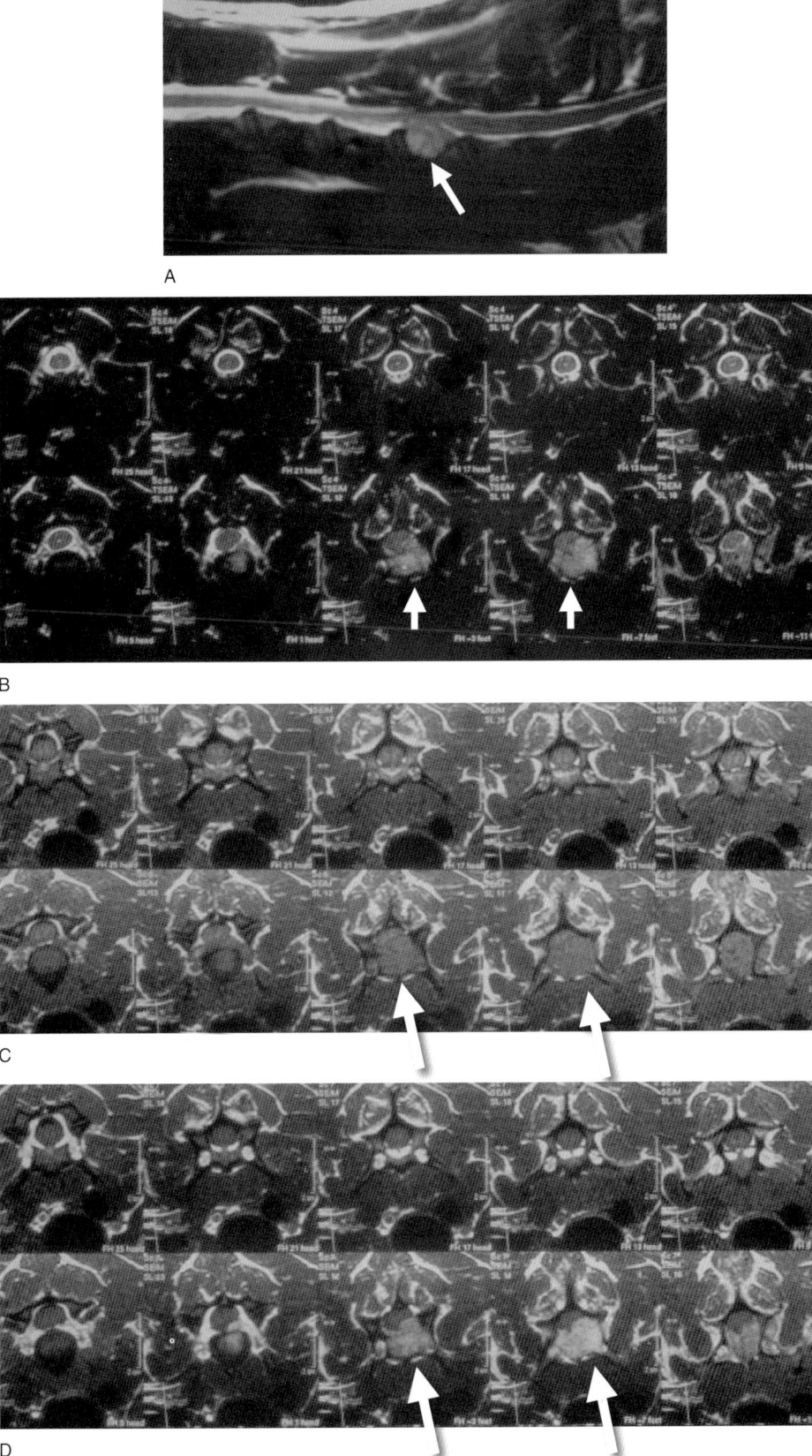

Figure 2.204. Sagittal (A) and transverse (B) T2-weighted MR images from a dog with a vertebral body tumor (arrows). Transverse T1-weighted MR images from similar levels before (C) and following (D) intravenous contrast administration from the same dog showing contrast enhancement of the vertebrae (arrows).

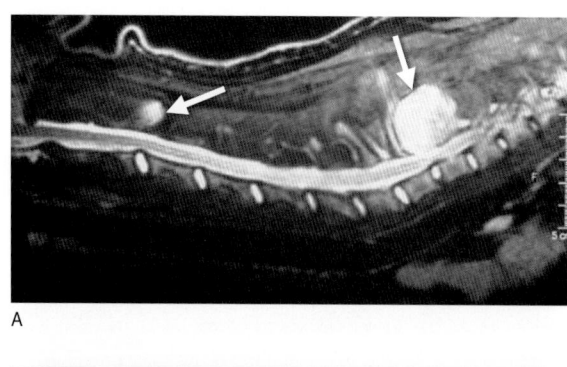

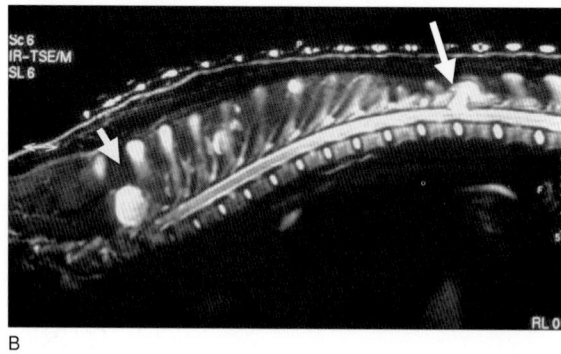

Figure 2.205. Sagittal T2-weighted MR images from a dog at the cervical (A) and thoracolumbar (B) levels with multiple cartilaginous exostoses (arrows).

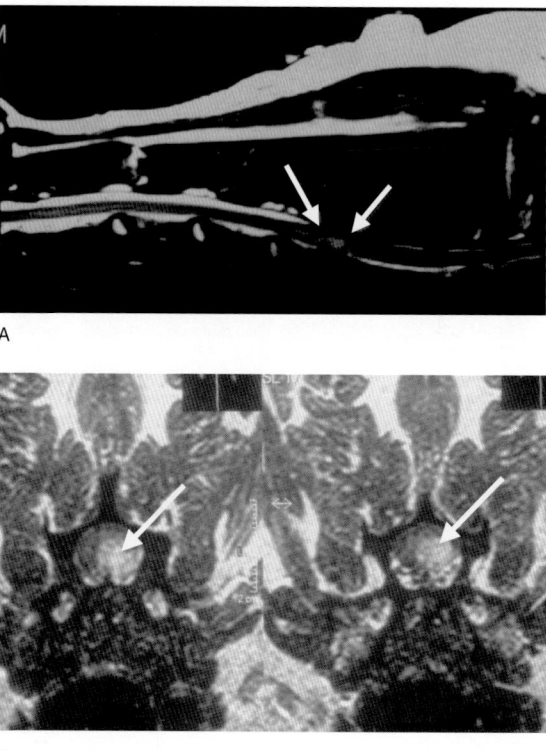

Figure 2.206. Sagittal T2-weighted MR image (A) from a dog with an intradural but extramedullary spinal tumor (arrows). (B) Transverse T1-weighted MR images from adjacent level through the tumor following intravenous contrast administration from the same dog showing contrast enhancement of the mass (arrow).

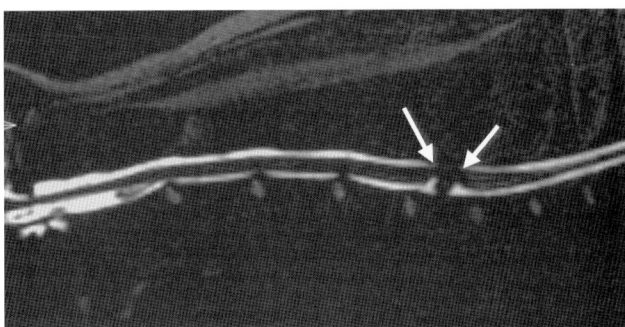

Figure 2.207. Myelogram effect MR image from a dog with an intradural but extramedullary spinal tumor (arrows).

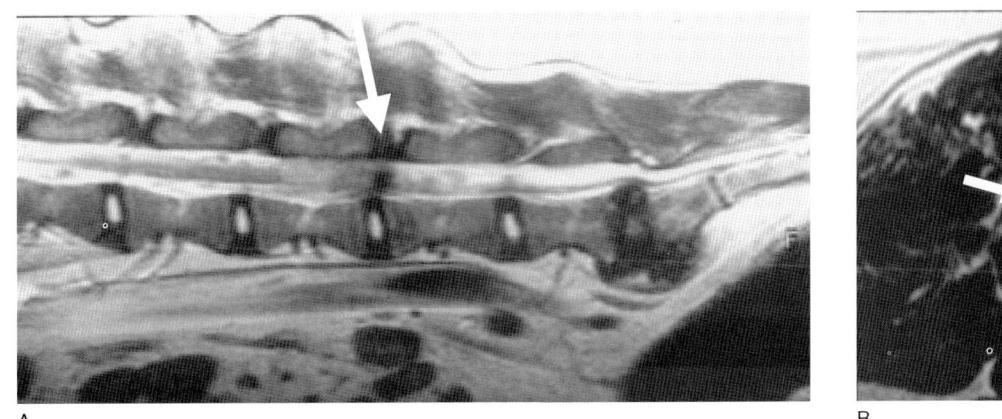

A

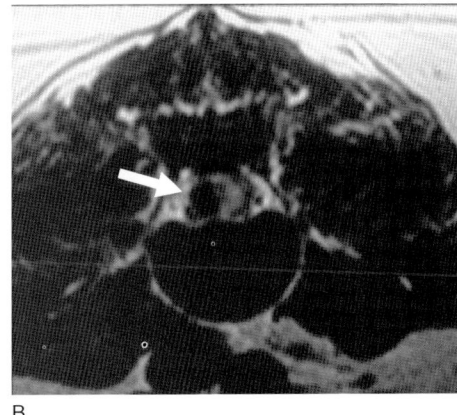

B

Figure 2.208. Sagittal (A) and transverse (B) T2-weighted MR images from a dog with a calcified meningioma (arrows).

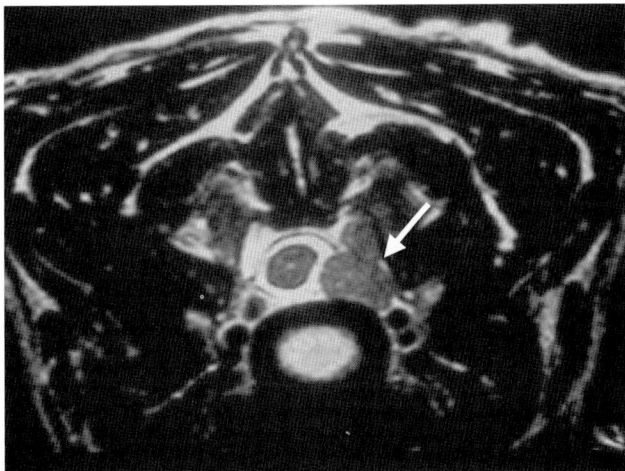

Figure 2.209. Transverse T2-weighted MR image from a dog with an extradural nerve sheath tumor (arrow).

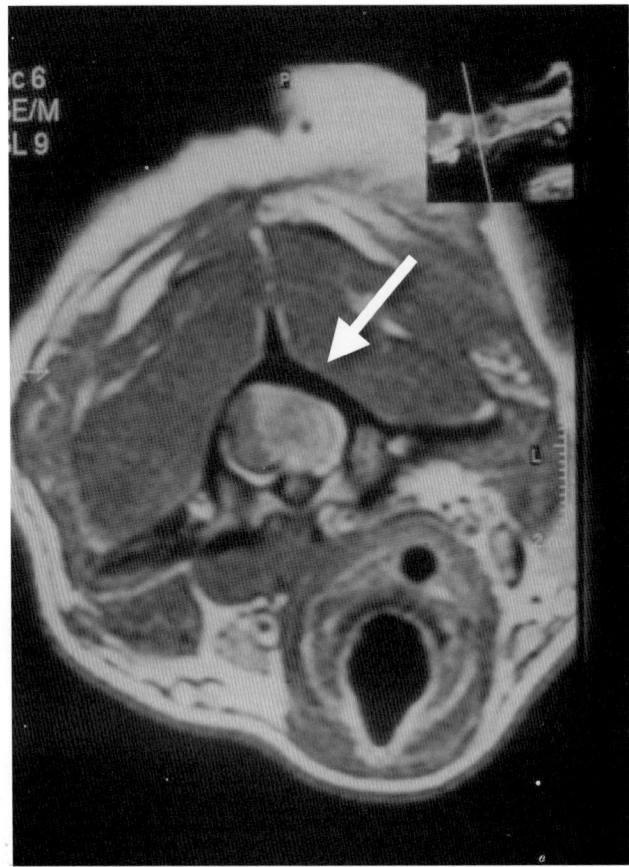

Figure 2.210. Transverse T1-weighted MR image following intravenous contrast administration from a dog showing contrast enhancement of a cervical meningioma (arrow).

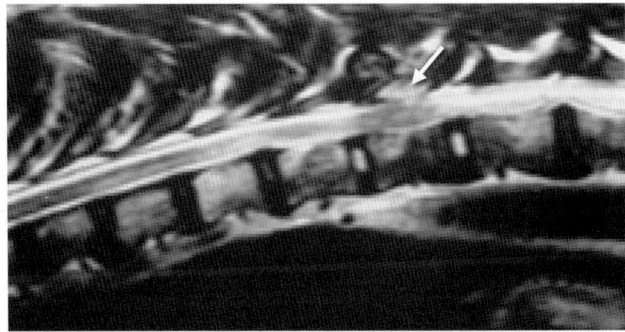

Figure 2.211. Sagittal T2-weighted MR image from a dog with an intramedullary spinal tumor (arrow).

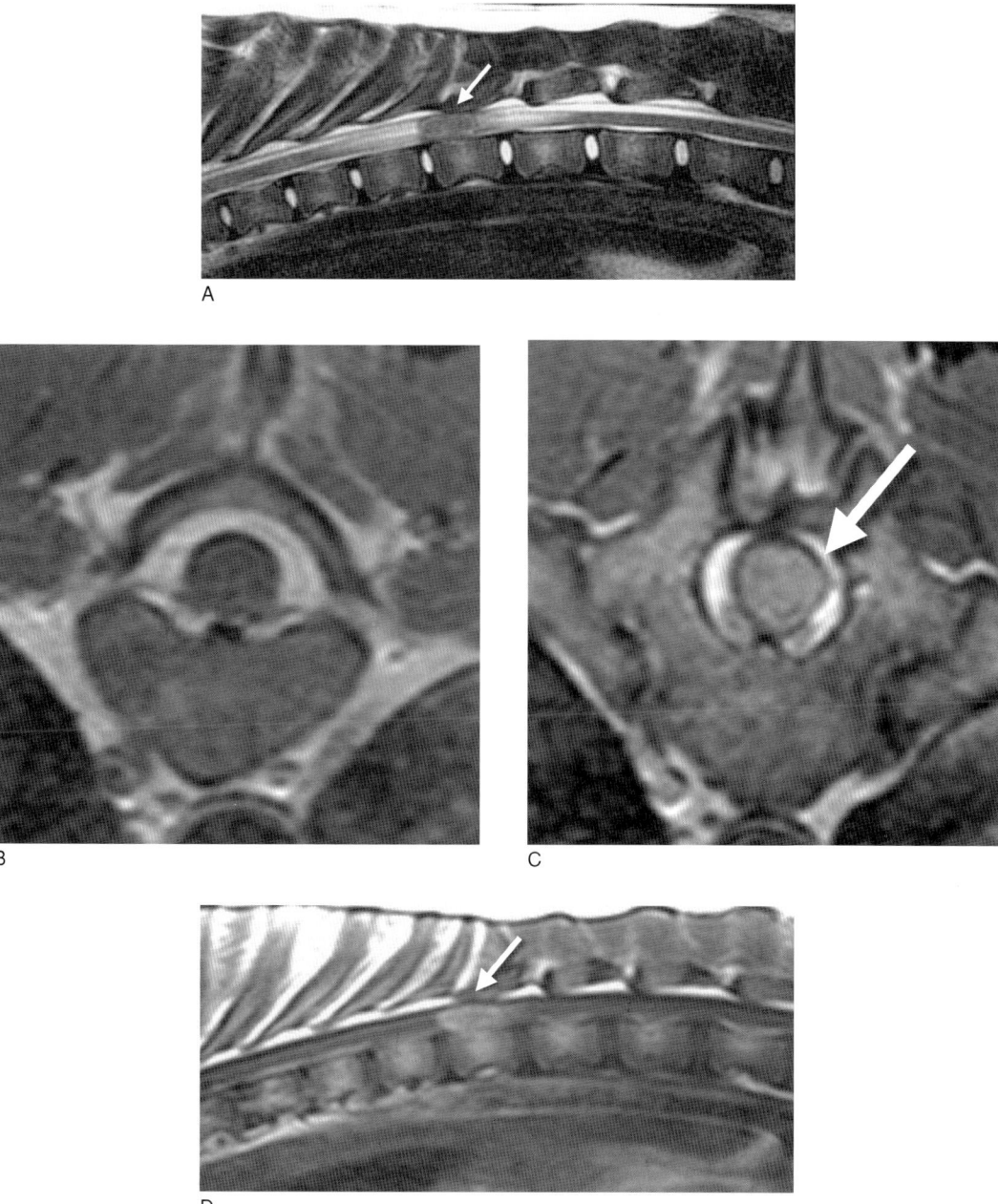

Figure 2.212.   Sagittal T2-weighted MR image (A) from a dog with an intradural but extramedullary spinal tumor (arrow). Histologic diagnosis was a nephroblastoma. Transverse T1-weighted MR images from adjacent levels from the same dog as in (A) before (B) and following (C) intravenous contrast administration showing contrast enhancement of the tumor (arrow). Sagittal T1-weighted MR image (D) from the same dog as in (A) following intravenous contrast administration showing contrast enhancement of the tumor (arrow).

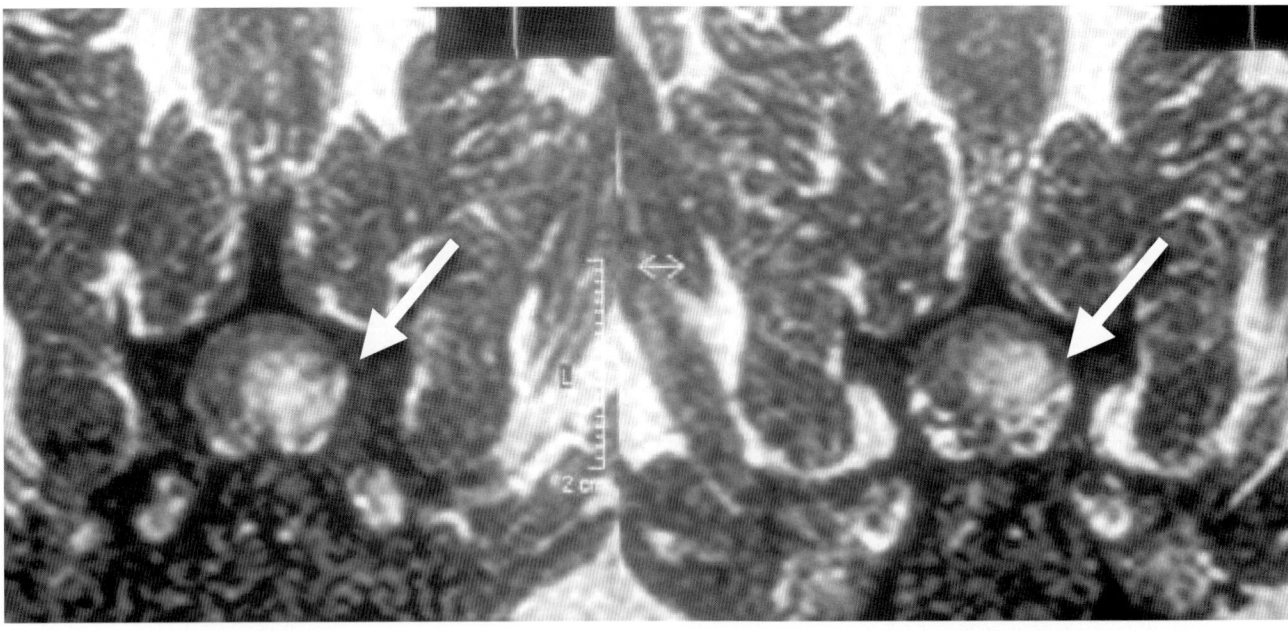

A

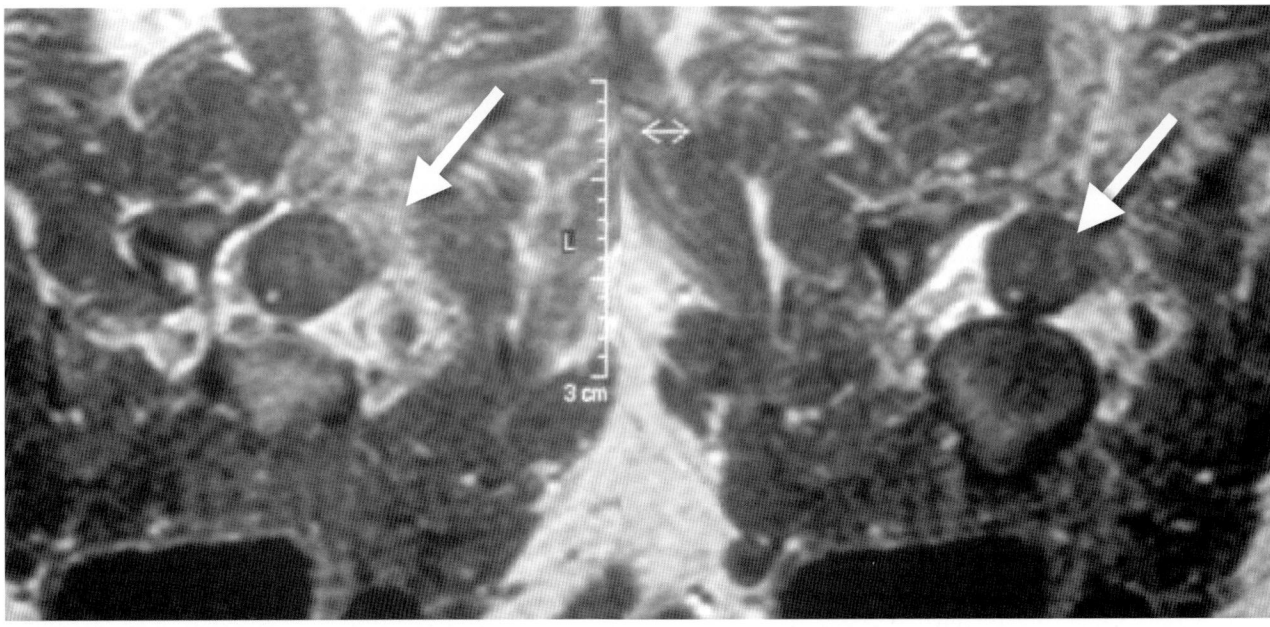

B

Figure 2.213.   (A) Transverse T1-weighted MR images from adjacent levels from the same dog as in Figure 2.206B following intravenous contrast administration showing contrast enhancement of a meningioma (arrows). (B) Transverse T1-weighted MR images from adjacent levels from the same dog immediately after surgical removal of the tumor following intravenous contrast administration showing no contrast enhancement in the region of the previous tumor (arrows).

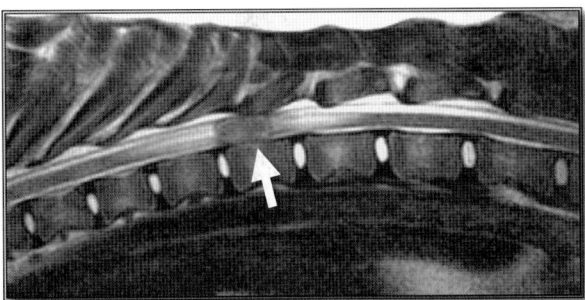

A

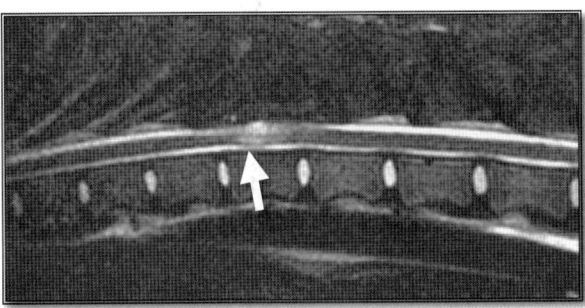

B

Figure 2.214. Sagittal T2-weighted MR images from the same dog as in Figure 2.212A before (A) and following surgical removal (B) of the tumor (arrow).

process. In general, in T1-weighted images, marrow signal should be roughly equivalent to disk material. In cases of diffuse marrow involvement, the disk spaces will show greater signal intensity than the vertebral marrow.

Tumors are typically vascular and invasive, disrupting the normal integrity of the BBB. Thus, intravenous injection of a contrast agent generally results in some degree of either diffuse or focal enhancement in the area affected by tumor. Contrast enhancement (intravenous gadolinium-DTPA) does not precisely define the tumor borders as neoplastic cells are generally found outside the enhanced portion of the mass. Gadolinium enhancement of tumors is inconsistent but, if present, may support a diagnosis of tumor. Other extradural disease processes, such as intervertebral disk herniation, may also show contrast enhancement on MR (Figure 2.135). Contrast enhancement characteristics alone, therefore, cannot be used as being pathognomonic for spinal neoplasia.

Intradural, extramedullary tumors often have a "golf-tee" appearance in the subarachnoid space similar to the appearance of these tumors on myelography. This golf-tee appearance is most evident in T2-weighted images as the CSF creating this appearance is white. These tumors may not be as obvious in sagittal

MR images as they may have little contrast difference with respect to the adjacent spinal cord and may be primarily located lateral to the spinal cord. Intravenous gadolinium administration usually results in enhancement of these tumors increasing their signal intensity in T1-weighted images. Dorsal and transverse contrast-enhanced images are helpful to detect this category of tumors.

Intramedullary tumors generally cause the spinal cord to be expanded. In T1-weighted images, most intramedullary neoplasms have diminished signal intensity with respect to the spinal cord. In T2-weighted images, they usually have a brighter (hyperintense) signal compared to spinal cord, which often reflects associated spinal cord edema or hemorrhage. Most tumors have a nonhomogeneous signal intensity and indistinct margins between tumor and surrounding normal cord.

CSF collected caudal to the location of a spinal tumor may show nonspecific increases in nucleated cells and protein. CSF can also be normal. Classically, CSF will show increases in protein content without concurrent increases in nucleated cell counts. Depending upon the severity and acuity of the clinical progression, CSF may show a variety of abnormalities including increases in protein content, increases in nucleated cell counts, or evidence of hemorrhage (with RBCs and erythrophagocytosis). Increases in protein and in nucleated cell counts in CSF are a reflection of inflammation, degeneration, or combination of these. Lymphocytes and monocytes are the predominant cell types present, however, neutrophils may also occasionally be present. Xanthochromia may accompany associated spinal or subarachnoid hemorrhage. Rarely, tumor cells will be evident on CSF cytologic analysis. This is most commonly found in instances of lymphoma, ependymoma, and carcinoma.

Multiple Cartilaginous Exostoses

Multiple cartilaginous exostoses are proliferations of bone and cartilage that are thought to result from aberrant growth displaced chondrocytes from the metaphyseal growth plates of bone. Subqeuently, this disease is most often seen in younger animals (<18 months of age). Dogs, cats, as well as other species including humans have been reported with this disease. The bony and cartilaginous proliferations often are numerous and can affect the long bones, ribs, or vertebrae. The bony protuberances may be palpable. If this bony proliferation affects the vertebrae, varying degrees of spinal pain, paresis, and/or paralysis may result. Radiographs of the affected bones often show proliferations of bone that are smooth, contoured, irregular, multilobulated.

With MR imaging, these vertebral lesions are expansile, irregular massses, and often involve the articular facets (Figure 2.205). The center of the mass has signal characteristics similar to medullary bone. A catilage cap (decreased signal intensity in a T2-weighted image) may be present at the periphery of the lesion. Surgical biopsy is necessary to definitively confirm the lesion.

Infectious/Inflammatory Diseases

Myelitis, encephalomyelitis, or meningoencephalomyelitis can result from a variety of infectious and noninfectious causes. Inflammation may occur anywhere along the spinal cord and can be focal or diffuse. In many animals with encephalitis and meningitis, the cardinal signs of systemic inflammatory processes such as the presence of a fever and increases in white blood cells in the leukogram may not be found, as localized inflammatory disease in the CNS may not elicit a systemic inflammatory response.

As some myelitis can result in or be associated with structural changes in the spinal cord, spinal cord imaging may be helpful in determining the extent and character of any regions of spinal cord inflammation (Figures 2.215 and 2.216). Survey radiographs are normal in cases of myelitis. Myelography may reveal a focally or diffusely swollen spinal cord. Rarely, with myelography, an irregular distribution of contrast agent in the subarachnoid space, or even contrast media becoming distributed into the spinal parenchyma may be seen. Computed tomographic scanning may show evidence of spinal cord disruption; however, MR imaging is more likely to show alterations in spinal cord parenchyma with myelitis. A variety of abnormalities may be evident on MR spinal imaging in cases of myeli-

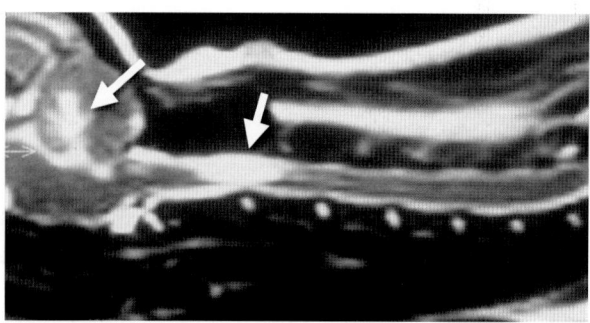

Figure 2.215. Sagittal T2-weighted MR image from a dog with inflammation of the cerebellum and the cervical spinal cord (arrows).

tis, including intramedullary spinal cord swelling (hyperintense signal), hemorrhage, or contrast enhancement. Multifocal discrete, anatomical lesions are often present within the nervous system, and may be especially conspicuous after intravenous contrast medium administration suggesting alterations in the BBB to the cerebral vasculature. Occasionally, myelitis will appear as a focal mass lesion on MR spinal imaging mimicking a spinal tumor or hematoma. Surgical biopsy, with aerobic, anaerobic, and fungal culturing of any collected lesions should provide for a more definitive diagnosis.

Diskospondylitis

Diskospondylitis is an infection in the IVD space and surrounding vertebral end plates and bodies. This disease can occur focally in any area of the spinal column or be present in multiple intervertebral disk sites. The most common class of infectious organisms associated with this disease is bacteria. Specific bacteria commonly associated with diskospondylitis are *Staphylococcus intermedius*, *Brucella canis*, and *Escherichia coli*. Rarely, fungal infections such as paecilomycosis and aspergillosis may be causative. Importantly, in situations of diskospondylitis, there are usually underlying processes that predispose to persistent bacteremia within the body. This may be due to persistent or recurrent infections in parts of the body (such as the skin, urinary tract, and prostate). Additionally, animals may have suppressed or otherwise abnormal immune responses that allow for persistent or unresolved bacteremias to continue. Immunosuppresion is commonly the result of exogenously administered corticosteroids.

Vertebral body osteomyelitis may result in similar clinical features. When present in the midlumbar vertebrae, osteomyelitis is often associated with a foreign body migration of a grass awn. In severe cases of osteomyelitis or diskospondylitis, a fistula may form from the vertebrae to the skin through the muscle and subcutaneous tissues. In the lumbar area, this fistula often is present in the lateral flank.

Diskospondylitis is usually evident on survey radiographic evaluations of the spine. Radiographic findings of lysis of the end plates of the vertebral bodies result in an irregular intervertebral disk, vertebral end plate margin. Within the surrounding vertebral structures, there is often sclerosis. Very early (i.e., <14 days) in the disease course, no radiographic abnormalities may be apparent. In the earlier stages of diskospondylitis, the intervertebral disk space appears widened as the disease erodes the vertebral end plate. As significant

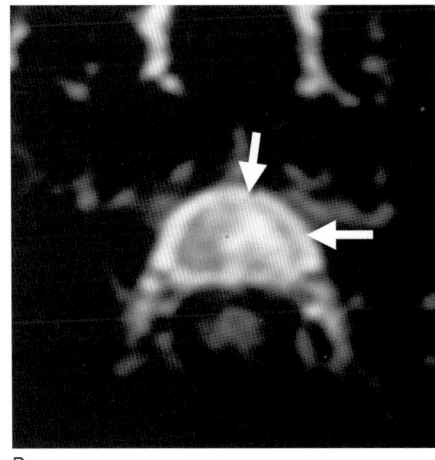

A   B

Figure 2.216. Sagittal (A) and transverse (B) T2-weighted MR images from a dog with inflammation of the cervical spinal cord (arrows).

amounts of bone are damaged over time, the adjacent vertebrae may collapse resulting in decreases in the intervertebral disk space. In rare instances, this disease may predispose one to vertebral luxation and fracture. These pathologic vertebral changes result in further collapse and malalignment of the spine.

Osteomyelitis can involve the vertebrae. On survey radiographs of affected animals, varying combinations of lysis and bony proliferation are present. These alterations primarily involve the vertebral body. The location of the vertebrae involvement (body vs. end plate) is used in differentiating vertebral osteomyelitis from diskospondylitis. Osteomyelitis results in combinations of bone lysis, new bone proliferation, and sclerosis. It is common that the vertebral body, lamina, facets, or dorsal spinous processes are also involved. In areas where grass awn migrations are endemic, osteomyelitis is often found in the ventral aspect of the middle lumbar (L2 through L4) vertebrae. This area is associated with the attachment of the diaphragm (and possible termination of foreign body migration) and is a common place for abscessation to occur.

Vertebral diskospondylitis and osteomyelitis may also be evident in MR studies (Figures 2.217–2.220). In the T2-weighted images, an increase in signal (hyperintense) is seen in the involved vertebral bodies or intervertebral disk area. Disruption of the low signal end plates in both T1 and T2 images is a hallmark of diskospondylitis/osteomyelitis that enables distinction of this entity from neoplasms, which rarely breach the end plates but frequently and extensively involve the marrow. Contrast enhancement is often present in the affected intervertebral disk space.

Spinal abscessation is rare in dogs and cats but can result from hematogenous infection or local penetrat-

ing trauma. Grass awn and porcupine quill migration may enter the spinal canal and result in focal infection. Actinomyces and Nocardia may be present in these locations. Fungal granulomas may also occur in the spinal canal. In some instances of diskospondylitis, the infectious process may extend from the disk into the perispinal tissues and fat. Diagnosis is supported by finding evidence of a compressive (most commonly extradural) or expansile lesion of the spinal cord in myelography, CT, or MR studies. CSF may show evidence of septic inflammation. If the abscess occurs extradurally, nonspecific increases in protein concentration and nucleated cell counts can occur. Occasionally, CSF will be normal.

External Trauma to the Spinal Cord

Spinal cord trauma is relatively common in small animals. This occurs either from exogenous or endogenous injury. Automobile-induced injury is the most common exogenous cause of trauma to the spine in small animals, with falls, trauma from falling objects, and projectile missile damage also occurring. Intervertebral disk extrusion remains the most common endogenous cause.

MR imaging is used to establish the presence of associated acute spinal pathology (Figures 2.221–2.224). When examination with MR is abnormal, the area affected may then be accessed by CT, if further clarification of vertebral involvement is necessary. CSF collected caudal to the lesion may show increases in RBCs, xanthochromia, and erythrophagocytosis. Increases in nucleated cells and protein concentration may be present with concurrent spinal cord inflammation (Figures 2.221–2.224).

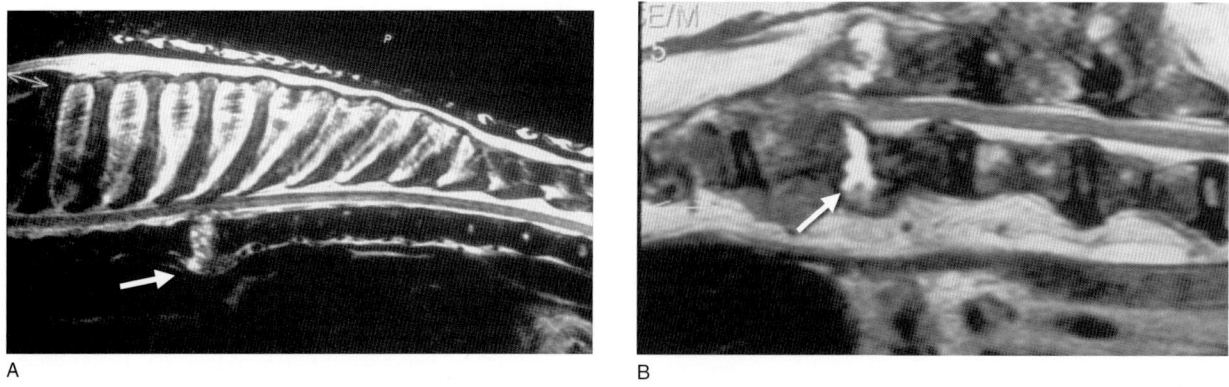

Figure 2.217.   Sagittal T2-weighted MR images from two dogs ((A) and (B)) with diskospondylitis (arrows).

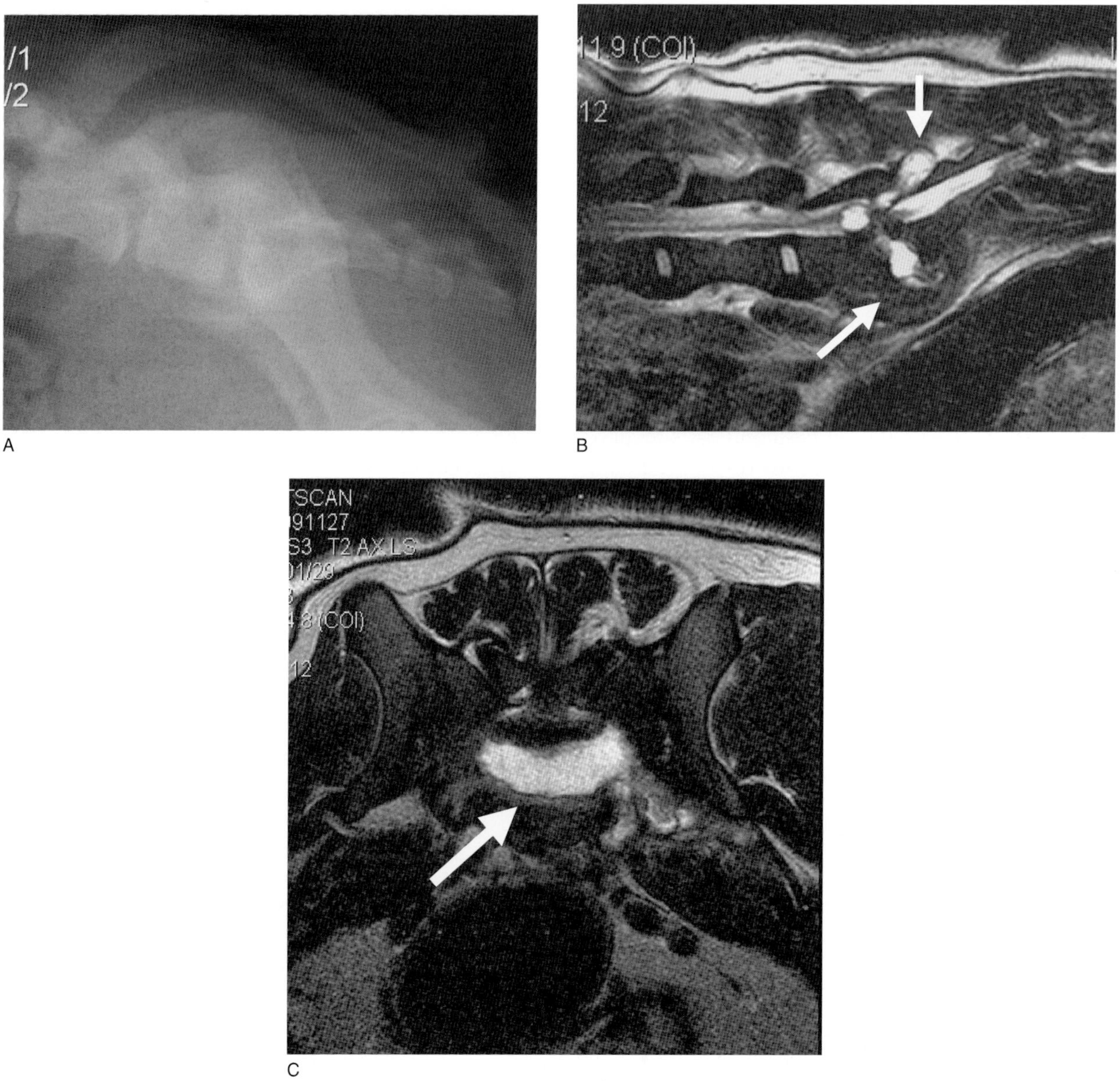

Figure 2.218.   Lateral radiograph (A), sagittal (B), and transverse (C) T2-weighted MR images from a dog with diskospondylitis (arrows) of the LS region.

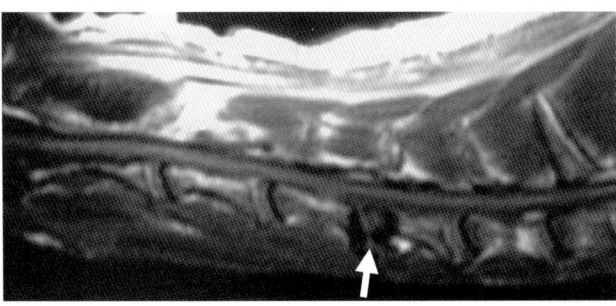

A

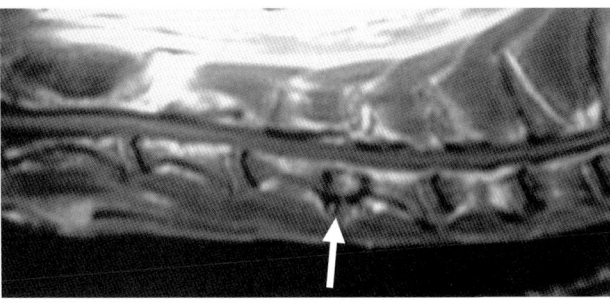

B

Figure 2.219. Sagittal T1-weighted MR images from a dog before (A) and following (B) intravenous contrast administration showing contrast enhancement of the intervertebral disk space with diskospondylitis (arrow).

Fibrocartilaginous Emboli

Ischemic myelopathy, or fibrocartilaginous emboli (FCE), is a disease entity diagnosed with increasing frequency in dogs over the last 15 years. This disease has been thought to result secondary to vascular thrombosis and infarction of the spinal cord with some pathologic evidence to support these conclusions. The spec-

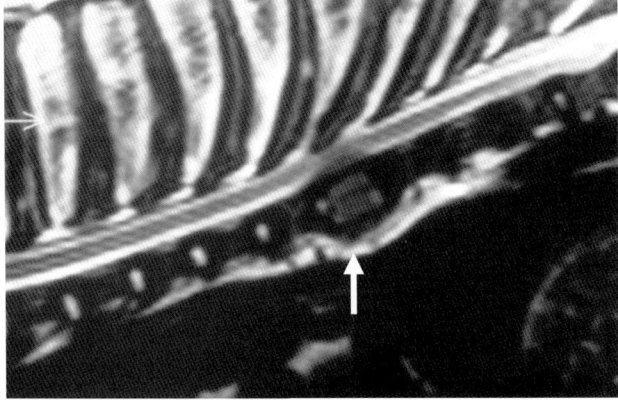

Figure 2.220. Sagittal T2-weighted MR image from a dog with vertebral body osteomyelitis due to fungal infection (arrow).

ulated cause of the infarction centers around fibrocartilage material, similar to that found in intervertebral disks, entering the vascular system and resulting in the embolization of the spinal cord vasculature. How this fibrocartilage enters the vascular system is unclear. Theories include disk extrusion into the vascular system, either directly or through neovascularization of the IVD associated with disk degeneration. It has also been suggested that the fibrocartilage actually arises from within the vascular system and subsequently becomes dislodged. A reasonable pathophysiologic explanation for this disease has been elusive.

Diagnosis is supported by the appropriate clinical signs and exclusion of other disease processes. Definitive diagnosis can only be made at necropsy. Myelography is often normal or may show cord swelling during the acute phases of the disease. Computed tomographic assessment may show similar changes as with myelography. An intramedullary spinal cord lesion is usually present on MR imaging of the affected spinal region (Figures 2.225–2.230). This abnormality usually has the appearance of edema or fluid (hyperintense or whiter signal in T2-weighted studies). The abnormality within the spinal cord is usually focal but may extend for a few disk spaces in the vicinity. These lesions may also contain imaging features suggestive of spinal cord hemorrhage. CSF, collected caudal to the lesion, may be normal or contain increases in nucleated cells and protein. A predisposition to formation of thrombi should be investigated with platelet counts, bleeding times, coagulation profiles, and antithrombin III measurements.

The antemortem diagnosis of FCE is somewhat confounded by the fact that similar clinical, myelographic, and CSF findings may occur in acute, noncompressive intervertebral disk herniation, vascular infarction, focal spinal hemorrhage, or myelitis. Intervertebral disk "explosions" have been previously reported in dogs. In these situations an otherwise normal disk is subjected to such acute and extreme pressure that the nucleus pulposus is rapidly transported into the spinal canal and impacts the spinal cord. The disk material, while causing significant spinal cord injury from the impact with the spinal cord is dissipated within the spinal canal and does not result in persistent spinal cord compression. The spinal injury related to these types of disk extrusions results more from spinal cord contusion than displacement of nucleus pulposus into the spinal cord parenchyma. In these dogs, in addition to the focal spinal cord edema and injury evident in MR studies, the associated nucleus pulposus of the intervertebral disk space may be distorted and irregular compared to adjacent or normal disk spaces (Figures 2.226–2.230).

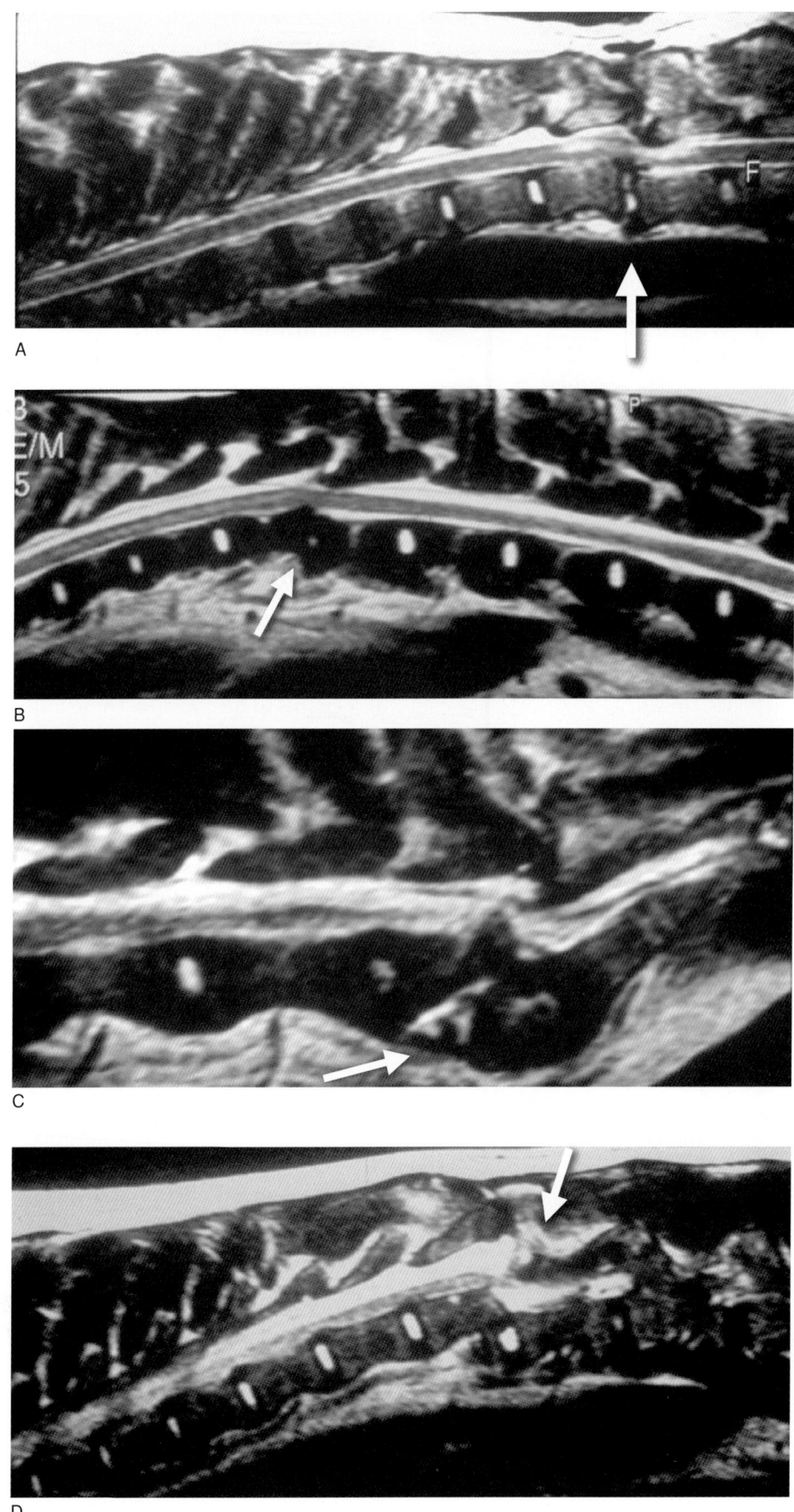

Figure 2.221. Sagittal T2-weighted MR images from four dogs with external spinal trauma (arrows).

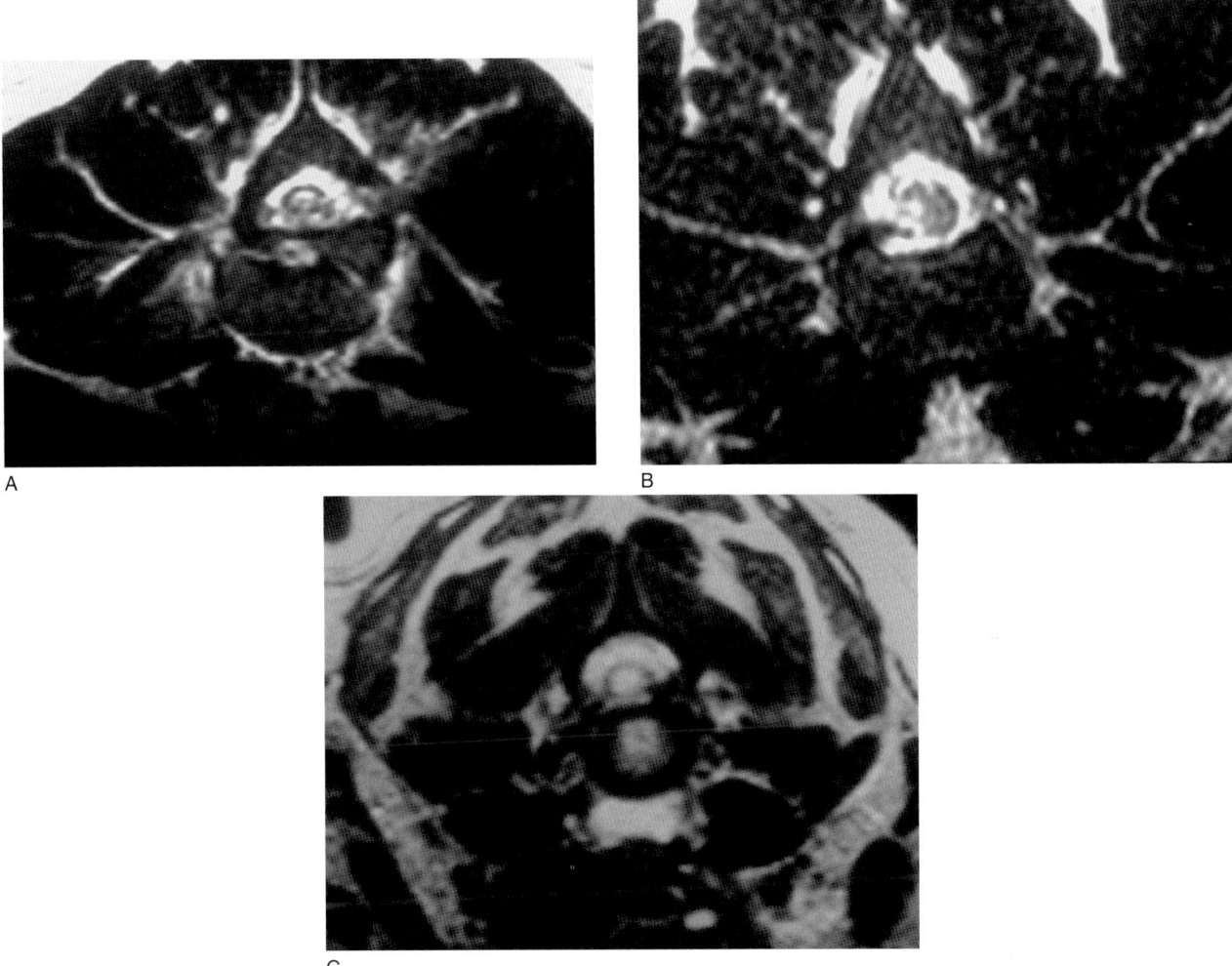

A

B

C

Figure 2.222. Transverse T2-weighted MR images from three dogs with external spinal trauma and associated fracture and/or associated intramedullary MR signal abnormalities.

Spinal Cord Hemorrhage or Hematoma

Spinal cord hemorrhage or hematoma may result in clinical signs of spinal cord dysfunction (Figures 2.231–2.233). Hemorrhage can occur at any level of the spinal cord. In most instances, extradural hematoma occurs from trauma, intervertebral disk extrusion, or underlying coagulopathies, platelet dysfunction, or vasculopathies. Extradural hematomas often appear as compressive spinal abnormalities. Intramedullary hematomas have also been reported. In rarer instances, focal spinal cord hemorrhage may result secondary to lumbar CSF collection (Figure 2.234).

Hemorrhagic CNS complications should be suspected in any animal with acute neurologic signs and associated signs of either thrombocytopenia or coagulopathy. In some instances, the nervous system signs will occur prior to any obvious systemic signs of a bleeding disorder. A thorough examination of the body for petechia is important, including the mucous membranes (especially of the penis, prepuce, and vulva) and the retina. Pallor, low-grade heart murmurs, weakness, and tachycardia are hallmark signs of coagulopathies with larger amounts of bleeding into body cavities. Thoracic auscultation for pleural fluid and abdominal palpation for hemoperitoneum is important. Radiographs and ultrasound may help when the physical examination is unrewarding but large amounts of internal bleeding are suspected. Remember that large amounts of blood can be lost through the gastrointestinal tract, and examination of the stool for hematochezia or melena is important.

Complete blood cell count, with special attention to red cell numbers and platelet counts, is important especially for the diagnosis of anemia and thrombocytopenia. Specific coagulation testing (bleeding time, PT, PTT,

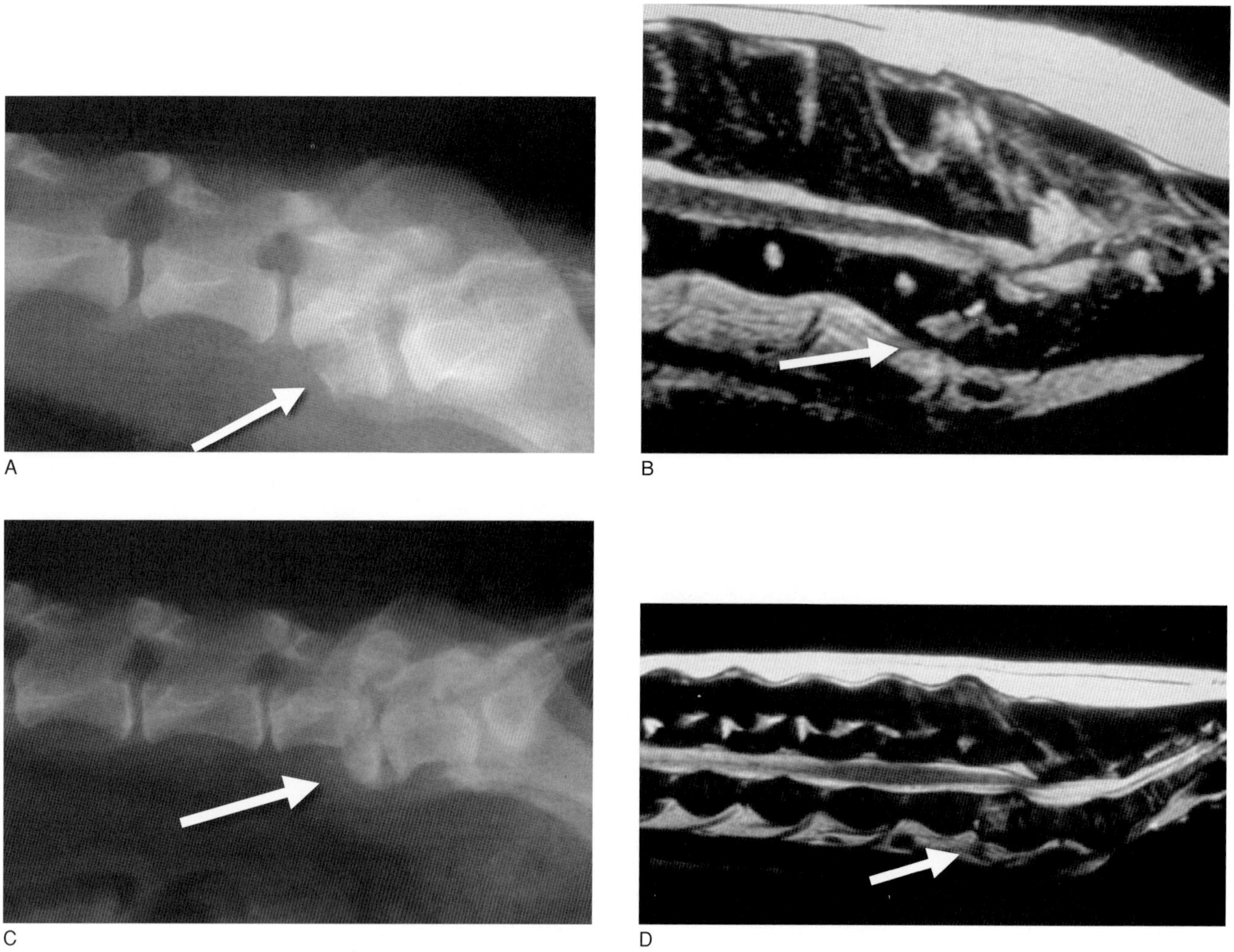

Figure 2.223.   Lateral radiograph ((A), (C)) and sagittal ((B), (D)) T2-weighted MR images from two dogs ((A), (B) and (C), (D)) with spinal fractures (arrows).

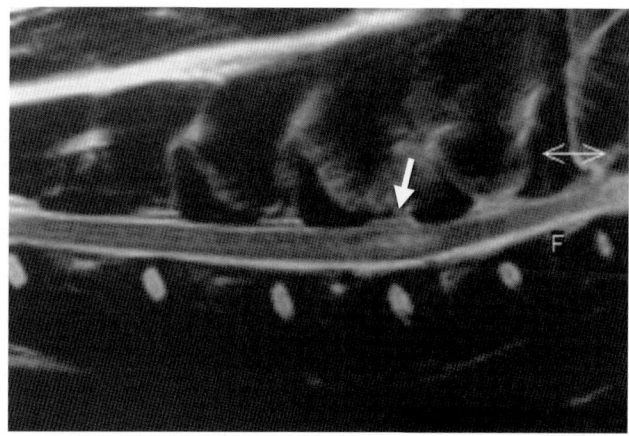

Figure 2.224.   Sagittal T2-weighted MR image from a dog with intramedullary MR signal abnormality associated with a gun shot injury (arrow).

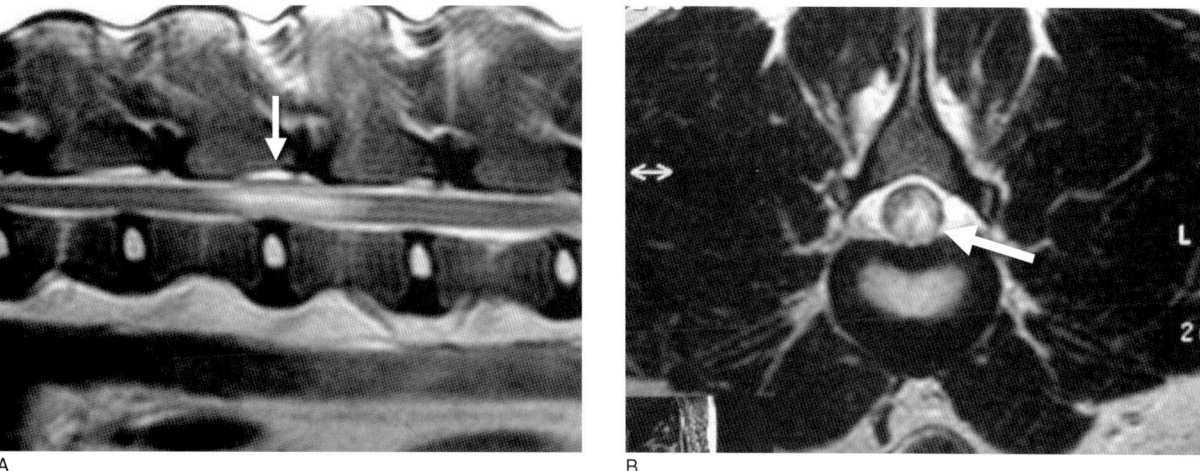

Figure 2.225.   Sagittal (A) and transverse (B) T2-weighted MR image from a dog with a fibrocartilagenous emboli (arrows).

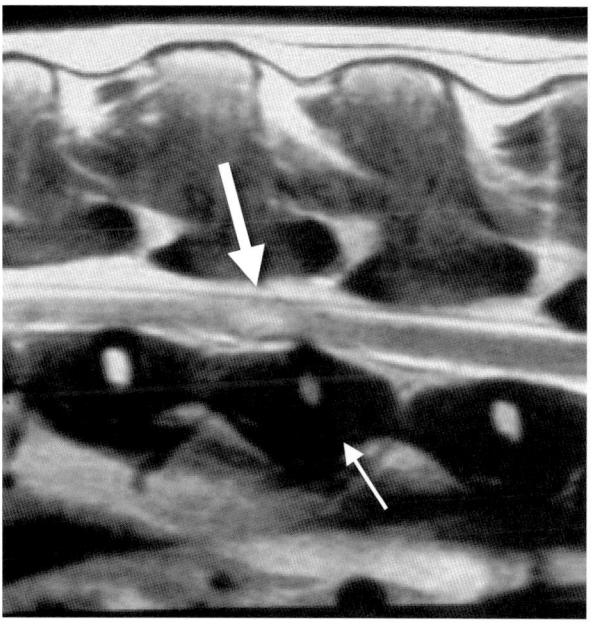

Figure 2.226.   Sagittal T2-weighted MR image from a dog with an acute intervertebral disk nucleus pulposus extrusion. Note the abnormal MR signal of the nucleus pulposus (small arrow) and the associated intraspinal cord signal abnormality (larger arrow).

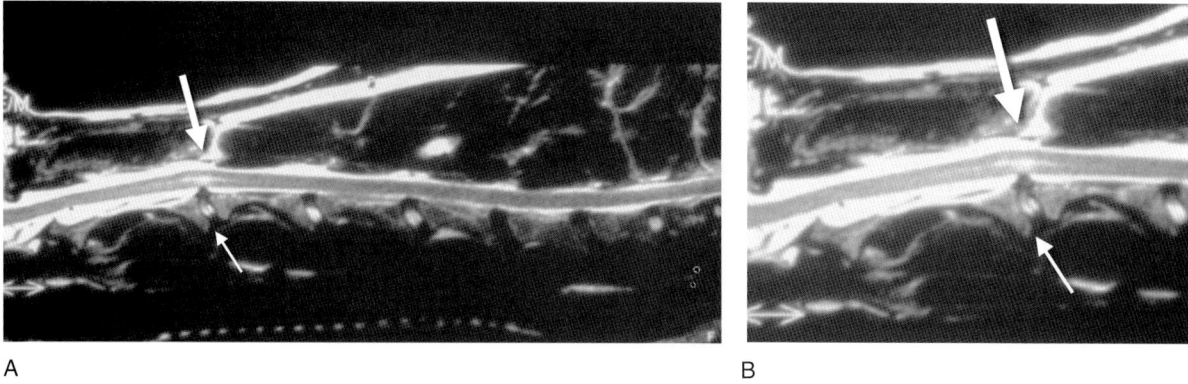

Figure 2.227.   Sagittal (A) T2-weighted MR image from a dog with an acute intervertebral disk nucleus pulposus extrusion at C2-3. Note the abnormal MR signal of the nucleus pulposus (small arrow) and the associated intraspinal cord signal abnormality (larger arrow). An enlarged view is shown in (B).

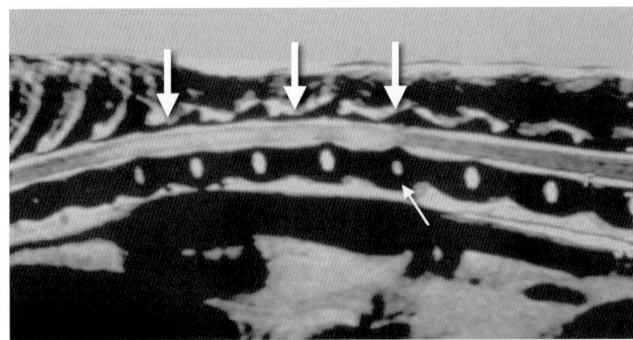

Figure 2.228.   Sagittal T2-weighted MR image from a dog with an acute intervertebral disk nucleus pulposus extrusion in the thoracolumbar area (small arrow). Note the extensive abnormal MR intraspinal cord signal abnormality (larger arrows).

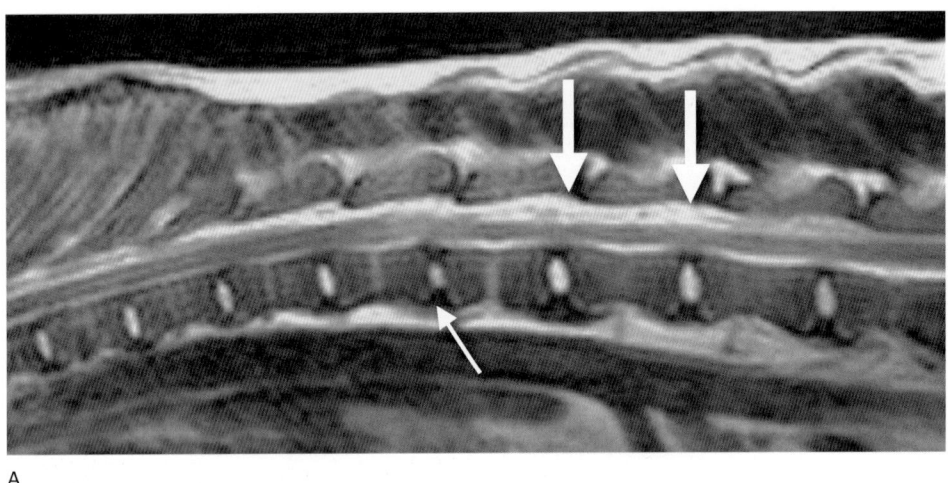

A

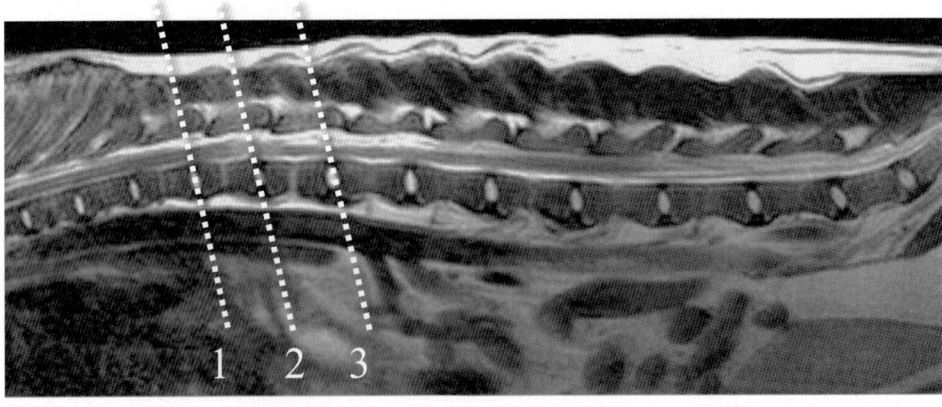

B

Figure 2.229.   Sagittal T2-weighted MR image (A) from a dog with an acute intervertebral disk nucleus pulposus extrusion in the thoracolumbar area (small arrow). Note the extensive abnormal MR extradural cord signal abnormality (larger arrows). (B) Same sagittal T2-weighted image showing the levels of the transverse planes (1, 2, 3) which correspond to (C) (1), (D) (2), and (E) (3).

C

D

E

Figure 2.229. (*Continued*) Note the normal nuclear signal of the intervertebral disks cranial (C) and caudal (E) compared to the abnormal one (D). Also note the extradural abnormal signal in (D) (arrows).

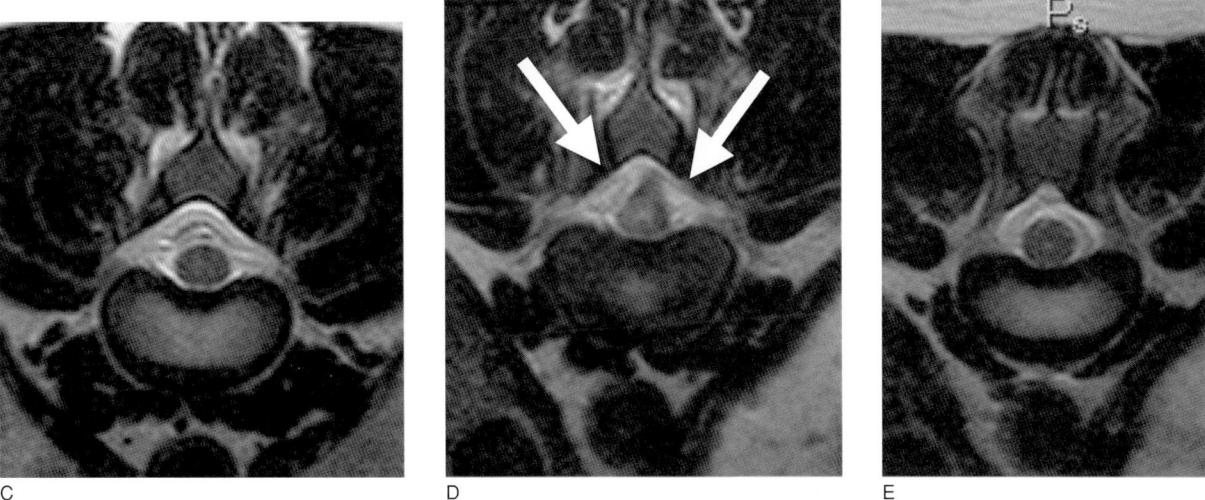

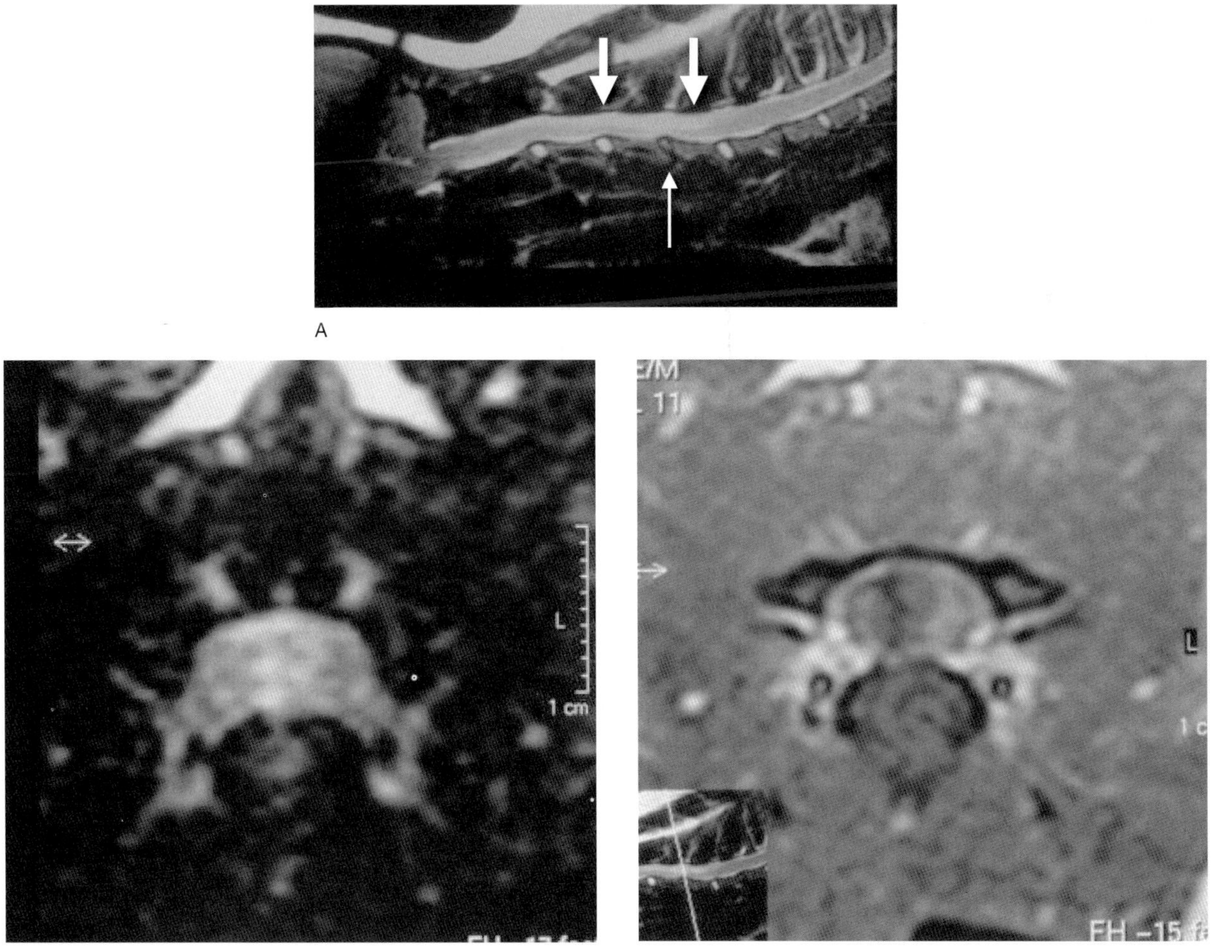

A

B

C

Figure 2.230. Sagittal T2-weighted MR image (A) from a dog with an acute intervertebral disk nucleus pulposus extrusion into the spinal cord. Note the abnormal MR signal of the nucleus pulposus (smaller arrow) and the extensive abnormal MR cord signal abnormality (larger arrows). Transverse T2-weighted (B) and T1-weighted (C) MR images from the same dog through the abnormal spinal cord at the level of the intervertebral disk extrusion. Note the hypointense curvilinear abnormal signal within the spinal cord in the T1-weighted study which was intraspinal abnormal intervertebral disk material.

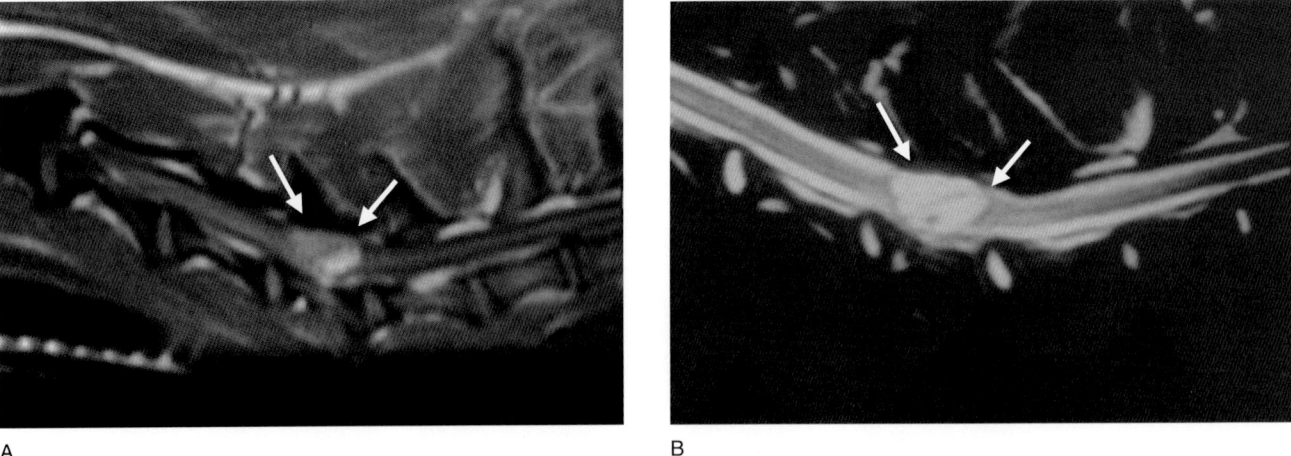

A   B

Figure 2.231.   Sagittal T1-weighted (A) and T2-weighted (B) MR images from a dog with a focal spinal hematoma (arrows).

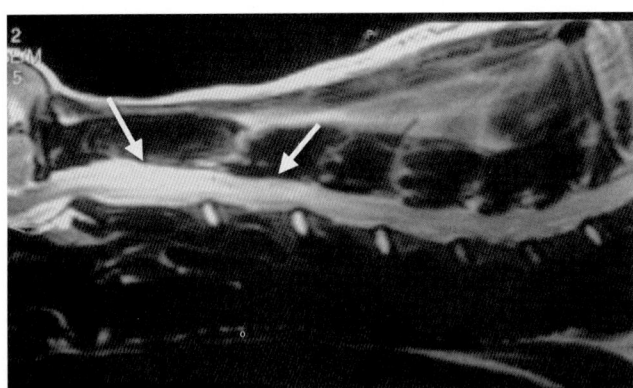

Figure 2.232.   Sagittal T2-weighted MR image from a dog with diffuse spinal hemorrhage (arrows).

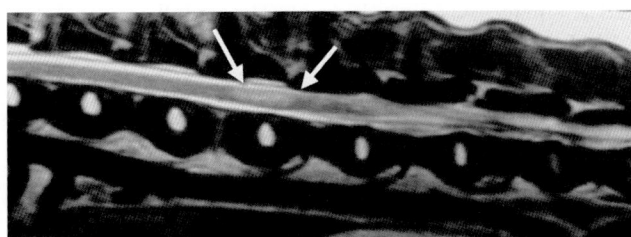

Figure 2.233.   Sagittal T2-weighted MR image from a dog with intramedullary and extradural spinal hemorrhage (arrows).

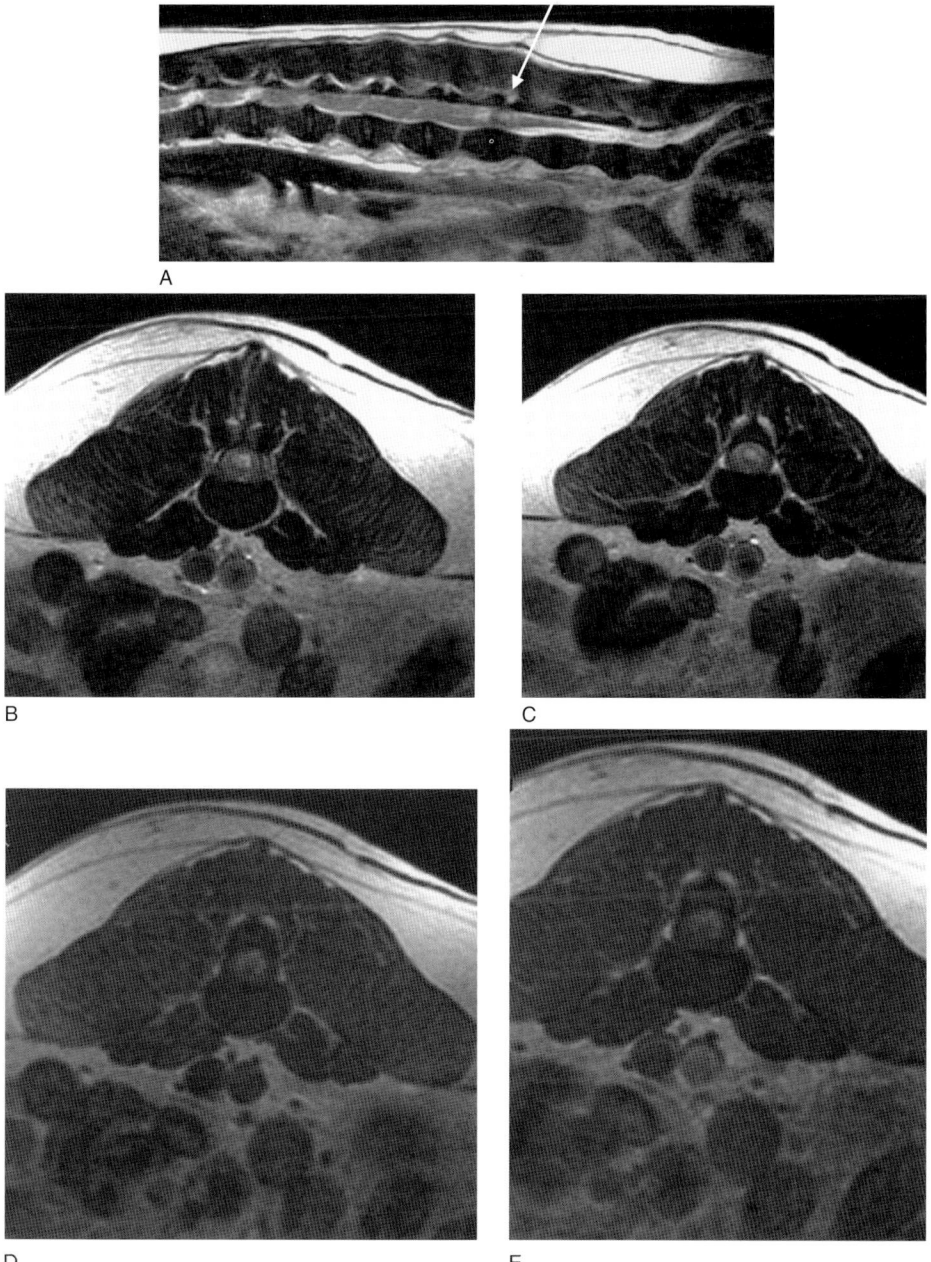

Figure 2.234.   Sagittal T2-weighted MR image (A) from a dog with intramedullary spinal abnormality subsequent to a lumbar cerebrospinal fluid collection (arrow). Transverse T2-weighted MR images ((B) and (C)) from the same dog at adjacent levels. Transverse T1-weighted MR images before (D) and following intravenous contrast administration (E) from the same dog at adjacent levels.

FDPs) is also commonly evaluated. Biochemical evidence of a predisposition to hypercoagulability such as proteinuria should be documented.

With most vascular diseases of the spinal cord survey spinal radiographs are normal. Myelography may reveal evidence of extradural or intramedullary abnormalities that distort the subarachnoid space. With extradural compression, the subarachnoid columns may be distorted inward toward the center of the spinal canal with myelographic evaluation. With intramedullary hematoma, the spinal cord appears focally enlarged.

Clarification of the cause of the clinical signs often requires advanced spinal imaging such as MR imaging (Figures 2.231–2.234). On MR, hemorrhage less than 12–24 h old may not be distinguishable from vasogenic edema. In the circulating blood, hemoglobin fluctuates between the oxyhemoglobin state and the deoxyhemoglobin state. The heme iron in both oxyhemoglobin and deoxyhemoglobin form is in the ferrous Fe^{2+} state. When hemoglobin is removed from the high-oxygen environment of the circulation, the heme iron undergoes oxidative denaturation to the ferric state (Fe^{3+}) forming methemoglobin. Continued oxidative denaturation forms ferric hemichromes (hemosiderin). As RBCs break down, the various forms of hemoglobin have changing paramagnetic properties influencing the appearance of the clot in the various images (T1- and T2-weighted). Besides the form of hemoglobin present, the signal intensities of a blood clot may vary depending on the operating field strength, the type of signal the operator chooses, and the technique (T1- vs. T2-weighted). Hemorrhage may also vary in appearance depending on where the bleed occurred, for example in the tissue (subdural vs. intraparenchymal vs. subarachnoid).

Artifacts

The common artifacts that influence the MR images of more standard pulse sequences have been discussed previously in Chapter 4 (Figures 2.235–2.248). Artifacts of image acquisition may result in misdiagnosis of clinical disease. The more common artifacts that result with spinal imaging are discussed further.

"Ghosts" are replica images that occur in the direction of the phase encoding. While this type of artifact may result for numerous reasons, motion may be the most common. Some of this motion may occur from within the normal structures of the patient such as CSF pulsation, blood flow through vessels, respiratory motion, and cardiac movements. Wrapping is where structures from outside the field of view are seemingly superimposed upon the region of interest. This is most often the result of aliasing where samples from a high frequency signal are not distinguished from samples of a much lower frequency. Flow of blood in vessels in or around the spine, and especially the venous sinus, may result in confusing MR imaging characteristics. In general, "faster" flowing blood will be hypointense or create a "flow void." In other instances, depending upon the direction and velocity of flow, iso- or hyperintense signal from vessels may result. Artifacts associated with blood flowing in arteries or veins around the spine may result in artifacts superimposed upon normal nervous tissue elements as well. Motion of flow of artifacts occurs along the phase-encoding axis.

Chemical shift artifact occurs along the frequency-encoding direction and results in misregistration between fat and water tissues. This misregistration most often results in a hypointense (darker) contour between these tissues and is most often present immediately adjacent to the spinal cord. This artifact can be confused with spinal cord compression, however, the discrete crescent shape associated with this artifact is usually apparent. Chemical shift artifact may be more apparent with MR units of higher magnetic strength.

Truncation artifacts are apparent as discrete lines that run parallel with the spinal cord and can be seen in sagittal images. These lines are hyperintense in T2-weighted images and occur usually at fat-CSF interfaces. These artifactual lines many mimic either central spinal cord gray matter or, more commonly, the central canal (Figure 2.193). Depending upon the width of this artifact, a misdiagnosis of hydromyelia may result. An absence of this apparent abnormality on the transverse image supports its artifactual nature.

Finally, another important factor that influences the utility of an MR examination of a clinically affected patient centers around overall image quality. Poor quality MR examinations result in an inability to gleam useful clinical information (Figure 2.249). Additionally, inappropriate neuroanatomical localization may result in misinterpretation of MR apparent abnormalities (Figure 2.250).

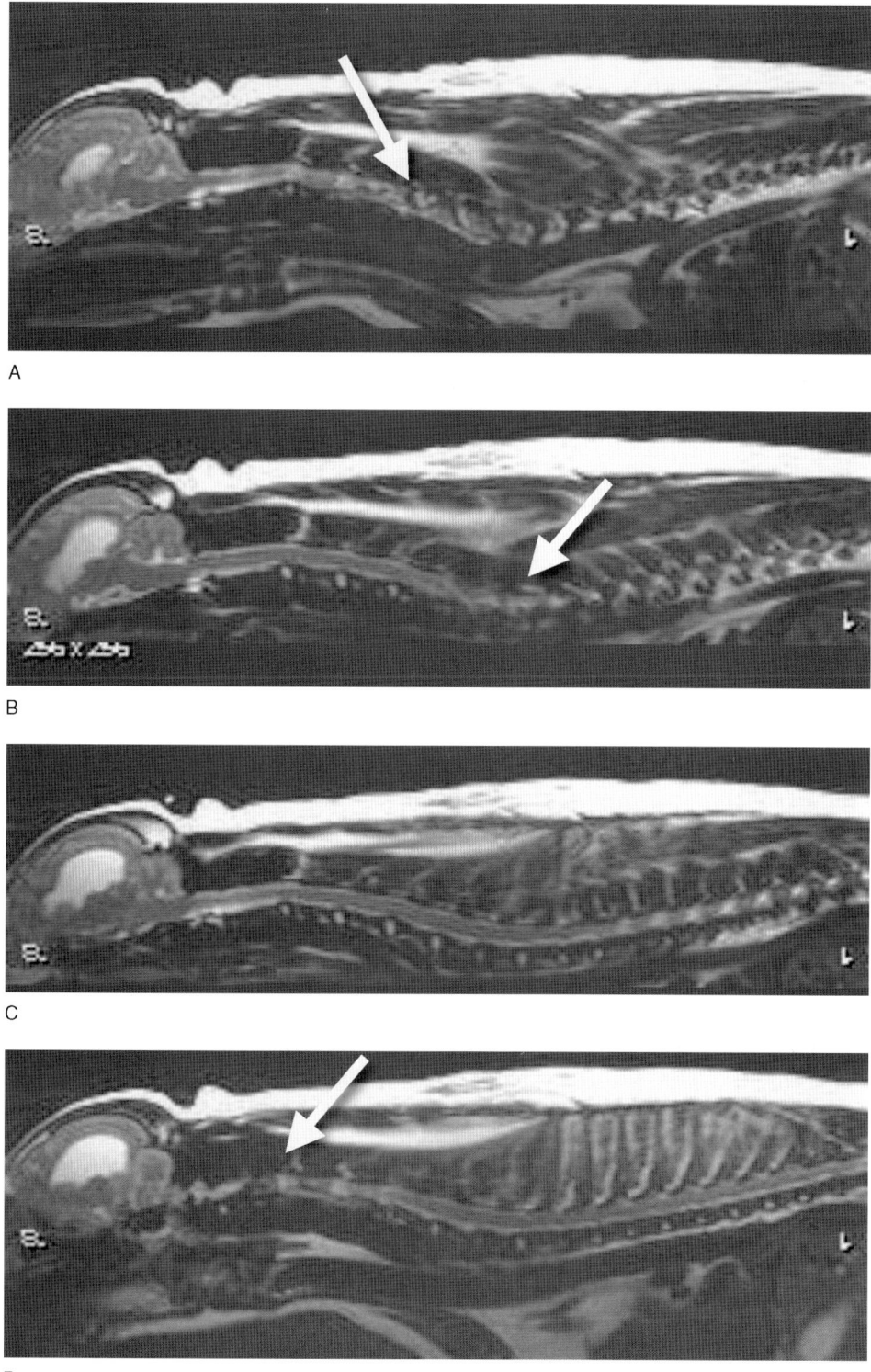

A

B

C

D

Figure 2.235. Sagittal and parasagittal T2-weighted MR images from a dog. Some of the parasagittal slices show the tangential nature of the slice plane (arrows).

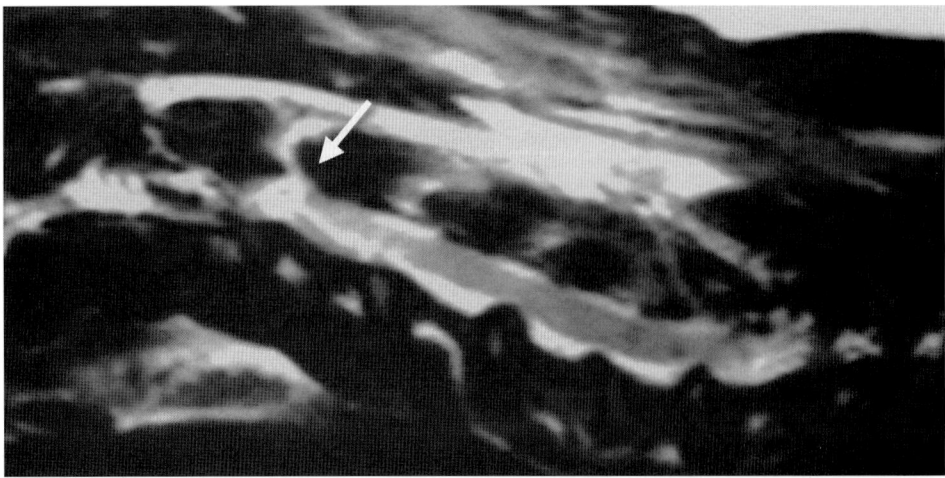

Figure 2.236. Sagittal T2-weighted MR image from a dog showing the tangential nature of the slice which caused distortion of the image (arrow).

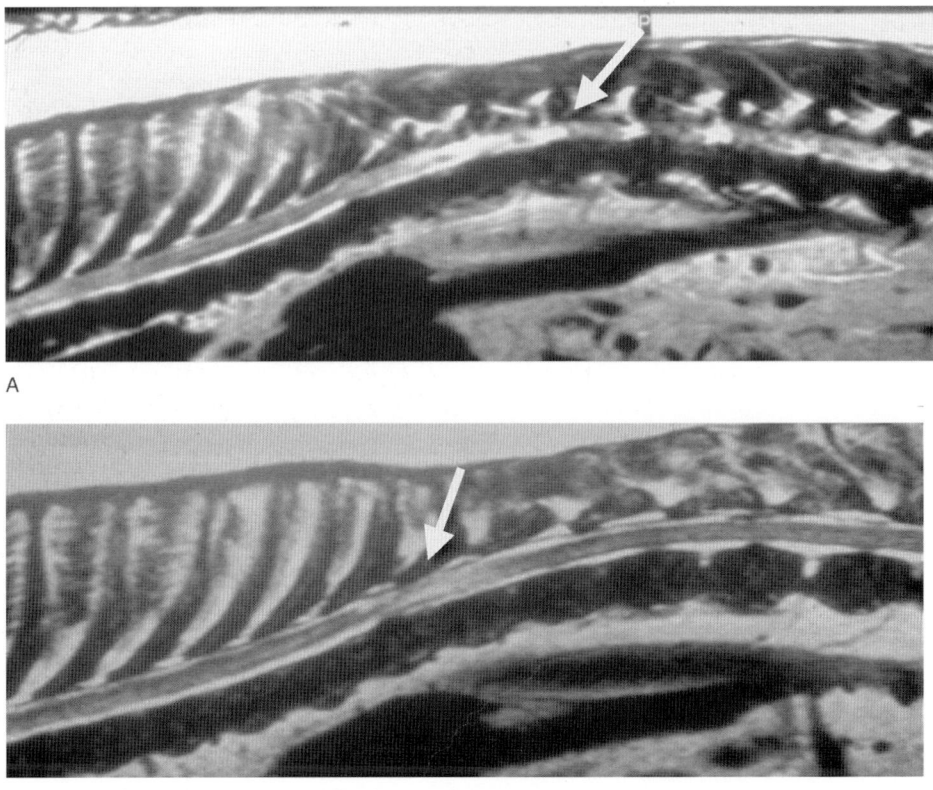

Figure 2.237. Sagittal T2-weighted MR images from a dog. The initially positioned image (A) showing the tangential nature of the slice (arrow). Once the animal was more appropriately positioned (B), the true lesion can more easily be identified (arrow).

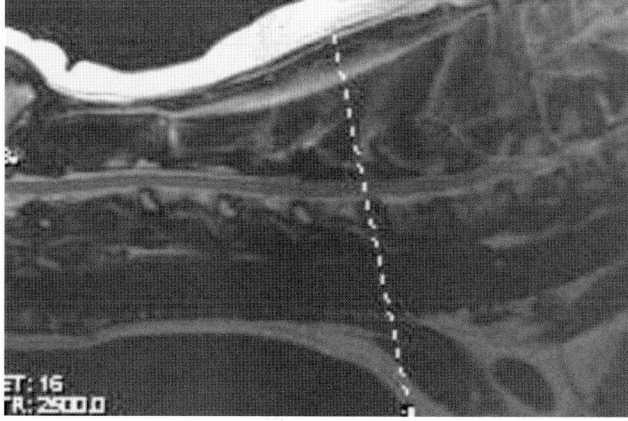

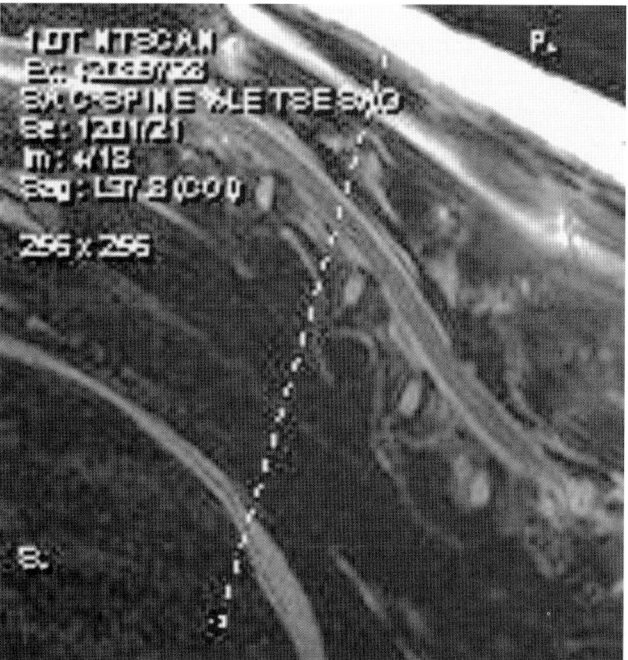

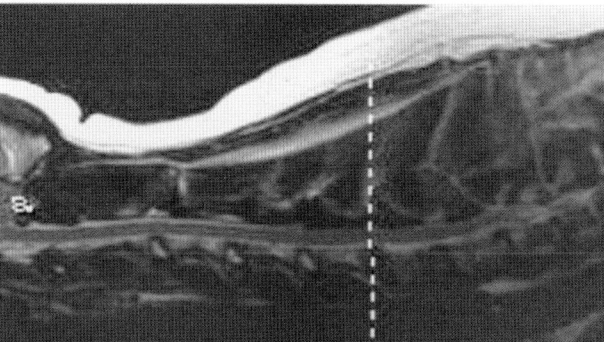

A

Figure 2.238. Sagittal T2-weighted MR images ((A) and (B)) from a dog showing the potential differing angles for the transverse slice plane (lines).

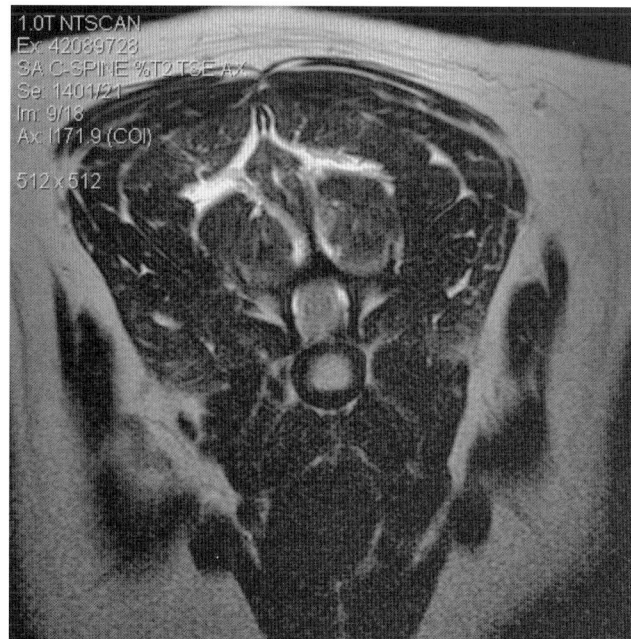

B

Figure 2.239. Sagittal (A) and transverse (B) T2-weighted MR images from a dog showing the "bleeding" appearance to the spinal cord due to the angulation of the slice ((A), line).

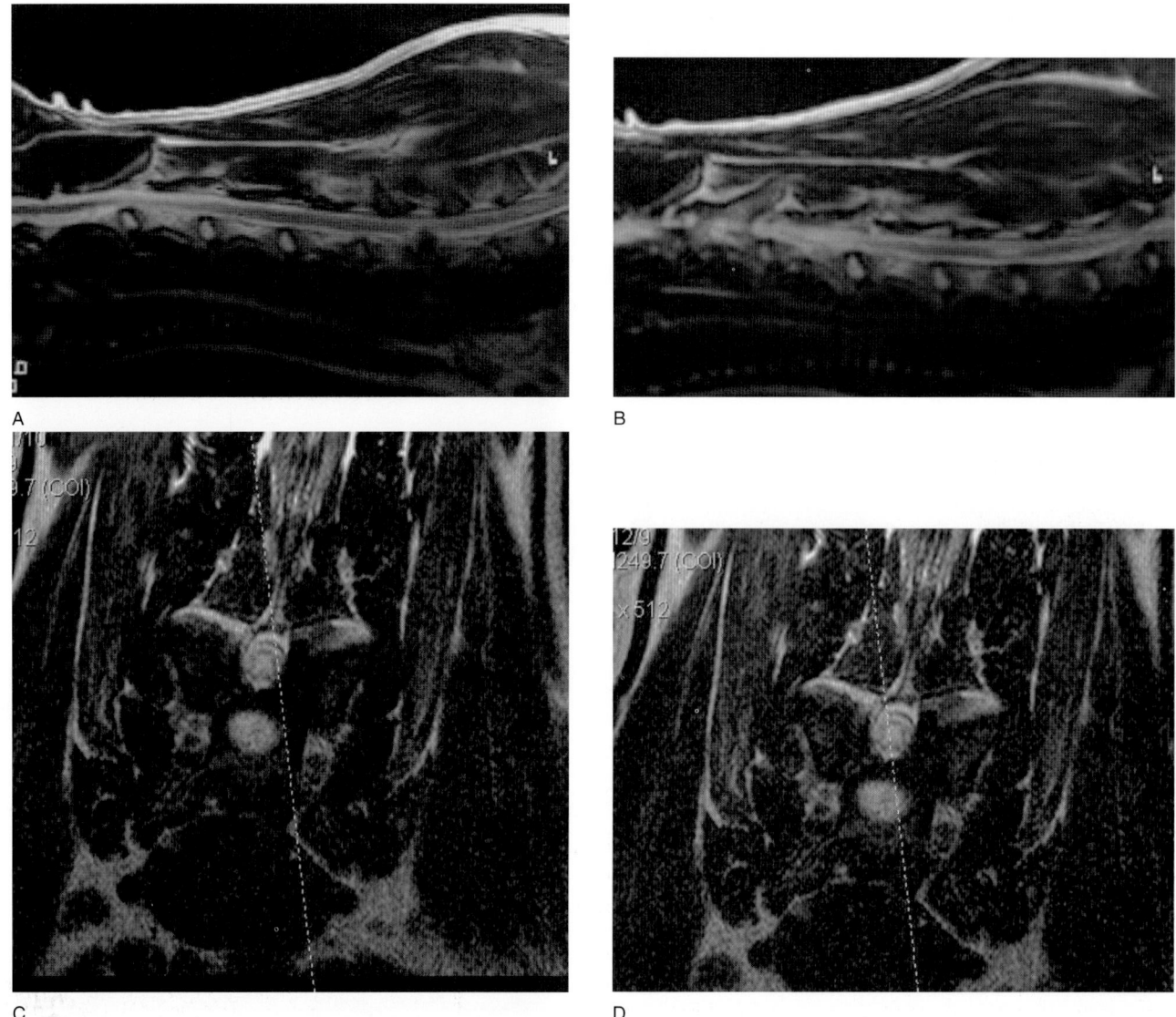

A

B

C

D

Figure 2.240. Sagittal (A), parasagittal (B), and transverse ((C) and (D)) T2-weighted MR images from a dog showing the differing appearance to the sagittal and parasagittal images due to the differing angulation of the slice place ((C) and (D), lines).

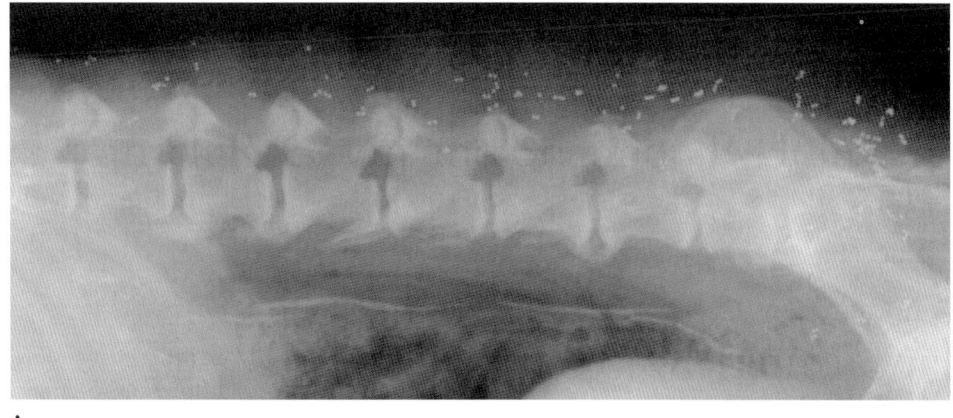

A

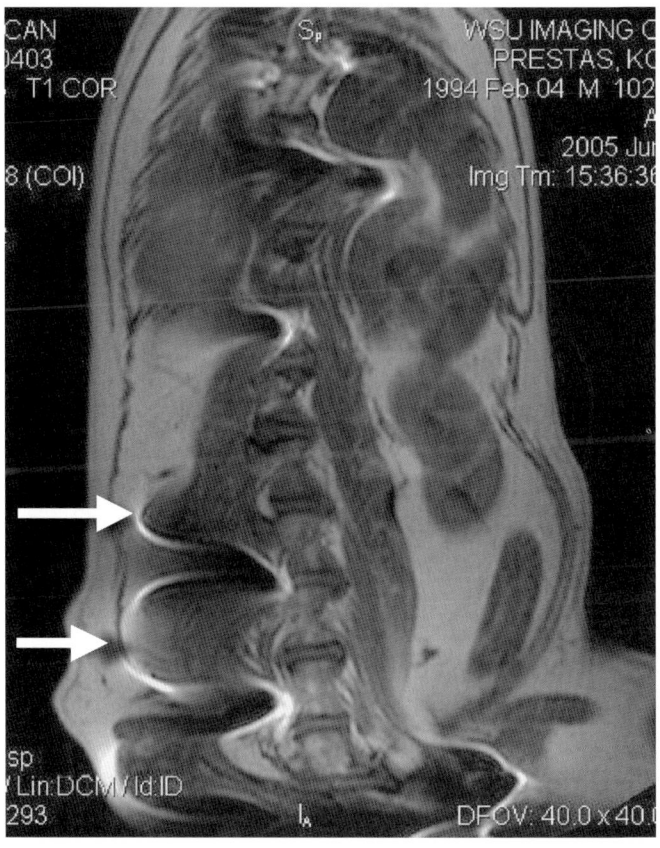

B

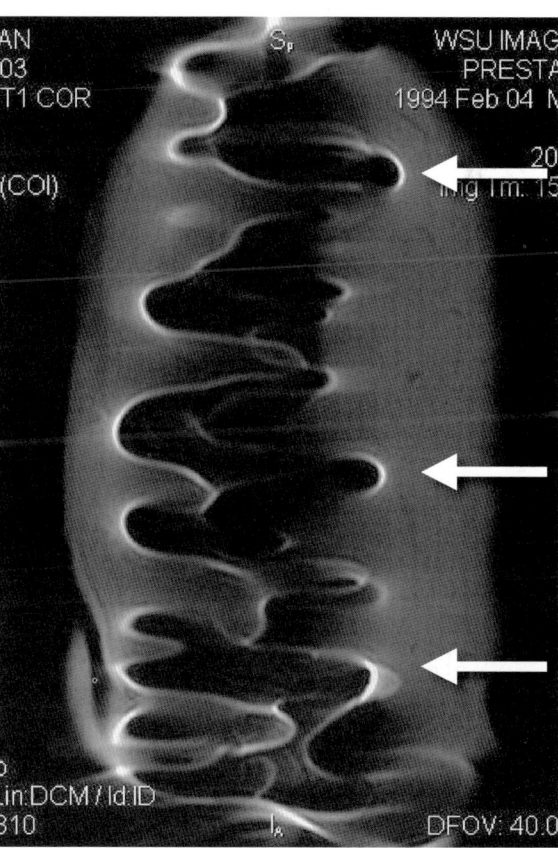

C

Figure 2.241. Lateral radiograph (A) image from a dog with gold bead implants along the spine. Dorsal plane, T1-weighted MR images ((B) and (C)) from the same dog at adjacent levels showing artifact produced by the gold beads (arrows).

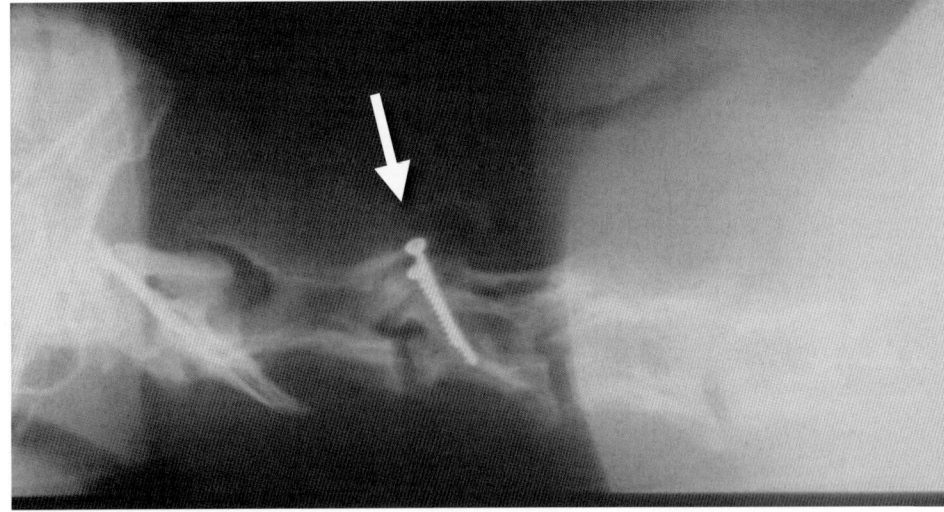

A

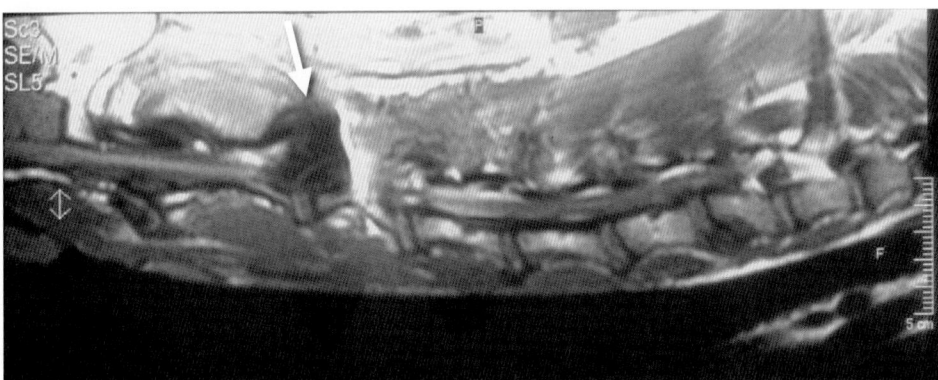

B

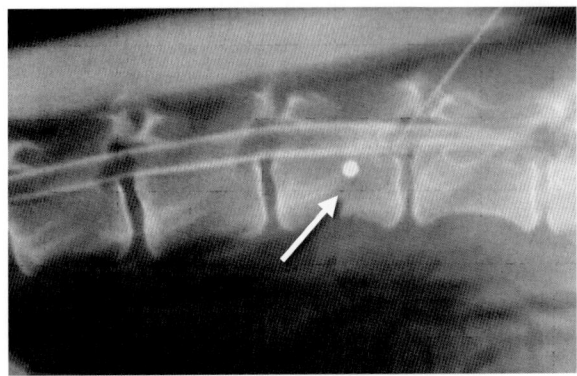

C

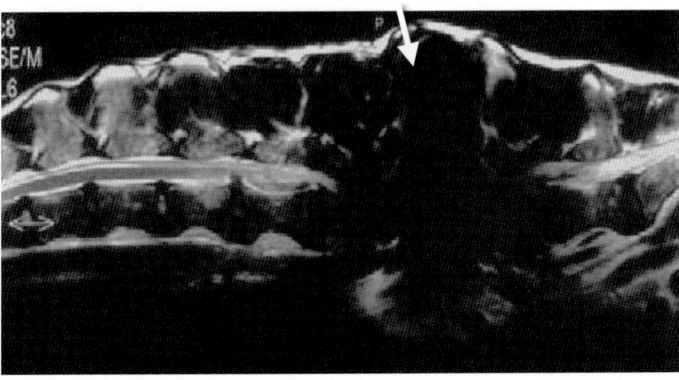

D

Figure 2.242.   Lateral radiograph (A) image from a dog with surgical screw implants in the cervical region. Sagittal plane T1-weighted MR image (B) from the same dog showing artifact produced by the screws (arrow). Lateral myelographic view (C) from a dog with a BB in the lumbar spinal region. Sagittal plane T2-weighted MR image (D) from the same dog showing artifact produced by the BB (arrow).

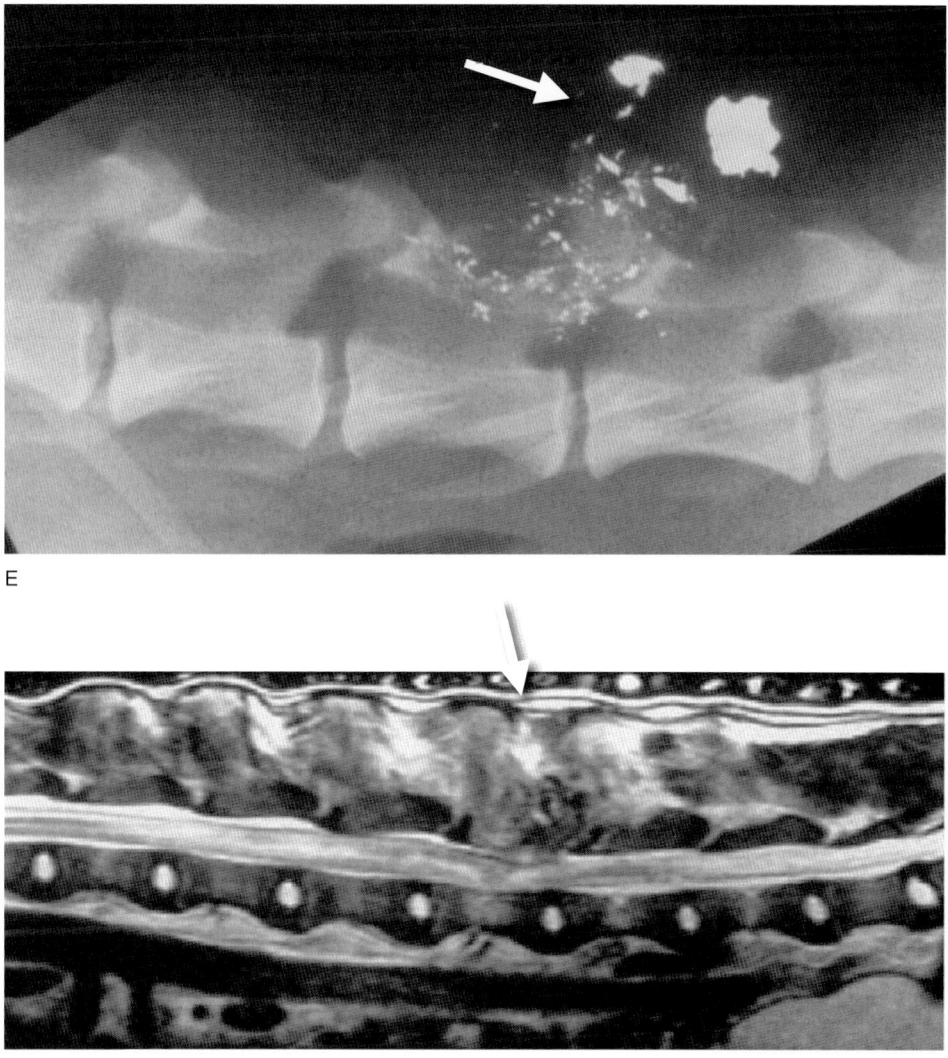

E

F

Figure 2.242. (*Continued*) Lateral radiographic view (E) from a dog with a gun shot lesion in the lumbar spinal region. Sagittal plane T2-weighted MR image (F) from the same dog showing no artifact produced by the lead projectile (arrow).

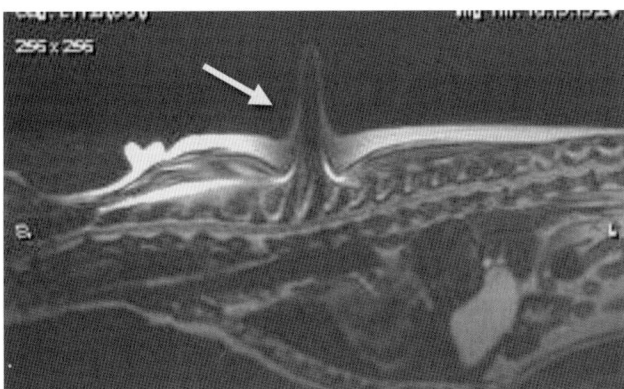

Figure 2.243. Sagittal T2-weighted MR image from a dog with an identification chip implanted subcutaneously in the dorsal cranial thoracic region. The artifact shown is the result of the metal within the chip (arrow).

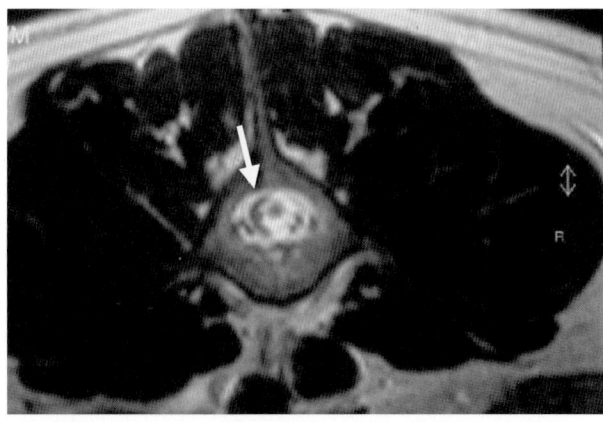

A

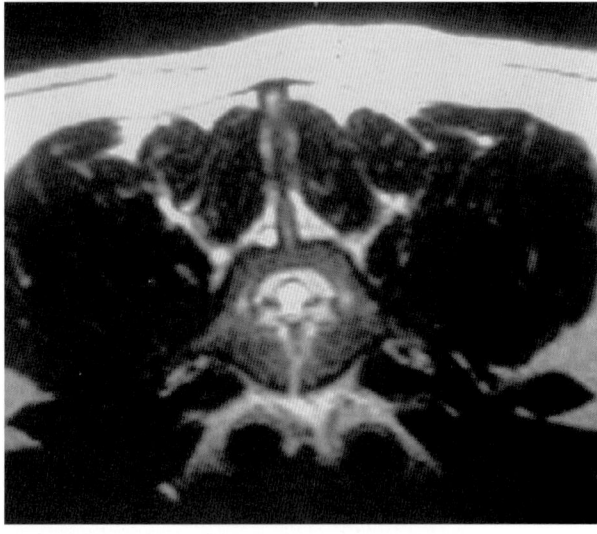

B

Figure 2.245. Transverse T2-weighted MR image (A) from a dog with chemical shift artifact (arrow). Transverse T2-weighted MR image (B) taken from the same dog after changing the phase and frequency direction when performing the image acquisition and subsequent elimination of the artifact.

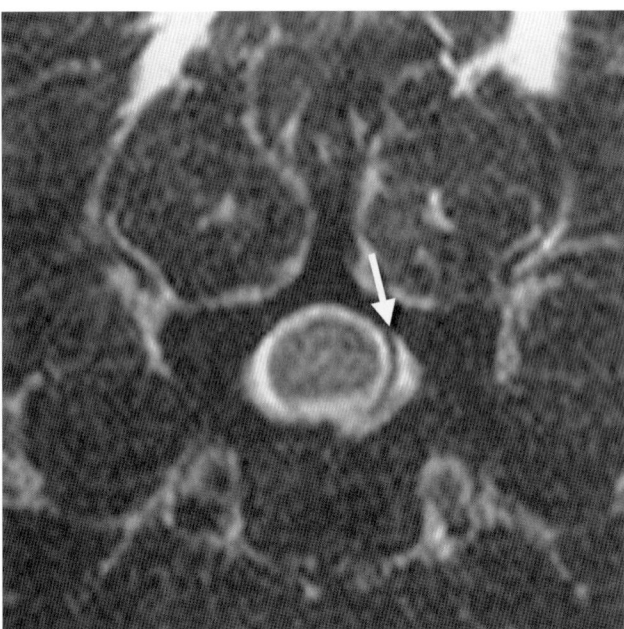

Figure 2.244. Transverse T2-weighted MR image from a dog with chemical shift artifact (arrow).

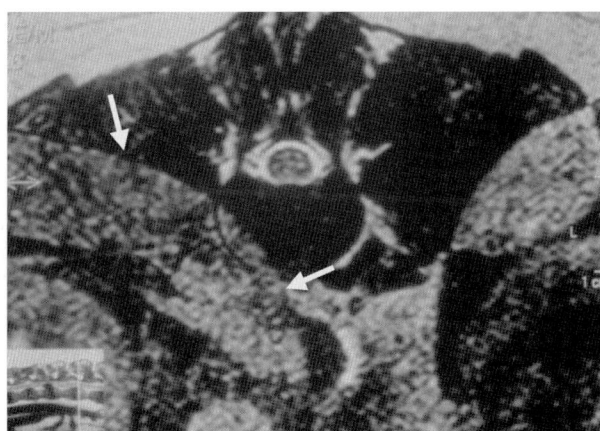

Figure 2.246. Transverse T2-weighted MR image from a dog with a wrapping artifact (arrows).

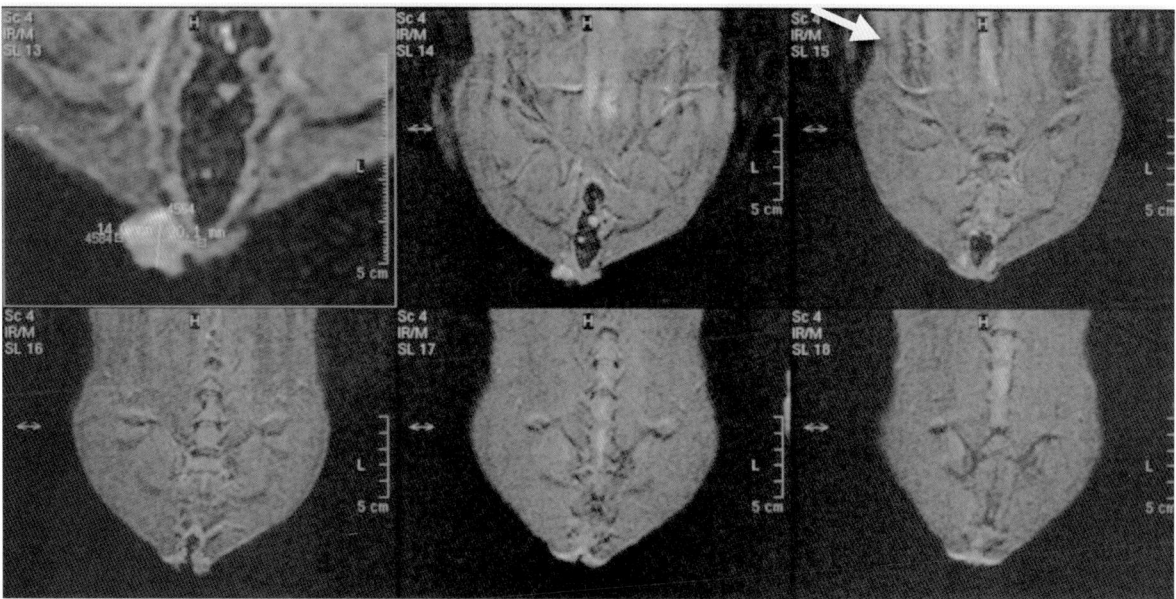

Figure 2.247.   Dorsal MR images from a dog with a motion artifact (arrow).

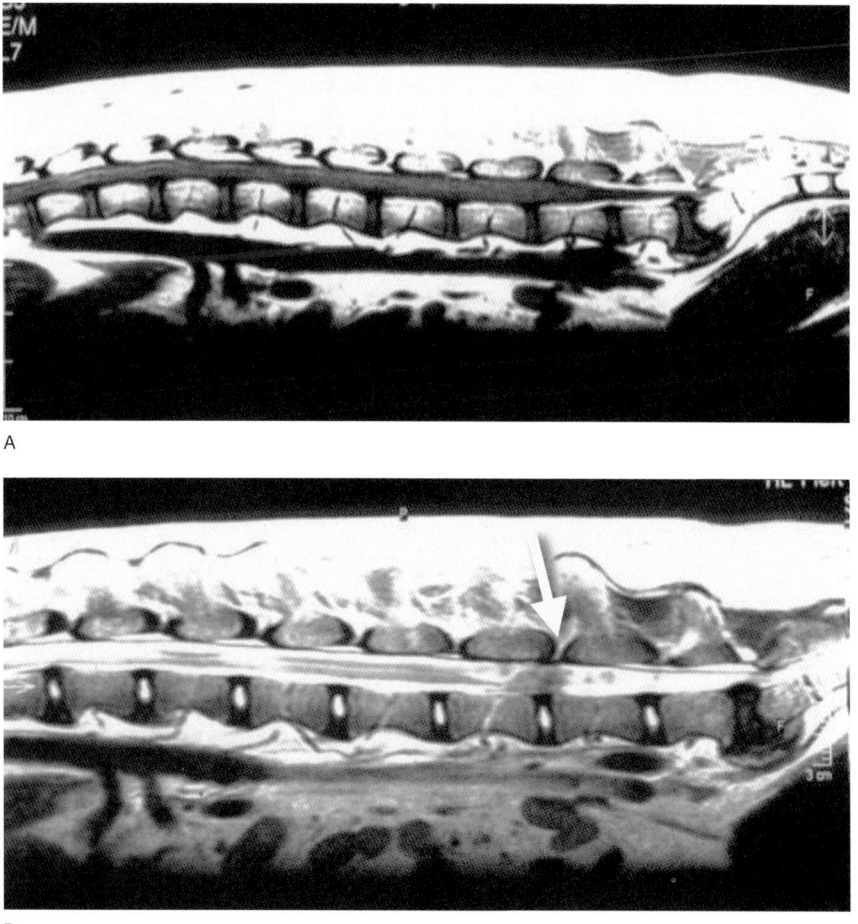

A

B

Figure 2.248.   Sagittal T1-weighted (A) and T2-weighted (B) MR images from a dog with a tumor (arrow) at L5-6 level. The tumor is easily missed on the T1-weighted image.

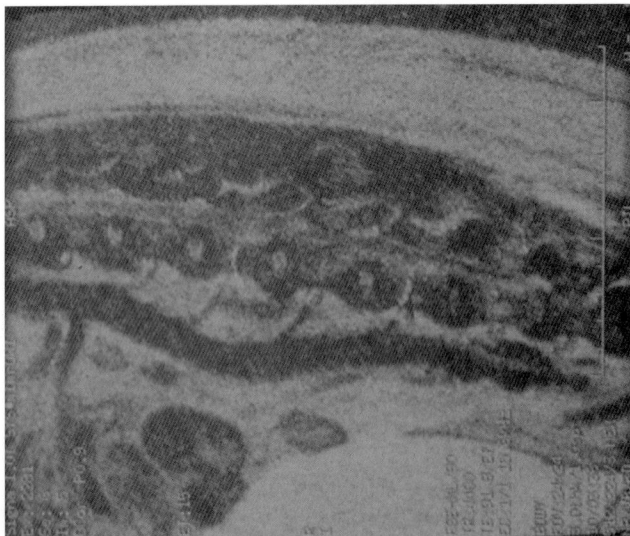

Figure 2.249.   Sagittal MR image from a dog, which is poor quality making objective assessment difficult.

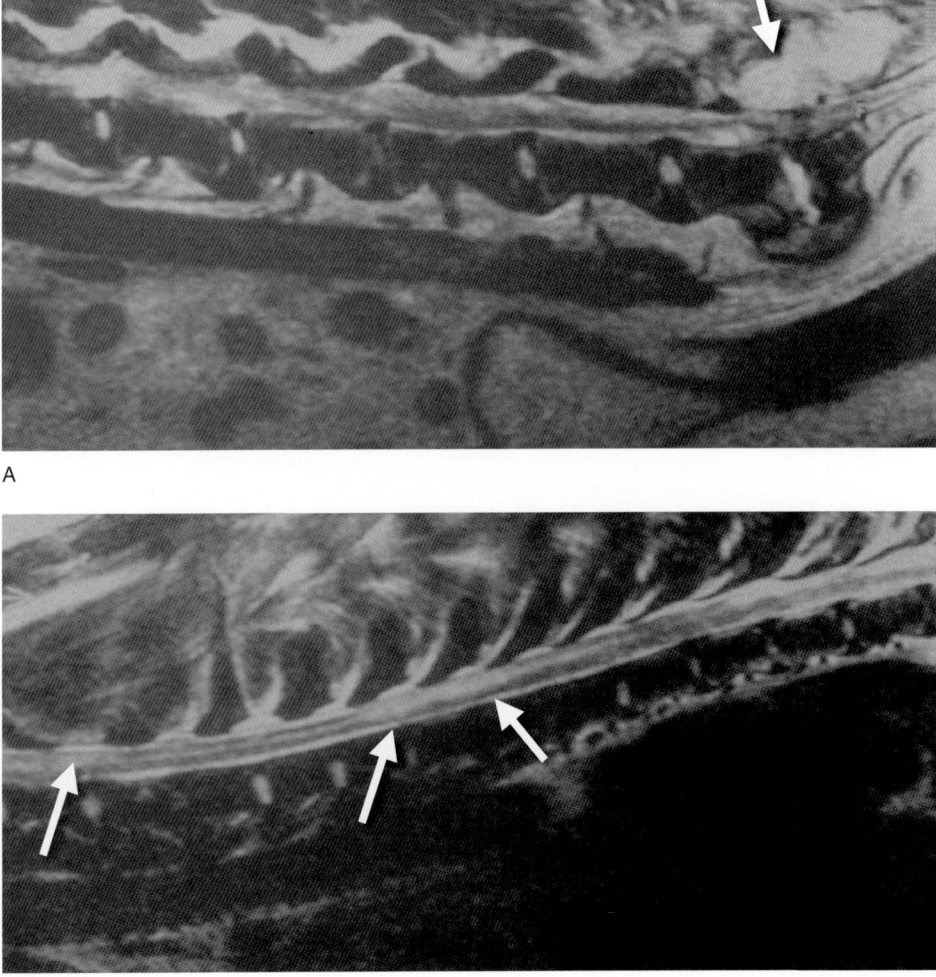

Figure 2.250.   Sagittal T2-weighted MR images from a dog that had a previous LS laminectomy and partial diskectomy ((A), arrow). The dog had a previous missed myelitis ((B), arrows).

MR Bibliography

Dogs

Abramson CJ, Garosi L, Platt SR, Dennis R, and McConnell JF. 2005. Magnetic resonance imaging appearance of suspected ischemic myelopathy in dogs. Vet Radiol Ultrasound 46(3):225–229.

Adams WH. 1999. The spine. Clin Tech Small Anim Pract 14(3):148–159.

Allam MW, Lee DG, Nulsen FE, and Fortune EA. 1952. The anatomy of the brachial plexus of the dog. Anat Rec 114:173–180.

al-Mefty O, Harkey HL, Marawi I, Haines DE, Peeler DF, Wilner HI, et al. 1993. Experimental chronic compressive cervical myelopathy. J Neurosurg 79(4):550–561.

An HS, Andreshak TG, Nguyen C, Williams A, and Daniels D. 1995. Can we distinguish between benign versus malignant compression fractures of the spine by magnetic resonance imaging? Spine 20(16):1776–1782.

An HS and Masuda K. 2006. Relevance of in vitro and in vivo models for intervertebral disc degeneration. J Bone Joint Surg Am 88(Suppl. 2):88–94.

An HS, Nguyen C, Haughton VM, Ho KC, and Hasegawa T. 1994. Gadolinium-enhancement characteristics of magnetic resonance imaging in distinguishing herniated intervertebral disc versus scar in dogs. Spine 19(18):2089–2094; discussion 2095.

Armbrust LJ, Hoskinson JJ, Biller DS, and Wilkerson M. 2004. Low-field magnetic resonance imaging of bone marrow in the lumbar spine, pelvis, and femur in the adult dog. Vet Radiol Ultrasound 45(5):393–401.

Benninger MI, Seiler GS, Robinson LE, Ferguson SJ, Bonel HM, Busato AR, et al. 2004. Three-dimensional motion pattern of the caudal lumbar and lumbosacral portions of the vertebral column of dogs. Am J Vet Res 65(5):544–551.

Benninger MI, Seiler GS, Robinson LE, Ferguson SJ, Bonel HM, Busato AR, et al. 2006. Effects of anatomic conformation on three-dimensional motion of the caudal lumbar and lumbosacral portions of the vertebral column of dogs. Am J Vet Res 67(1):43–50.

Besalti O, Ozak A, Pekcan Z, Tong S, Eminaga S, and Tacal T. 2005. The role of extruded disk material in thoracolumbar intervertebral disk disease: a retrospective study in 40 dogs. Can Vet J 46(9):814–820.

Besalti O, Pekcan Z, Sirin YS, and Erbas G. 2006. Magnetic resonance imaging findings in dogs with thoracolumbar intervertebral disk disease: 69 cases (1997–2005). J Am Vet Med Assoc 228(6):902–908.

Bodner DR, Delamarter RB, Bohlman HH, Witcher M, Biro C, and Resnick MI. 1990. Urologic changes after cauda equina compression in dogs. J Urol 143(1):186–190.

Bohn AA, Wills TB, West CL, Tucker RL, and Bagley RS. 2006. Cerebrospinal fluid analysis and magnetic resonance imaging in the diagnosis of neurologic disease in dogs: a retrospective study. Vet Clin Pathol 35(3):315–320.

Cantile C, Baroni M, Tartarelli CL, Campani D, Salvadori C, and Arispici M. 2003. Intramedullary hemangioblastoma in a dog. Vet Pathol 40(1):91–94.

Carlson GD, Gorden CD, Oliff HS, Pillai JJ, and LaManna JC. 2003. Sustained spinal cord compression: part I: time-dependent effect on long-term pathophysiology. J Bone Joint Surg Am 85-A(1):86–94.

Cauzinille L and Kornegay JN. 1992. Acquired syringomyelia in a dog. J Am Vet Med Assoc 201(8):1225–1228.

Cerda-Gonzalez S and Olby NJ. 2006. Fecal incontinence associated with epidural spinal hematoma and intervertebral disk extrusion in a dog. J Am Vet Med Assoc 228(2):230–235.

Chambers JN, Selcer BA, Sullivan SA, and Coates JR. 1997. Diagnosis of lateralized lumbosacral disk herniation with magnetic resonance imaging. J Am Anim Hosp Assoc 33(4):296–299.

Chen AV, Bagley RS, West CL, Gavin PR, and Tucker RL. 2005. Fecal incontinence and spinal cord abnormalities in seven dogs. J Am Vet Med Assoc 227(12):1945–1951, 1928.

Cherubini GB, Cappello R, Lu D, Targett M, Wessmann A, and Mantis P. 2004. MRI findings in a dog with discospondylitis caused by Bordetella species. J Small Anim Pract 45(8):417–420. Erratum in: 2004 J Small Anim Pract 45(9):viii.

Chuma A, Kitahara H, Minami S, Goto S, Takaso M, and Moriya H. 1997. Structural scoliosis model in dogs with experimentally induced syringomyelia. Spine 22(6):589–594.

Churcher RK and Child G. 2000. Chiari 1/syringomyelia complex in a King Charles Spaniel. Aust Vet J 78(2):92–95.

Coates JR. 2000. Intervertebral disk disease. Vet Clin North Am Small Anim Pract 30(1):77—110.

da Costa RC, Parent JM, Partlow G, Dobson H, Holmberg DL, and Lamarre J. 2006. Morphologic and morphometric magnetic resonance imaging features of Doberman Pinschers with and without clinical signs of cervical spondylomyelopathy. Am J Vet Res 67(9):1601–1612.

da Costa RC, Parent JM, Poma R, and Duque MC. 2004. Cervical syringohydromyelia secondary to a brainstem tumor in a dog. J Am Vet Med Assoc 225(7):1061–1064, 1048.

da Costa RC, Poma R, Parent JM, Partlow G, and Monteith G. 2006. Correlation of motor evoked potentials with magnetic resonance imaging and neurologic findings in Doberman Pinschers with and without signs of cervical spondylomyelopathy. Am J Vet Res 67(9):1613–1620.

Daniel GB, Edwards DF, Harvey RC, and Kabalka GW. 1995. Communicating hydrocephalus in dogs with congenital ciliary dysfunction. Dev Neurosci 17(4):230–235.

Davies ES, Fransson BA, and Gavin PR. 2004. A confusing magnetic resonance imaging observation complicating surgery for a dermoid cyst in a Rhodesian Ridgeback. Vet Radiol Ultrasound 45(4):307–309.

de Haan JJ, Shelton SB, and Ackerman N. 1993. Magnetic resonance imaging in the diagnosis of degenerative lumbosacral stenosis in four dogs. Vet Surg 22(1):1–4.

Dennis R. 2005. Assessment of location of the celiac and cranial mesenteric arteries relative to the thoracolumbar spine using magnetic resonance imaging. Vet Radiol Ultrasound 46(5):388–390.

De Risio L, Sharp NJ, Olby NJ, Munana KR, and Thomas WB. 2001. Predictors of outcome after dorsal decompressive laminectomy for degenerative lumbosacral stenosis in dogs: 69 cases (1987–1997). J Am Vet Med Assoc 219(5):624–628.

De Risio L, Thomas WB, and Sharp NJ. 2000. Degenerative lumbosacral stenosis. Vet Clin North Am Small Anim Pract 30(1):111–132.

Forterre F, Kaiser S, Garner M, Stadie B, Matiasek K, Schmahl W, et al. 2006. Synovial cysts associated with cauda equina syndrome in two dogs. Vet Surg 35(1):30–33.

Fukuda S, Nakamura T, Kishigami Y, Endo K, Azuma T, Fujikawa T, et al. 2005. New canine spinal cord injury model free from laminectomy. Brain Res Brain Res Protoc 14(3):171–180.

Galloway AM, Curtis NC, Sommerlad SF, and Watt PR. 1999. Correlative imaging findings in seven dogs and one cat with spinal arachnoid cysts. Vet Radiol Ultrasound 40(5):445–452.

Ganey T, Libera J, Moos V, Alasevic O, Fritsch KG, Meisel HJ, et al. 2003. Disc chondrocyte transplantation in a canine model: a treatment for degenerated or damaged intervertebral disc. Spine 28(23):2609–2620.

Gemmill TJ. 2004. What is your diagnosis? Spondylosis of the lumbosacral junction. J Small Anim Pract 45(4):177, 219–220.

Glyde M, Doyle R, McAllister H, Campoy L, and Callanan JJ. 2004. Magnetic resonance imaging in the diagnosis and surgical management of sacral osteochondrosis in a mastiff dog. Vet Rec 155(3):83–86.

Gnirs K, Ruel Y, Blot S, Begon D, Rault D, Delisle F, et al. 2003. Spinal subarachnoid cysts in 13 dogs. Vet Radiol Ultrasound 44(4):402–408.

Gonzalo-Orden JM, Altonaga JR, Orden MA, and Gonzalo JM. 2000. Magnetic resonance, computed tomographic and radiologic findings in a dog with discospondylitis. Vet Radiol Ultrasound 41(2):142–144.

Grunenfelder FI, Weishaupt D, Green R, and Steffen F. 2005. Magnetic resonance imaging findings in spinal cord infarction in three small breed dogs. Vet Radiol Ultrasound 46(2):91–96.

Harkey HL, al-Mefty O, Marawi I, Peeler DF, Haines DE, and Alexander LF. 1995. Experimental chronic compressive cervical myelopathy: effects of decompression. J Neurosurg 83(2):336–241.

Hopkins AL, Garner M, Ackerman N, Chrisman CL, and Eskin T. 1995. Spinal meningeal sarcoma in a Rottweiler puppy. J Small Anim Pract 36(4):183–186.

Ito D, Matsunaga S, Jeffery ND, Sasaki N, Nishimura R, Mochizuki M, et al. 2005. Prognostic value of magnetic resonance imaging in dogs with paraplegia caused by thoracolumbar intervertebral disk extrusion: 77 cases (2000–2003). J Am Vet Med Assoc 227(9):1454–1460.

Itoh T, Nishimura R, Matsunaga S, Kadosawa T, Mochizuki M, and Sasaki N. 1996. Syringomyelia and hydrocephalus in a dog. J Am Vet Med Assoc 209(5):934–936.

Jones JC, Banfield CM, and Ward DL. 2000. Association between postoperative outcome and results of magnetic resonance imaging and computed tomography in working dogs with degenerative lumbosacral stenosis. J Am Vet Med Assoc 216(11):1769–1774.

Jurina K and Grevel V. 2004. Spinal arachnoid pseudocysts in 10 Rottweilers. J Small Anim Pract 45(1):9–15.

Kim HJ, Chang HS, Choi CB, Song YS, Kim SM, Lee JS, et al. 2005. Infiltrative lipoma in cervical bones in a dog. J Vet Med Sci 67(10):1043–1046.

Kinzel S, Wolff M, Buecker A, Krombach GA, Stopinski T, Afify M, et al. 2005. Partial percutaneous discectomy for treatment of thoracolumbar disc protrusion: retrospective study of 331 dogs. J Small Anim Pract 46(10):479–484.

Kippenes H, Gavin PR, Bagley RS, Silver GM, Tucker RL, and Sande RD. 1999. Magnetic resonance imaging features of tumors of the spine and spinal cord in dogs. Vet Radiol Ultrasound 40(6):627–633.

Kippenes H, Gavin PR, Parsaei H, Phillips MH, Cho PS, Leathers CW, et al. 2003. Spatial accuracy of fractionated IMRT delivery studies in canine paraspinal irradiation. Vet Radiol Ultrasound 44(3):360–366.

Kirberger RM, Jacobson LS, Davies JV, and Engela J. 1997. Hydromyelia in the dog. Vet Radiol Ultrasound 38(1):30–38. Erratum in: 1997 Vet Radiol Ultrasound 38(3):238.

Kobayashi S, Meir A, Baba H, Uchida K, and Hayakawa K. 2005. Imaging of intraneural edema by using gadolinium-enhanced MR imaging: experimental compression injury. AJNR Am J Neuroradiol 26(4):973–980.

Kobayashi S, Uchida K, Takeno K, Baba H, Suzuki Y, Hayakawa K, et al. 2006. Imaging of cauda equina edema in lumbar canal stenosis by using gadolinium-enhanced MR imaging: experimental constriction injury. AJNR Am J Neuroradiol 27(2):346–353.

Kobayashi S, Yoshizawa H, Hachiya Y, Ukai T, and Morita T. 1993. Vasogenic edema induced by compression injury to the spinal nerve root. Distribution of intravenously injected protein tracers and gadolinium-enhanced magnetic resonance imaging. Spine 18(11):1410–1424.

Kraft SL, Mussman JM, Smith T, Biller DS, and Hoskinson JJ. 1998. Magnetic resonance imaging of presumptive lumbosacral discospondylitis in a dog. Vet Radiol Ultrasound 39(1):9–13.

Levitski RE, Chauvet AE, and Lipsitz D. 1999. Cervical myelopathy associated with extradural synovial cysts in 4 dogs. J Vet Intern Med 13(3):181–186.

Levitski RE, Lipsitz D, and Chauvet AE. 1999. Magnetic resonance imaging of the cervical spine in 27 dogs. Vet Radiol Ultrasound 40(4):332–341.

Lipscomb VJ and Muir P. 2000. Magnetic resonance imaging of a dog with sciatic nerve root signature. Vet Rec 147(14):393–394.

Lipsitz D, Levitski RE, Chauvet AE, and Berry WL. 2001. Magnetic resonance imaging features of cervical stenotic myelopathy in 21 dogs. Vet Radiol Ultrasound 42(1):20–27.

Mayhew PD, Kapatkin AS, Wortman JA, and Vite CH. 2002. Association of cauda equina compression on magnetic resonance images and clinical signs in dogs with degenerative lumbosacral stenosis. J Am Anim Hosp Assoc 38(6):555–562.

McConnell JF, Garosi LS, Dennis R, and Smith KC. 2003. Imaging of a spinal nephroblastoma in a dog. Vet Radiol Ultrasound 44(5):537–541.

McDonnell JJ, Knowles KE, deLahunta A, Bell JS, Lowrie CT, and Todhunter RJ. 2003. Thoracolumbar spinal cord compression due to vertebral process degenerative joint disease in a family of Shiloh Shepherd dogs. J Vet Intern Med 17(4):530–537.

McDonnell JJ, Tidwell AS, Faissler D, and Keating J. 2005. Magnetic resonance imaging features of cervical spinal cord meningiomas. Vet Radiol Ultrasound 46(5):368–374.

Naughton JF, Tucker RL, and Bagley RS. 2005. Radiographic diagnosis–paraspinal abscess in a dog. Vet Radiol Ultrasound 46(1):23–26.

Nguyen CM, Ho KC, Yu SW, Haughton VM, and Strandt JA. 1989. An experimental model to study contrast enhancement in MR imaging of the intervertebral disk. AJNR Am J Neuroradiol 10(4):811–814.

Okada M, Koie H, Kitagawa M, Kanayama K, Sato T, Yamamura H, et al. 2006. MRI findings of haematomyelia in a dog with spontaneous systemic haemorrhage. Aust Vet J 84(9):332–335.

Olby N, Munana K, De Risio L, Sebestyen P, and Hansen B. 2002. Cervical injury following a horse kick to the head in two dogs. J Am Anim Hosp Assoc 38(4):321–326.

Olsewski JM, Schendel MJ, Wallace LJ, Ogilvie JW, and Gundry CR. 1996. Magnetic resonance imaging and biological changes in injured intervertebral discs under normal and increased mechanical demands. Spine 21(17):1945–1951.

Ono A, Harata S, Takagaki K, and Endo M. 1998. Proteoglycans in the nucleus pulposus of canine intervertebral discs after chondroitinase ABC treatment. J Spinal Disord 11(3):253–260.

Otani K, Arai I, Mao GP, Konno S, Olmarker K, and Kikuchi S. 1997. Experimental disc herniation: evaluation of the natural course. Spine 22(24):2894–2899.

Penderis J and Dennis R. 2004. Use of traction during magnetic resonance imaging of caudal cervical spondylomyelopathy ("wobbler syndrome") in the dog. Vet Radiol Ultrasound 45(3):216–219.

Penderis J, Schwarz T, McConnell JF, Garosi LS, Thomson CE, and Dennis R. 2005. Dysplasia of the caudal vertebral articular facets in four dogs: results of radiographic, myelographic and magnetic resonance imaging investigations. Vet Rec 156(19):601–605.

Platt SR, Dennis R, Murphy K, and de Stefani A. 2005. Hematomyelia secondary to lumbar cerebrospinal fluid acquisition in a dog. Vet Radiol Ultrasound 46(6):467–471.

Platt SR, McConnell JF, and Bestbier M. 2006. Magnetic resonance imaging characteristics of ascending hemorrhagic myelomalacia in a dog. Vet Radiol Ultrasound 47(1):78–82.

Purdy PD, Duong RT, White CL, III, Baer DL, Reichard RR, Pride GL, Jr, et al. 2003. Percutaneous translumbar spinal cord compression injury in a dog model that uses angioplasty balloons: MR imaging and histopathologic findings. AJNR Am J Neuroradiol 24(2):177–184.

Purdy PD, White CL, III, Baer DL, Frawley WH, Reichard RR, Pride GL, Jr, et al. 2004. Percutaneous translumbar spinal cord compression injury in dogs from an angioplasty balloon: MR and histopathologic changes with balloon sizes and compression times. AJNR Am J Neuroradiol 25(8):1435–1442.

Ramirez O, III and Thrall DE. 1998. A review of imaging techniques for canine cauda equina syndrome. Vet Radiol Ultrasound 39(4):283–296.

Rappard G, Metzger GJ, Weatherall PT, and Purdy PD. 2004. Interventional MR imaging with an endospinal imaging coil: preliminary results with anatomic imaging of the canine and cadaver spinal cord. AJNR Am J Neuroradiol 25(5):835–839.

Rossi F, Seiler G, Busato A, Wacker C, and Lang J. 2004. Magnetic resonance imaging of articular process joint geometry and intervertebral disk degeneration in the caudal lumbar spine (L5-S1) of dogs with clinical signs of cauda equina compression. Vet Radiol Ultrasound 45(5):381–387.

Rusbridge C, Greitz D, and Iskandar BJ. 2006. Syringomyelia: current concepts in pathogenesis, diagnosis, and treatment. J Vet Intern Med 20(3):469–479.

Rusbridge C and Knowler SP. 2003. Hereditary aspects of occipital bone hypoplasia and syringomyelia (Chiari type I malformation) in Cavalier King Charles spaniels. Vet Rec 153(4):107–112.

Rusbridge C, MacSweeny JE, Davies JV, Chandler K, Fitzmaurice SN, Dennis R, et al. 2000. Syringohydromyelia in Cavalier King Charles spaniels. J Am Anim Hosp Assoc 36(1):34–41.

Sale CS, Skerritt GC, and Smith KC. 2004. Spinal nephroblastoma in a crossbreed dog. J Small Anim Pract 45(5):267–271.

Sande RD. 1992. Radiography, myelography, computed tomography, and magnetic resonance imaging of the spine. Vet Clin North Am Small Anim Pract 22(4):811–831.

Sanders SG, Bagley RS, and Gavin PR. 2002. Intramedullary spinal cord damage associated with intervertebral disk material in a dog. J Am Vet Med Assoc 221(11):1594–1596, 1574–1575.

Sanders SG, Bagley RS, Gavin PR, Konzik RL, and Cantor GH. 2002. Surgical treatment of an intramedullary spinal cord hamartoma in a dog. J Am Vet Med Assoc 221(5):659–661, 643–644.

Schouman-Claeys E, Frija G, Cuenod CA, Begon D, Paraire F, and Martin V. 1990. MR imaging of acute spinal cord injury: results of an experimental study in dogs. AJNR Am J Neuroradiol 11(5):959–965.

Schulz KS, Walker M, Moon M, Waldron D, Slater M, and McDonald DE. 1998. Correlation of clinical, radiographic, and surgical localization of intervertebral disc extrusion in small-breed dogs: a prospective study of 50 cases. Vet Surg 27(2):105–111.

Seiler G, Hani H, Scheidegger J, Busato A, and Lang J. 2003. Staging of lumbar intervertebral disc degeneration in nonchondrodystrophic dogs using low-field magnetic resonance imaging. Vet Radiol Ultrasound 44(2):179–184.

Sessums KB and Ducote JM. 2006. What is your diagnosis? Spinal arachnoid cysts. J Am Vet Med Assoc 228(7):1019–1020. No abstract available.

Sether LA, Nguyen C, Yu SN, Haughton VM, Ho KC, Biller DS, et al. 1990. Canine intervertebral disks: correlation of anatomy and MR imaging. Radiology 175(1):207–211.

Silver GM, Bagley RS, Gavin PR, and Kippenes H. 2001. Radiographic diagnosis: cartilaginous exostoses in a dog. Vet Radiol Ultrasound 42(3):231–234.

Skeen TM, Olby NJ, Munana KR, and Sharp NJ. 2003. Spinal arachnoid cysts in 17 dogs. J Am Anim Hosp Assoc 39(3):271–282.

Smith PM and Jeffery ND. 2005. Spinal shock–comparative aspects and clinical relevance. J Vet Intern Med 19(6):788–793.

Steffen F, Berger M, and Morgan JP. 2004. Asymmetrical, transitional, lumbosacral vertebral segments in six dogs: a characteristic spinal syndrome. J Am Anim Hosp Assoc 40(4):338–344.

Swensen SJ, Keller PL, Berquist TH, McLeod RA, and Stephens DH. 1985. Magnetic resonance imaging of hemorrhage. AJR Am J Roentgenol 145(5):921–927.

Taga A, Taura Y, Nakaichi M, Wada N, and Hasegawa T. 2000. Magnetic resonance imaging of syringomyelia in five dogs. J Small Anim Pract 41(8):362–365.

Taga A, Taura Y, Nishimoto T, Takiguchi M, and Higuchi M. 1998. The advantage of magnetic resonance imaging in diagnosis of cauda equine syndrome in dogs. J Vet Med Sci 60(12):1345–1348.

Takagi S, Kadosawa T, Ohsaki T, Hoshino Y, Okumura M, and Fujinaga T. 2005. Hindbrain decompression in a dog with scoliosis associated with syringomyelia. J Am Vet Med Assoc 226(8):1359–1363, 1347.

Tanaka H, Nakayama M, Ori J, and Takase K. 2005. Usefulness of intraoperative ultrasonography for two dogs with spinal disease. J Vet Med Sci 67(7):727–730.

Tanaka H, Nakayama M, and Takase K. 2006. Intraoperative spinal ultrasonography in two dogs with spinal disease. Vet Radiol Ultrasound 47(1):99–102.

Tartarelli CL, Baroni M, and Borghi M. 2005. Thoracolumbar disc extrusion associated with extensive epidural haemorrhage: a retrospective study of 23 dogs. J Small Anim Pract 46(10):485–490.

Thomas WB. 2000. Diskospondylitis and other vertebral infections. Vet Clin North Am Small Anim Pract 30(1):169–182.

Tidwell AS, Specht A, Blaeser L, and Kent M. 2002. Magnetic resonance imaging features of extradural hematomas associated with intervertebral disc herniation in a dog. Vet Radiol Ultrasound 43(4):319–324.

Ueno H, Morimoto M, Kobayashi Y, Hizume T, Murayama N, and Uzuka Y. 2006. Surgical and radiotherapy treatment of a spinal cord ependymoma in a dog. Aust Vet J 84(1–2):36–39.

Ueno H, Shimizu J, Uzuka Y, Kobayashi Y, Hirokawa H, Ueno E, et al. 2005. Fibrocartilaginous embolism in a chondrodystrophoid breed dog. Aust Vet J 83(3):142–144.

van Klaveren NJ, Suwankong N, De Boer S, Van Den Brom WE, Voorhout G, Hazewinkel HA, et al. 2005. Force plate analysis before and after dorsal decompression for treatment of degenerative lumbosacral stenosis in dogs. Vet Surg 34(5):450–456.

Webb AA, Pharr JW, Lew LJ, and Tryon KA. 2001. MR imaging findings in a dog with lumbar ganglion cysts. Vet Radiol Ultrasound 42(1):9–13.

Westworth DR, Vernau KM, Cullen SP, Long CD, Van Halbach V, and LeCouteur RA. 2006. Vascular anomaly causing subclavian steal and cervical myelopathy in a dog: diagnosis and endovascular management. Vet Radiol Ultrasound 47(3):265–269.

Yamada K, Nakagawa M, Kato T, Shigeno S, Hirose T, Miyahara K, et al. 2001. Application of short-time magnetic resonance examination for intervertebral disc diseases in dogs. J Vet Med Sci 63(1):51–54.

Yamada K, Tanabe S, Ueno H, Oinuma A, Takahashi T, Miyauchi S, et al. 2001. Investigation of the short-term effect of chemonucleolysis with chondroitinase ABC. J Vet Med Sci 63(5):521–525.

Young B, Klopp L, Albrecht M, and Kraft S. 2004. Imaging diagnosis: magnetic resonance imaging of a cervical wooden foreign body in a dog. Vet Radiol Ultrasound 45(6):538–541.

Cats

Adams WH. 1999. The spine. Clin Tech Small Anim Pract 14(3):148–159.

Asperio RM, Marzola P, Zibellini E, Villa W, Sbarbati A, Osculati F, et al. 1999. Use of magnetic resonance imaging for diagnosis of a spinal tumor in a cat. Vet Radiol Ultrasound 40(3):267–270.

Coates JR. 2000. Intervertebral disk disease. Vet Clin North Am Small Anim Pract 30(1):77–110.

De Risio L, Thomas WB, and Sharp NJ. 2000. Degenerative lumbosacral stenosis. Vet Clin North Am Small Anim Pract 30(1):111–132.

Galloway AM, Curtis NC, Sommerlad SF, and Watt PR. 1999. Correlative imaging findings in seven dogs and one cat with spinal arachnoid cysts. Vet Radiol Ultrasound 40(5):445–452.

Garosi L, de Lahunta A, Summers B, Dennis R, and Scase T. 2006. Bilateral, hypertrophic neuritis of the brachial plexus in a cat: magnetic resonance imaging and pathological findings. J Feline Med Surg 8(1):63–68. Epub 2005 Oct 6.

Lu D, Lamb CR, Wesselingh K, and Targett MP. 2002. Acute intervertebral disc extrusion in a cat: clinical and MRI findings. J Feline Med Surg 4(1):65–68.

MacKay AD, Rusbridge C, Sparkes AH, and Platt SR. 2005. MRI characteristics of suspected acute spinal cord infarction in two cats, and a review of the literature. J Feline Med Surg 7(2):101–107.

McConnell JF and Garosi LS. 2004. Intramedullary intervertebral disk extrusion in a cat. Vet Radiol Ultrasound 45(4):327–330.

Mikszewski JS, Van Winkle TJ, and Troxel MT. 2006. Fibrocartilaginous embolic myelopathy in five cats. J Am Anim Hosp Assoc 42(3):226–233.

Pattany PM, Puckett WR, Klose KJ, Quencer RM, Bunge RP, Kasuboski L, et al. 1997. High-resolution diffusion-weighted MR of fresh and fixed cat spinal cords: evaluation of diffusion coefficients and anisotropy. AJNR Am J Neuroradiol 18(6):1049–1056.

Sanders S, Bagley RS, Tucker RL, and Nelson NR. 1999. Radiographic diagnosis: focal spinal cord malacia in a cat. Vet Radiol Ultrasound 40(2):122–125.

Tani K, Taga A, Itamoto K, Iwanaga T, Une S, Nakaichi M, et al. 2001. Hydrocephalus and syringomyelia in a cat. J Vet Med Sci 63(12):1331–1334.

Magnetic Resonance Imaging of Peripheral Nerve Disease

Rodney S. Bagley, Patrick R. Gavin, and Shannon P. Holmes

In comparison to MR imaging of the brain and spinal cord, the peripheral nervous system (PNS) has been less frequently imaged with MR. Imaging of the PNS has usually been relegated to imaging of neoplastic processes or other infiltrative diseases, as these PNS diseases are those that tend to affect peripheral nerve structure by enlarging the nerves. The sequences and quality of images historically collected have been less than adequate to determine disease in normal sized nerves. As MR imaging advances, with improved spacial resolution and sequence acquisition, more information may be gained regarding the anatomical abnormalities affecting the PNS.

As the peripheral nerves are a component of the lower motor neuron, and peripheral nerves innervate muscles, disease of the muscle may, in some settings, result in clinical signs that may overlap with those associated with the PNS. Therefore, in addition to anatomical alterations on peripheral nerve, abnormalities of muscle may be associated with, or lend clues to, underlying peripheral nerve disease. MR abnormalities of muscle may also be associated with primary musculoskeletal diseases. The MR appearance of these types of muscle abnormalities is discussed more thoroughly in those chapters of this book that describe musculoskeletal imaging. In this chapter, the primary emphasis will be on imaging of peripheral nerve neoplastic and other infiltrative processes, and on those muscle abnormalities that may be associated with, or mimic, PNS diseases.

ANATOMICAL CONSIDERATIONS

The PNS includes any nerve myelinated by a Schwann cell (deLahunta 1983; Jenkins 1978; King 1987; Kitchell

1993). Schwann cells begin myelinating peripheral nerves to the limbs at the intervertebral foramen of the vertebral column. Using this strict definition, other components of the peripheral nerve, such as the cell body of the motor neuron in the ventral gray matter of the spinal cord, the synapse, or the effector organ, would not be included in the PNS. Functionally, however, a lesion of the peripheral nerve or cell body would result in identical clinical signs as a lesion in the peripheral nerve. Therefore, the term "PNS" functionally includes all components from the cell body to the effector organ. In addition, sensory components of these nerve structures would also be included in the PNS.

In essence, the PNS forms the final link between the central integrating pathways of the nervous system and the body structures necessary to ultimately perform a specific function. Without this connection, regardless of what initiating events occur in the CNS, the function will not be completed. These structures are sometimes referred to as the final common pathway for expression of nervous system function.

This suggests that the ultimate effect of any nervous system function is delivered to the body organs and limbs through the PNS and for structures of the head, the CNs. The PNS is responsible for projecting information to (afferent, sensory) and from (efferent, motor) the CNS.

With regards to a sensory nerve, the cell body is often found in a ganglion outside the CNS. Receptors recognize stimuli and project this information in dendritic processes toward the cell body. Once information is projected toward the cell body, axons from the cell body enter the spinal cord through the dorsal nerve root. Sensory axons may then be projected in the CNS pathways in the spinal cord, or may terminate on additional neuronal elements within the spinal cord.

Neuronal cell bodies responsible for movement are found primarily in the ventral gray matter of the spinal cord. These neurons tend to be relatively larger cells with larger, myelinated axons such as alpha fibers. These motor neuron cell elements may be stimulated by local neurons in the spinal cord or from the terminations of axons descending from more cranial in the CNS, such as the brain and brain stem. In this way, the components of the CNS may signal movement in the muscles of the limb, for example. Local axons from the dorsal root ganglion cells may also terminate on these motor neurons allowing for local spinal reflex functions.

Peripheral Nerve Pathophysiology

Disease processes affecting the peripheral nerves and associated cell bodies can be many and varied (Summers 1995). Many of these diseases, however, result in a finite number of alterations in the neuronal cell body, axon, or synapse. Pathophysiologic alterations may be physiologic or anatomical. The ultimate consequence, however, is disruption of neural impulse generation or destruction of neural elements. A *neuropraxia* is an interruption in function and conduction in the nerve, usually associated with a lesion of the myelin without severe axonal involvement. Neuropraxia is the least severe of the types of nerve damage or dysfunction, which also usually equates to the greatest likelihood of reversal and clinical improvement. *Axonotmesis* suggests separation and damage of some axons. Again, this usually occurs through mechanical disruption, but may also result from diseases of the axon. Some regeneration of axons may occur, so this type of injury may be somewhat reversible. Improvement in function will depend upon the magnitude of the axon loss (i.e., percentage of axonal damage). *Neurotmesis* is complete severance of all structures of the nerve and is the most severe form of injury. The likelihood of regeneration is less with neurotmesis as compared to neuropraxia or axonotmesis.

Peripheral Nerve MR Imaging

Because of the quality and resolution of MR imaging in current clinical practice, MR imaging of peripheral nerve disease is primarily limited to imaging of peripheral nerve neoplastic diseases. As MR imaging is progressing, improved imaging of other peripheral nerve diseases is on the horizon.

Specific Diseases

Neoplastic Neuropathies

Of the neoplastic diseases nerve sheath tumors (Schwannoma, neurofibroma, neurofibrosarcoma)

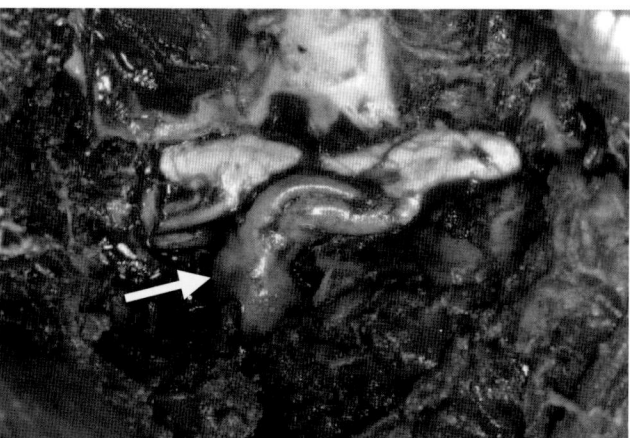

Figure 2.251. Gross view of a nerve sheath tumor (arrow) following hemilaminectomy.

commonly involve the peripheral nerves (Figure 2.251). Any peripheral nerve, including the CNs, may be involved. These types of peripheral nerve neoplastic infiltrations, however, may be difficult to see on routine MR sequences (T1 and T2 sequences) (Figures 2.252–2.254). The difficulty occurs due to the signal from fat and blood vessels throughout the muscles that are usually surrounding the nerve of interest (see Chapter 6, Figures 6.9–6.11). Therefore, fat-suppression sequences such as STIR may allow for a better delineation of these neoplastic processes (Figure 2.253).

Other factors that influence the ease at which these processes can be identified and localized include the variable course of the peripheral nerves as they course through the muscle that they innervate. Therefore, the nerve may travel in various planes throughout its course. Orientation of the MR scanning planes to follow the course of the peripheral nerves is often necessary to see discrete peripheral nerve enlargement.

When the exiting peripheral nerves are neoplastic at either the spinal canal, foramen, or immediately distal to their exit of the foramen, these processes may be identified with spinal MR imaging. If the peripheral nerve tumor is present within the dura, an intradural, extramedullary appearance or "golf-tee" appearance in the subarachnoid space similar to the appearance of these tumors on myelography may be seen. This "golf-tee" appearance is most evident in T2-weighted images as the CSF creating this appearance is white. A myelographic effect sequence (long T2-sequence) may also more easily show this type of "golf-tee" shaped appearance (see Section 2, Figure 2.207).

These tumors may not be as obvious in sagittal MR images as they may have little contrast difference with respect to the adjacent spinal cord and may be primarily

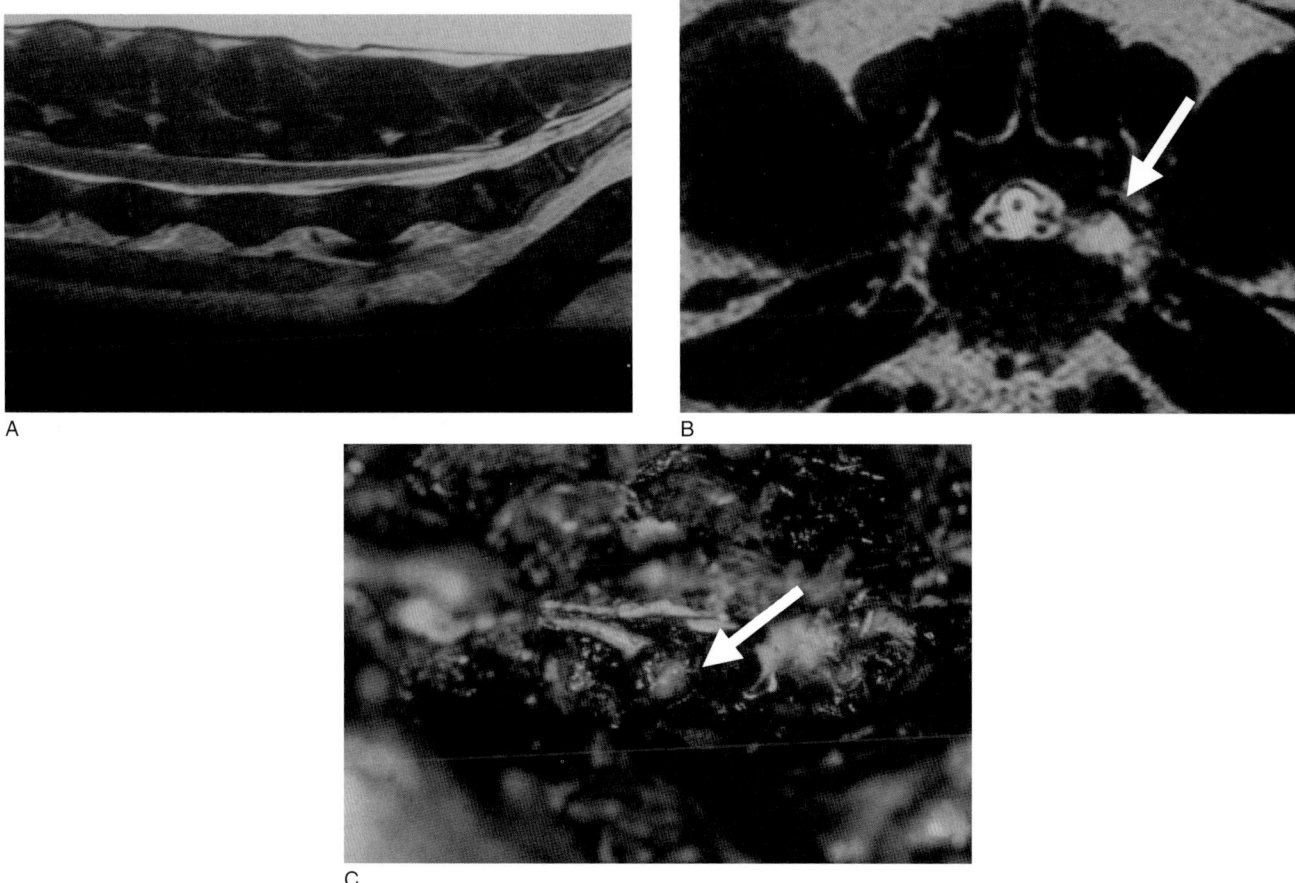

Figure 2.252. Sagittal T2-weighted MR image (A) from a dog with a pelvic limb leg-carrying lameness. No abnormalities are noted in this plane. Transverse T2-weighted MR image (B) from the same dog at the L7-S1 intervertebral foramen showing a focal mass within the exiting peripheral nerve (arrow). View at surgery (C) (hemilaminectomy) of the mass (arrow). Histologic diagnosis was a neuroma.

located lateral to the spinal cord (Figure 2.252). Intravenous gadolinium administration usually results in enhancement of these tumors increasing their signal intensity in T1-weighted images (Figure 2.254). Dorsal and transverse contrast-enhanced images are the images helpful to detect this category of tumors. In some instances, if the tumor infiltrates or originates in the spinal cord gray matter, an intramedullary expansile lesion will be seen. Often either within the lesion or within the spinal cord surrounding (including proximal and distal to) the lesion there will be associated hyperintense signal within the spinal cord parenchyma on T2-weighted sequences. This most likely represents edema, and may be restricted primarily to the gray matter or more centralized regions of the spinal cord.

Tumors may have a variety of appearances with MR imaging, and need to be differentiated from other spinal disease processes such as intervertebral disk herniation. Tumors are typically vascular and invasive, disrupting the normal integrity of the BBB. Thus, intravenous in-

jection of a contrast agent generally results in some degree of either diffuse or focal enhancement in the area affected by tumor. Contrast enhancement (intravenous gadolinium-DTPA) does not precisely define the tumor borders as neoplastic cells are generally found outside the enhanced portion of the mass. Gadolinium enhancement of tumors is inconsistent but, if present, may support a diagnosis of tumor. Other extradural disease processes, such as intervertebral disk herniation, may also show contrast enhancement on MR. Contrast enhancement characteristics alone, therefore, cannot be used as being pathognomonic for neoplasia.

In the spinal canal external to the dura, peripheral nerve tumors, depending upon the slice plane may also have more of an extradural appearance. In some instances, normal structures such as the vessels (venous sinus) can be mistaken for a peripheral nerve neoplasm.

Affected dogs often present for a lameness that, in some instances, may have been present for a prolonged time prior to presentation. Often dogs are initially

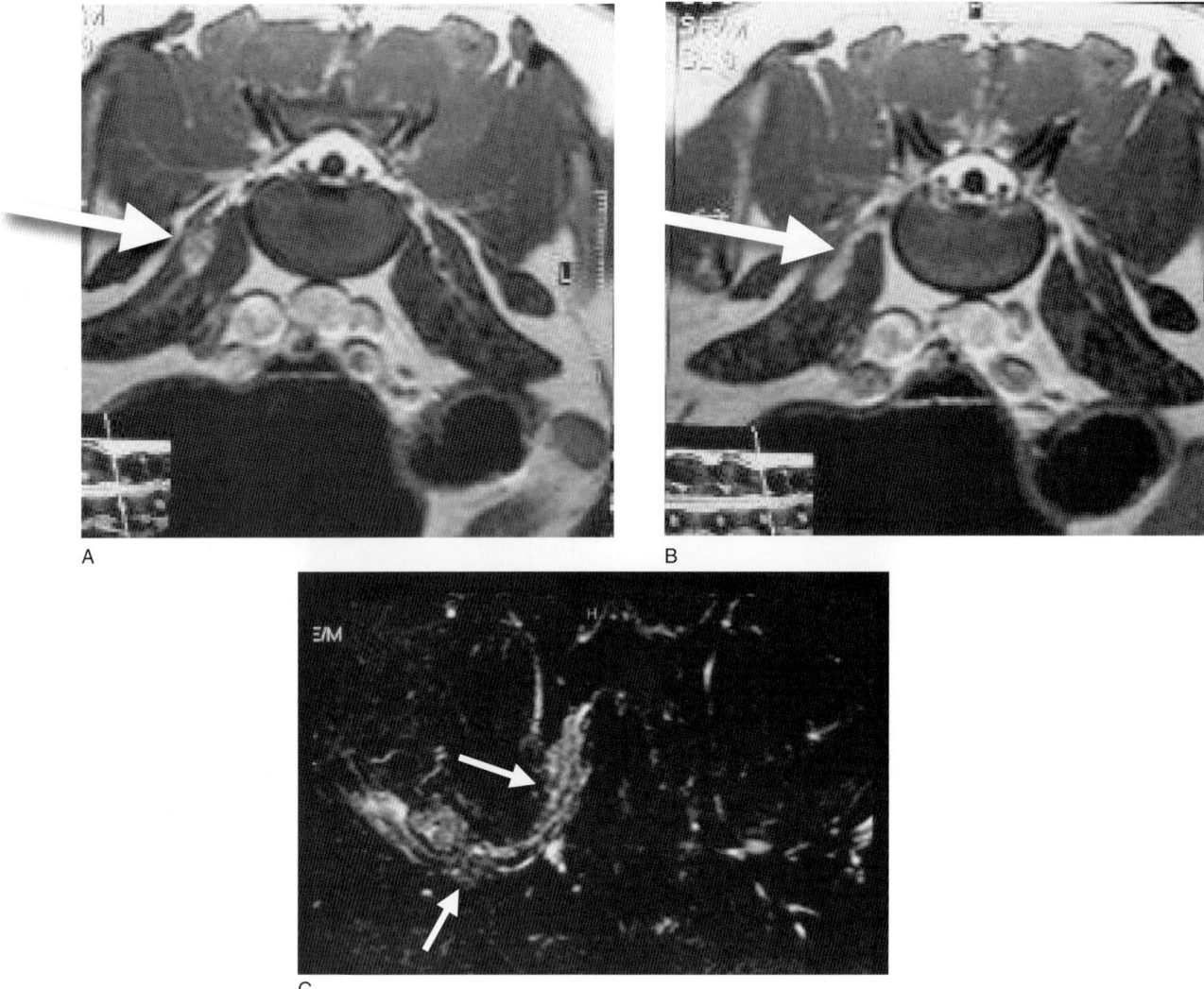

Figure 2.253. Transverse T1-weighted MR images ((A) and (B)) following intravenous contrast administration from adjacent levels (L6-7) from a dog with a unilateral pelvic limb lameness. There is a tumor of the sciatic nerve present (arrow). Dorsal STIR MR image (C) from the same dog as in (A) showing the tumor (arrows).

diagnosed with arthritis or another orthopedic disease which they may, in fact, have serendipitious evidence of, as many affected animals are older. Clinical clues include atrophy of selected thoracic limb muscles and pain upon local palpation of the nerve. In some instances, a discrete mass can be palpated in the nerve. Animals that are extremely painful may require general anesthesia for adequate palpation.

If the tumor results in denervation of associated muscles, these muscles may atrophy and appear smaller in MR images. Often, as well, denervated muscle appears hyperintense on T2 sequences and, occasionally, T1 sequences.

Other neoplastic processes may infiltrate along peripheral nerves. Lymphoma and other hematological neoplasia are more likely to do so. The MR characteristics of these neoplastic processes are often similar to their appearance in other body tissues, and may also not be able to be distinguished from nerve sheath tumor.

Infectious Neuritis

Diseases such as toxoplasmosis and *Neospora caninium* may result in infiltration and enlargement of peripheral nerves. These enlarged peripheral nerves may have a similar MR appearance to neoplastic peripheral nerve disease. In some instance, neospora in particular, may result in multifocal bulbous enlargement of exiting peripheral nerves and nerve roots within the spinal canal.

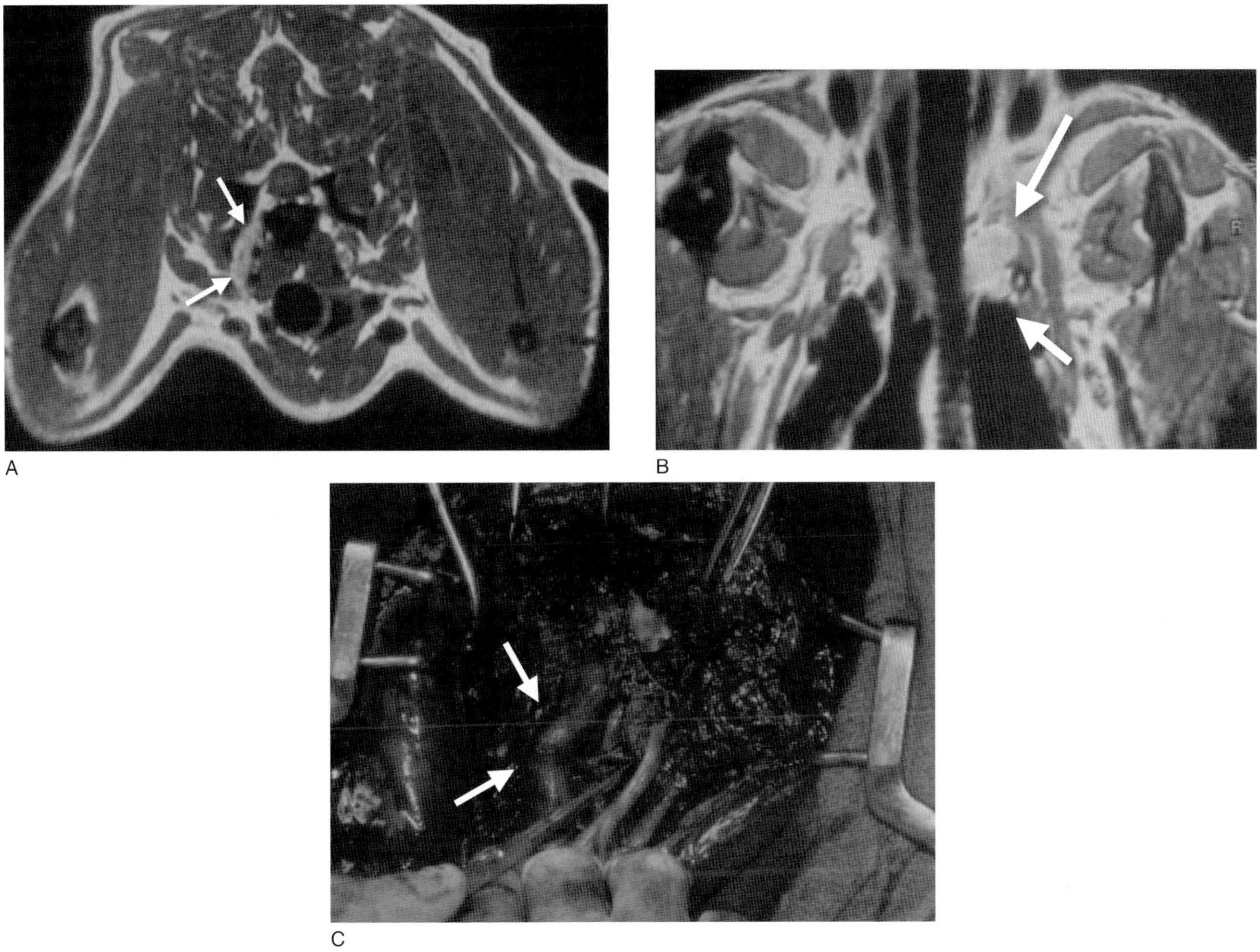

Figure 2.254. Transverse (A) and dorsal (B) T1-weighted MR images from a dog with thoracic limb lameness following intravenous contrast administration showing contrast enhancement of a peripheral nerve tumor (arrows). Gross view (C) of a nerve sheath tumor (arrows) following brachial plexus exploratory surgery.

Disease of Muscle

Paraspinal muscles may have abscessation, which is often associated with migrating foreign material (such as grass awns of porcupine quills). Abscesses with muscle often result in multifocal hyperintense (on T2) or hypointense (on T1) irregular regions suggesting focal pockets of fluid accumulation. These muscles may be subsequently enlarged, and often have varying degrees of enhancement following intravenous contrast administration.

It is also possible to see focal hyperintense signal on T2-weighted sequences in the paraspinal muscle surrounding some regions of intervertebral disk extrusion. Biopsy of these muscles usually reveals no obvious pathology. The reason for this signal change therefore is not known, but most likely represents some degree of muscle injury associated with shifts of the verte-

bral structures following the IVD extrusion. In some instances, similar changes may occur in other muscle groups and may be the result of muscle injury occurring during the process of the animal falling, possibly as the result of the acute paralysis or paresis. Some of this muscle change may also be the result of muscle damage during subsequent recumbency. A similar appearance may also be present in paraspinal muscles in instances of exogenous spinal injury.

Traumatic Neuropathies and Myopathies

Brachial plexus avulsion may result in alterations in the MR appearance of the spinal cord and associated limb muscles. As the nerve damage with brachial plexus avulsion usually occurs at the level of the smaller nerve rootlets adjacent to the spinal cord, images of this region may show focal intraspinal hyperintensity in T2-weighted images, which most likely reflects associated spinal cord edema, hemorrhage, or inflammation. Focal enlargement may be seen in the region of the nerve rootlets, possibly the result of similar pathogenic mechanisms associated with the traumatic disruption of these nerve rootlets. In addition, hemorrhage may occur in the subarachnoid space. This hemorrhage may result in a variety of appearance on MR sequences similar to what has previously been discussed for the appearance of spinal hemorrhage in the spinal disease chapter (see Section 2). Hemorrhage may be more easily discernable on diffusion-weighted sequences.

Depending upon when in relation to the traumatic event the limb is imaged, limb muscles may be atrophied and become hyperintense in T2-weighted images similar to other denervated muscles.

Muscle thrombosis, embolism, and infarction may result from a variety of vascular insults. The MR appearance of muscle damaged in such a way can have either an isotense or hyperintense appearance on T2-weighed sequences. Focal or diffuse muscle hemorrhage may also be more easily discernable on diffusion-weighted sequences.

MR Bibliography

Dogs

Abraham LA, Mitten RW, Beck C, Charles JA, and Holloway SA. 2003. Diagnosis of sciatic nerve tumour in two dogs by electromyography and magnetic resonance imaging. Aust Vet J 81(1–2):42–46.

Brofman PJ and Thrall DE. 2006. Magnetic resonance imaging findings in a dog with caudal aortic thromboembolism and ischemic myopathy. Vet Radiol Ultrasound 47(4):334–338.

Bush WW, Throop JL, McManus PM, Kapatkin AS, Vite CH, and Van Winkle TJ. 2003. Intravascular lymphoma involving the central and peripheral nervous systems in a dog. J Am Anim Hosp Assoc 39(1):90–96.

Drost WT, Bahr RJ, Henry GA, and Campbell GA. 1999. Aortoiliac thrombus secondary to a mineralized arteriosclerotic lesion. Vet Radiol Ultrasound 40(3):262–266.

Endo H, Taru H, Nakamura K, Koie H, Yamaya Y, and Kimura J. 1999. MRI examination of the masticatory muscles in the gray wolf (Canis lupus), with special reference to the M. temporalis. J Vet Med Sci 61(6):581–586.

Ferreira AJ, Peleteiro MC, Correia JH, Jesus SO, and Goulao A. 2005. Small-cell carcinoma of the lung resembling a brachial plexus tumour. J Small Anim Pract 46(6):286–290.

Grosslinger K, Lorinson D, Hittmair K, Konar M, and Weissenbock H. 2004. Iliopsoas abscess with iliac and femoral vein thrombosis in an adult Siberian husky. J Small Anim Pract 45(2):113–116.

Kathmann I, Bottcher ICh, von Klopmann T, Gerdwilker A, and Tipold A. 2006. Chronic inflammatory demyelinating polyradiculoneuropathy with hypertrophy of cervicothoracal nerve roots in a dog. Schweiz Arch Tierheilkd 148(6):297–302.

Kornegay JN, Sharp NJ, Bartlett RJ, Van Camp SD, Burt CT, Hung WY, et al. 1990. Golden retriever muscular dystrophy: monitoring for success. Adv Exp Med Biol 280:267–272.

Lipscomb VJ and Muir P. 2000. Magnetic resonance imaging of a dog with sciatic nerve root signature. Vet Rec 147(14):393–394.

Platt SR, Graham J, Chrisman CL, Collins K, Chandra S, Sirninger J, et al. 1999. Magnetic resonance imaging and ultrasonography in the diagnosis of a malignant peripheral nerve sheath tumor in a dog. Vet Radiol Ultrasound 40(4):367–371.

Platt SR and McConnell F. 2002. What is your diagnosis? Malignant nerve sheath tumour. J Small Anim Pract 43(3):103, 139–140.

Stepnik MW, Olby N, Thompson RR, and Marcellin-Little DJ. 2006. Femoral neuropathy in a dog with iliopsoas muscle injury. Vet Surg 35(2):186–190.

Strong M, Hruska J, Czyrny J, Heffner R, Brody A, and Wong-Chung J. 1994. Nerve palsy during femoral lengthening: MRI, electrical, and histologic findings in the central and peripheral nervous systems—a canine model. J Pediatr Orthop 14(3):347–351.

Tucker DW, Olsen D, Kraft SL, Andrews GA, and Gray AP. 2000. Primary hemangiosarcoma of the iliopsoas muscle eliciting a peripheral neuropathy. J Am Anim Hosp Assoc 36(2):163–167.

Cats

Garosi L, de Lahunta A, Summers B, Dennis R, and Scase T. 2006. Bilateral, hypertrophic neuritis of the brachial plexus in a cat: magnetic resonance imaging and pathological findings. J Feline Med Surg 8(1):63–68. Epub 2005 Oct 6.

Mellanby RJ, Jeffery ND, Baines EA, Woodger N, and Herrtage ME. 2003. Magnetic resonance imaging in the diagnosis of lymphoma involving the brachial plexus in a cat. Vet Radiol Ultrasound 44(5):522–525.

Vite CH, McGowan JC, Braund KG, Drobatz KJ, Glickson JD, Wolfe JH, et al. 2001. Histopathology, electrodiagnostic testing, and magnetic resonance imaging show significant peripheral and central nervous system myelin abnormalities in the cat model of alpha-mannosidosis. J Neuropathol Exp Neurol 60(8):817–828.

CHAPTER THREE

ORTHOPEDIC

Patrick R. Gavin and Shannon P. Holmes

Our physician colleagues utilize MR more for orthopedic disease than for any other body system. The superior soft tissue contrast, especially for defining pathologic change, has greatly improved diagnoses, treatment options, and therapeutic outcomes for their patients. Similar advances are beginning to be recognized in veterinary medicine. For decades, we have been fixated on the skeletal system for the diagnosis of orthopedic abnormalities. We forgot that it is the *musculo*-skeletal system, complete with tendons and ligaments, nerves, blood vessels, fascia and synovial membranes, along with bones, that make up the entire complex tissue affected by orthopedic injuries. Previously MR was thought to be a poor imaging modality for osseous structures. It is now recognized that MR has exquisite sensitivity and specificity for osseous abnormalities, most of which cannot be delineated by other imaging modalities. Nuclear scintigraphy has excellent sensitivity, but lacks specificity.

MR imaging is increasingly being used in the diagnosis of lamenesses suspected to involve the shoulder region. The specific cause of shoulder lameness is often difficult to diagnose on the basis of the previously standard diagnostic assessments (i.e., physical examination including palpation and conventional radiography). Arthroscopy with direct visualization has added information as to intra-articular abnormalities, however, is invasive. Additionally, many of the diseases that affect the shoulder are not primarily intra-articular and, therefore, are more likely to be seen with MR imaging providing for a more global assessment of the shoulder region.

The most often requested magnetic resonance study in veterinary orthopedics today is for the diagnosis of shoulder lameness. Shoulder lameness is difficult to diagnose based on conventional examination, including palpation and radiography. Often, the profession has resorted to arthroscopy as a diagnostic procedure, which may be appropriate if it is an intra-articular abnormality. Many of the diseases that affect the shoulder are not intra-articular and, therefore, are best visualized with MR.

IMAGING TECHNIQUE

An MR evaluation of the shoulder region must be appropriately broad in order to image the important anatomy of upper thoracic limb lameness, without compromising spatial resolution. As a lameness could result from disease of the spinal cord and associated peripheral nerves (including the brachial plexus), the scapula, humerus, shoulder joint capsule, joint surfaces, associated muscles, tendons, and ligaments, and adjacent soft tissue and vasculature. It is preferable, therefore, when imaging the shoulder region to at least run screening images of the caudal cervical and cranial thoracic spine and brachial plexus. We have found that optimum image quality of many of the musculo-skeletal structures is obtained by placing the animal in lateral recumbent position with the affected limb downward. This is especially important when a surface coil is being utilized. The limb is positioned in normal anatomical angulation, which results in an approximate 90° angle at the shoulder, elbow, stifle, and tarsus. The body weight of the animal usually eliminates motion of the limb region from breathing. This necessitates rolling the animal over for bilateral studies, but the extra effort has proven valuable. An attempt to image both limbs at once should be avoided as the FOV is too large and the slice orientation and volume averaging will not be identical for the two limbs. These factors can result in erroneous interpretation.

Standard imaging sequences utilized to examine the shoulder include high-resolution T1-weighted sequences to define anatomic abnormalities. However, our imaging protocols most heavily rely on STIR or fat-suppressed proton density sequences for the detection of disease. T2-weighted sequences are necessary to prevent misinterpretation from magic angle artifact (see Chapter 1, Section 4: Artifacts), unless the MR unit is capable of acquiring more T2-weighted (TE ≥ 35–40 ms) proton density fat-suppressed sequences. An ideal shoulder imaging protocol would include a sagittal T2-weighted sequence of the cervical and

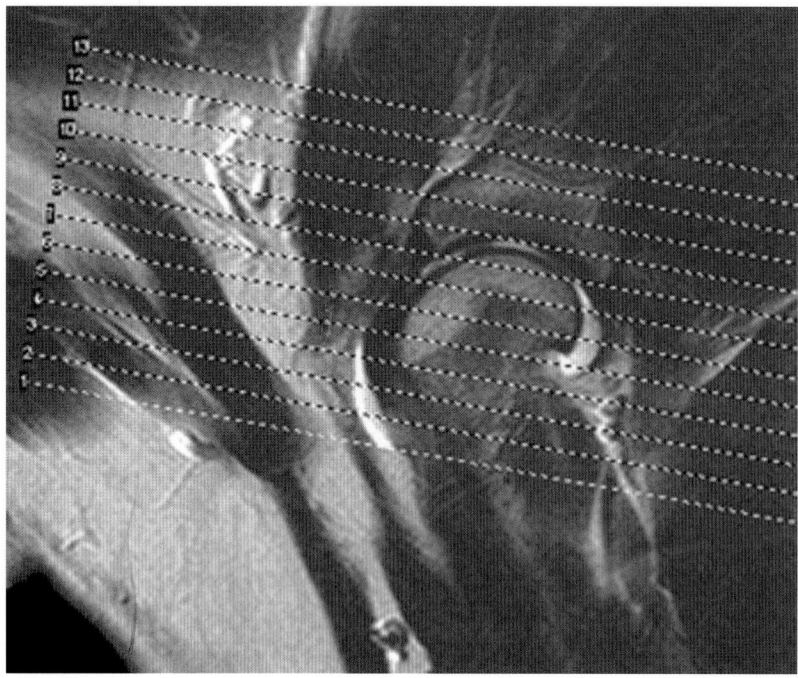
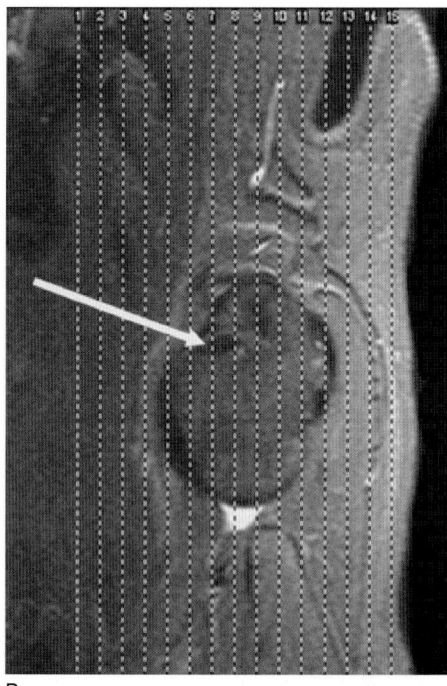

A   B

Figure 3.1. Normal scanning planes. It is important for the angles of the scan planes to hold constant. Imaging of the shoulder relies most heavily on the transverse and sagittal scan planes. (A) T2-weighted image in the sagittal plane with the transverse slice planes superimposed (parallel white dashed lines). The transverse plane is oriented perpendicular to the biceps tendon at the level of the intertubercular groove. (B) T2-weighted, fat-suppressed transverse image with the sagittal slice planes superimposed. The orientation of the sagittal plane is aligned with the biceps tendon (white arrow) and cranially from the midpoint of the intertubercular groove through the midpoint of the humeral head caudally. Accurately planning this scan plan can be more challenging when the biceps is displaced medially out of the intertubercular groove.

cranial thoracic spine, a STIR dorsal sequence of the spinal cord through the ventral aspect of the brachial plexus region (a STIR dorsal plane is planned dorsal relative to the spine), and a combination of multiplanar sequences through the shoulder joint. Our current protocol obtains images in all three planes of the shoulder using fat-suppressed proton density sequences, a T2 sagittal and dual echo axial of the shoulder joint. Other imaging centers prefer to use sagittal sequences with T1-weighting, STIR or proton density fat saturation, and T2-weighting. Transverse imaging (i.e., transverse to the biceps tendon within the bicipital groove) of STIR sequences or T2-weighting generally complete the sequence. Field of view should be scaled according to the animal's body size to provide clear visualization of the shoulder. If contrast enhancement is deemed necessary, the contrast is administered and post-contrast studies are acquired in the sagittal and other planes as needed. In general, however, contrast studies are not required.

Familiarity with normal shoulder anatomy (Figures 3.1–3.3) is critical for identification of pathologic changes. Virtually all structures of the shoulder joint can be visualized with MR. There is clear visualization of the insertion of the supraspinatus and infraspinatus muscles on the medial and lateral aspect of the grater tubercle respectively. The origin and path of the biceps tendon is readily apparent. The integrity of the tendon should be evaluated on long TE sequences as the tendon angle often results in a magic angle artifact. The joint capsule and synovial fluid are easily seen. The thin articular cartilage is seen between the synovial fluid and the subchondral bone. The glenohumeral ligaments are difficult to see in isolation from the larger tendons and ligaments forming the collateral support of the shoulder joint. Secondary changes at the site of insertion are used as sentinel indicators that pathologic changes may be present. Even though the transverse humeral ligament is small this ligament can be imaged in the axial plane, if images are acquired

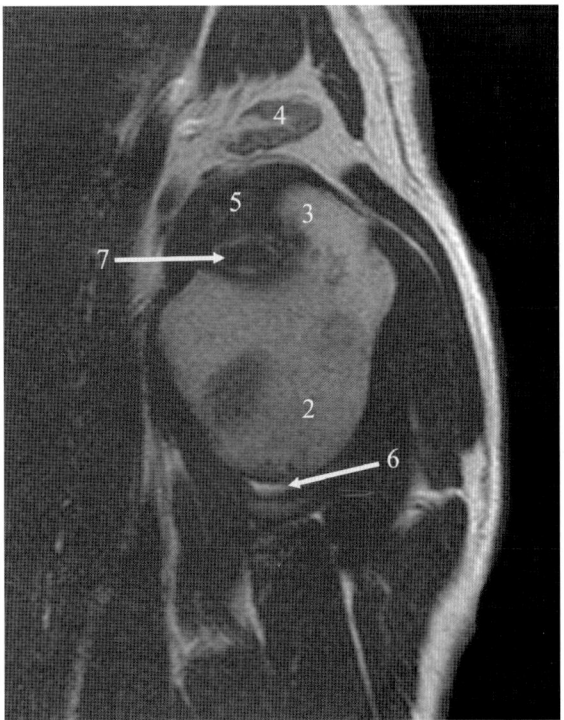
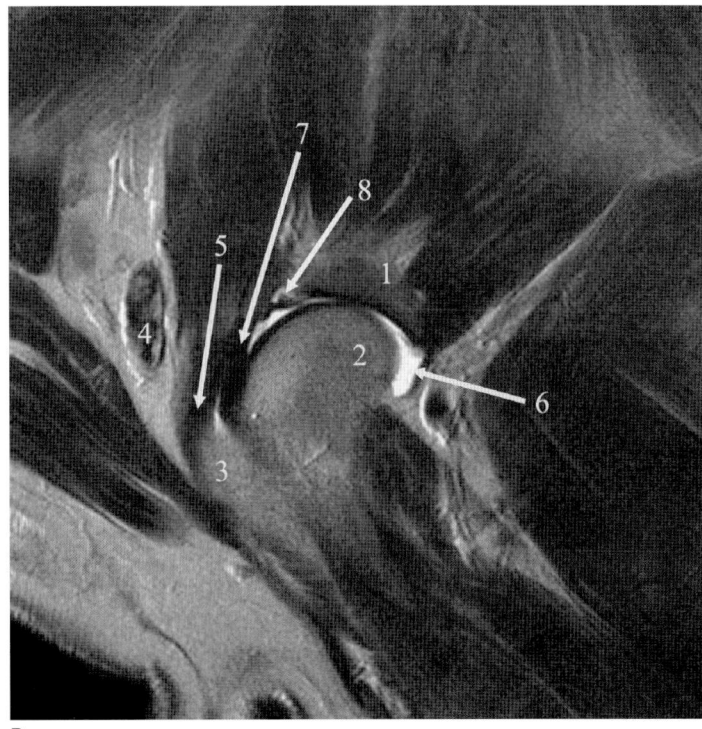

A   B

Figure 3.2. Normal shoulder anatomy. T2-weighted transverse (A) and sagittal (B) images of the shoulder. All osseous and soft tissues are easily visualized, with a few exceptions. The transverse humeral ligament is extremely thin, and requires an axial slice plane oriented perpendicular to the long axis of the humerus. Because the glenohumeral ligaments are so thin and intimately associated with the joint capsule, they cannot be seen as distinct structures. (1) glenoid cavity, (2) humeral head, (3) greater tubercle, (4) superficial cervical lymph node, (5) supraspinatus tendon insertion, (6) joint capsule with synovial fluid in caudal pouch, (7) biceps tendon near origin, (8) glenoid labrum.

perpendicular to the long axis of the biceps tendon (Figure 3.1).

Abnormalities of the Shoulder Joint Complex

Prior to the use of MR, bicipital tenosynovitis appeared to be the most frequently diagnosed condition of the dog shoulder. The condition does occur, but incidence of this disease recognized on MR is less common and perhaps even uncommon relative to other pathologic changes seen on MR examinations in our experience. The most common abnormality present in the shoulder joint to date in animals undergoing MR imaging has been supraspinatus tendinitis.

The insertion of the supraspinatus tendon on the medial aspect of the greater tubercle undergoes apparent repetitive trauma resulting in a proliferative mass of collagen that causes secondary impingement on the biceps tendon. This pathological change results in a high signal intensity on STIR or T2 or proton sequences and is best seen with fat-suppression sequences. There is medial displacement of the biceps tendon from its normal position within the intertubercular groove and flattening the tendon. The T1-weighted images often have fatty replacement at the myotendinous junction of the supraspinatus tendon. Therefore, it is easy to see why many clinicians feel these animals have bicipital tenosynovitis on a physical examination and arthroscopy/arthrotomy. The supraspinatus damage appears to result in secondary compression of the biceps tendon. With MR, this extracapsular defect is clearly defined, as well as the degenerative secondary changes on the greater tubercle. In this instance, the MR definition of supraspinatus tendinitis has altered the clinical therapeutic course in management of shoulder lameness (Figures 3.4–3.6).

Other abnormalities of the shoulder that have been identified with MR include tumors of the scapula and

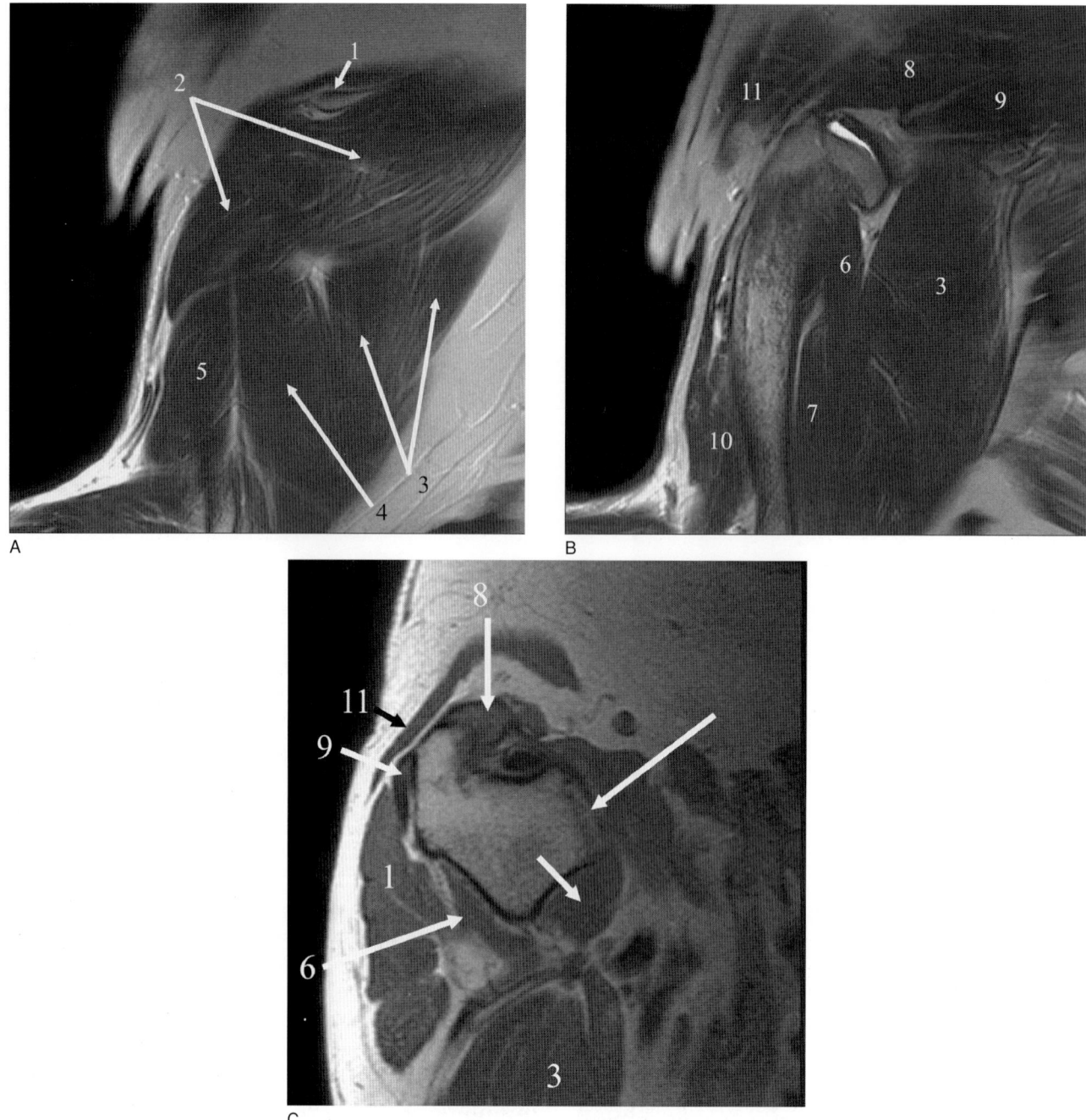

Figure 3.3. Normal shoulder musculature. The extrinsic muscles are important in the assessment of the shoulder, since their function is essential for shoulder stability. A large field of view scan in the sagittal plane is often helpful in anatomically localizing specific muscles. Normal tendons, muscles, and cortical bone have low (i.e., black) signal intensity on T1, T2 and PD sequences, whereas muscle becomes intermediate signal intensity on STIR or SPIR sequences. (A–B) T2-weighted sagittal images in series from lateral to medial. (C) PD-weighted transverse images at the level of the proximal intertubercular groove. (1) Acromion, (2) deltoid muscle, (3) triceps muscle, long head, (4) triceps muscle, lateral head, (5) brachialis, (6) triceps muscle, accessory head, (7) triceps muscle, medial head, (8) supraspinatus muscle, (9) infraspinatus muscle, (10) biceps muscle, (11) cleidobrachialis.

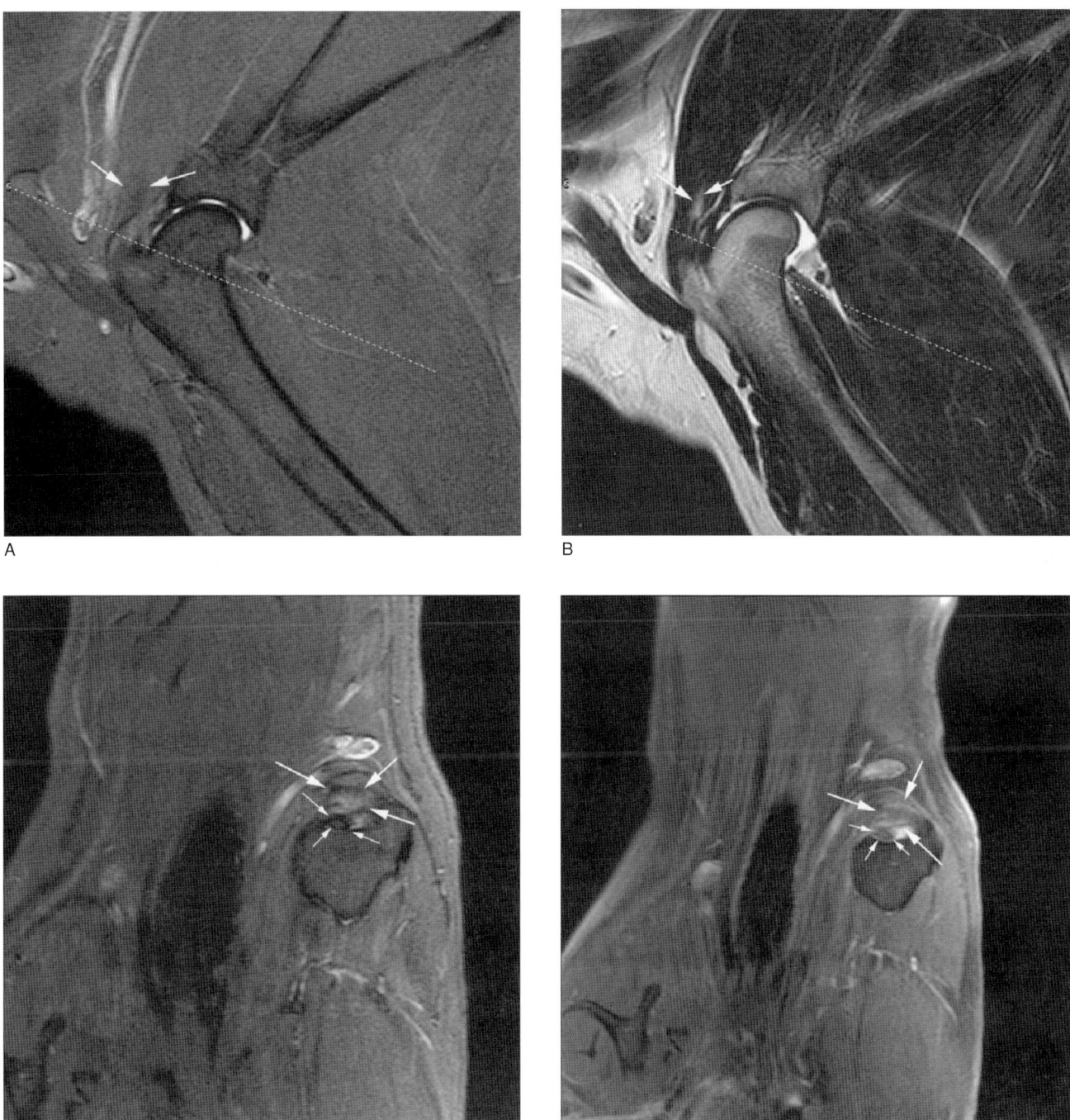

Figure 3.4.   Supraspinatus tendinitis. (A) STIR sequence in the sagittal plane. Arrows point to an area of fat at the myotendinous junction that is dark on the STIR sequence. The dotted line shows the position of transverse image 3C. (B) T2-weighted image through the same site as A. Note on this T2-weighted image the fat is bright where there has been tearing at the myotendinous junction with fatty replacement. (C) STIR-weighted transverse sequence. The marked hyperintensity of the immature collagen from the ruptured supraspinatus tendon is shown with the large arrows. Small arrows show displacement of the biceps tendon from this proliferative mass out of its normal bicipital groove. (D) T1-weighted, post-contrast, fat-suppressed image. There is no enhancement of the proliferative lesions seen on the STIR sequence at the insertion of the supraspinatus. Displaced tendon is seen. There is mild enhancement of the synovial lining.

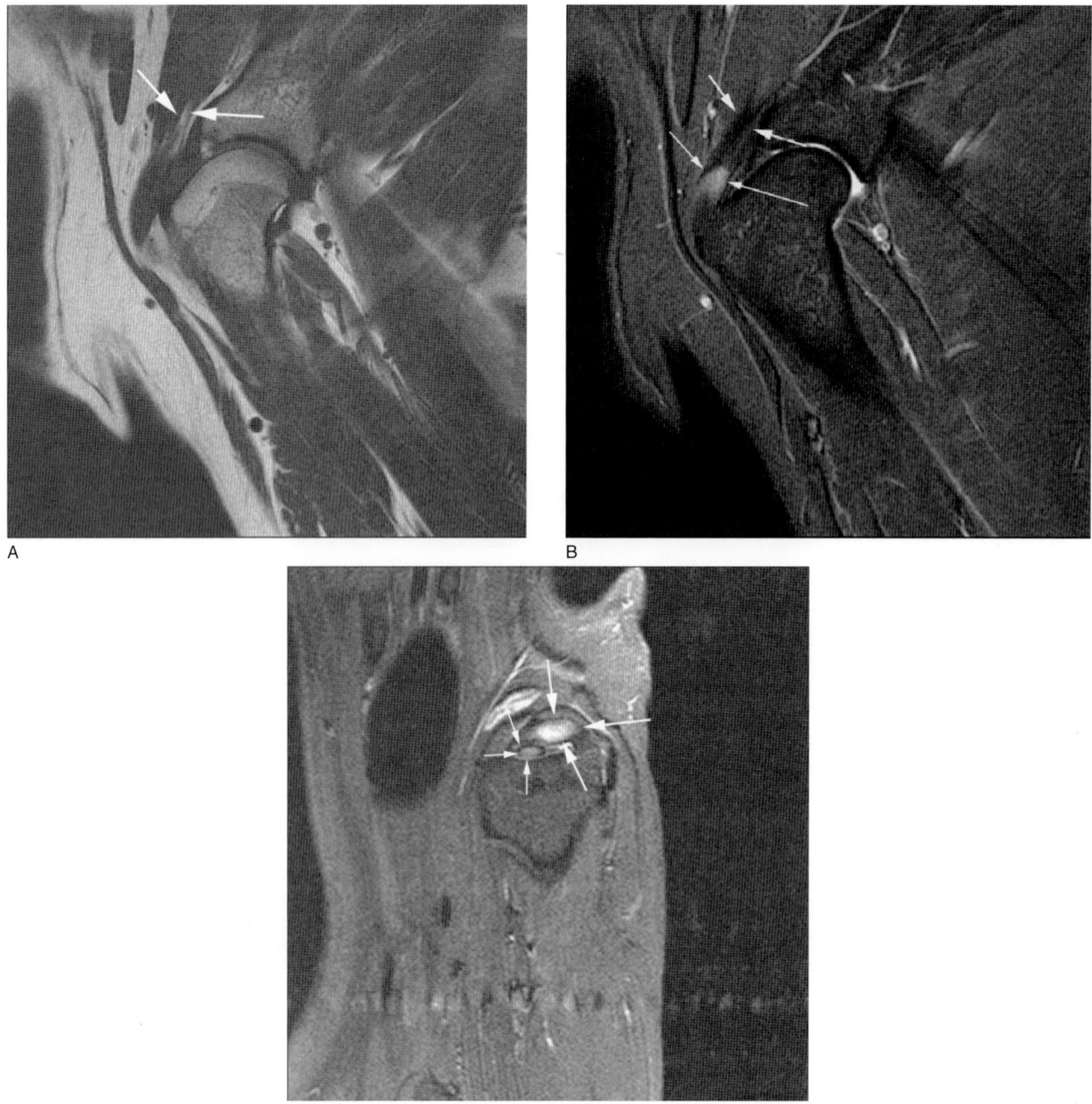

Figure 3.5. Another case of supraspinatus tendinitis. There is fat in the myotendinous region as seen on the T2-weighted A and the STIR sequence, B. (A) T1-weighted sagittal image. Arrows indicate fat at the myotendinous junction. (B) The proliferative lesion from immature collagen at the tearing of the insertion of the supraspinatus tendon on the greater tubercle is seen with the small arrows on 9B. (C) Transverse image—the hyperintensity is shown with the large arrows for the tearing of the supraspinatus, and the small arrows show the displacement of the biceps tendon.

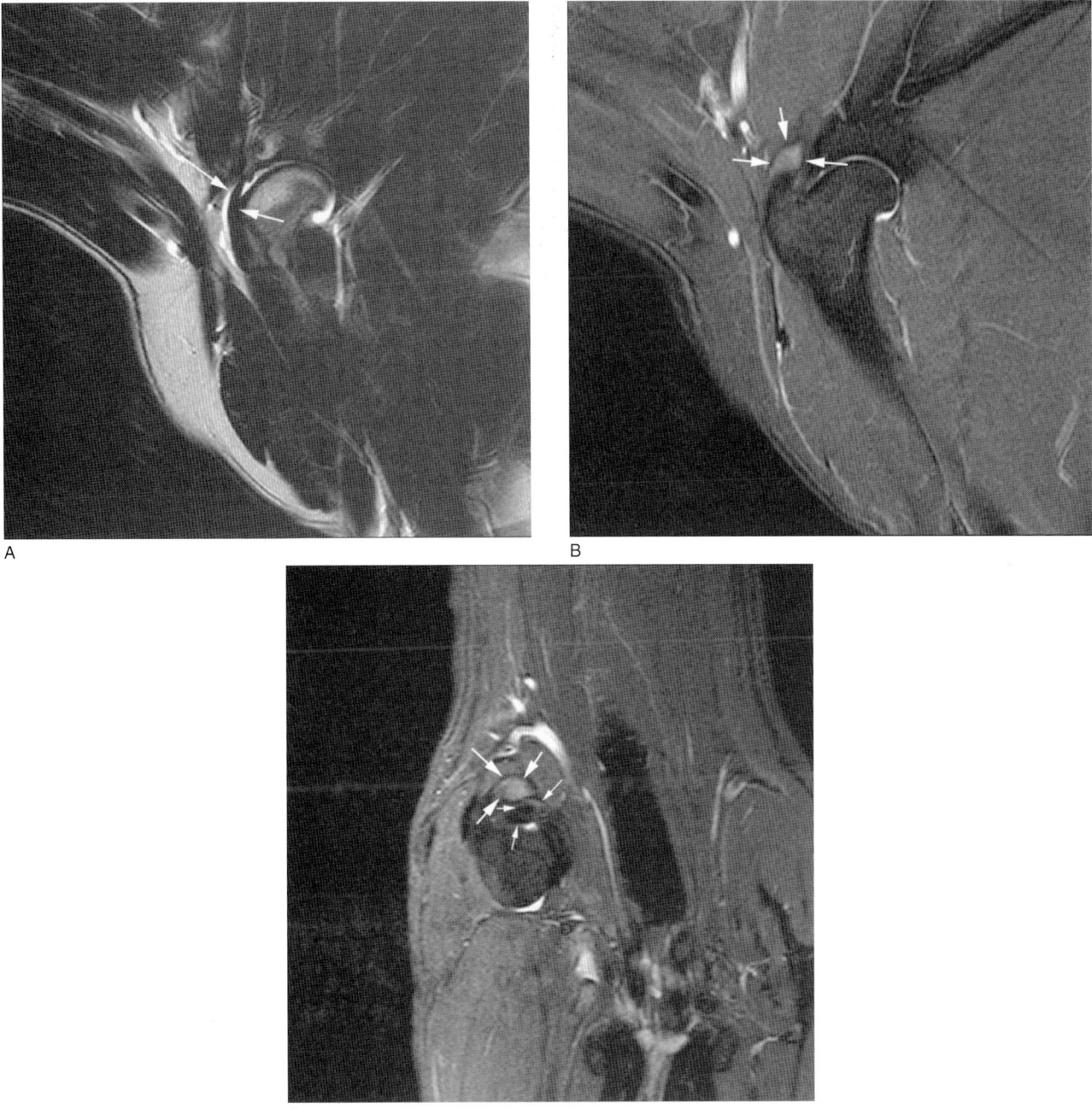

Figure 3.6. Supraspinatus tendinitis. (A) T2-weighted sagittal sequence showing a normal appearance to the biceps tendon with some fluid around it. (B) STIR sagittal sequence showing the hyperintensity at the tearing of the supraspinatus at the insertion. (C) Transverse imaging showing the hyperintensity of the torn supraspinatus and the normal appearance to the biceps tendon (small arrows).

proximal humerus (Figures 3.7 and 3.8), bicipital tenosynovitis (Figure 3.9), medial glenohumeral ligament abnormalities with instability, brachial plexus avulsion (Figure 3.10), infraspinatus contracture, and the less common infraspinatus tendinopathy (Figure 3.11). Changes in signal intensities are similar for these diseases as the cellular pathologic changes in the tendons are similar for these traumatic diseases. The use of STIR or T2 fat-suppressed sequences provide an excellent screening image as the background structures are hypointense (darker) and lesions are hyperintense (whiter) signal intensities. The use of the higher resolution proton density and T1-weighted sequences helps define the anatomic structures that are affected. The use of contrast enhancement sequences generally adds limited additional diagnostic information in order to justify the increased anesthesia time associated with this procedure.

Brachial Plexus Disease

The recognition of brachial plexus abnormalities is much more common with the advent of MR than previously thought. The use of the large field-of-view STIR sequence allows for detection of small lesions that can then be followed with T2-weighted sequences in the transverse plane and T1 before and after contrast as necessary (Figure 3.12). The large FOV STIR sequence allows screening of the nerves of the thoracic limb from the elbow to the spine. With this imaging technique, abnormalities appear as "light bulbs" on a dark background. The challenge associated with these types of lesions is distinguishing the adjacent normal vascular structures from abnormal, enlarged, hyperintense nerves.

While MR provides excellent delineation of the macroscopic extent of disease, histopathologic correlation has shown that the microscopic extent of peripheral nerve disease is usually underestimated. Extension of the macroscopic disease process through the intervertebral foramen and into the spinal canal should be determined as this information may affect therapeutic decisions (Figure 3.12). Unfortunately, extension of peripheral nerve disease into the foraminal region is sometimes not apparent on MR imaging studies even though it is present in the animal. If there is any concern regarding the proximal extent of a brachial plexus neoplastic disease, appropriate imaging of the associated spinal segments and exiting peripheral nerve rootlets should be performed.

Muscle Abnormalities

In addition to the more chronic tendinous and ligamentous diseases, acute muscle tears have been identified as the source of shoulder lameness (Figures 3.13 and 3.14). Muscle tears are generally seen with sufficient time interval from the traumatic event to have formation of methemoglobin. As covered in Chapter 2, methemoglobin will have a high signal intensity of T1, T2, and proton density sequences. Fat is also intense on these sequences, but fat in the muscle would null out on the STIR or fat-suppressed sequences while the methemoglobin would remain bright. These types of lesions require rest and rehabilitation, rather than surgical intervention. Soft tissue lesion such as these demonstrate the importance of obtaining the correct diagnosis through advanced imaging and promotes the consideration of proper treatment options with presumably better therapeutic outcomes.

Shoulder Joint Abnormalities

Abnormalities of the shoulder joint surfaces such as osteochondrosis can easily be missed on a radiographic examination due to the curvature of the humeral head. Joint surface abnormalities, however, are usually readily apparent on MR studies (Figure 3.15). The epiphysis has a high (hyperintense) signal intensity in non-fat-suppressed images, and the defect is clearly seen as a change in contour and signal intensity. There is decreased signal intensity on all sequences deep to the lesion indicating a sclerotic subchondral bone. If any cartilaginous flaps are seen and active inflammation is present in the bone, those will be seen on the STIR or T2 fat-saturated sequences as an area of high signal intensity.

The Elbow Joint Region

The elbow region has been evaluated less frequently to date compared to the shoulder joint. Due to the relatively small size of the joint, adequate imaging of this joint was initially less than ideal. With new MR technology and better receiver coils, however, better images of this joint are possible. The anatomic structures including the coronoid processes are clearly seen. The congruity of the joints can be evaluated as the sequences can be acquired in all planes. The transverse and dorsal plane images are set to the axis of the radius and ulna.

Currently, many veterinarians and veterinary surgeons rely heavily on computed tomography for the

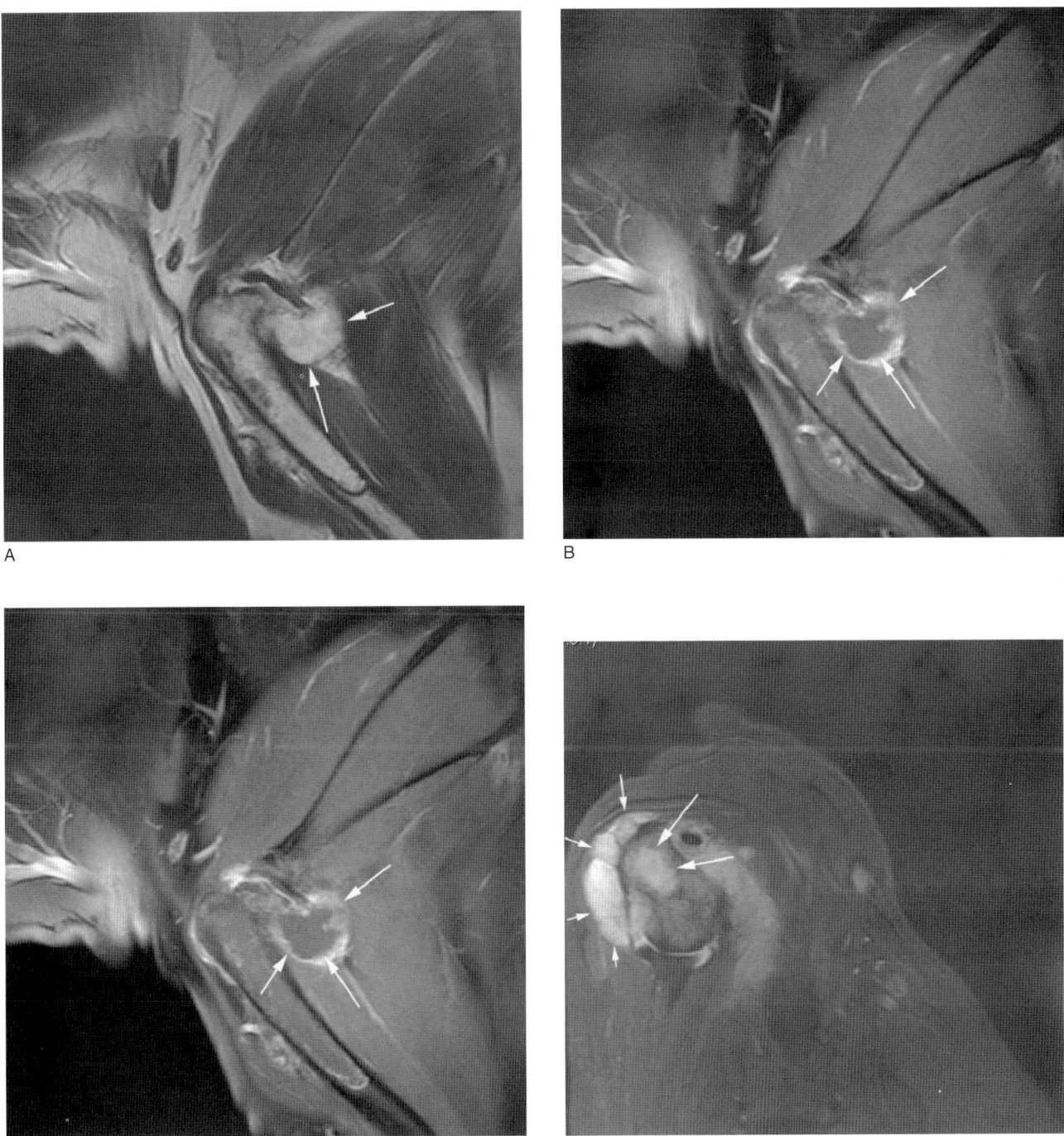

A

B

C

D

Figure 3.7. (A) T2-weighted sagittal sequence depicting mass in the caudal aspect of the joint. (B) STIR sequence in the sagittal plane. Hyperintensity of the mass in the caudal aspect can be seen, as well as the cranial aspect of the proximal humerus and within the proximal humerus. STIR sequences create fat suppression and the entire humerus should be of low signal intensity. (C) T1-weighted post-contrast sagittal image. Enhancement of the periphery of the mass can be seen on the caudal aspect, as noted by the arrows, as well as within the medullary cavity and slightly on the cranial aspect of the humerus. (D) Post-contrast transverse image. The contrast enhancement of the mass can be seen outside of the humerus with the small arrows and within the body of the humerus (large arrows). This mass is a sarcoma and was not visible radiographically.

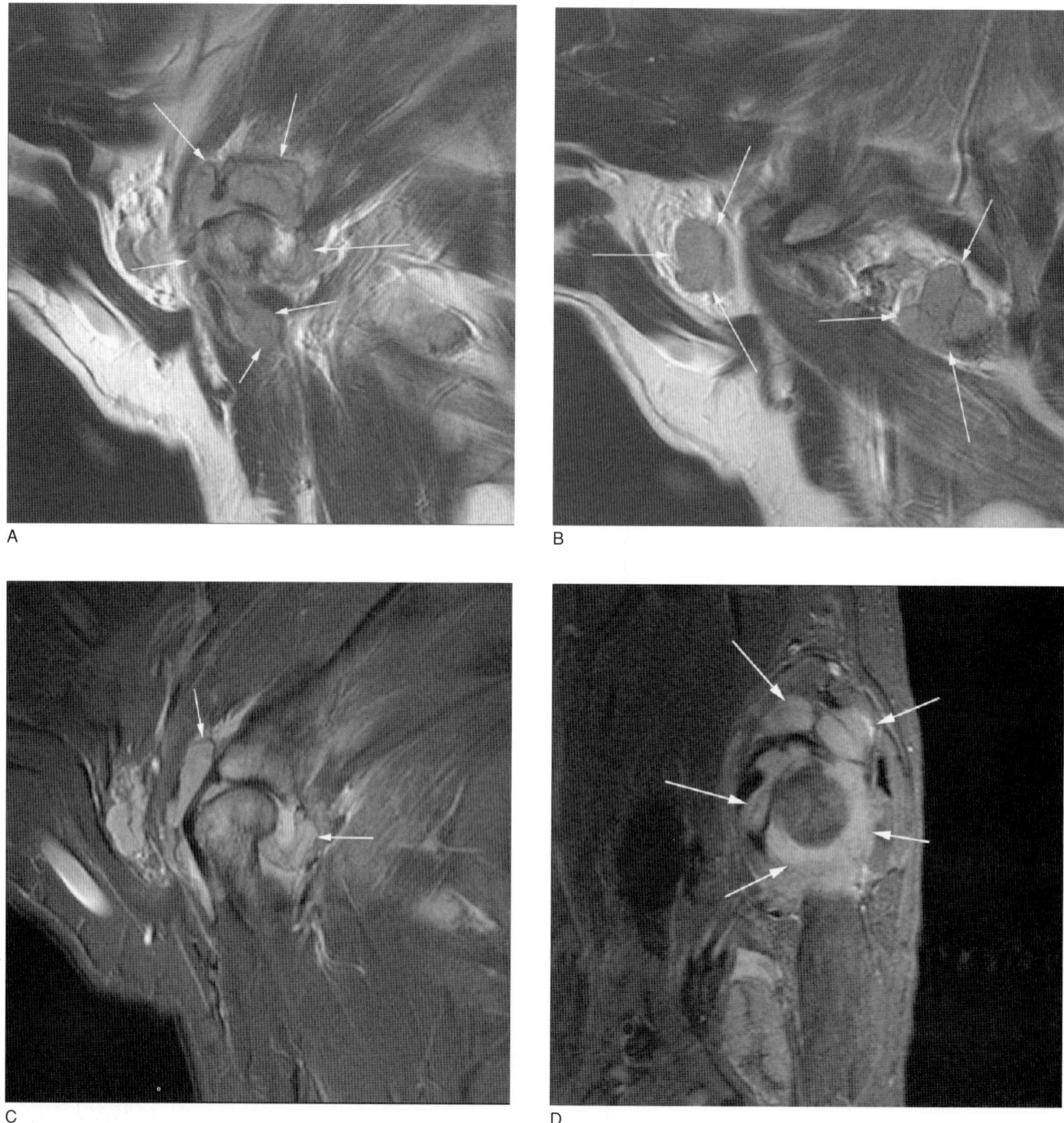

Figure 3.8. (A) T2-weighted sagittal image shows a mass in the region of the shoulder joint. Mass appears to involve the scapula as well as the proximal humerus. (B) T2-weighted sagittal image on the medial aspect of the shoulder joint. Arrows point to enlarged superficial cervical (prescapular) and axillary lymph nodes. (C) T1-weighted, post-contrast, fat-suppressed image. The mass can be seen exterior to the joint as well as within the distal scapula and proximal humerus. (D) Transverse image through the shoulder joint showing the presence of the mass outside of the normal confines of the shoulder joint. The mass was proven to be a synovial cell sarcoma.

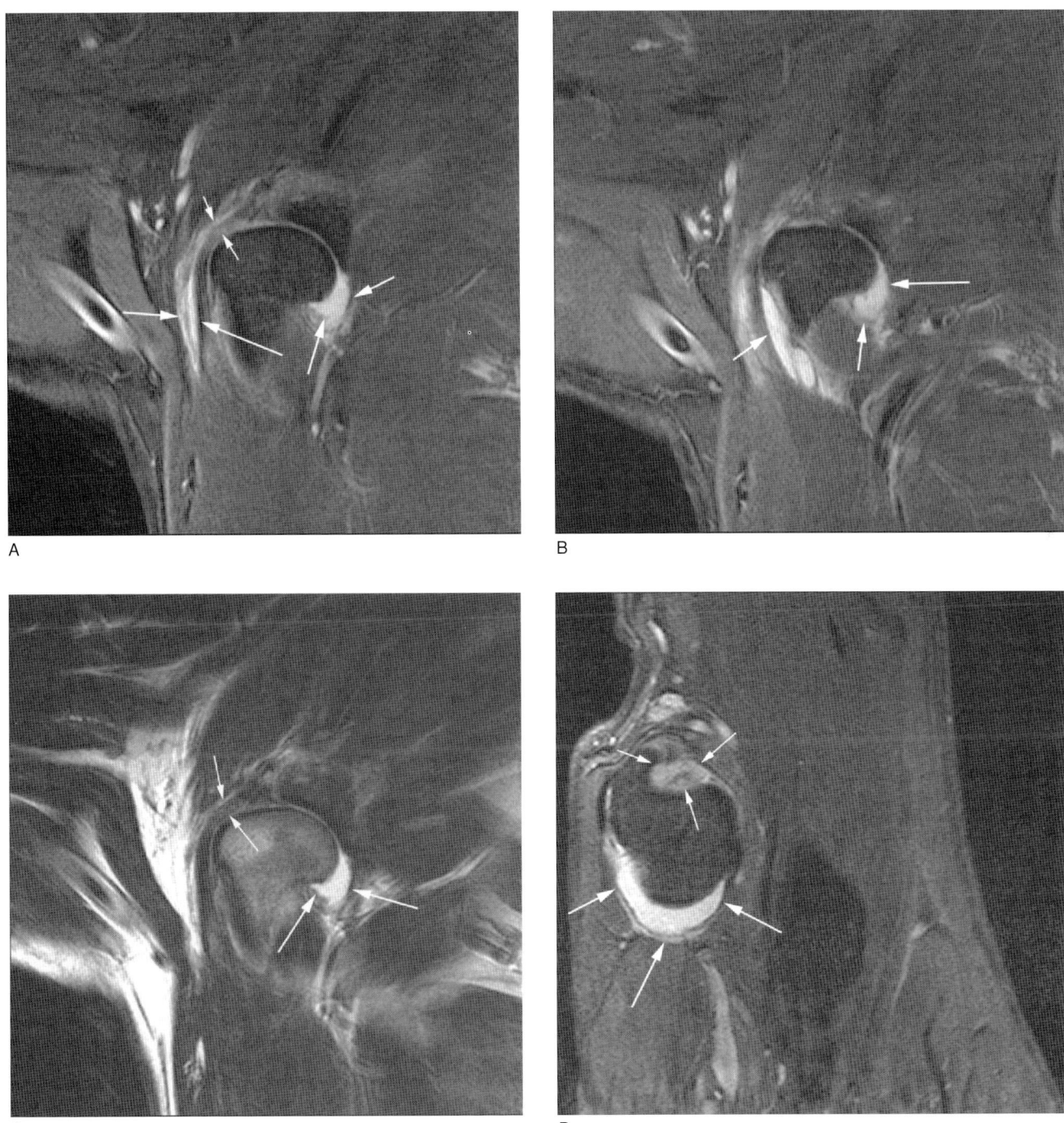

A

B

C

D

Figure 3.9. Bicipital tenosynovitis. (A) and (B) STIR sequences in the sagittal planes on adjacent slices. Small arrows show the presence of hyperintensity in the proximal biceps tendon on (A). The distal portion of the tendon is seen on (B). The hyperintensity is suspect on STIR-weighted sequences due to magic angle artifact. (C) T2-weighted sagittal sequence in the same plane as (A). The hyperintensity of the biceps tendon is seen. Therefore, this finding has been confirmed on a T2-weigthed image that was not artifactual. There is mild joint effusion. (D) STIR transverse image. The marked synovitis can be seen, as indicated by the small arrows, and the joint distention by the large arrows.

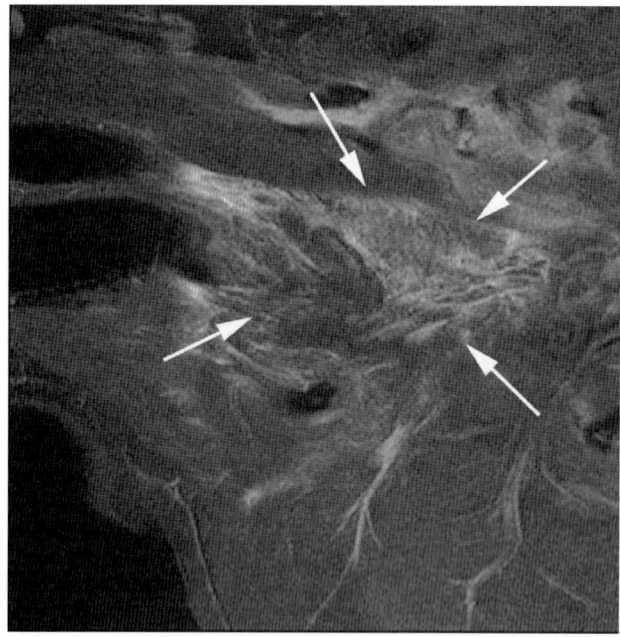
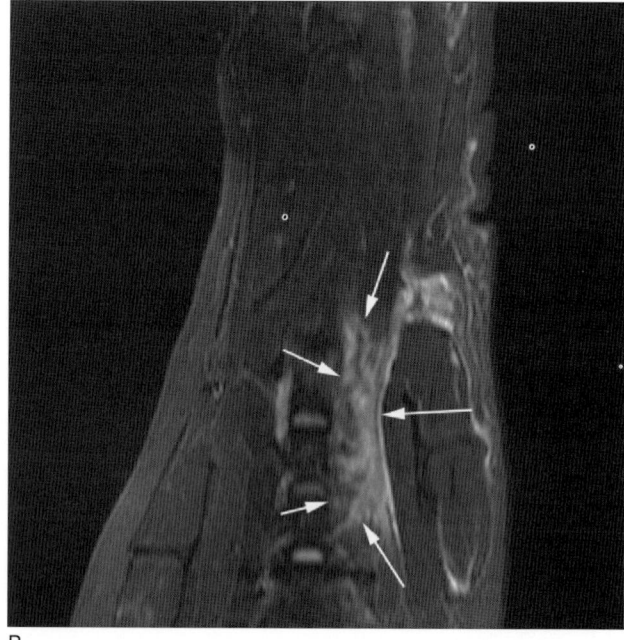

A   B

Figure 3.10. Brachial plexus avulsion. (A) STIR sequence in the parasagittal plane to the left of midline. (B) STIR dorsal plane image. The hyperintensity to the left of the spinal column is between the spinal column and scapula is readily seen. This is confirmed to be an avulsion of the brachial plexus from a traumatic incident.

diagnosis of fragmented medial coronoid process, a condition all too common in the active and sporting breeds. Orthopedic surgeons recognized that canine elbow dysplasia is a far more complex syndrome, which is typically related to more abnormalities than those just involving the medial coronoid process. Many of these are associated with other soft tissue abnormalities, and therefore can go unrecognized on CT examinations of the elbow.

Images of the normal elbow depict all anatomical structures clearly (Figure 3.16). Many clinicians will request bilateral studies to utilize the non-affected limb as a control for the affected limb. While this can be useful, familiarity with normal MR anatomy precludes the necessity for this second study. It is important to recognize, however, that elbow diseases can be bilateral and therefore, bilateral imaging studies are often appropriate. Confusion can occur, as many abnormal conditions are bilaterally symmetric from an imaging standpoint, while the animal may be more, or exclusively affected in a single limb. Bilateral studies should be performed if there is a clinical indication for diagnosis, prognosis, or treatment.

Abnormalities of the elbow that have been diagnosed with MR include fragmented coronoid process (Figure 3.17). The fragment is best seen on the proton density or T2 fat saturated or STIR sequences as the synovial fluid dissects along the fissure. Trauma to the insertion

of the triceps tendon on the olecranon (Figure 3.18) is seen as a loss of integrity of the tendon in T1 images and poorly marginated T2 hyperintensity from the inflammatory response, and there can be methemoglobin present as increased signal on T1 prior to contrast.

Osteoarthritis (Figure 3.19) of the elbow is a common condition, and the MR appearance of joint effusion as seen on the T2-weighted sequences and osteophytes on the periarticular margins with contrast enhancement of the synovial lining is seen and helps rule out more serious conditions. Neoplastic conditions of the elbow are not common, but are readily detected on a standard MR examination. Damage to the origin of the deep digital flexor tendon at the level of the medial epicondyle of the humerus can be seen (Figure 3.20). There is a high T2-weighted signal intensity of the peritendinous structures best seen on the STIR sequence to null out the adjacent subcutaneous fat signal. The tendon is enlarged on the sequences due to the typical unorganized attempts to repair the damaged collagen fibers.

PELVIC REGION

MR studies of the pelvic region are often indicated in animals due to the complexity of the soft tissue structures in this region. It is best to place the animal in

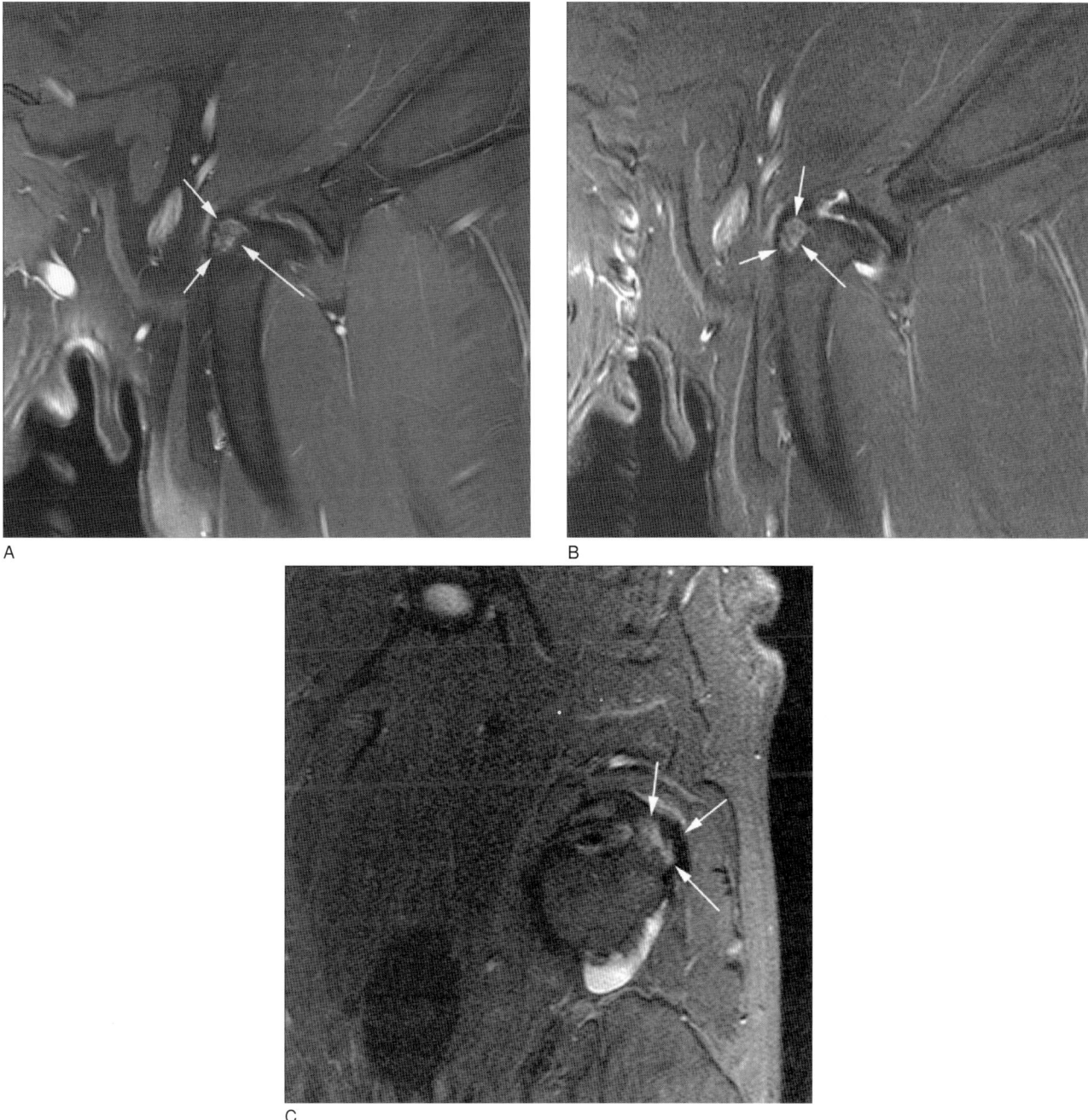

A

B

C

Figure 3.11. (A) STIR sequence showing hyperintensity to the lateral aspect of the greater tubercle. (B) Slightly different plane from (A), showing the lesion in the greater tubercle and some fluid within the shoulder joint. (C) Transverse image showing the hyperintensity in the proximal humerus underneath the infraspinatus tendon. In this case, the lesion of the infraspinatus insertion is causing more bone edema from avulsion of the fibers at their insertion. The anatomical difference between supraspinatus and infraspinatus diseases is readily seen.

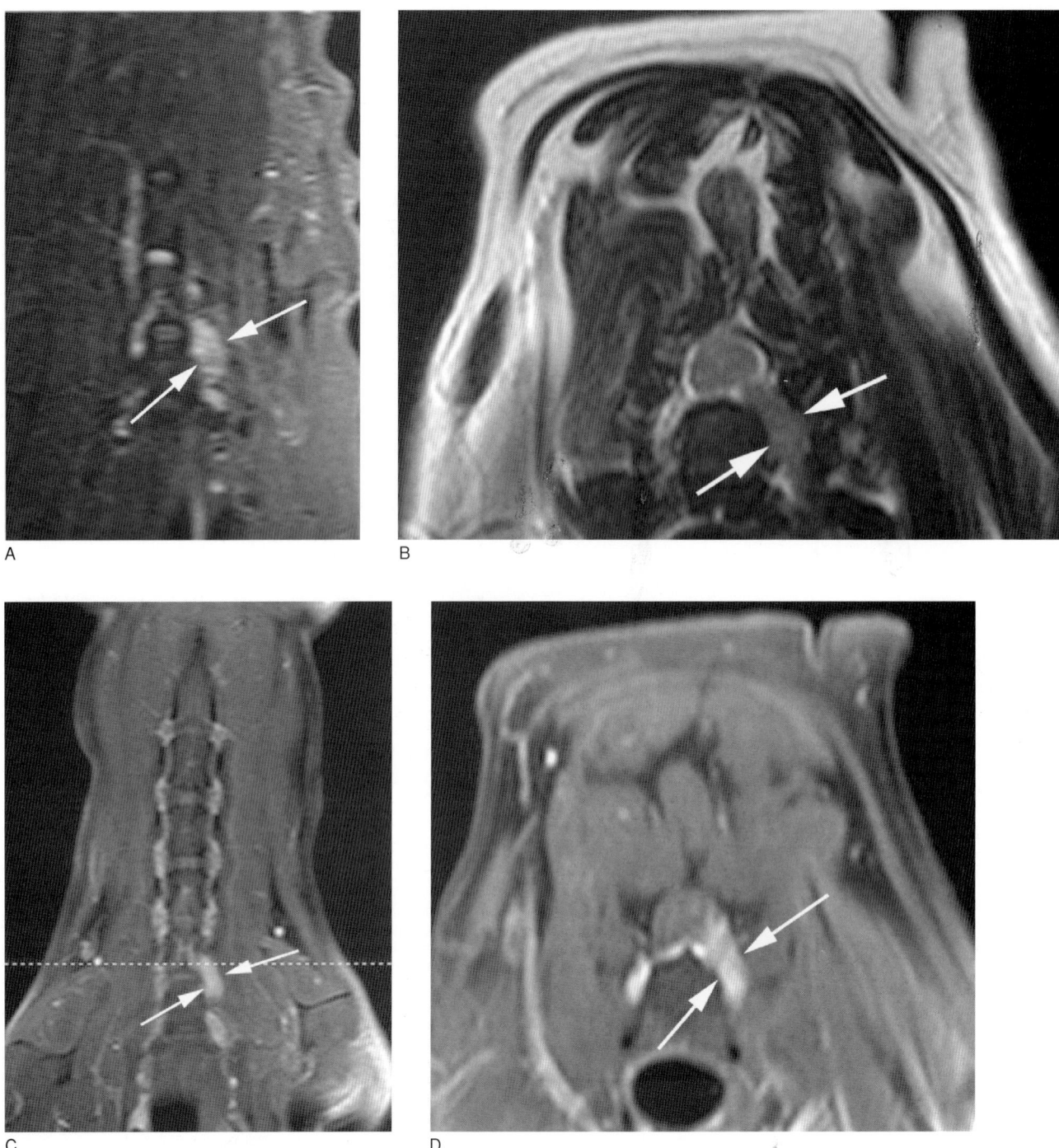

Figure 3.12.   Brachial plexus lesion. (A) Large FOV STIR dorsal image. Hyperintense area lateral to the spine is indicated with arrows. (B) T2-weighted transverse image showing an enlargement in the intervertebral foramen. (C) T1-weighted, post-contrast, fat-suppressed dorsal plane image. The line indicates the plane of section of D. (D) T1-weighted, post-contrast, fat-suppressed image showing increased signal intensity in the region of the nerve root. Tentative diagnosis—enlarged nerve root, seventh cervical nerve. Finding is compatible with either neuritis or nerve sheath tumor.

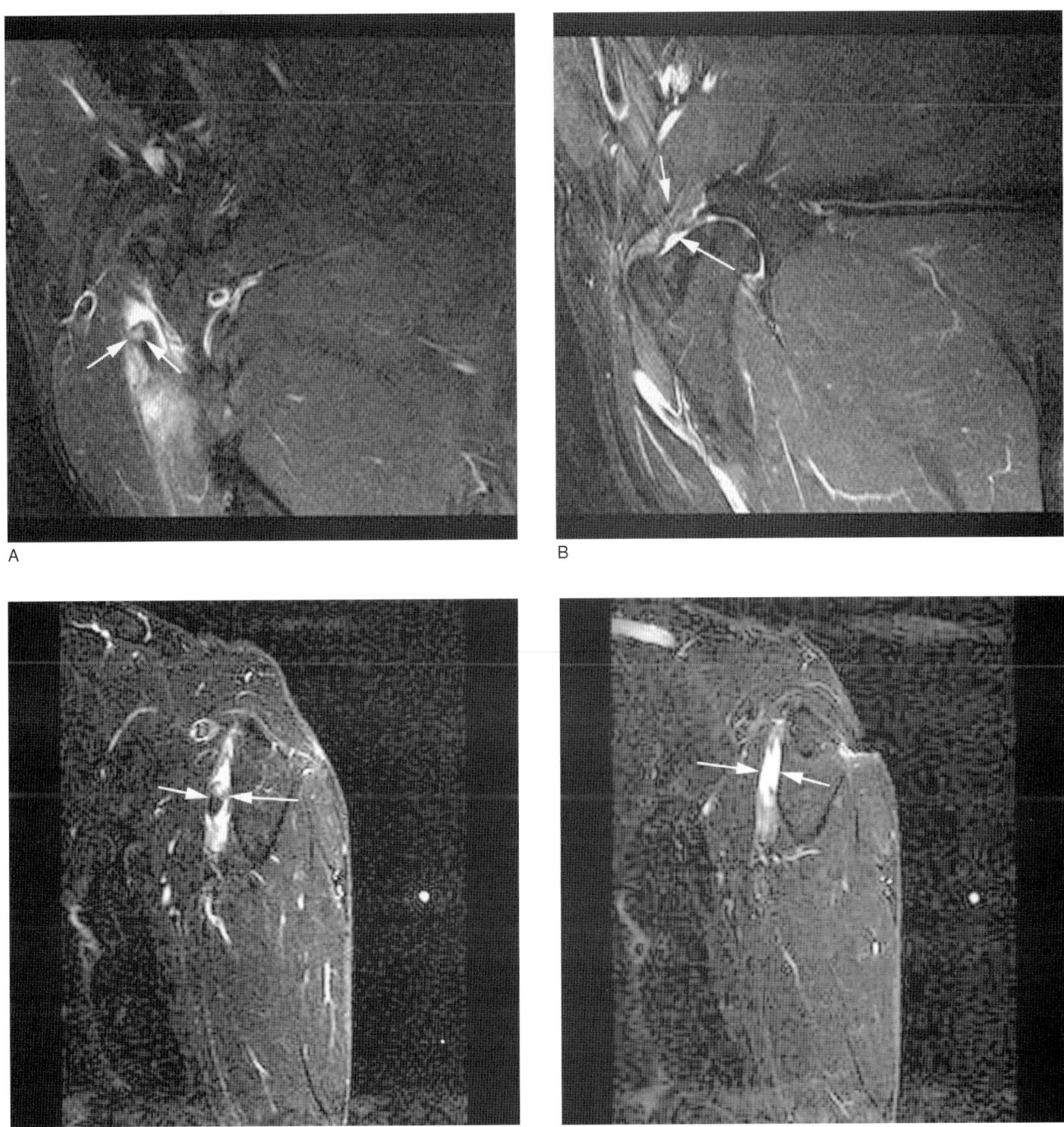

Figure 3.13.   Avulsion of the biceps tendon. (A) T2-weighted sagittal sequence. The arrows point to the end of the biceps tendon surrounded by fluid. (B) STIR sequence showing the lack of a biceps tendon in its normal location, which would be between the arrows. (C) Transverse image through the end of the biceps tendon at the level seen in (A). (D) Just proximal to the end showing only the fluid within the sheath of the tendon with no tendon being present.

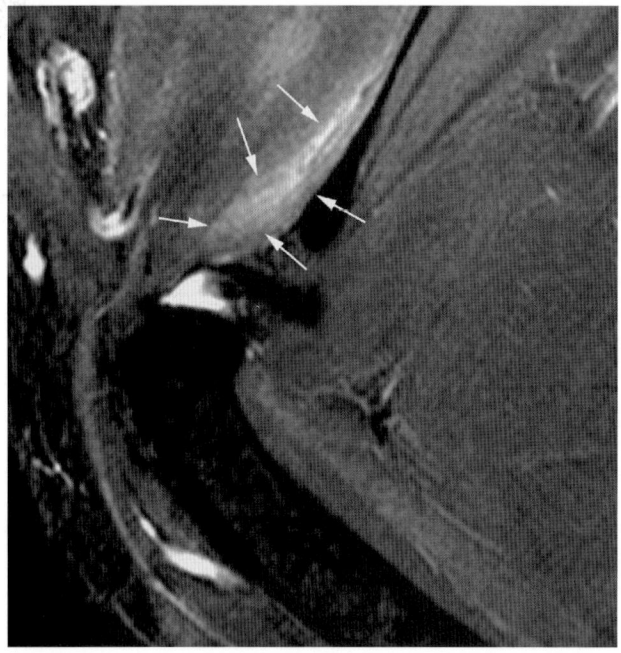
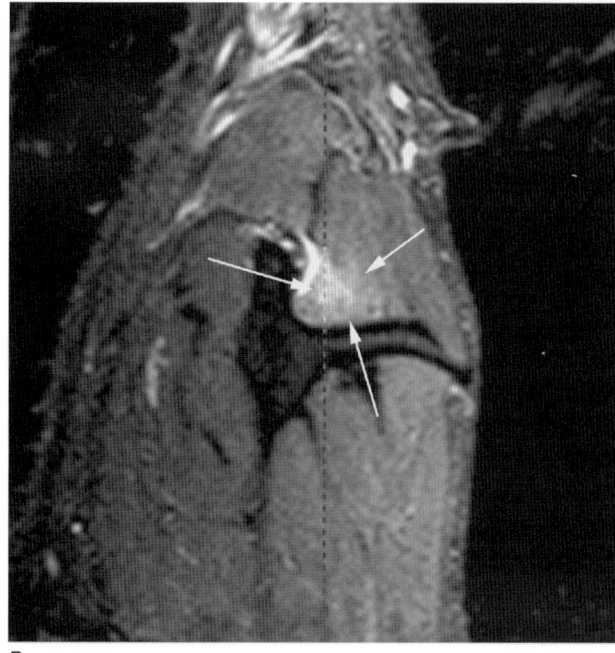

A

B

Figure 3.14. (A) Traumatic tear to the supraspinatus muscle is seen on the STIR sagittal sequence. (B) STIR transverse sequence showing this tear in the supraspinatus muscle. The dotted line shows the plane of section of (A).

dorsal recumbent position and use a field of view that encompasses the entire pelvic region, typically defined as the region from approximately L5 to the anus, and laterally to include both gluteal musculature and coxofemoral joints. The standard imaging protocol of the pelvis using MR includes acquisition of all planes using fat-suppressed sequences, like STIR or fat-suppressed proton density sequences. In addition, some information, albeit limited, can be gained from the visualization of the degree of contrast enhancement of the lesions. In general, however, it is better to acquire multiple sequences with different weighting, in various planes and without contrast rather than to rely heavily on the contrast enhancement properties of the abnormal tissue. Contrast enhancement is beneficial, however, may be helpful distinguish benign from infectious lesions of the lumbosacral joint complex.

A surprising number of tumors of the skeleton and surrounding soft tissues in the pelvic region have been found with MR imaging that were previously undetectable (Figures 3.21 and 3.22). All planes are readily acquired utilizing fat-suppressed sequences including STIR or fat-suppressed proton density sequences. The lesions are readily seen as hyperintense abnormalities on a dark (hypointense) background structures. Contrast enhancement, however, should not be used as an absolute criterion for the presence of neoplastic tissue.

Osteoarthritis of the coxofemoral joint can have marked enhancement of the synovial membrane and large areas of cellulitis and synovitis (Figure 3.23). While the degree of change is obvious, it is possible that septic arthritis or even synovial cell sarcoma could have a similar appearance. The degree of soft tissue inflammation is common with osteoarthritis and should not be overinterpreted as evidence of neoplasia.

Magnetic resonance is the best imaging modality for the accurate diagnosis of iliopsoas muscle tears. This condition appears to be overdiagnosed clinically based on physical examination and ultrasonographic findings, but when present the muscle abnormalities are clearly seen (Figure 3.24). The muscle tear is high signal on STIR or T2 and may have methemoglobin hyperintensity on T1 prior to contrast, and the resulting inflammation will be enhanced with contrast studies.

NERVE SHEATH TUMORS

While the brachial plexus is the most commonly affected site with tumors of the nerve sheath, the second most common site is within the pelvic region. Tumors of the femoral and sciatic nerves are more common than previously thought with reapplication of MR and its

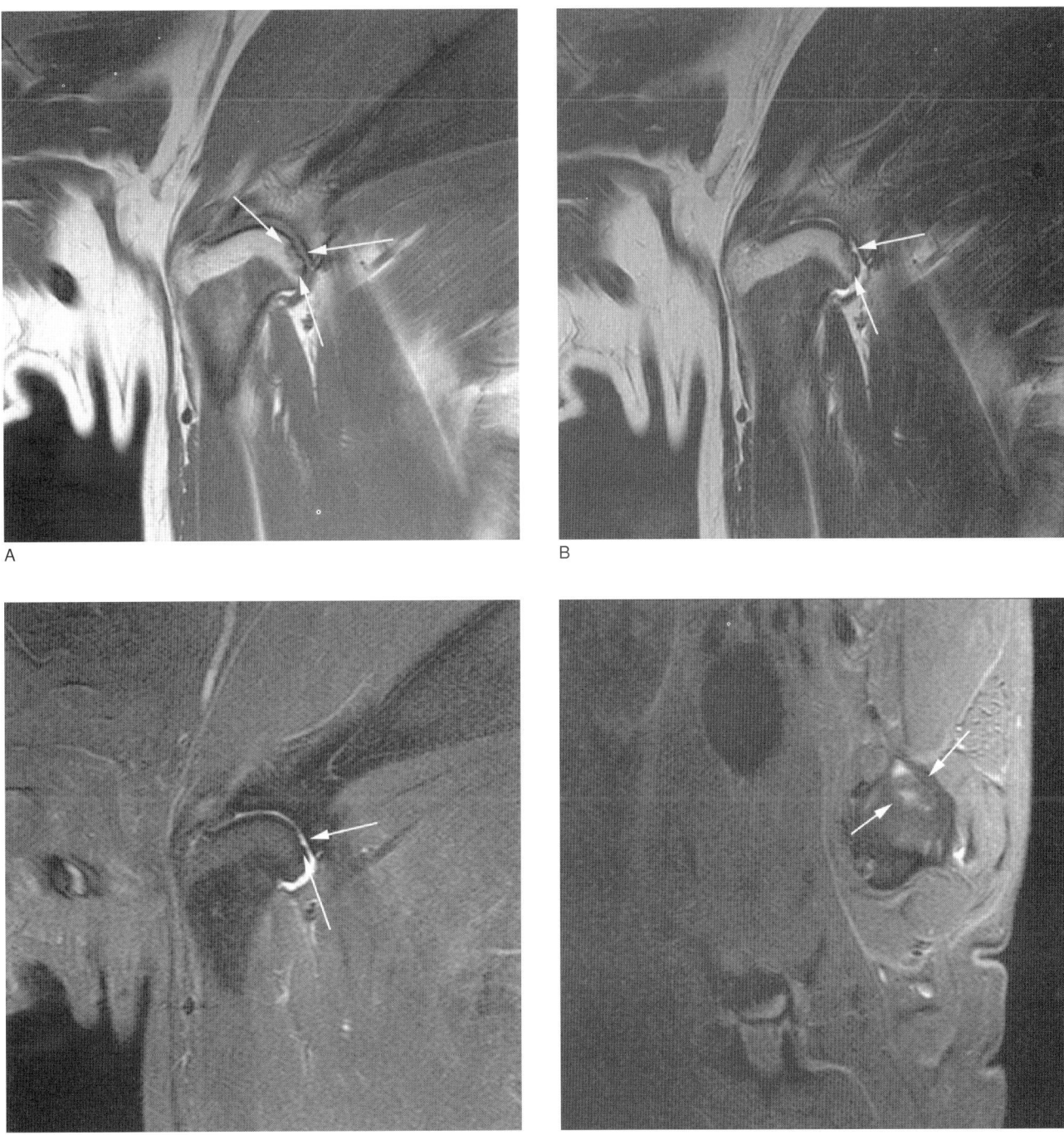

Figure 3.15.   Osteochondrosis. (A) T1-weighted image. The hyperintensity of the epiphysis is commonly seen. There is more fat signal within the epiphysis compared to the diaphysis. (B) T2-weighted image in the similar plane. (C) STIR sequence in the similar plane. Note how a small flap can be seen in (C). This was not visible in the other two sequences. There is no significant subchondral edema, indicating this is not an active lesion, but quiescent. The area of erosion at the head of the humerus can be seen on (B). Again, there is no surrounding subchondral edema, and this not an active inflammatory lesion at this time. This lesion was not seen on a good quality radiographic examination. Radiographic exams can fail to see these small lesions due to obliquity and the improper tangent projection. (D) Transverse STIR sequence through the articular surface of the humerus.

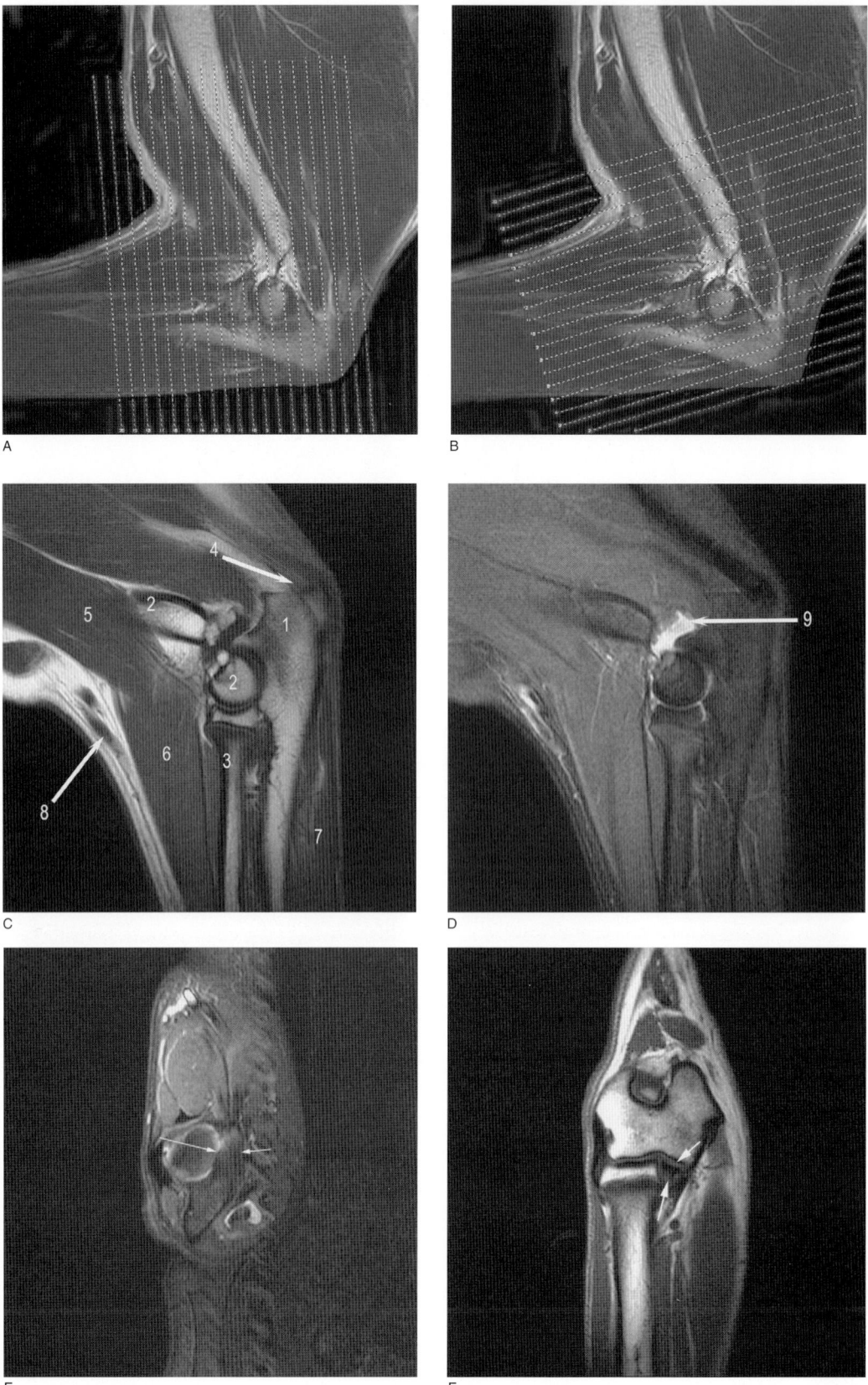

Figure 3.16. Normal elbow. The hyperintensity of the proximal radius is seen in this young patient. Note how the physeal plate is readily seen. (A) T2-weighted image in sagittal plane. (1) Olecranon process of ulna, (2) humerus, (3) radius, (4) triceps muscles with arrow indicating tendinous insertion, (5) biceps muscle, (6) extensor muscles, (7) flexor muscles, (8) cephalic vein. (B) STIR image in sagittal plane. Note the normal amount of synovial fluid (9) within the elbow joint. The congruity of the humeral ulnar articulation is well seen. (C) T1-weighted appearance of the normal medial coronoid process in the sagittal plane. (D) STIR-weighted sagittal sequence showing the normal medial coronoid process. (E) Gradient recalled echo (GRE) transverse image of a normal medial coronoid process. (F) Transverse STIR sequence through the medial coronoid process, as shown by the arrows. Note the flow of artifact from the cubital vein going in a top to bottom direction. (G) Dorsal plane through the coronoid process as shown with the arrow.

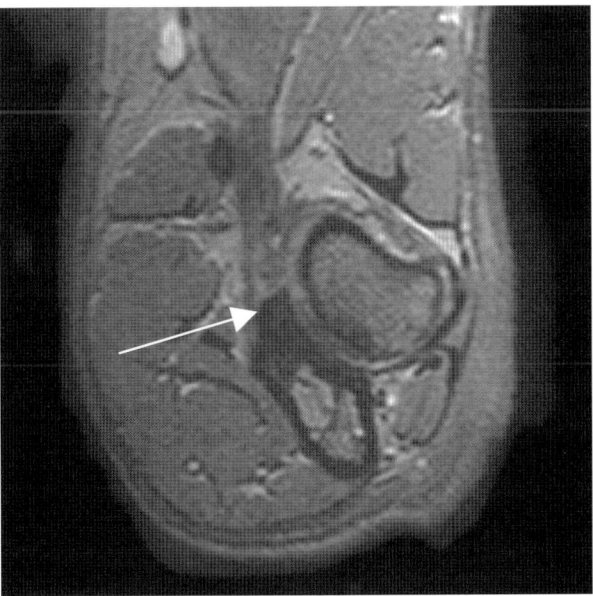

G

Figure 3.16.   *(Continued)*

superior soft tissue contrast. While any nerve can undergo a malignant transformation, it has been our experience that the brachial plexus is the most common, followed by the sciatic nerve, and thirdly the femoral nerve. It is, therefore, our protocol that all animals with pelvic limb abnormalities, generally referred to the lumbosacral spine, be screened for nerve sheath tumors using a large field-of-view STIR sequence in a plane planned dorsal to the spine. Any abnormalities can be followed up with transverse imaging, including before and after the administration of contrast agent. Examples of these lesions are given in Chapters 2 (Section 3) and 7.

STIFLE JOINT

The stifle joint is one of the most commonly imaged human joints utilizing magnetic resonance. By comparison, the veterinary community has been relatively slow to adopt with imaging modality for the assessment of lameness localized to this joint. The menisci, cranial and caudal cruciate ligaments, collateral ligaments, tendon of the long digital extensor, the infrapatellar fat body, and the synovial fluid and membrane are all clearly seen. The osseous components are clearly seen and the cartilage can be visualized in larger patients. We have looked at stifle MR studies in a retrospective fashion and found a large percentage of these animals fail to have abnormalities that were suspected during phys-

ical examination and radiographic examination. Some cases are normal or have something that was not seen in the soft tissues (Figure 3.25). The presence or absence of joint effusion is readily apparent on MR. While many of the diseases have similar changes on the various sequences, the clear depiction of the anatomy allows for numerous diagnoses. Obviously, there are times when biopsy and histopathology or direct visualization is needed for confirmation of the lesions. We have also found a large number of instances where two or more different disease processes are occurring concurrently; most commonly, this clinical scenario includes stifle osteoarthrosis with a neoplastic process that is not evident on radiographic examination.

The most common disease within the canine stifle remains damage to the cranial cruciate ligament. Most of the patients submitted for MR do not have complete tears with obvious drawer signs. The animals submitted for MR tend to have relatively stable stifles and presumed joint effusion based on stifle radiographs; thus, the presumptive diagnosis is a partial tear of the cranial cruciate ligament. These partial tears are diagnosed based on loss of the normal linearity of the collagen fibers that span the entire length from origin to insertion. Damage to the collagen fibers results in inflammation spreading of these fibers, especially at their origins and insertions. These lesions are then readily seen on MR studies as increased signal intensity in the normally hypointense ligament origins and insertions, especially with STIR, T2, or proton density studies with

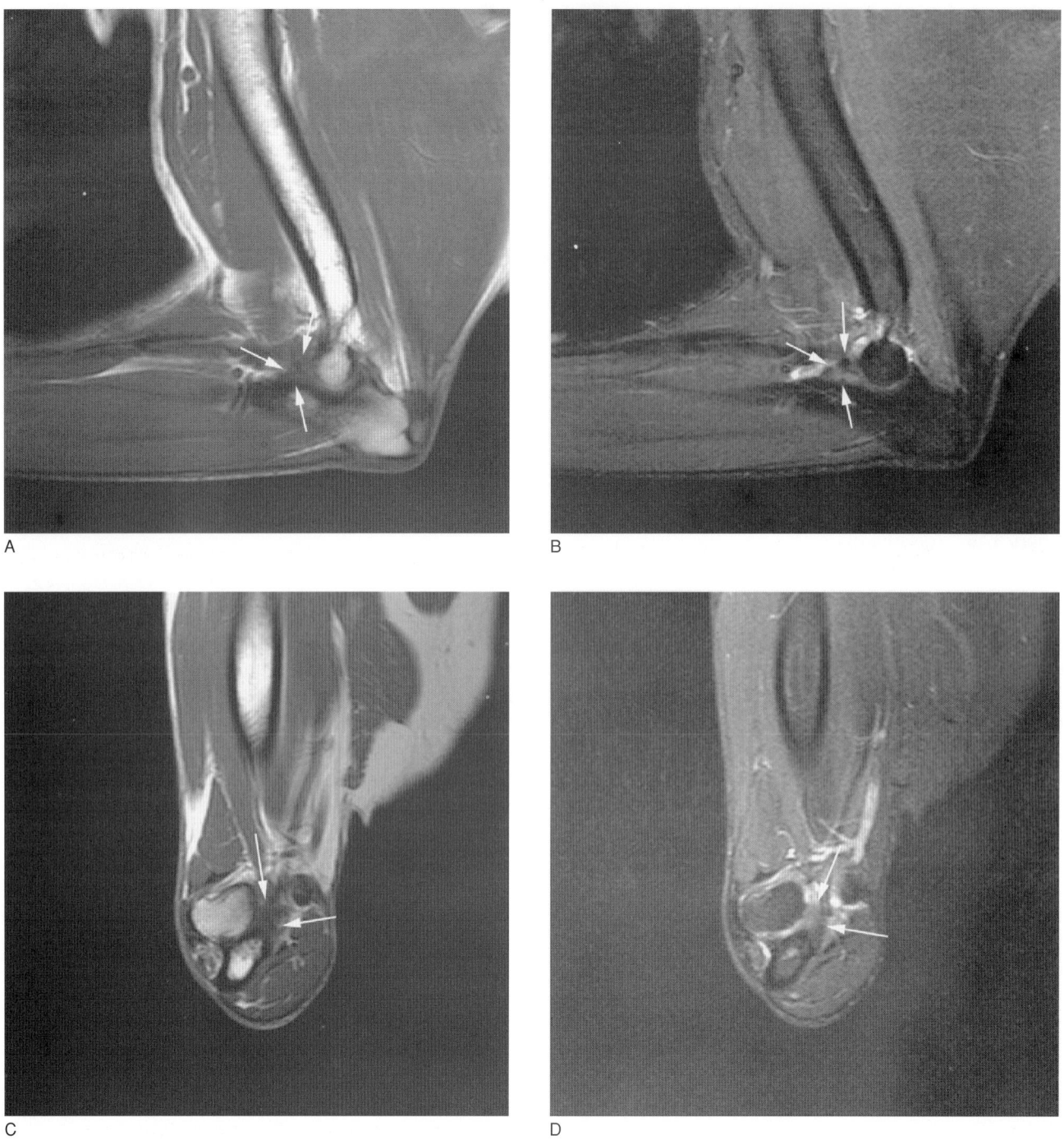

Figure 3.17. Fragmented medial coronoid process. (A) Fragmentation of the medial coronoid process as seen on a T1-weighted sagittal sequence. (B) STIR sagittal sequence showing this fragmented medial coronoid process. (C) T1-weighted transverse showing this fragmentation. (D) STIR-weighted transverse sequence showing this same fragmentation.

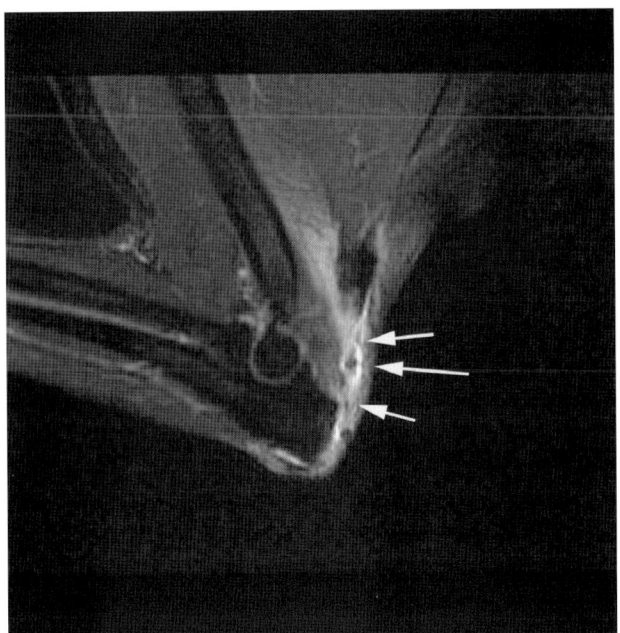

Figure 3.18. Avulsion of the triceps tendon from the olecranon. The high signal intensity identified with the arrows is presumed hemorrhage and edematous fluid. The dark tendon can be seen proximal to that area.

fat suppression. The origin of the cranial cruciate ligament is fan shaped and it often has a higher signal intensity due to volume averaging of the origin and the synovial fluid; knowledge of this fact should help prevent overinterpretation of damage to the cranial cruciate ligament. The caudal cruciate ligament is more of a thick rope-like structure and is uniformly dark on all sequences. Examples or partial tears to cranial cruciate ligaments are given (Figures 3.26 and 3.27). However, one should again be reminded that other conditions occur, including traumatic muscle tears (Figure 3.28), synovial cell sarcomas (Figure 3.29), and other conditions (Figures 3.30–3.32). Again, the signal intensities are similar (high on T2 and STIR) but the clear anatomic depiction allows the conditions to be cataloged differently.

The radiographic abnormality that most have trusted prior to this time to diagnose stifle disease has been apparent joint effusion with displacement of the infrapatellar fat body. While this can be overinterpreted, it can also be transient and not necessarily associated with severe clinical disease. In addition, some animals are found to be normal on MR imaging evaluations that were suspected based on physical examination of having stifle disease. Even in dogs with clinical abnormalities reflected of stifle disease, a large percentage of these animals have abnormalities that are not generally attributable to cranial cruciate ligament damage. Diseases that are found in addition to this diagnosis are damage to the medial and lateral meniscus. In these instances, synovial fluid dissects in the meniscal tear and this abnormality is readily apparent. In general, however, it is best to confirm all lesions on more than one plane to prevent errors due to volume averaging artifacts. Other diseases that have been diagnosed in a retrospective review of 60 stifle MR examinations include disruption of the long digital extensor tendon, caudal cruciate ligament damage, synovial cell sarcoma, traumatic muscle tears, simple osteoarthritis, and patellar cartilaginous damage.

TARSUS AND CARPUS REGIONS

Many diseases of the tarsus have previously been diagnosed with radiography or, more recently, CT. Some improvements of the diagnosis of common conditions such as osteochondrosis of the talus have occurred with the use of CT. However, again there are soft tissue abnormalities that are not seen with these low soft tissue contrast techniques and are best seen with MR. With conditions such as osteochondrosis, the lesion is easily seen with MR, but a secondary effect on the flexor tendons is also identified. The secondary arthritic reaction results in proliferation of soft tissues and deformity of the deep digital flexor tendon in the region of the sustentaculum tali. This reaction is considered a contributing component of the lameness associated with this abnormality (Figure 3.33). Tumor and foreign bodies are also well visualized with MR (Figures 3.34 and 3.35). The precise localization of a foreign body in the distal limb greatly facilitates surgical removal. Foreign bodies are dark on all sequences and are surrounded by fluid. These lesions are often seen as well or better on the STIR sequence than on the T1 post-contrast studies even if fat suppression is used. The overdependence of veterinary radiologists on post-contrast studies is probably based on experience with other modalities and CT in particular. The strength of MR is the visualization of the chemistry of the tissue allows for diagnoses without contrast. Post-contrast studies have value, but they should be judged against the cost. The cost includes the agent, technician and equipment time, and increased anesthetic time.

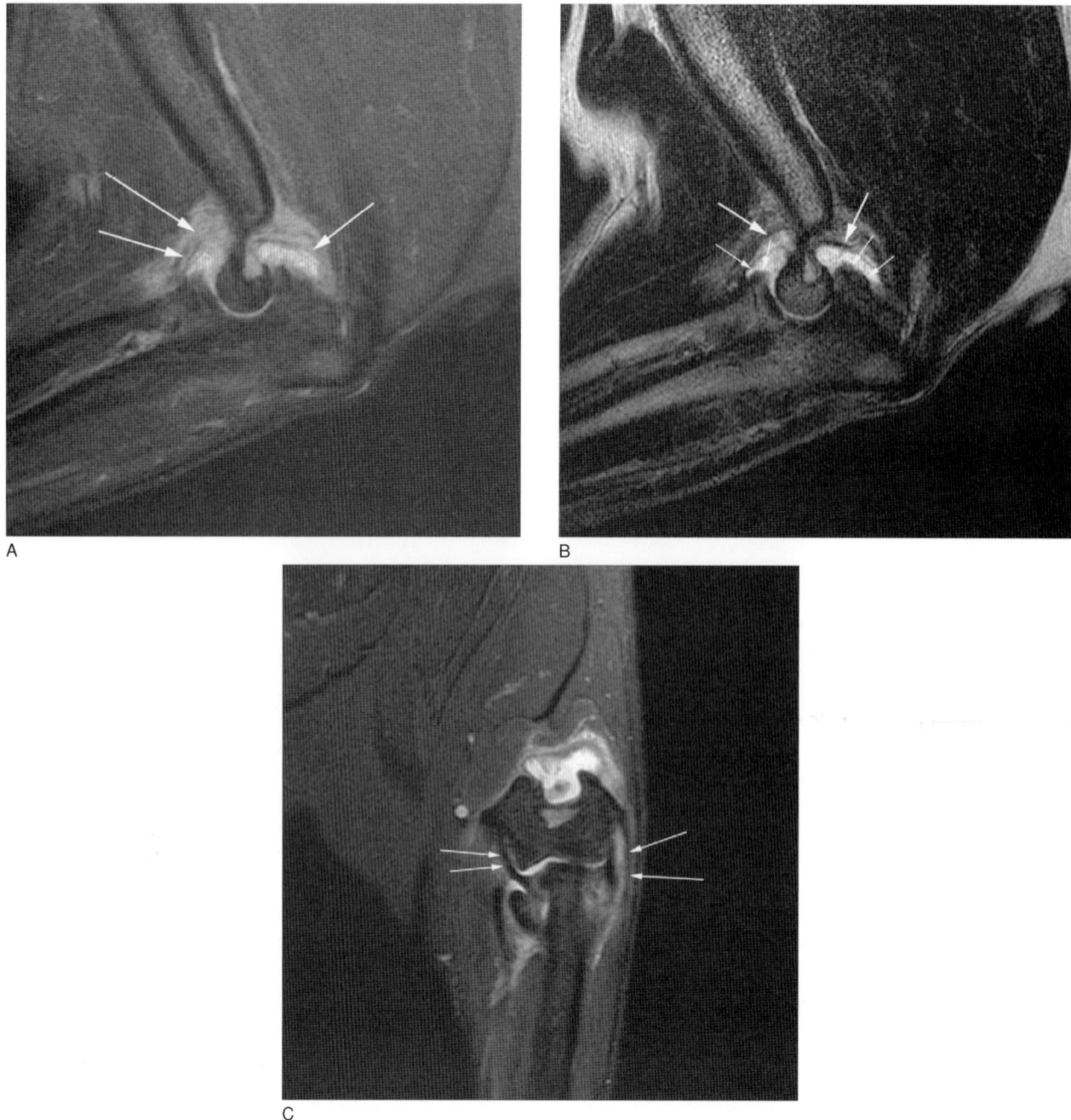

Figure 3.19. (A) Sagittal STIR sequence. Arrows indicate the joint effusion and inflammation. (B) T2-weighted sagittal image in the same plane as (A). Large arrows indicate joint effusion. Small arrows point to osteophytes on the radius and anconeal process. (C) Normal medial collateral ligament hyperintensity, lateral collateral ligament on STIR dorsal plane image.

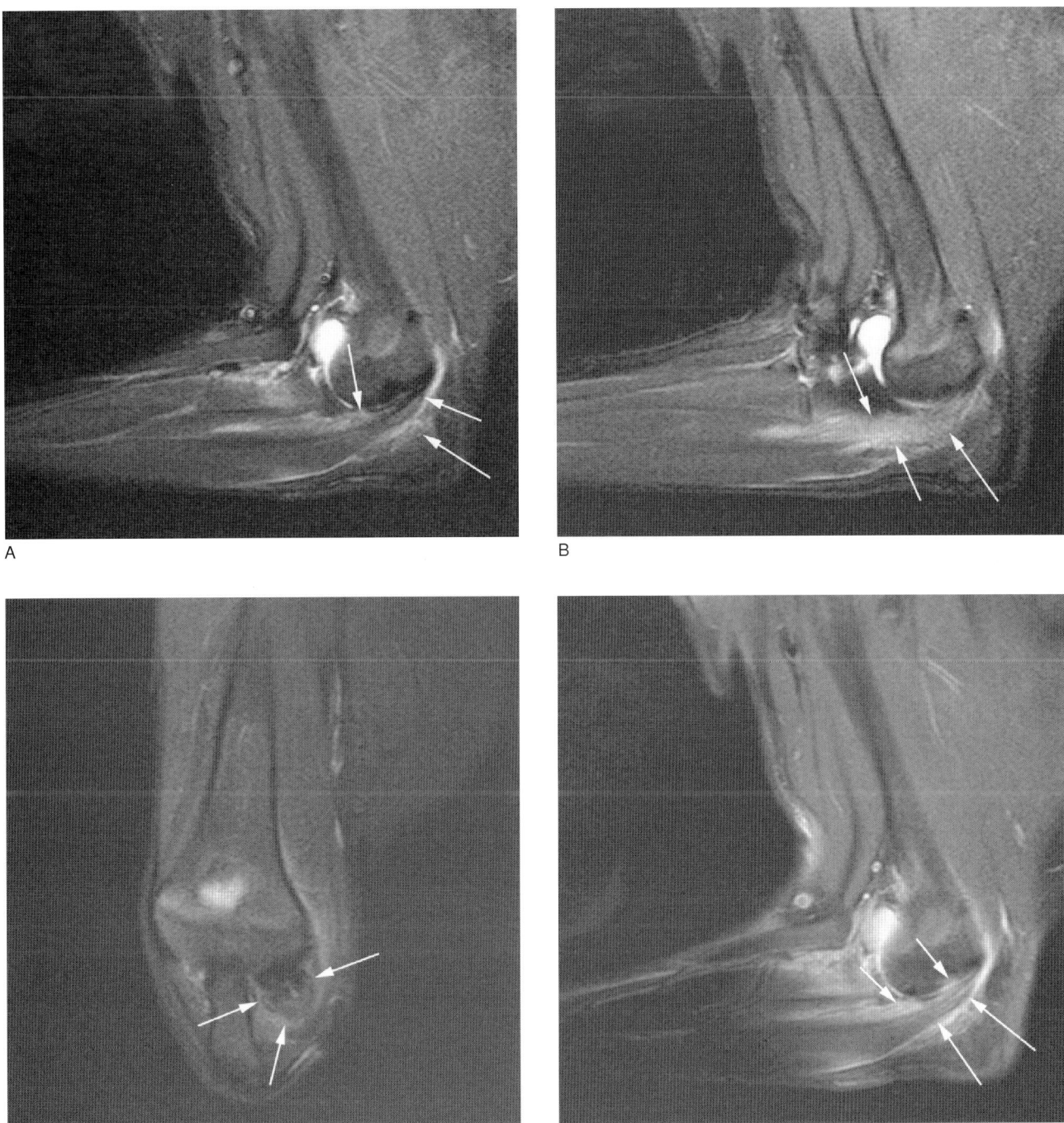

Figure 3.20.   Deep digital flexor tendinitis. (A) STIR sagittal image. Arrows point to hyperintensity peripheral to the digital flexor origin. (B) Adjacent slice showing the peritendinous increased signal intensity compatible with an inflammatory reaction. (C) Transverse STIR image showing enlarged, abnormal deep digital flexor tendon at its origin from the medial epicondyle. (D) Sagittal T1-weighted, post-contrast, fat-suppressed image showing contrast enhancement in the peritendinous tissues. Also enhancement of the joint capsule of the elbow.

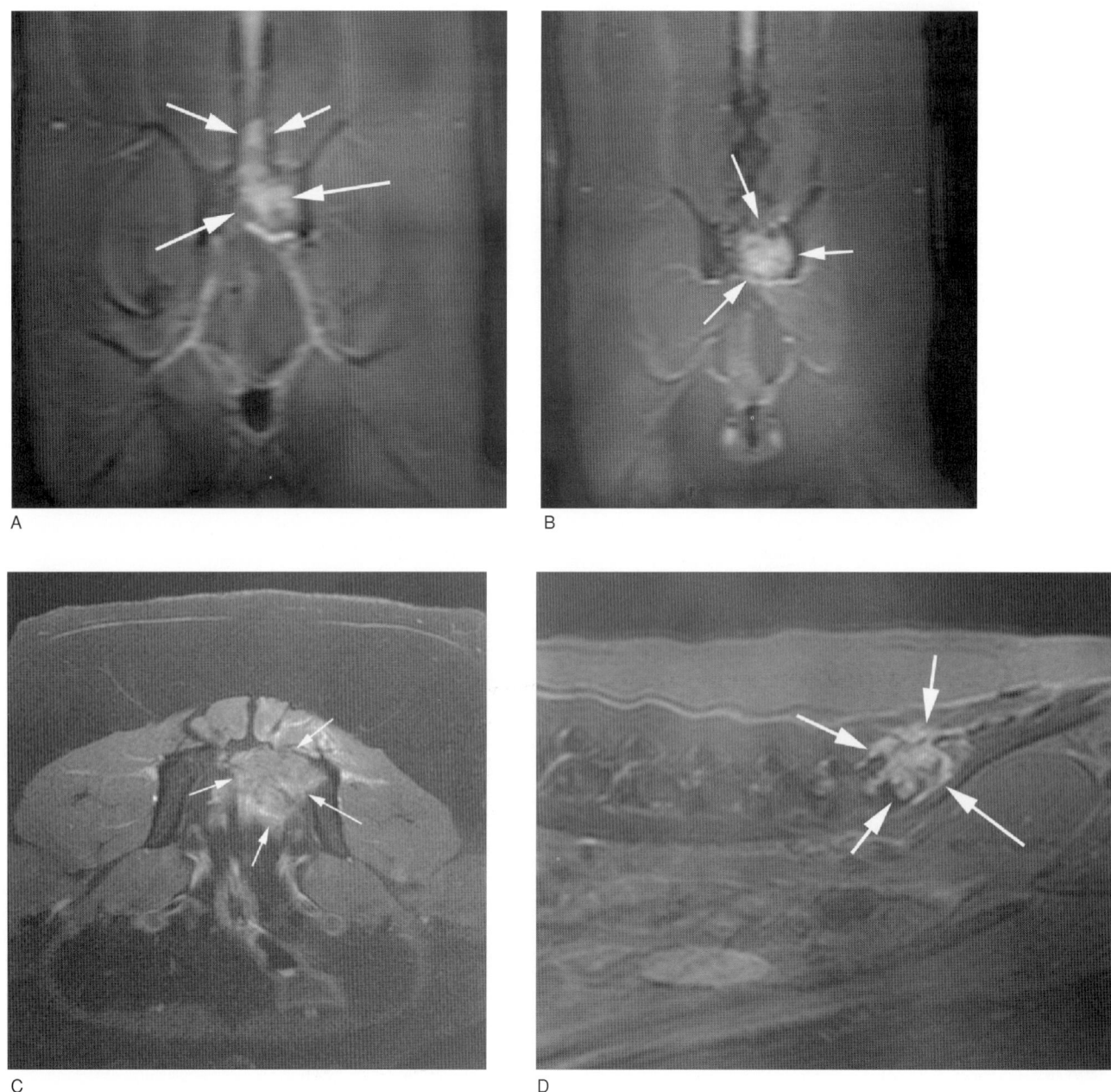

Figure 3.21. Tumor of the sacrum invading the spinal canal. (A) STIR sequence in the dorsal plane. Mass can be seen in the left sacrum extending into the spinal canal. (B) STIR sequence slightly dorsal. (C) Transverse STIR sequence. The mass can be seen invading the left portion of the sacrum. (D) Sagittal STIR sequence showing the mass in the left sacrum.

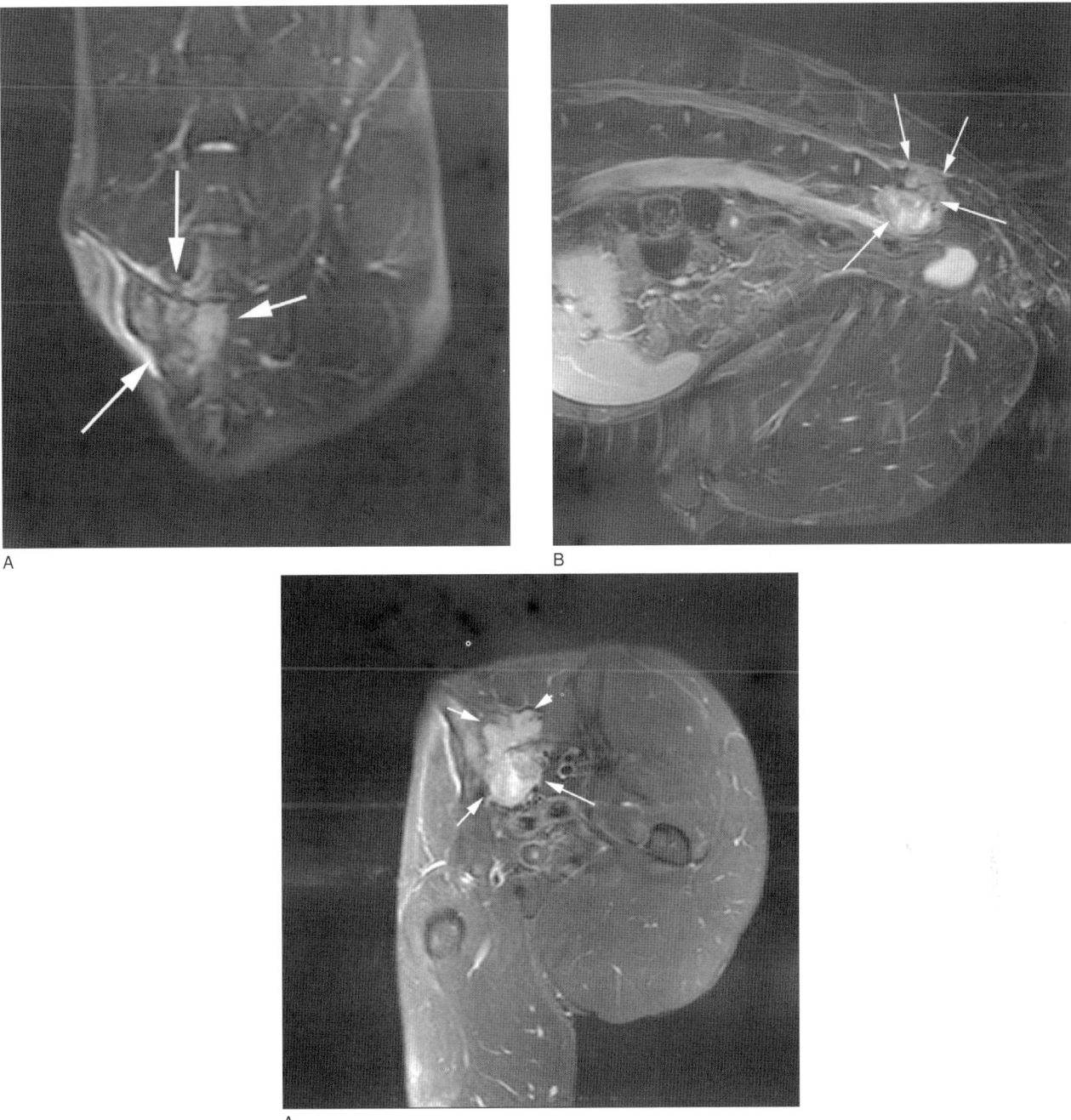

Figure 3.22. Sacral mass. (A) STIR dorsal plane sequence showing the mass affecting the right sacrum. (B) STIR sagittal sequence showing the mass in the sacrum and ventral to the body of the sacrum in the caudal aspect of L7. This image shows the mass invading the spinal canal. (C) Transverse sequence showing the mass within the sacrum and invading the spinal canal in the sacral region.

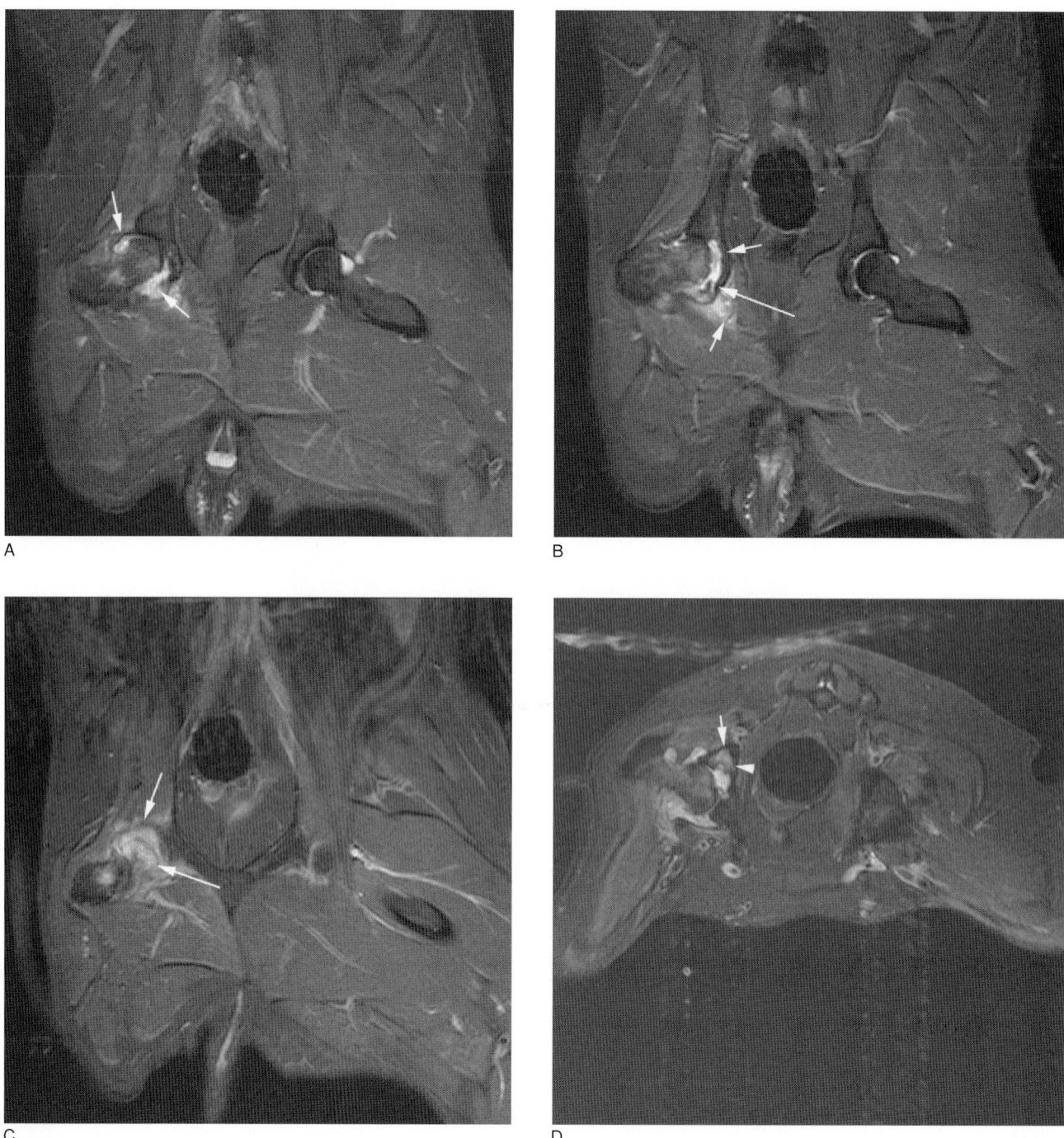

Figure 3.23. Osteoarthritis of the coxofemoral joint. (A–D) STIR-weighted sequences in the dorsal plane and adjacent slices. Hyperintensity can be seen of the synovial fluid. Some hyperintensity can be seen within the skeleton. On biopsy this was proven to be an inflammatory condition. The amount of soft tissue change has never been well appreciated from our radiographic experiences. This is a typical appearance of an active osteoarthritis.

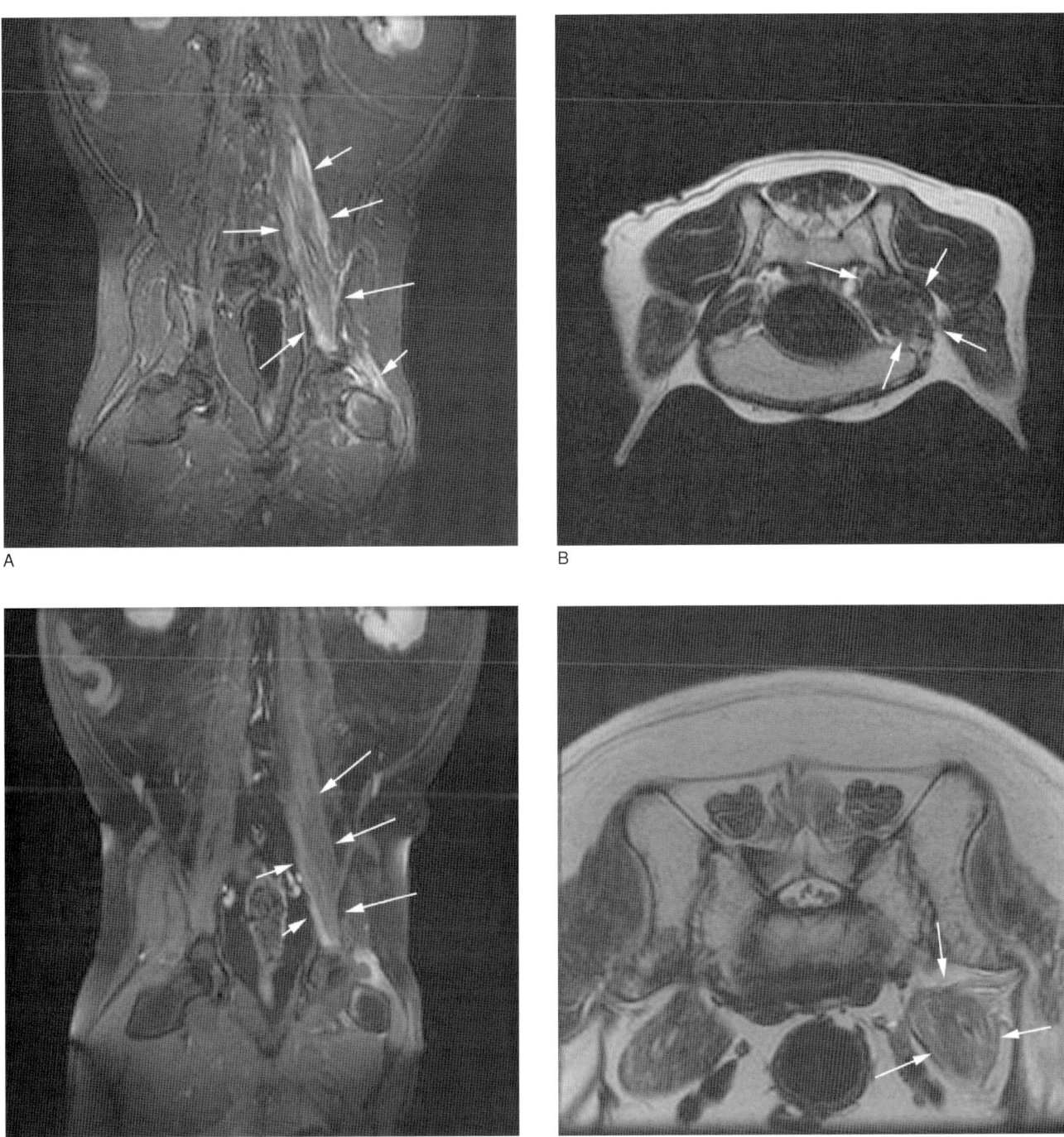

Figure 3.24. Rupture of the iliopsoas muscle. (A) STIR sequence in the dorsal plane. The hyperintensity of the iliopsoas is well seen, including down to its insertion at the lesser trochanter of the proximal femur. (B) T2-weighted transverse sequence showing the enlargement of the iliopsoas muscle at the level of the sacrum. (C) T1-weighted, fat-suppressed, post-contrast study showing mild enhancement of the iliopsoas muscle in places, and lack of enhancement in others. (D) T1-weighted, post-contrast image without fat suppression. The mild hyperintensity of the iliopsoas muscle is seen compared to the contralateral side.

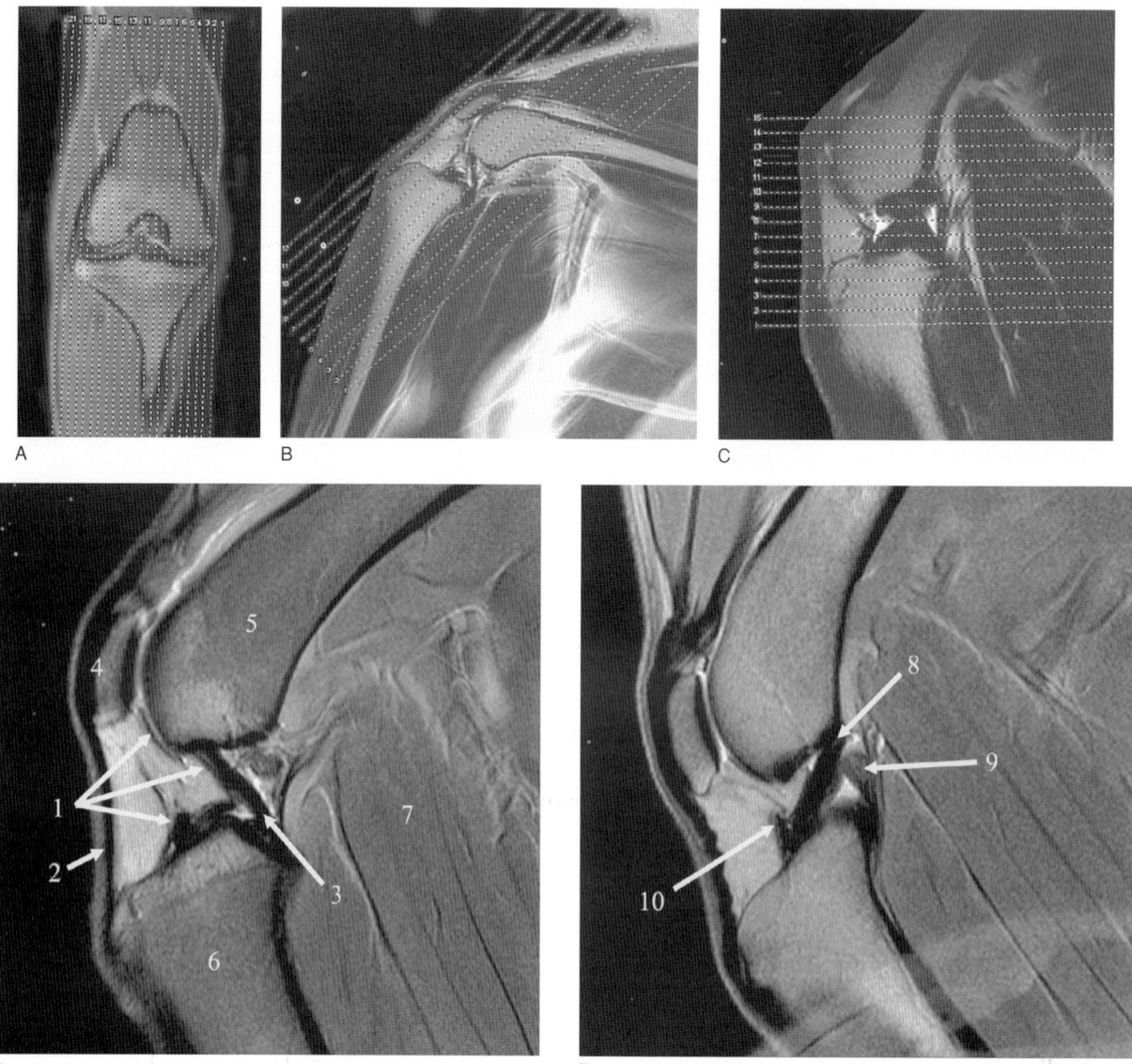

Figure 3.25. Normal stifle. (A) PD-weighted fat-suppressed coronal image with the sagittal slice planes superimposed (parallel white dashed lines). The sagittal plane is oriented parallel to the medial collateral ligament. We found that no additional information regarding the integrity of the cranial cruciate ligament (CCL) is gained by aligning the sagittal plane with the CCL as it travels from lateral to medial. (B) T2-weighted sagittal image with the coronal slice planes superimposed (parallel white dashed lines), which is aligned parallel to the patellar tendon. (C) T2-weighted sagittal image with the transverse slice planes superimposed (parallel white dashed lines), which is aligned perpendicular to the patellar tendon. (D), (E) T2-weighted sagittal images near the midline of the stifle joint. The cranial cruciate ligament is typically not as well seen as the caudal cruciate ligament due to its structure where it starts off as a fan-shaped structure prior to becoming a more round ligamentous structure. The caudal cruciate ligament is always better seen on standard images. (1) Infrapatellar fat pad—caudal extent immediately adjacent to cruciate ligaments, (2) patellar tenon, (3) caudal cruciate ligament, (4) patella, (5) femur, (6) tibia, (7) gastrocnemius muscles, (8) cranial cruciate ligament, (9) meniscofemoral ligament, (10) transverse ligament. Note the fold-over artifact over the bottom of the image in (E). (F), (G) A normal meniscus (11), like tendons and ligaments, has uniform low signal intensity on all imaging sequences and alterations in the shape and/or signal intensity should be regarded as pathologic change. When viewed at the level of the midbody of the femoral condyles, it will have a typical "bowtie" appearance. The synovial fluid (12) is typically best assessed on T2-weighted sequences. The articular cartilage (13) can be seen with both images, and is typically best seen on fat-suppressed imaging sequences. Cartilage imaging is generally considered extremely challenging, even in human patients who have thicker cartilage. Changes in the subchondral bone in fat-suppressed images have proven reliable indicators of cartilage damage, even if not visualized. (H)–(J) PD-weighted, fat-suppressed images in the transverse (H), and coronal (I) plane, and a T2-weighted parasagittal image. The unlabeled arrows demark the medial collateral ligament in (I) and (J).

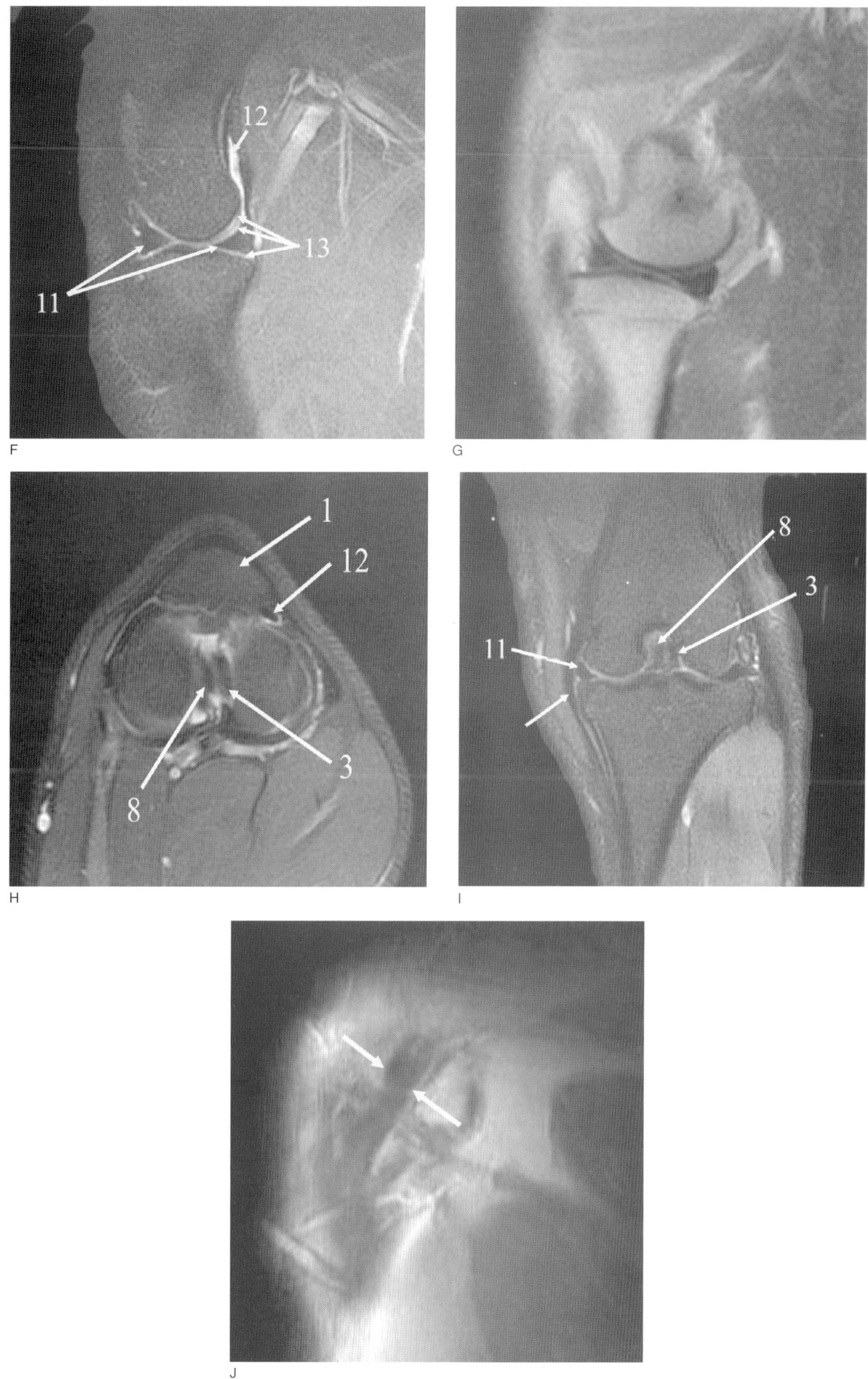

Figure 3.25. (*Continued*)

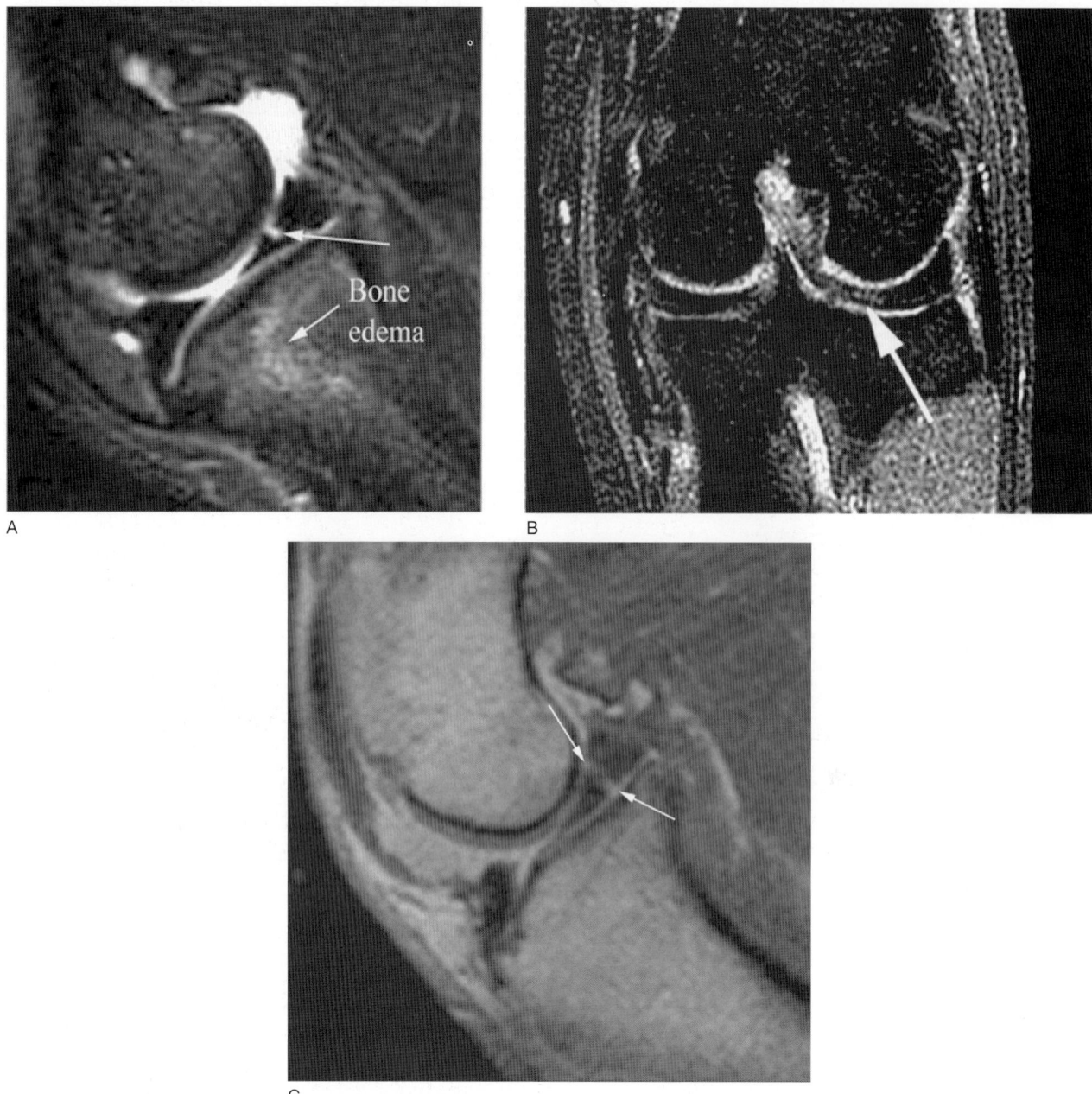

Figure 3.26.   Torn meniscus. (A) STIR sequence. The fluid is bright and can easily be seen within the torn meniscus. (B) Dorsal plane image. Again, while this image was made with a 0.5 T machine, there is still adequate resolution to see the increased signal intensity within the meniscus. (C) T1-weighted image. While the torn meniscus can be seen, it is much more difficult than that of (A).

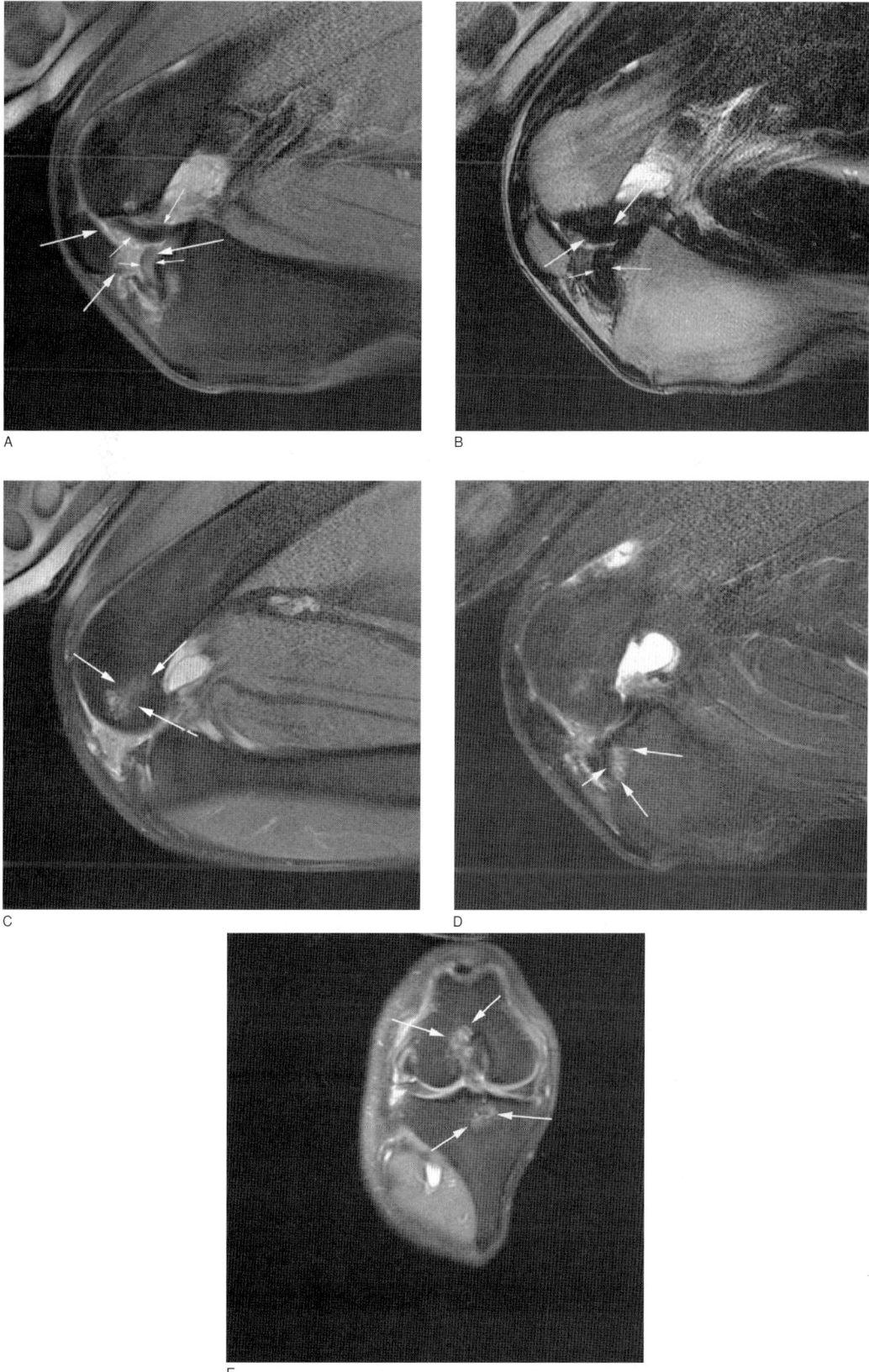

Figure 3.27. Partial tear of the cranial cruciate ligament. (A) The large arrows show joint effusion and displacement of the infrapatellar fat body. Small arrows show the normal appearance to the caudal cruciate ligament and a hyperintensity to the cranial cruciate ligament. (B) T2-weighted sequence in the same plane. Large arrows show the caudal cruciate ligament and the small arrows show the cranial cruciate ligament. (C) This image shows the hyperintensity within the proximal femur at the origin of the cranial cruciate ligament. (D) Image showing the hyperintensity of the proximal tibia at the insertion of the cranial cruciate ligament. (E) Dorsal plane, proton density, fat suppressed showing the hyperintensity at both the origin and insertion of the cranial cruciate ligament. This was confirmed as a partial tear in the cranial cruciate ligament.

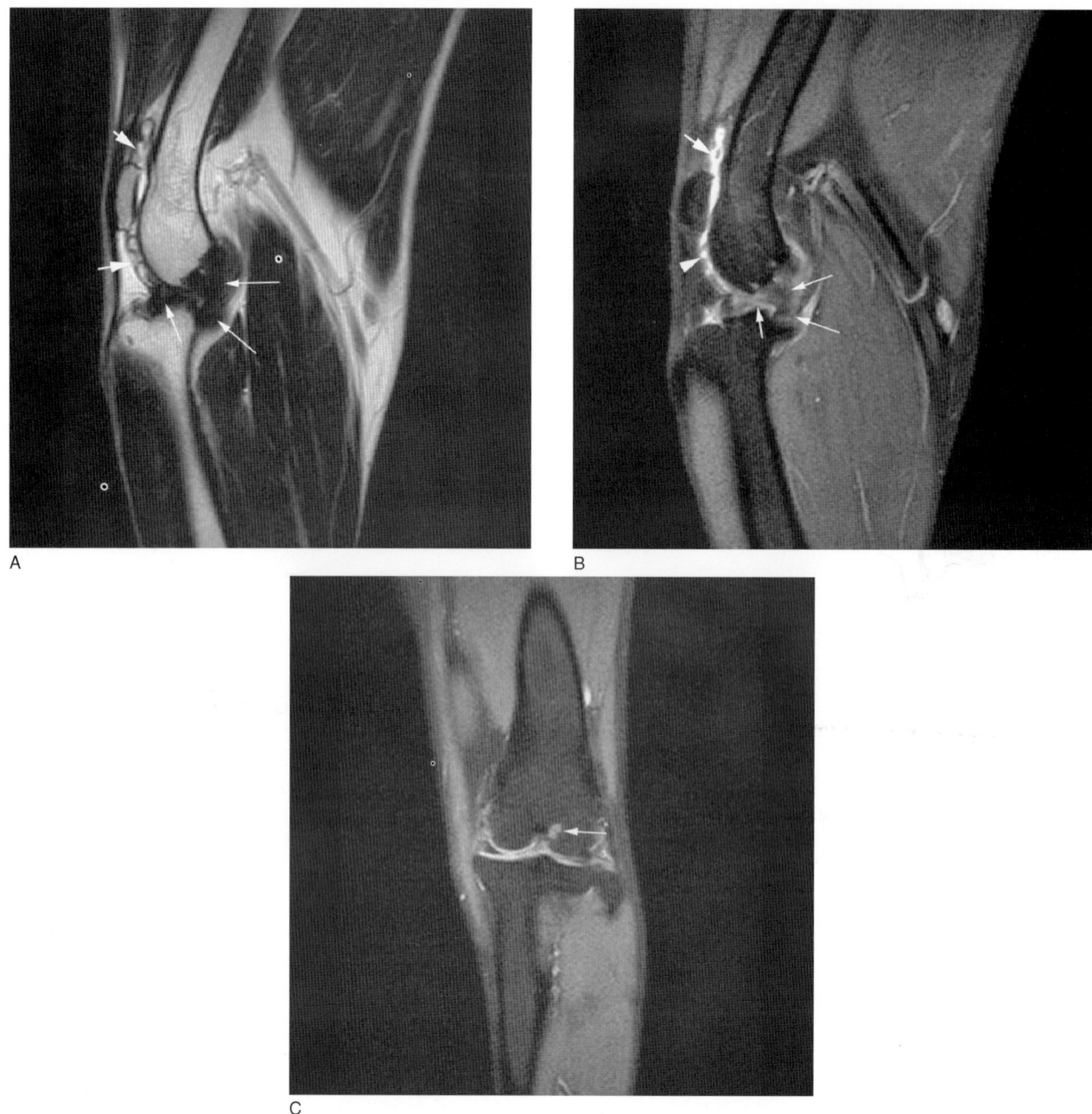

Figure 3.28. (A) T2 sagittal, large arrow indicate joint effusion and synovitis, small arrows point to lack of CrCL visualization and stretching of CaCL. Note cranial displacement of the tibia relative to normal position. (B) Proton density fat suppressed sagittal image depicting same structures seen in A. (C) PD fat sat dorsal plane image with edema at origin of the CrCL.

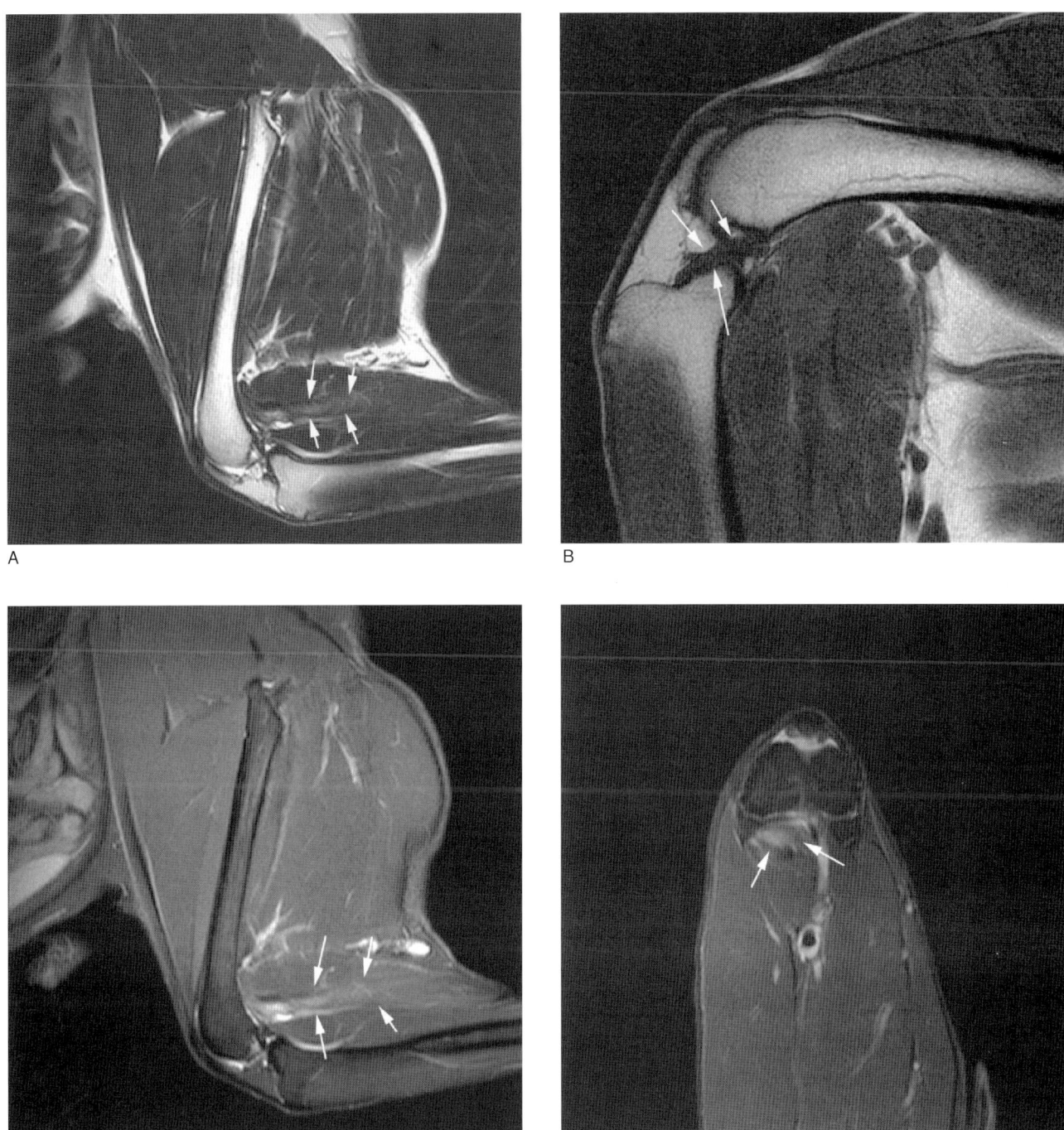

Figure 3.29.   Patient with an acute hind limb lameness, referable to the stifle and thought to be a cruciate ligament rupture. (A) T2-weighted image showing a hyperintensity within the gastrocnemius muscle. (B) T2-weighted image showing a perfectly normal appearance to the cranial cruciate ligament, and a normal appearance to the infrapatellar fat body. (C) STIR sequence in the same plane as (A). (D) Transverse image showing hyperintensity of the gastrocnemius muscle caudal to the proximal femur. This study correctly shows the presence of a torn gastrocnemius muscle with no involvement of the stifle joint. This animal did not have to undergo surgery based on a radiographic and clinical examination that had cranial cruciate ligament rupture as its primary differential diagnosis.

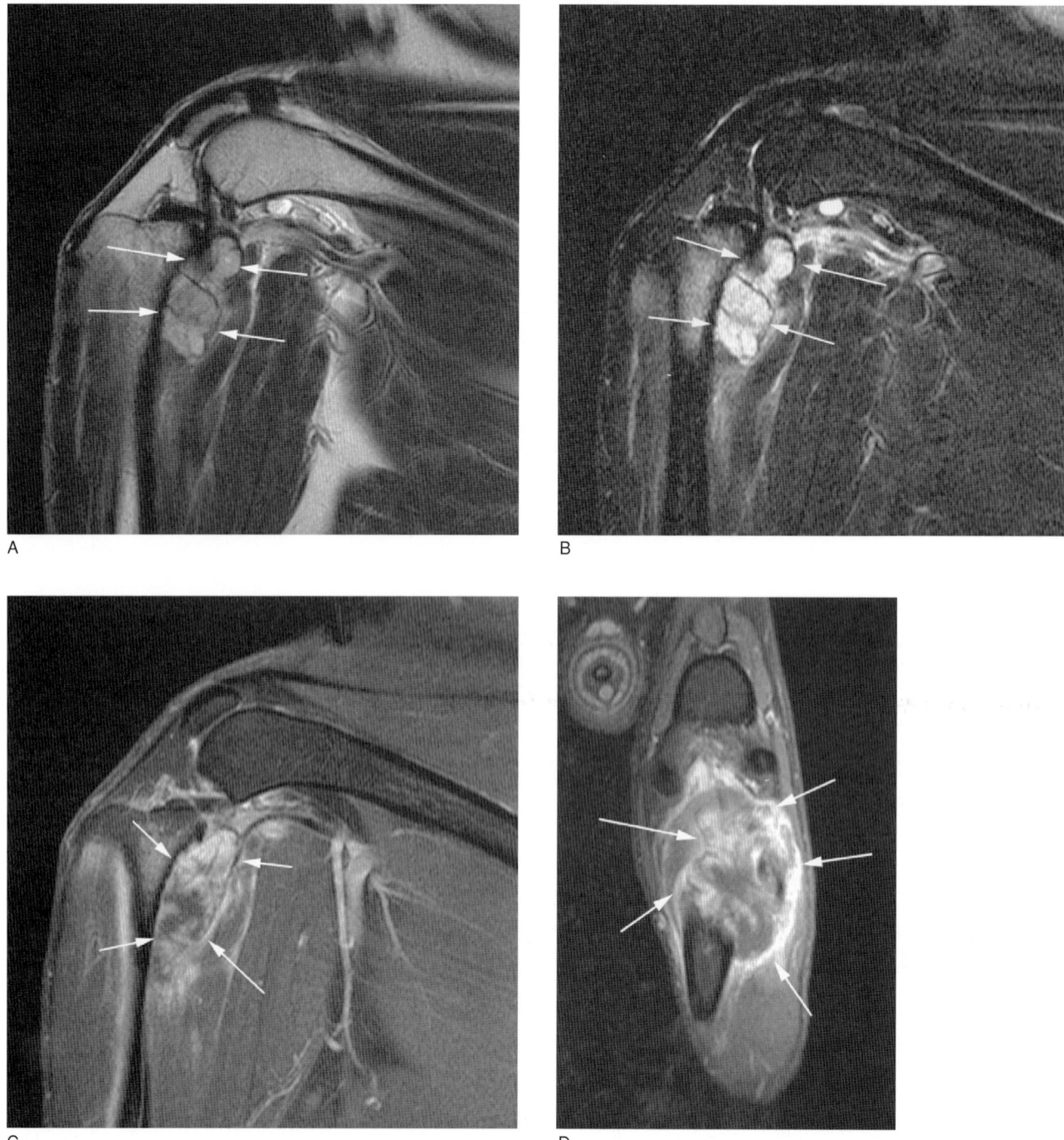

Figure 3.30. Young Labrador with acute hind limb lameness, thought to be a cranial cruciate ligament rupture. (A) T2-weighted sagittal image showing a mass at the caudal aspect of the proximal tibia. (B) STIR sequence showing the same mass. Note how the cranial and caudal cruciate ligaments and the infrapatellar fat body are all normal. (C) T1-weighted, fat-suppressed, post-contrast study showing marked and heterogenous enhancement of this mass. (D) Transverse image through this mass. Mass was histologically proven to be a synovial cell sarcoma. Again, in this young Labrador, there was active and field trial competition and was thought to be a cruciate ligament rupture based on radiographic exam and physical examination. MR provided the differential diagnosis of a mass. The imaging study allowed the dog to have a proper surgical removal, which in this case involved amputation of this hind limb after an extensive metastatic survey proved negative.

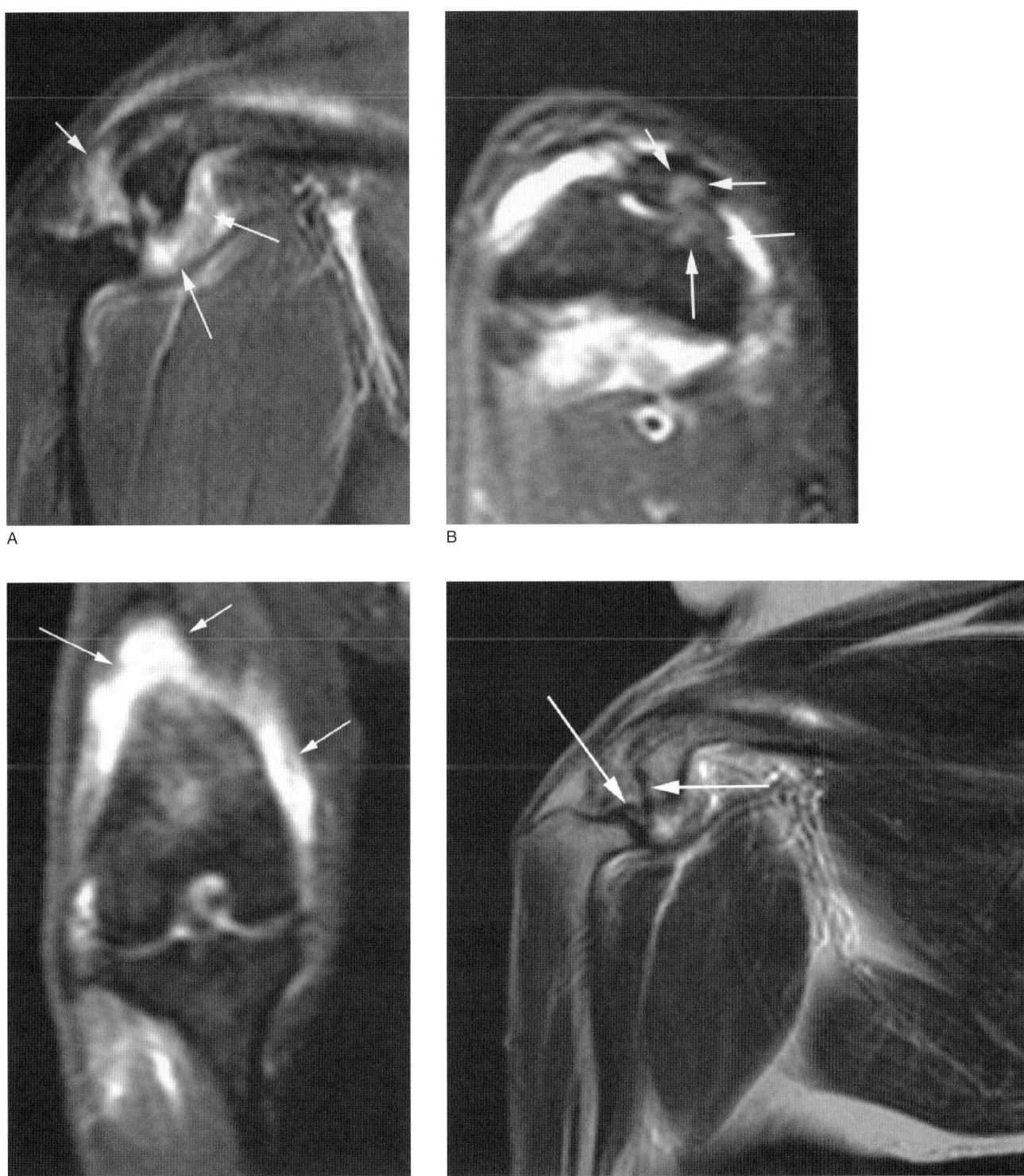

Figure 3.31. Medial patellar luxation. (A)–(C) STIR images in sagittal, transverse, and dorsal plane respectively. Arrows on A and C point to the synovial fluid distention. Arrows on B point to the bone edema in the patella and media ridge of the trochlea. (D) T2 sagittal image, the cranial arrow points to the normal cranial cruciate ligament and the caudal arrow points to the normal caudal cruciate ligament.

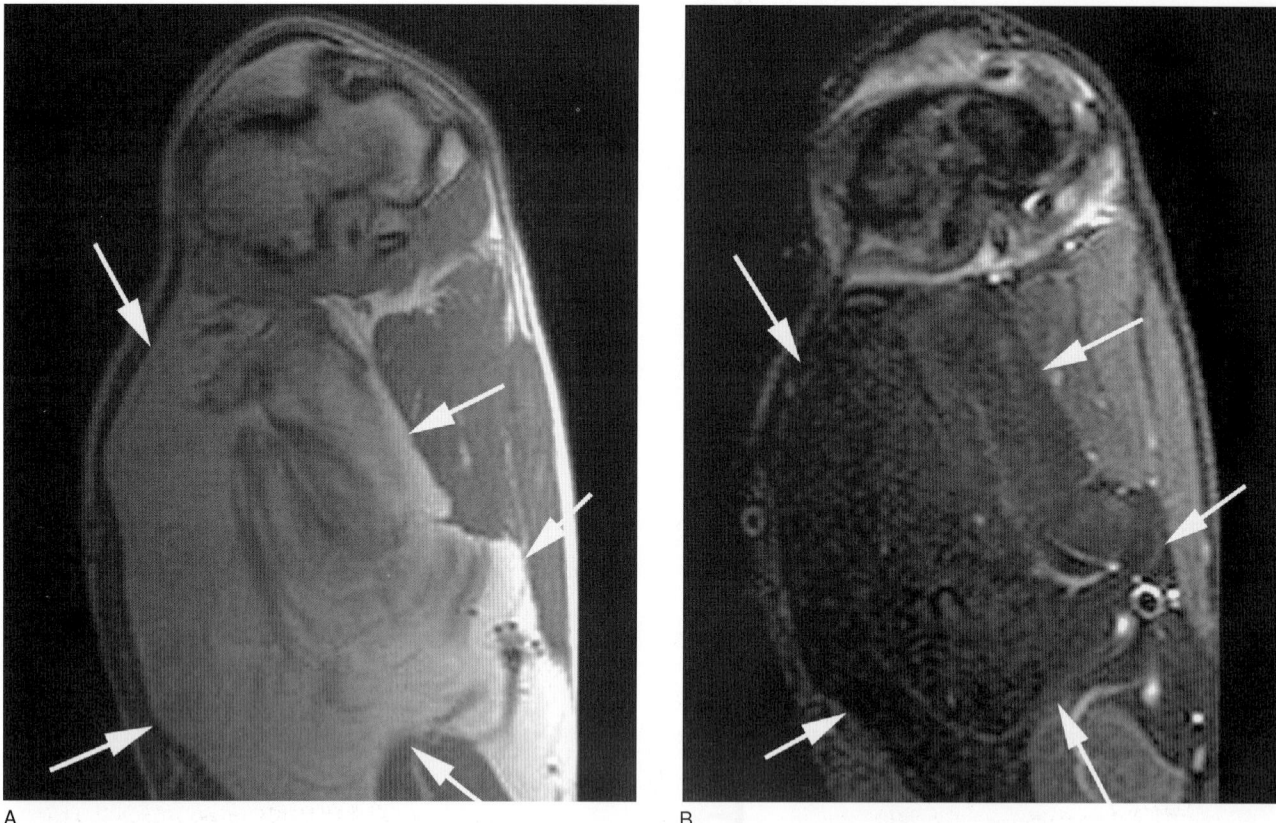

Figure 3.32. Infiltrative lipoma. (A) T2-weighted transverse image of the thigh in the region of the stifle. The arrows point to an infiltrative lipoma in the muscle facial planes. (B) STIR sequence and the arrows point to the nulled signal from the fat of the lipoma.

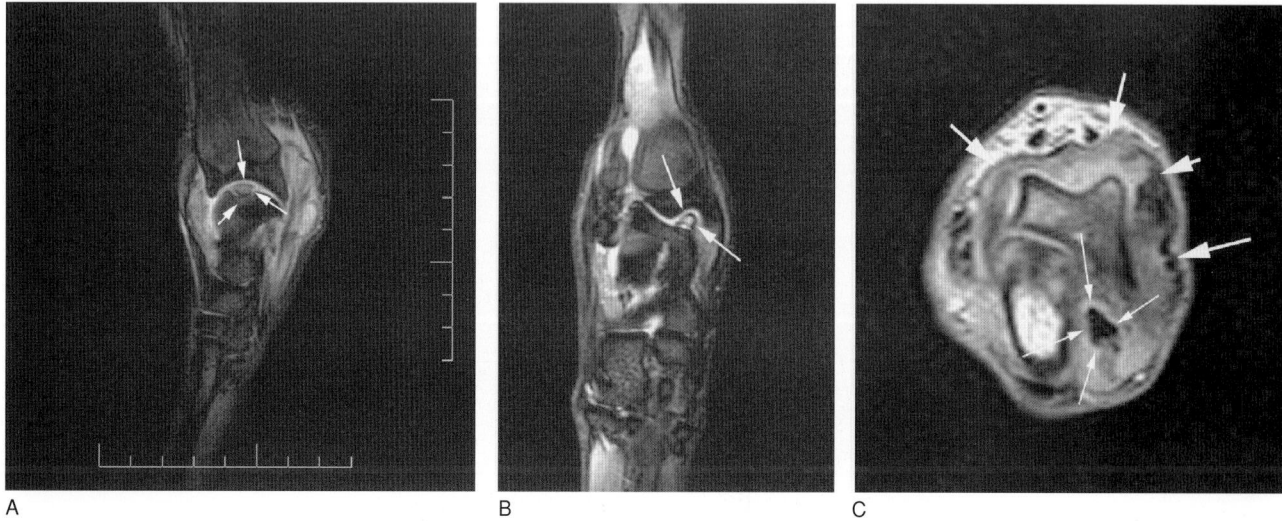

Figure 3.33. Tarsal OCD. (A) Sagittal STIR sequence. The osteochondral fragment is readily seen as indicated by the arrows and the hyperintensity around the joint is from the synovitis. (B) T2-weighted dorsal plane image showing the hyperintensity of the medial trochlea of the talus, associated with the OCD lesion. (C) Marked synovitis and joint distension is seen as shown by the large arrows. The small arrows show the presence of the deep digital flexor tendon being squeezed into an arrowhead shape out of its normal oblong shape as it rides over the sustentaculum tali. This imaging has allowed better understanding of the secondary effects of osteochondrosis on the deep digital flexor tendon.

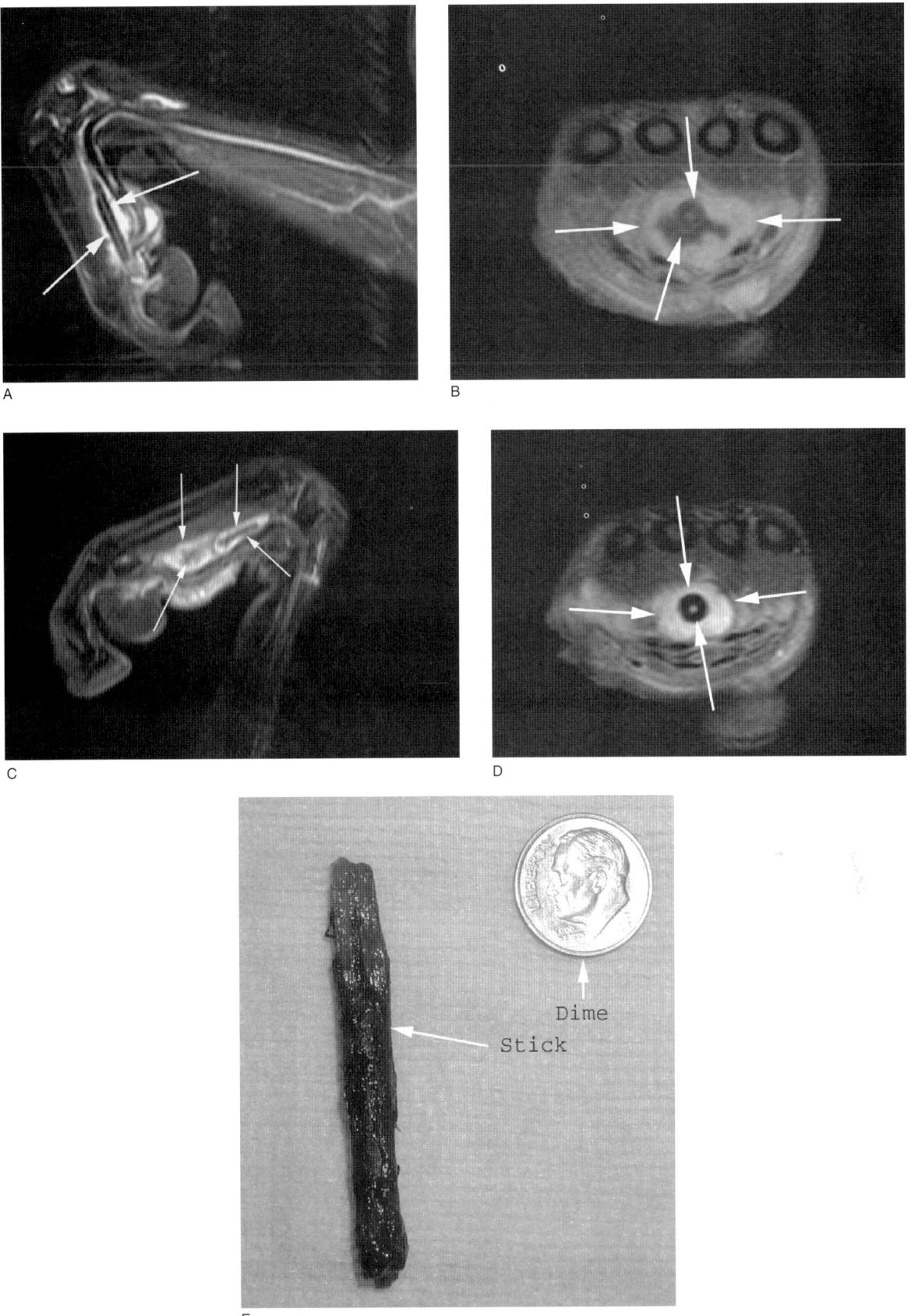

Figure 3.34. Foreign body within the carpus. This animal had two previous surgeries and only small pieces of wood were found. MR exam allowed for the clear visualization of a foreign material deep to the flexor tendons in the metacarpal region. The arrows point to the wood foreign body. (A), (C) STIR sequences in the sagittal and transverse planes, respectively. (B), (D) T1-weighted post-contrast studies in the same planes. Note how the contrast images really do not show the lesion as well as the STIR sequences. Contrast often provides minimal information on magnetic resonance studies. Strength of magnetic resonance is visualized in the varying stages of chemistry through sequence selection. (E) Photograph of the stick that was removed at surgery.

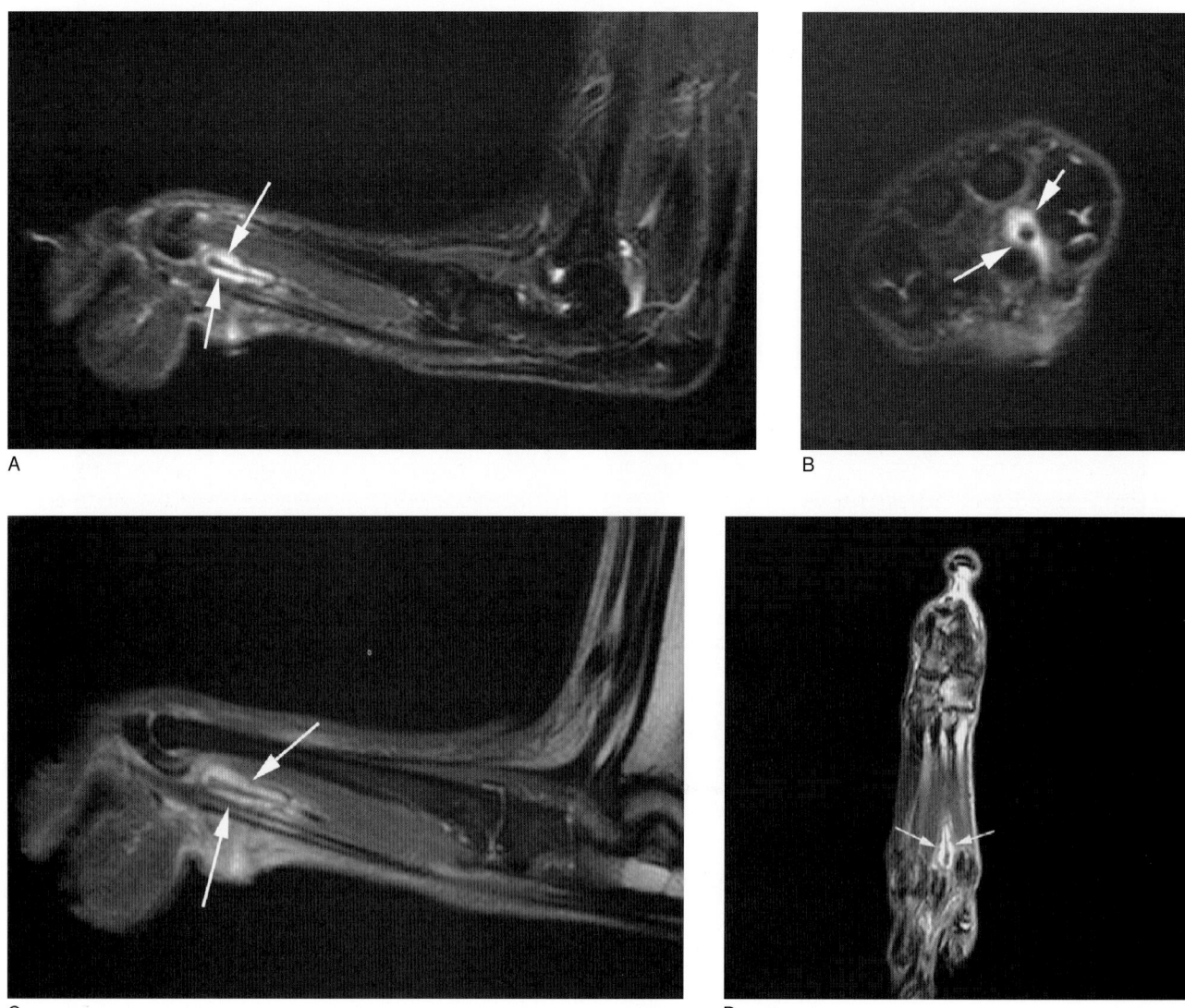

A

B

C

D

Figure 3.35. Foreign body in the metatarsal region. (A), (B) STIR sequences in the sagittal and transverse planes, respectively. Foreign body with fluid around it is well seen. (C), (D) T1-weighted images post-contrast. Part (C) has better fat suppression than that seen in (D). Again, note how the contrast does not improve visualization and is necessary in these types of studies.

BIBLIOGRAPHY

Alhadlaq HA, Xia Y, Moody JB, and Matyas JR. 2004. Detecting structural changes in early experimental osteoarthritis of tibial cartilage by microscopic magnetic resonance imaging and polarised light microscopy. Ann Rheum Dis 63(6):709–717.

Arnoczky SP, Cooper TG, Stadelmaier DM, and Hannafin JA. 1994. Magnetic resonance signals in healing menisci: an experimental study in dogs. Arthroscopy 10(5):552–557.

Azer NM, Winalski CS, and Minas T. 2004. MR imaging for surgical planning and postoperative assessment in early osteoarthritis. Radiol Clin North Am 42(1):43–60.

Baird DK, Hathcock JT, Kincaid SA, Rumph PF, Kammermann J, Widmer WR, et al. 1998. Low-field magnetic resonance imaging of early subchondral cyst-like lesions in induced cranial cruciate ligament deficient dogs. Vet Radiol Ultrasound 39(3):167–173.

Baird DK, Hathcock JT, Rumph PF, Kincaid SA, and Visco DM. 1998. Low-field magnetic resonance imaging of the canine stifle joint: normal anatomy. Vet Radiol Ultrasound 39(2):87–97.

Baird DK, Kincaid SA, Hathcock JT, Rumph PF, Kammerman J, and Visco DM. 1999. Effect of hydration on signal intensity of gelatin phantoms using low-field magnetic resonance imaging: possible application in osteoarthritis. Vet Radiol Ultrasound 40(1):27–35.

Banfield CM and Morrison WB. 2000. Magnetic resonance arthrography of the canine stifle joint: technique and applications in eleven military dogs. Vet Radiol Ultrasound 41(3):200–213.

Bischofberger AS, Konar M, Ohlerth S, Geyer H, Lang J, Ueltschi G, et al. 2006. Magnetic resonance imaging, ultrasonography and histology of the suspensory ligament origin: a comparative study of normal anatomy of warmblood horses. Equine Vet J 38(6):508–516.

Carrig CB. 1997. Diagnostic imaging of osteoarthritis. Vet Clin North Am Small Anim Pract 27(4):777–814.

Davis GJ, Kapatkin AS, Craig LE, Heins GS, and Wortman JA. 2002. Comparison of radiography, computed tomography, and magnetic resonance imaging for evaluation of appendicular osteosarcoma in dogs. J Am Vet Med Assoc 220(8):1171–1176.

De Smet AA, Dueland RT, and Dubielzig RR. 1993. Case report 775. Canine osteosarcoma with associated avascular necrosis and sequestrum formation. Skeletal Radiol 22(2):146–149.

Evans PM, Gassel A, and Huber M. 2004. What is your diagnosis? Synovial cell sarcoma. J Am Vet Med Assoc 224(4):511–512.

Fitch RB, Wilson ER, Hathcock JT, and Montgomery RD. 1997. Radiographic, computed tomographic and magnetic resonance imaging evaluation of a chronic long digital extensor tendon avulsion in a dog. Vet Radiol Ultrasound 38(3):177–181.

Franci P, Leece EA, and Brearley JC. 2006. Post anaesthetic myopathy/neuropathy in horses undergoing magnetic resonance imaging compared to horses undergoing surgery. Equine Vet J 38(6):497–501.

Fransson BA, Gavin PR, and Lahmers KK. 2005. Supraspinatus tendinosis associated with biceps brachii tendon displacement in a dog. J Am Vet Med Assoc 227(9):1429–1433, 1416.

Ganey T, Libera J, Moos V, Alasevic O, Fritsch KG, Meisel HJ, et al. 2003. Disc chondrocyte transplantation in a canine model: a treatment for degenerated or damaged intervertebral disc. Spine 28(23):2609–2620.

Goodfellow M and Platt S. 2003. What is your diagnosis? Chrondroblastic osteosarcoma. J Small Anim Pract 44(11):479, 515–516.

Grosslinger K, Lorinson D, Hittmair K, Konar M, and Weissenbock H. 2004. Iliopsoas abscess with iliac and femoral vein thrombosis in an adult Siberian husky. J Small Anim Pract 45(2):113–116.

Hayes AM, Dennis R, Smith KC, and Brearley MJ. 1999. Synovial myxoma: magnetic resonance imaging in the assessment of an unusual canine soft tissue tumour. J Small Anim Pract 40(10):489–494.

Hoskinson JJ and Tucker RL. 2001. Diagnostic imaging of lameness in small animals. Vet Clin North Am Small Anim Pract 31(1):165–180, vii.

Janach KJ, Breit SM, and Kunzel WW. 2006. Assessment of the geometry of the cubital (elbow) joint of dogs by use of magnetic resonance imaging. Am J Vet Res 67(2):211–218.

Kaiser S, Cornely D, Golder W, Garner MT, Wolf KJ, Waibl H, et al. 2001. The correlation of canine patellar luxation and the anteversion angle as measured using magnetic resonance images. Vet Radiol Ultrasound 42(2):113–118.

Keller MD, Galloway GJ, and Pollitt CC. 2006. Magnetic resonance microscopy of the equine hoof wall: a study of resolution and potential. Equine Vet J 38(5):461–466.

Kippenes H and Johnston G. 1998. Diagnostic imaging of osteochondrosis. Vet Clin North Am Small Anim Pract 28(1):137–160.

Kirberger RM and Fourie SL. 1998. Elbow dysplasia in the dog: pathophysiology, diagnosis and control. J S Afr Vet Assoc 69(2):43–54.

Kornegay JN, Sharp NJ, Bartlett RJ, Van Camp SD, Burt CT, Hung WY, et al. 1990. Golden retriever muscular dystrophy: monitoring for success. Adv Exp Med Biol 280:267–272.

Lahm A, Uhl M, Erggelet C, Haberstroh J, and Mrosek E. 2004. Articular cartilage degeneration after acute subchondral bone damage: an experimental study in dogs with histopathological grading. Acta Orthop Scand 75(6):762–767.

Lee JM, Choi SH, Park HS, Lee MW, Han CJ, Choi JI, et al. 2005. Radiofrequency thermal ablation in canine femur: evaluation of coagulation necrosis reproducibility and MRI-histopathologic correlation. Am J Roentgenol 185(3):661–667.

Lipsitz D, Levitski RE, Chauvet AE, and Berry WL. 2001. Magnetic resonance imaging features of cervical stenotic myelopathy in 21 dogs. Vet Radiol Ultrasound 42(1):20–27.

Martig S, Konar M, Schmokel HG, Rytz U, Spreng D, Scheidegger J, et al. 2006. Low-field MRI and arthroscopy of meniscal lesions in ten dogs with experimentally induced cranial cruciate ligament insufficiency. Vet Radiol Ultrasound 47(6):515–522.

Mazur WJ and Lazar T. 2005. What is your diagnosis? Chondrosarcoma. J Am Vet Med Assoc 226(8):1301–1302.

Mrosek EH, Lahm A, Erggelet C, Uhl M, Kurz H, Eissner B, et al. 2006. Subchondral bone trauma causes cartilage matrix degeneration: an immunohistochemical analysis in a canine model. Osteoarthr Cartil 14(2):171–178.

Nadel SN, Debatin JF, Richardson WJ, Hedlund LW, Senft C, Rizk WS, et al. 1992. Detection of acute avascular necrosis of the femoral head in dogs: dynamic contrast-enhanced MR imaging vs spin-echo and STIR sequences. Am J Roentgenol 159(6):1255–1261.

Nakamura T, Matsumoto T, Nishino M, Tomita K, and Kadoya M. 1997. Early magnetic resonance imaging and histologic findings in a model of femoral head necrosis. Clin Orthop Relat Res (334):68–72.

Nolte-Ernsting CC, Adam G, Buhne M, Prescher A, and Gunther RW. 1996. MRI of degenerative bone marrow lesions in experimental osteoarthritis of canine knee joints. Skeletal Radiol 25(5):413–420.

Nordberg CC and Johnson KA. 1999. Magnetic resonance imaging of normal canine carpal ligaments. Vet Radiol Ultrasound 40(2):128–136.

Platt SR, McConnell JF, Garosi LS, Ladlow J, de Stefani A, and Shelton GO. 2006. Magnetic resonance imaging in the diagnosis of canine inflammatory myopathies in three dogs. Vet Radiol Ultrasound 47(6):532–537.

Schaefer SL and Forrest LJ. 2006. Magnetic resonance imaging of the canine shoulder: an anatomic study. Vet Surg 35(8):721–728.

Shubitz LF and Dial SM. 2005. Coccidioidomycosis: a diagnostic challenge. Clin Tech Small Anim Pract 20(4):220–226.

Smith M, Murray R, Dyson S, Mair T, and Boswell J. 2006. Magnetic resonance imaging study in horses. Vet Rec 159(19):643.

Smith MR, Wright IM, and Smith RK. 2007. Endoscopic assessment and treatment of lesions of the deep digital flexor tendon in the navicular bursae of 20 lame horses. Equine Vet J 39(1):18–24.

Snaps FR, Balligand MH, Saunders JH, Park RD, and Dondelinger RF. 1997. Comparison of radiography, magnetic resonance imaging, and surgical findings in dogs with elbow dysplasia. Am J Vet Res 58(12):1367–1370.

Snaps FR, Park RD, Saunders JH, Balligand MH, and Dondelinger RF. 1999. Magnetic resonance arthrography of the cubital joint in dogs affected with fragmented medial coronoid processes. Am J Vet Res 60(2):190–193.

Snaps FR, Saunders JH, Park RD, Daenen B, Balligand MH, and Dondelinger RF. 1998. Comparison of spin echo, gradient echo and fat saturation magnetic resonance imaging sequences for imaging the canine elbow. Vet Radiol Ultrasound 39(6):518–523.

Stepnik MW, Olby N, Thompson RR, and Marcellin-Little DJ. 2006. Femoral neuropathy in a dog with iliopsoas muscle injury. Vet Surg 35(2):186–190.

Suga K, Yuan Y, Ogasawara N, Okada M, and Matsunaga N. 2003. Visualization of normal and interrupted lymphatic drainage in dog legs with interstitial MR lymphography using an extracellular MR contrast agent, gadopentetate dimeglumine. Invest Radiol 38(6):349–357.

Tidwell SA, Graham JP, Peck IN, and Berry CR. 2007. Incidence of pulmonary embolism after non-cemented total hip arthroplasty in eleven dogs: computed tomographic pulmonary angiography and pulmonary perfusion scintigraphy. Vet Surg 36(1):37–42.

Turan E, Bolukbasi O, and Omeroglu A. 2007. The effect of the tarsal joint positions on the tibial nerve motor action potential latency in dog: electrophysiological and anatomical studies. Dtsch Tierarztl Wochenschr 114(1):20–24.

van Bree H, Degryse H, Van Ryssen B, Ramon F, and Desmidt M. 1993. Pathologic correlations with magnetic resonance images of osteochondrosis lesions in canine shoulders. J Am Vet Med Assoc 202(7):1099–1105.

van Bree H, Van Ryssen B, Degryse H, and Ramon F. 1995. Magnetic resonance arthrography of the scapulohumeral joint in dogs, using gadopentetate dimeglumine. Am J Vet Res 56(3):286–288.

Wallack ST, Wisner ER, Werner JA, Walsh PJ, Kent MS, Fairley RA, et al. 2002. Accuracy of magnetic resonance imaging for estimating intramedullary osteosarcoma extent in preoperative planning of canine limb-salvage procedures. Vet Radiol Ultrasound 43(5):432–441.

Widmer WR, Buckwalter KA, Braunstein EM, Visco DM, and O'Connor BL. 1991. Principles of magnetic resonance imaging and application to the stifle joint in dogs. J Am Vet Med Assoc 198(11):1914–1922.

Yabe K, Yoshida K, Yamamoto N, Nishida S, Ohshima C, Sekiguchi M, et al. 1997. Diagnosis of quinolone-induced arthropathy in juvenile dogs by use of magnetic resonance (MR) imaging. J Vet Med Sci 59(7):597–599.

Young B, Klopp L, Albrecht M, and Kraft S. 2004. Imaging diagnosis: magnetic resonance imaging of a cervical wooden foreign body in a dog. Vet Radiol Ultrasound 45(6):538–541.

Zarucco L, Wisner ER, Swanstrom MD, and Stover SM. 2006. Image fusion of computed tomographic and magnetic resonance images for the development of a three-dimensional musculo-skeletal model of the equine forelimb. Vet Radial Ultrasound 47(6):553–562.

CHAPTER FOUR

MAGNETIC RESONANCE IMAGING OF ABDOMINAL DISEASE

Patrick R. Gavin and Shannon P. Holmes

Magnetic resonance studies of the abdomen can provide exquisite anatomical detail of organ systems. In animals, these studies are aided by general anesthesia, which reduces motion from the gastrointestinal tract. Sequences found to be of most use include T2-weighted images (especially with fat-suppression), STIR sequences, and T1-weighted images before and after contrast administration. If possible, T1-weighted images also benefit from fat-suppression due to the large amount of intra-abdominal fat in most veterinary patients. In general, respiratory gaiting is not required and if flow or respiratory motion artifact becomes a problem with interpretation, simply swapping the phase and frequency encoding directions will allow for complete visualization of the abdominal viscera (Figure 4.1).

For imaging of the abdominal structures, the animal is most commonly placed in a dorsally recumbent position.

NORMAL ABDOMINAL ANATOMY

Abdominal structures can be distinguished based on location and imaging characteristics. Fat saturation techniques are generally used due to the large amount of fat in the abdomen. Various imaging planes may be necessary to image the complex geometry of some of the abdominal structures. In dogs larger than 20 kg body weight, slice thicknesses of 1 cm are appropriate.

The organs will be similar in appearance to the gross anatomical features, and those features are as important as signal characteristics. The appearance has many vari-

ables, and the TR and TE have major effects as well as spin echo versus gradient echo sequences. The following is a general guideline. The normal liver is relatively hyperintense on T1 sequences and isointense on T2-weighted sequences. The differing lobes are usually of the same signal intensity. Within the liver, the gall bladder is present as a discrete, semicircular hyperintense structure (relative to the signal of the liver parenchyma) on T2-weighted sequences. Utilizing various imaging planes, the location of the biliary system including the common and cystic bile ducts can also be determined.

Vascular structures associated with the liver are easily seen and appear as hypointense or hyperintense on T1 and T2, respectively. The normal pancreas is slightly hyperintense to liver on T1 sequences and isointense to liver on T2-weighted sequences. The normal spleen is hypointense to liver on T1 sequences and hyperintense to liver on T2-weighted sequences.

The kidneys have a more complex appearance with MR imaging. The normal kidney cortex is markedly hyperintense to liver on T1 sequences and very hyperintense to liver and isointense to spleen on T2-weighted sequences. The medullary region is moderately hyperintense to liver on T1 sequences and more similar in appearance to renal cortex only more hyperintense on T2-weighted sequences.

The urinary bladder has low signal intensity on T1 sequences and is very hyperintense on T2-weighted sequences. This appearance is primarily the result of the signal from the urine.

The adrenal glands are isointense to renal cortex on T1 sequences and isointense to renal cortex on T2-weighted sequences. These structures are present immediately adjacent to the relatively hypointense vena cava, which is tubular in appearance and relatively circular in transverse plane imaging sequences.

273

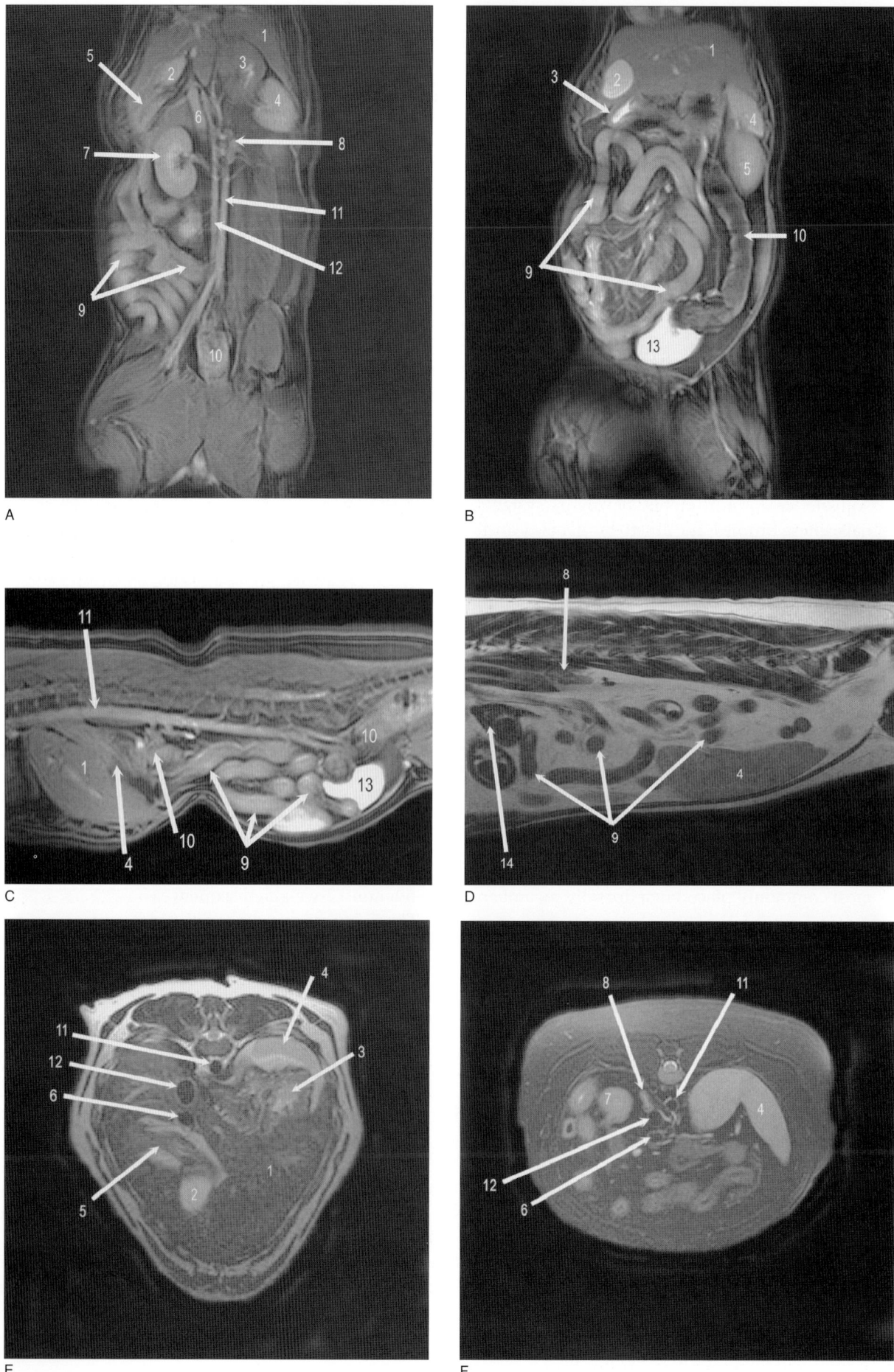

Figure 4.1.

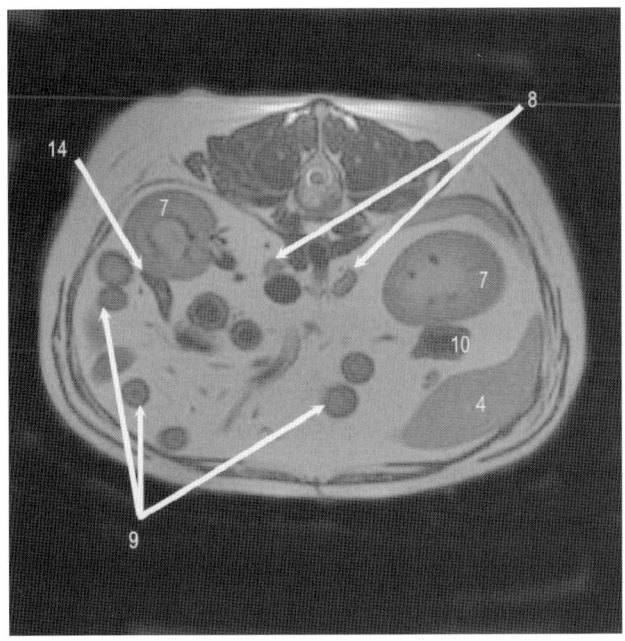

G

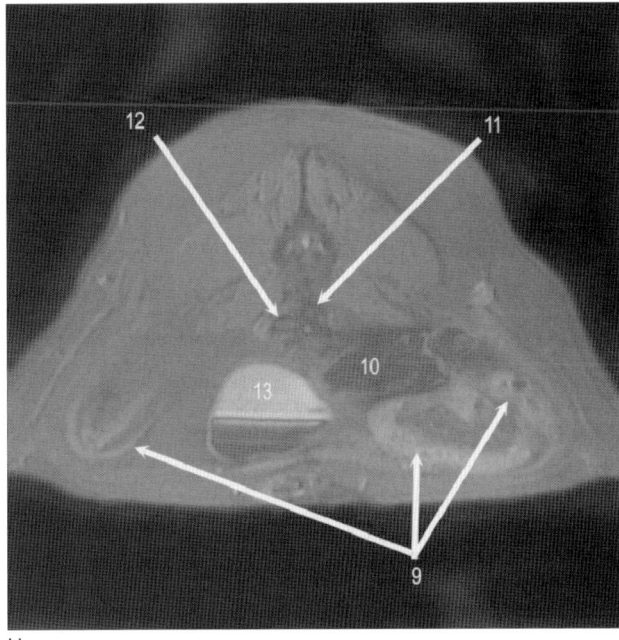

H

Figure 4.1. Normal Anatomy. (A), (B) Coronal T2-weighted fat-suppressed images. (C) Sagittal T2-weighted fat-suppressed image. (D) Sagittal T2-weighted image; notice the subcutaneous and intra-abdominal fat is hyperintense. (E), (G) Transverse T2-weighted images. (F), (H) Transverse T2-weighted fat-suppressed images. (1) liver, (2) gallbladder, (3) stomach, (4) spleen, (5) duodenum, (6) portal vein, (7) kidney, (8) adrenal gland, (9) small intestines, (10) colon, (11) descending aorta, (12) caudal vena cava, (13) urinary bladder, (14) pancreas.

The normal intestinal structures are isointense to spleen on T1 sequences and on T2-weighted sequences.

In the caudal abdomen, the reproductive structures may be imaged. Normal ovaries are mildly hyperintense on T1 sequences and moderately hyperintense on T2-weighted sequences. The uterus is isointense on T1 sequences and hyperintense on T2-weighted sequences.

The normal prostate is isointense on T1 sequences and hyperintense on T2-weighted sequences.

The major abdominal vascular structures of the aorta and caudal vena cava are variable on T1 sequences and on T2-weighted sequences due to flow and phase encoding direction. Knowledge of normal anatomy allows for clear visualization of these vessels and other large vessels including the portal vein.

In some instances, the lymphatic system is apparent. The chylous ducts are hypointense on T1 sequences and hyperintense on T2-weighted sequences. Normal lymph nodes are isointense on T1 sequences and hyperintense on T2-weighted sequences.

The omentum is usually not readily apparent as a discrete structure, however, contributes to the relative fat signal in various regions of the abdomen.

ABNORMALITIES OF THE LIVER AND ASSOCIATED STRUCTURES

Lesions are readily appreciated, generally as a hyperintensity on T2-weighting in the liver and spleen. Contrast enhancement is of limited benefit unless arterial, as well as venous, studies are performed. If arterial and venous studies are performed on hepatic and splenic lesions, the correct diagnosis of benign from malignant disease is reported to be over 90%.

The liver studies are performed to determine whether lesions involve the vena cava or portal vein (Figure 4.2). Liver studies are also used to detect relatively smaller primary tumors or metastases (Figure 4.3). Lesions that should not be confused with neoplastic processes are the hypointensities seen within the spleen on virtually all sequences. These hypointensities are not macroscopic or microscopic structural lesions. We have performed histopathology of these "lesions" and no abnormalities have been detected (Figure 4.4). To date, we have been unable to prove their chemical composition, but all indications are they represent iron storage sites.

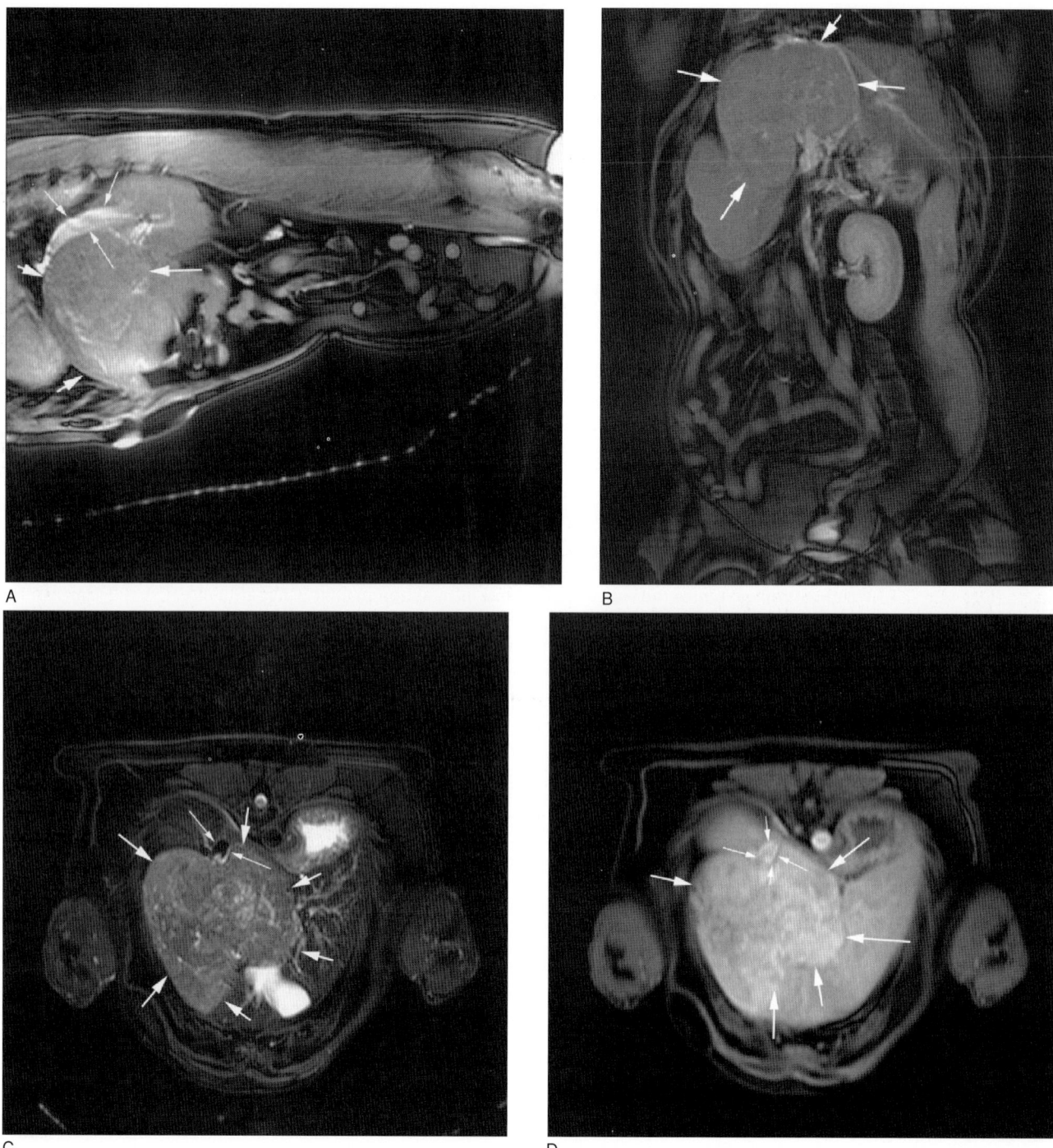

Figure 4.2. (A) Sagittal T2-weighted fat-suppressed gradient echo image with a large hepatic mass indicated by the large arrows. The small arrows indicate the vena cava. The vena cava does not appear to be compressed. (B) Dorsal T2-weighted fat-suppressed gradient echo of the liver mass ventral to the vena cava. Note the mass has a similar appearance to the remaining liver on this sequence. (C) Transverse STIR image. The large arrow indicates the mass and the small arrows the vena cava. Note the difference in appearance between the mass and the remaining liver on this sequence. (D) Transverse post-contrast T1-weighted fat-suppressed gradient echo image of the mass in the same position as (C). Note how the contrast does not make visualization better in this case and the best definition of the mass is in (C).

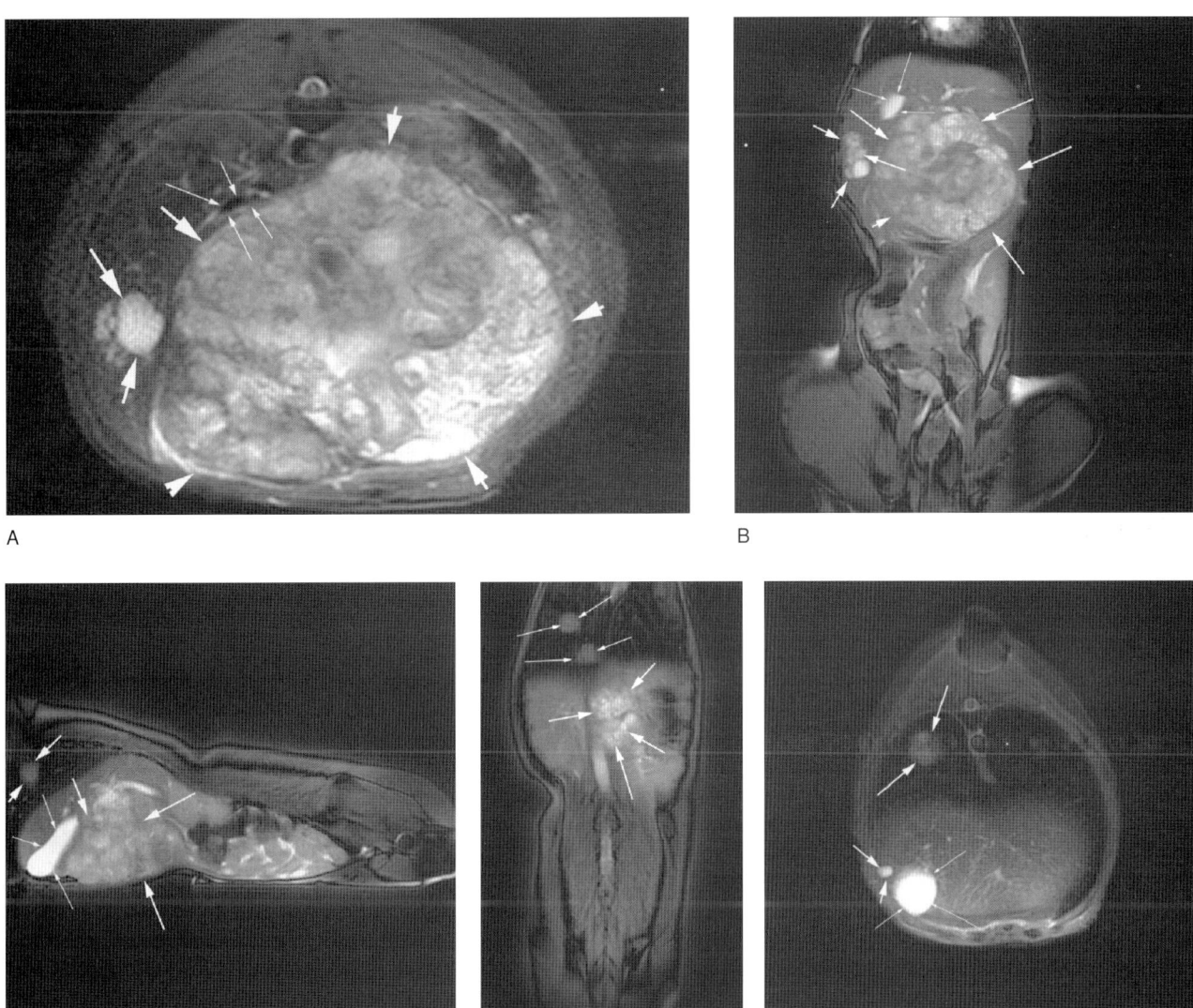

Figure 4.3. (A) Transverse T2-weighted gradient echo image showing a large hepatic mass as outlined by large arrows. Note this large mass is in the left lateral and medial lobes. A smaller mass is seen in the right lateral lobe. Small arrows indicate the displaced caudal vena cava. (B) T2-weighted gradient echo sequence in the dorsal plane. Arrows show the same masses as seen before. Small arrows point to the neck of the gall bladder. (C) T2-weighted gradient echo in the sagittal plane. Large arrows show the mass in the left lateral liver encroaching well beyond midline. Small arrows indicate the gall bladder. Arrows in the thorax indicate a spherical lesion compatible with a pulmonary metastasis. (D) T2-weighted gradient echo dorsal to (B). Small arrows point to two lesions within the thorax. The more lateral cranial lesion is seen on (C); the medial lesion is not detected in the previous images. Both lesions are compatible with metastatic lesions. Biopsy would be needed for confirmation. (E) T2-weighted, gradient echo, transverse plane rostral to (A). The small arrows show the gall bladder. Large arrows next to the gall bladder show the presence of a very small mass, presumed to be a probable metastasis to the liver. Arrows in the thorax point to a spherical lesion compatible with metastasis.

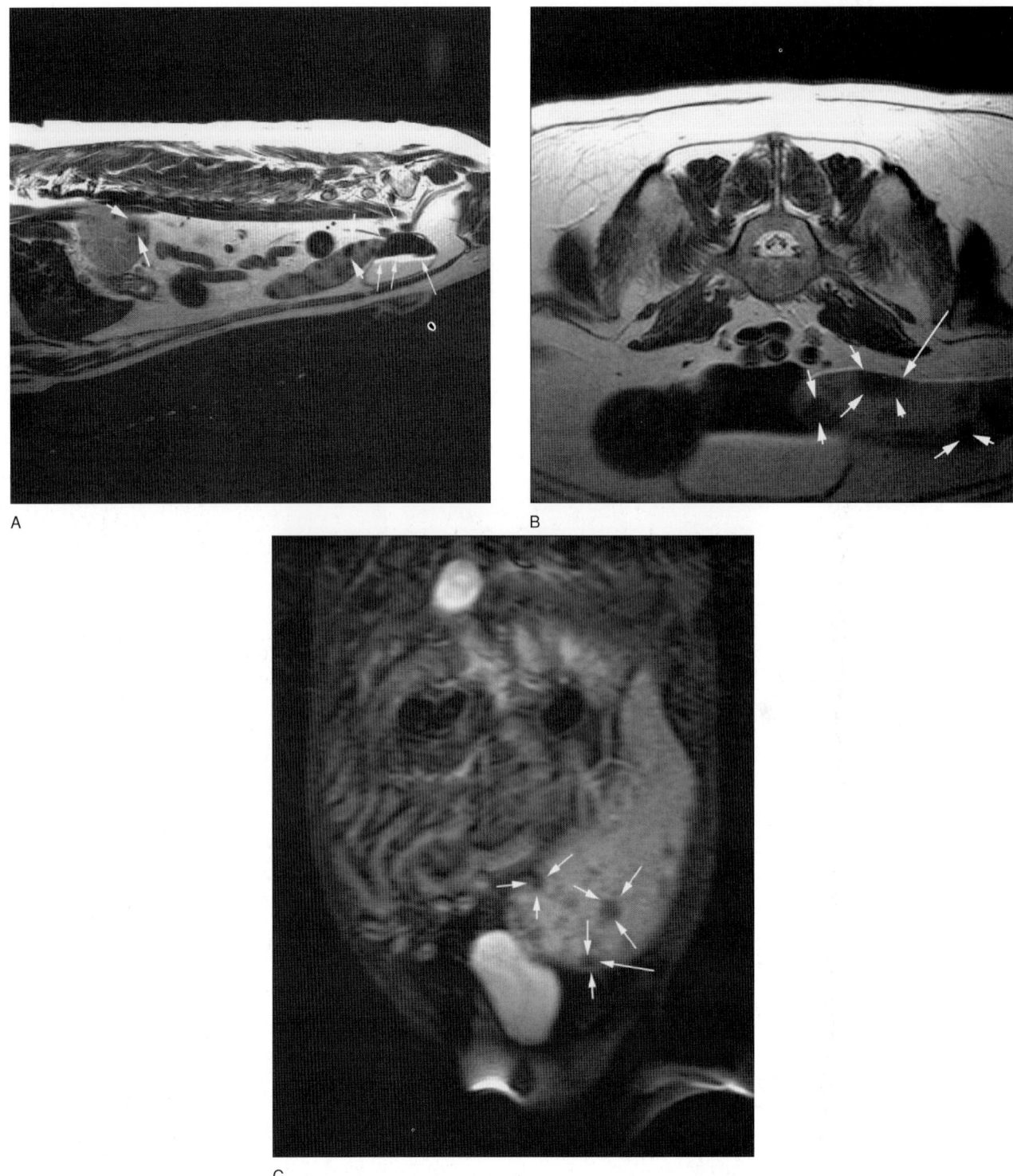

Figure 4.4. (A) T2-weighted sagittal image. All images were post-contrast, as the brain had been studied prior to the abdomen. Large arrows point to the hypointense lesions within the spleen. These lesions are not visible ultrasonographically, on gross pathology, or on histopathology. Therefore, they must represent some form of chemical change, probably related to iron storage. Small arrows point to the artifact seen with high concentrations of gadolinium within the urinary bladder following contrast. It must be remembered that the patient was scanned in dorsal recumbency and hence, the highest concentrations of gadolinium are in the dorsal portions of the urinary bladder. (B) T2-weighted transverse imaging showing the hypointense lesions within the spleen, compatible with iron storage. (C) T2-weighted gradient echo sequence in the dorsal plane showing the same hypointense lesions within the spleen. These lesions are hypointense in all image sequences.

ABNORMALITIES OF THE KIDNEYS AND ADRENAL GLANDS

Renal and adrenal studies are readily performed with magnetic resonance imaging. Cases where ultrasonography has been unable to give a clear diagnosis are good candidates for MRI due to the superior resolution and contrast (Figure 4.5). Adrenal tumors can invade the vena cava. Definite invasion of the vena cava can be difficult to ascertain from other imaging modalities. The

ability of magnetic resonance imaging to clearly image the structure in all three major planes allows for clear definition of invasion (Figure 4.6). These studies can aid in deciding whether lesions are infiltrative which may influence surgical excisability. Studies in the humans have found that with techniques to ascertain lipid content, the fat containing adrenal masses are generally benign with a high degree of specificity. Adrenal tumors that are clinically inapparent have also been found when imaging the thoracolumbar spine. Tumors may be single or bilateral (Figures 4.7 and 4.8).

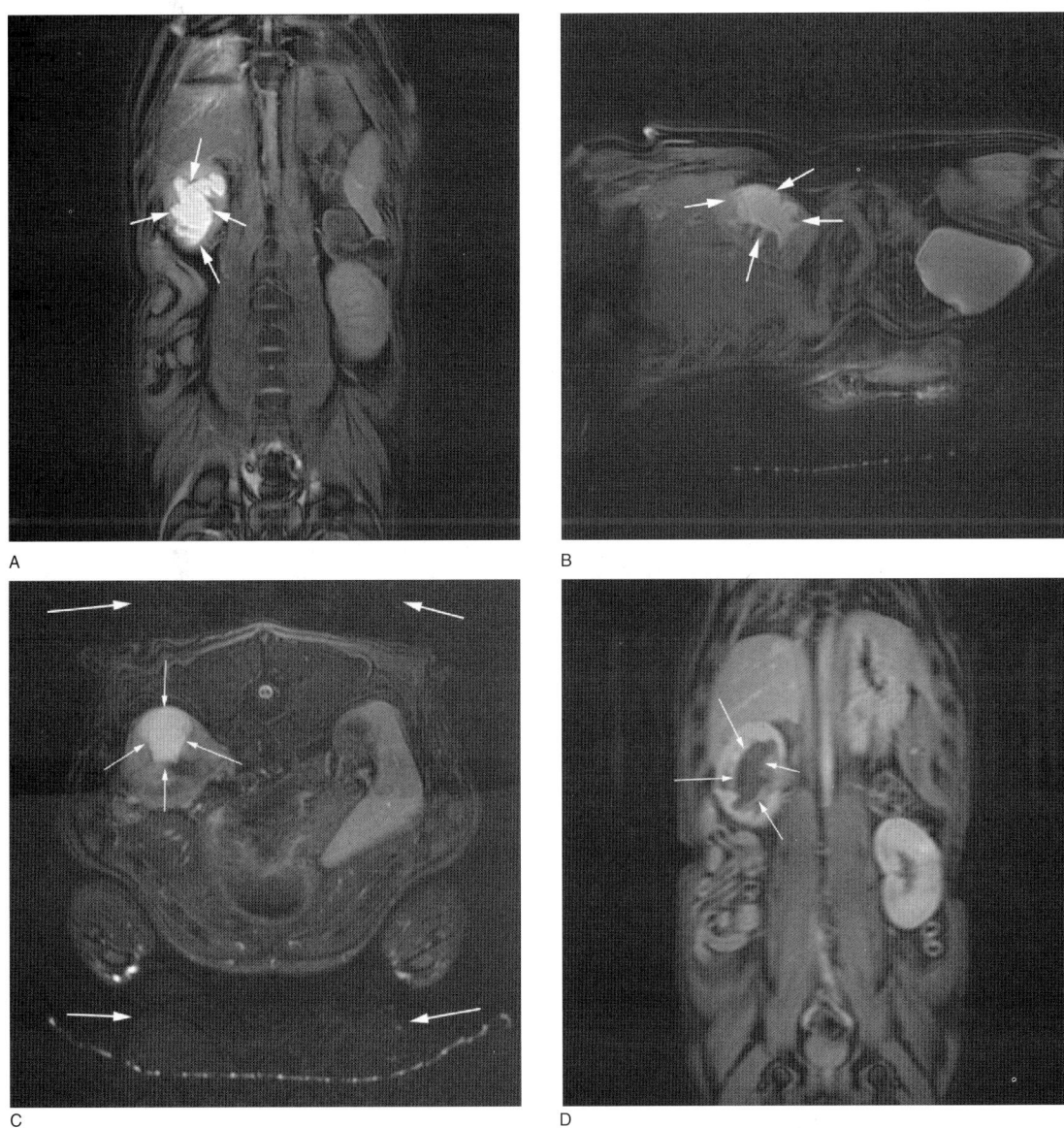

Figure 4.5. Case was followed with ultrasonography. A "lesion" was seen in the right kidney that appeared to be getting larger. Patient was referred for MRI. (A)–(C) T2-weighted gradient echo sequences in the dorsal, sagittal, and transverse planes, respectively. A large hyperintense lesion in the right renal pelvis compatible with hydronephrosis is highlighted with arrows. (D) T1-weighted, post-contrast, gradient echo sequence. The previous hyperintensity on T2-weighting is now a uniform hypointensity on T1-weighting, compatible with a fluid of low cellularity or hydrogen content.

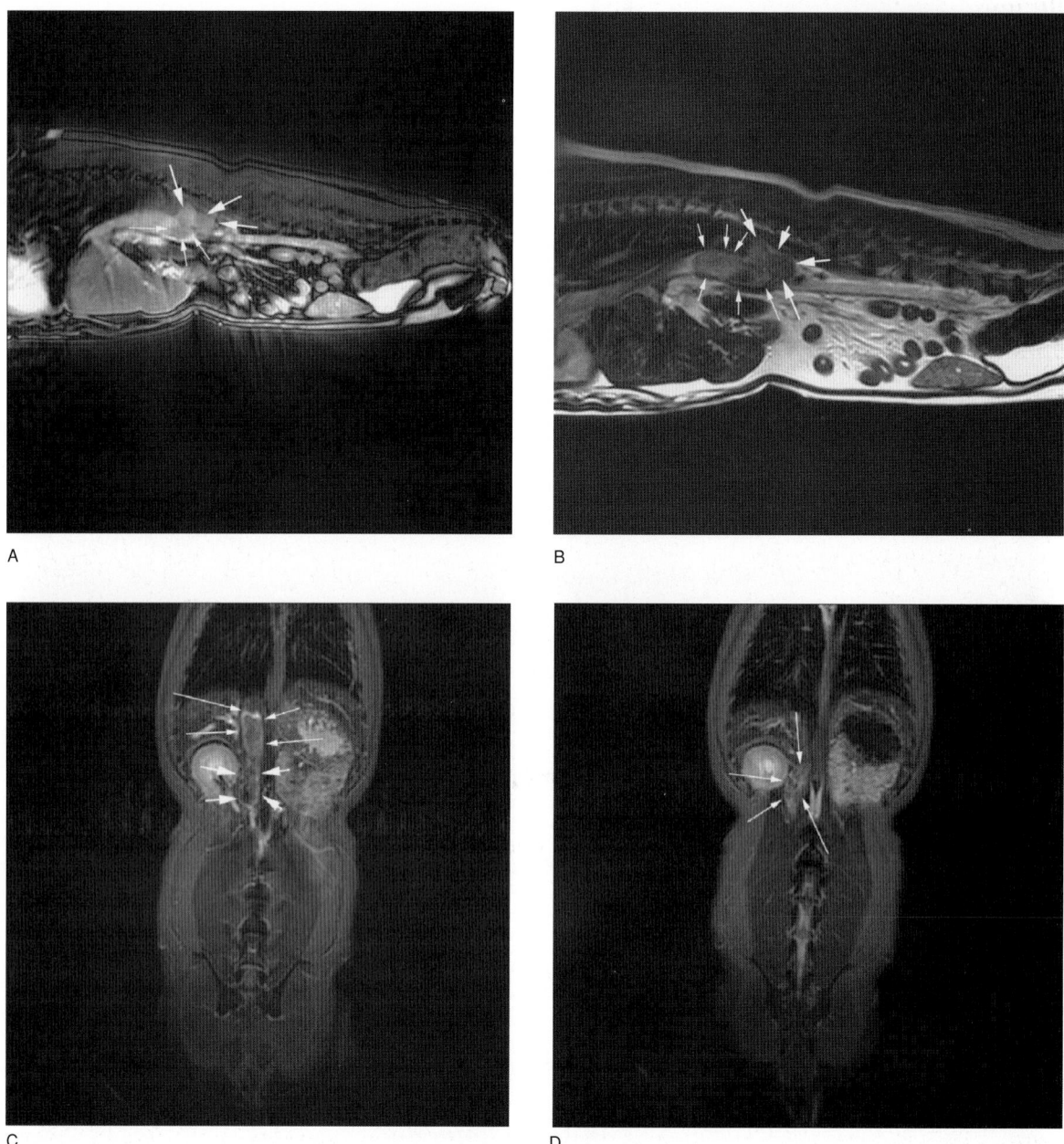

Figure 4.6. (A) T2-weighted gradient echo sequence in the sagittal plane. Large arrows show an adrenal mass. Small arrows show the mass invading the caudal vena cava. (B) T2-weighted, spin-echo sagittal image. Note the improved detail of spin-echo sequences over gradient echo sequences. All the material present within the caudal vena cava may not be tumor. Some of it may represent thrombus formation. (C) T2-weighted gradient echo sequence in the dorsal plane. Mass invading the vena cava is highlighted with arrows. (D) T2-weighted gradient echo sequence in the dorsal plane, dorsal to (C). Enlarged right adrenal is readily seen.

Figure 4.7. (A) T2-weighted STIR sequence in the dorsal plane. Large arrows highlight an enlarged left adrenal gland. Small arrows show flow artifact going outside the patient. It must be remembered that this flow artifact would also be superimposed on the patient. All of these sequences are obtained post-contrast and, therefore, some of the image intensities will be altered. Note the right kidney has a low signal intensity and it should be higher on a STIR sequence. The low signal intensity is probably due to high concentrations of gadolinium within the kidney. $\longrightarrow$ (B) T2-weighted, gradient echo, fat-suppressed sequence in the sagittal plane. The large left adrenal is highlighted. (C) T2-weighted, gradient echo, fat-suppressed image in the dorsal plane. Note how there is less motion artifact in a gradient echo sequence than in the STIR sequence due to a much shortened acquisition time. (D) T2-weighted gradient echo, fat-suppressed sequence in the transverse plane. Large adrenal is seen. The aorta and vena cava are indicated with large arrows. Note there is no vascular involvement present.

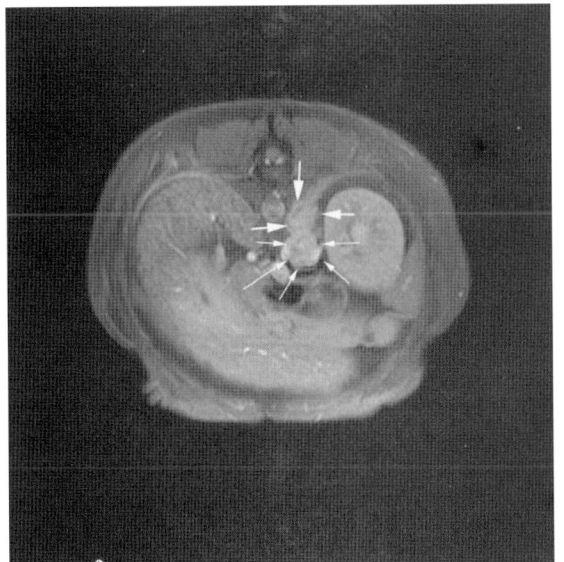

E

Figure 4.6. (*Continued*) (E) T1-weighted gradient echo sequence, transverse plane image. Large arrows show the large right adrenal gland. Small arrows show the invasion into the vena cava. A small portion of the lumen of the vena cava is still patent with a lack of signal intensity indicating blood flow.

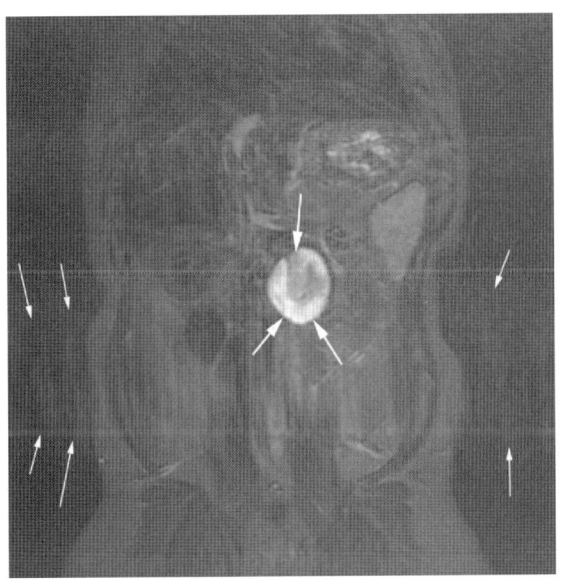

A

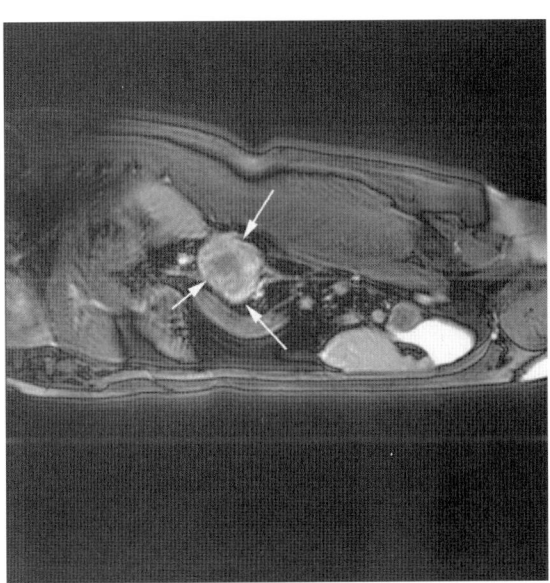

B

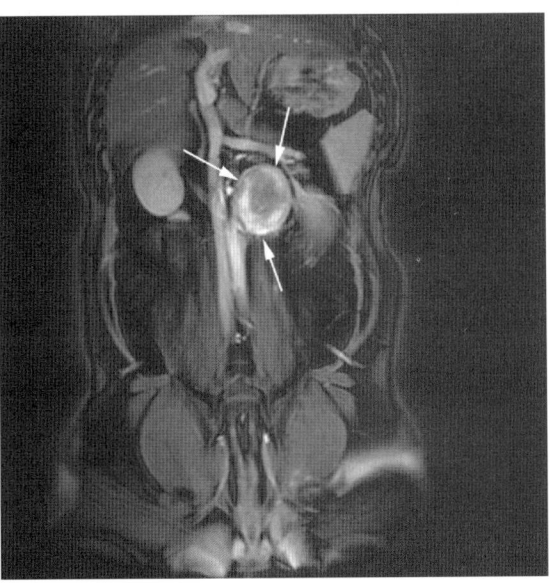

C

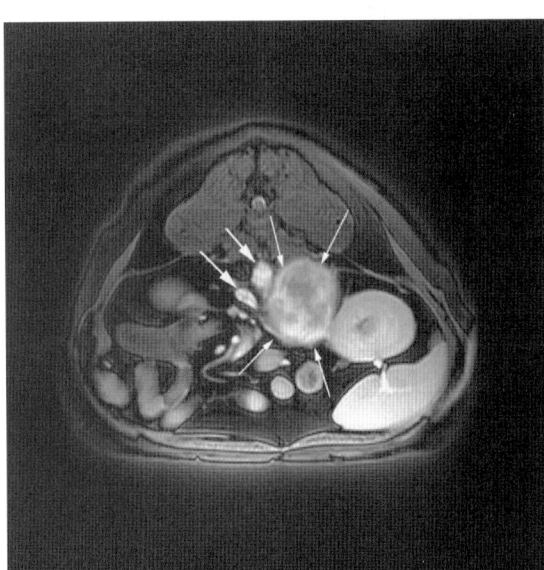

D

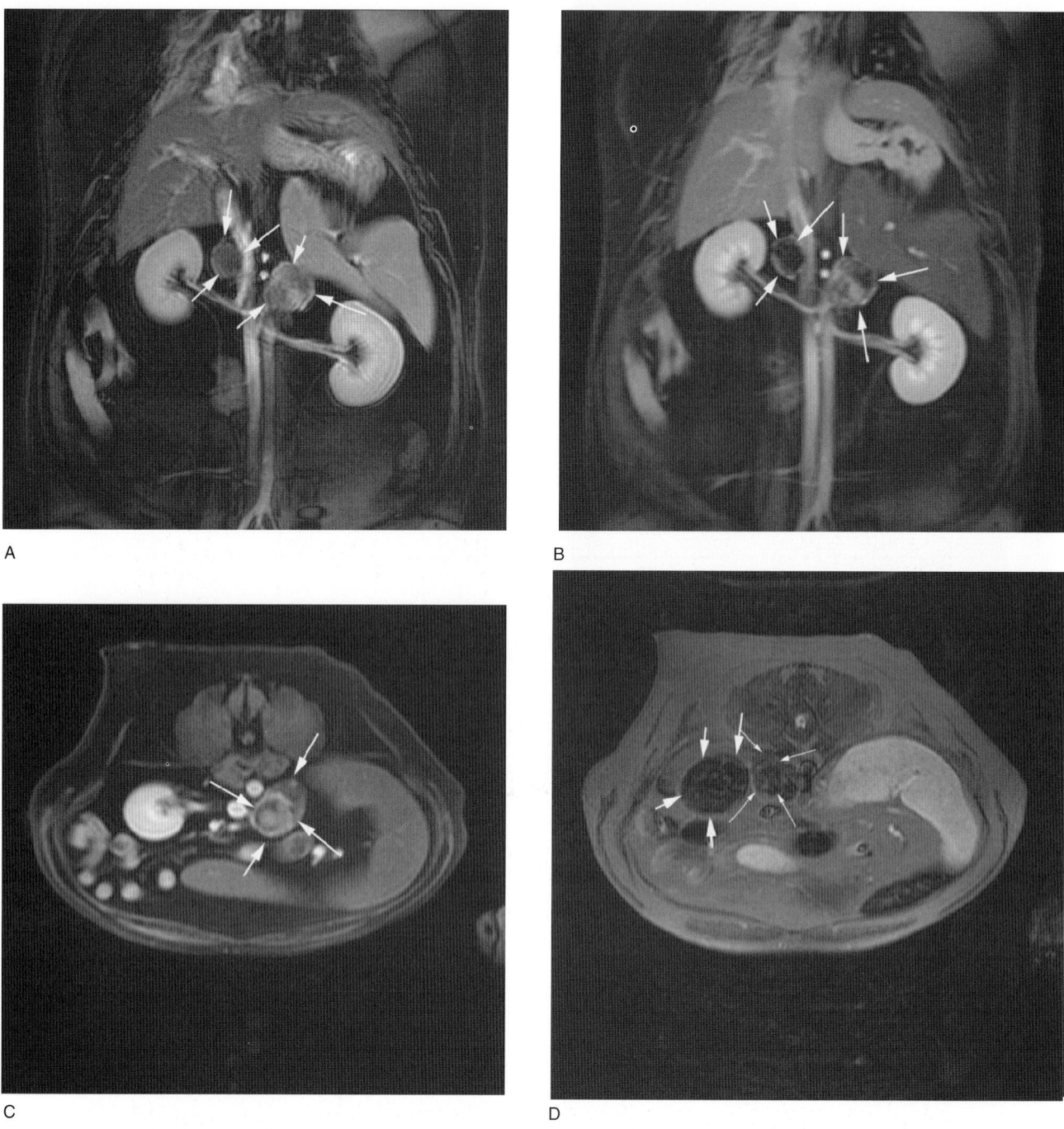

A

B

C

D

Figure 4.8. Bilateral adrenal masses. All of these lesions are post-contrast. (A) T2-weighted, gradient echo, fat-suppressed image in the dorsal plane. Left and right adrenal masses are seen. (B) T1-weighted, gradient echo, post-contrast, fat-suppressed image. (C) T2-weighted gradient echo sequence in the transverse plane. In this transverse section, only the enlarged left adrenal is seen. (D) STIR sequence in the transverse plane. The large arrows show the low signal intensity in the kidney. This is probably artifactual due to high gadolinium concentrations. The small arrows show the enlarged right adrenal gland. The low signal intensities in the adrenal glands could represent fat in these fat-suppressed images or could represent artifacts due to high gadolinium concentration. This is an inherent problem when scanning other parts of the body after contrast has already been administered.

Figure 4.9. Patient with high insulin levels and hypoglycemia. (A) T2-weighted, gradient echo sequence, fat-suppressed, dorsal plane image. Arrows indicate a spherical mass that appears to be in the liver. However, due to volume average artifact, this mass could also be within the adjacent pancreas. (B) STIR sequence, transverse plane. Same mass is seen in the transverse plane. Again, volume average artifact could make this mass appear to be within the hepatic parenchyma while residing in the adjacent pancreas. (C) STIR-weighted sequence in the dorsal plane showing the same mass. (D) Another section of the STIR sequence. Another mass was detected closer to midline. This may represent an enlarged lymph node. (E) T2-weighted, gradient-echo sequence, fat-suppressed image in the sagittal plane. The mass seen in Figure 4.9 (D) is depicted here.

OTHER ASSOCIATED ORGANS

Other organs have been imaged on occasion. These include the pancreas in the search for small, non-ultrasonographically detectable insulinomas. To date, the majority of these insulinomas have been detected; however, there have been cases of presumed insulinoma based on serum insulin levels that have evaded MR detection (Figure 4.9). MR can be utilized to visualize gastrointestinal abnormalities, including masses.

The MR often helps determine resectability of lesions within the pelvis due to the inability of ultrasound to provide a complete examination in this area.

MR can be used to study lesions of the genitourinary tract, but to date, most lesions have been found in a serendipitous fashion. Magnetic resonance can be used for superior visualization of tumors such as transitional cell carcinomas in the bladder. The use of a FLAIR sequence will allow a T2 image of the tumor while nulling out the signal from the urine (Figure 4.10).

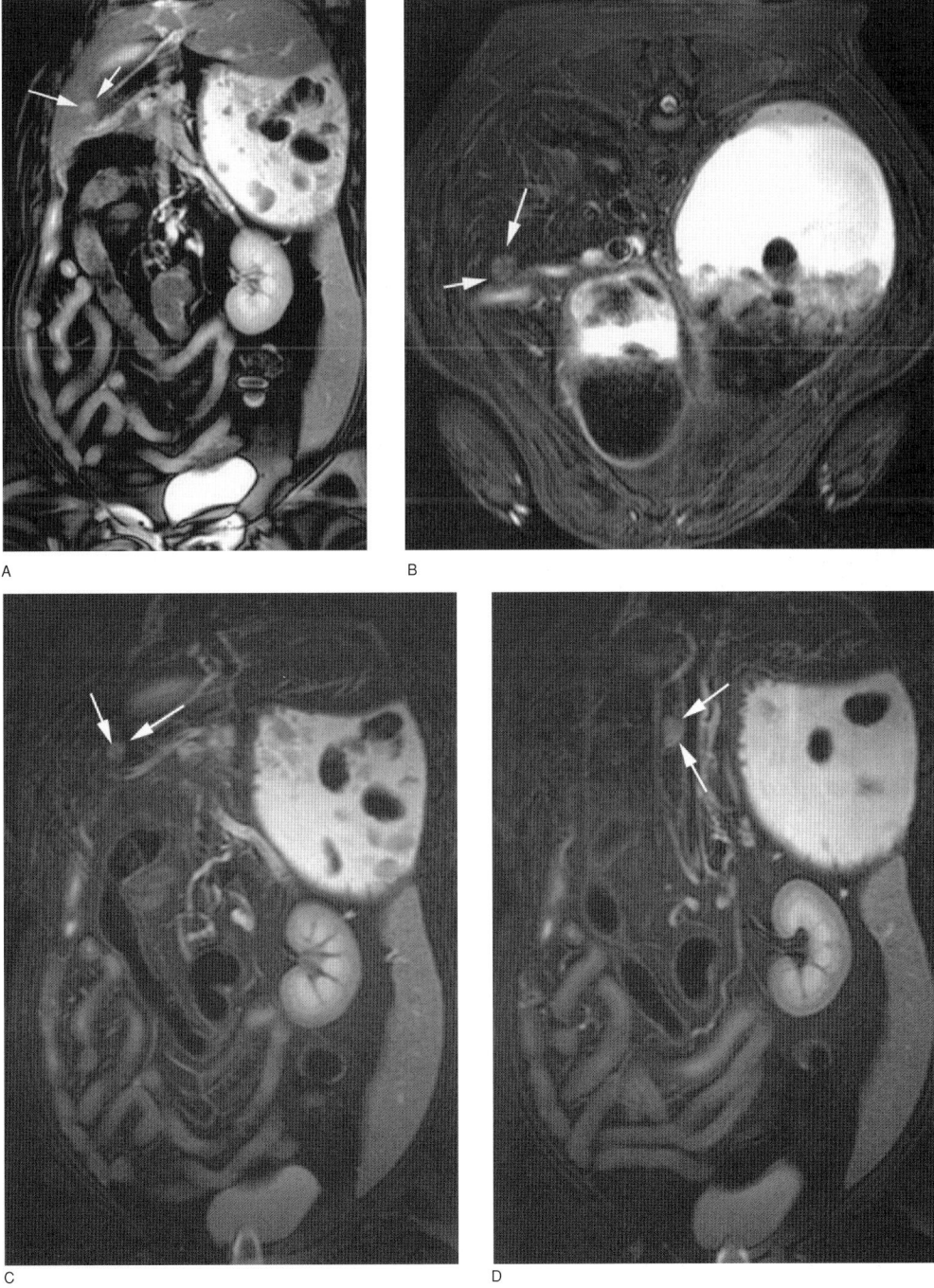

A

B

C

D

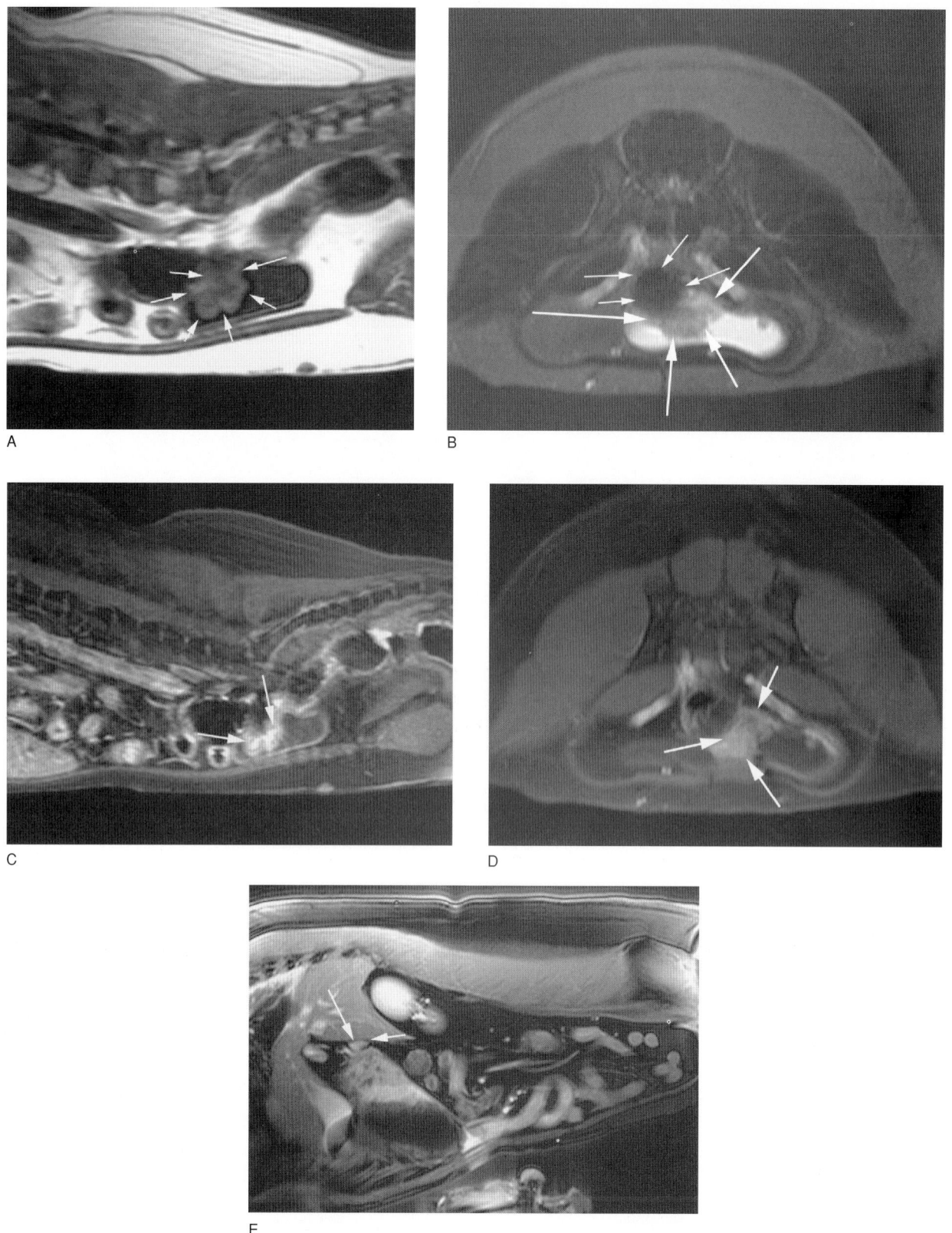

Figure 4.10. Transitional cell carcinoma. (A) FLAIR inversion recovery sequence. This allows for nulling of the urine and improved visualization of the mass. (B) T2-weighted, gradient echo sequence, fat-saturated, transverse image. Urine is bright. Mass is less intense than the urine. Small arrows show the presence of the colon. (C) T1-weighted, post-contrast fat-suppressed image. Contrast enhancement of the mass is readily seen. (D) T1-weighted, gradient echo sequence, fat-suppressed, transverse image. Excellent visualization of the mass is obtained. MR is often used in research purposes for definitive measurement of the volume of lesions to ascertain therapeutic efficacy.

Portosystemic Shunts

Both CT and MR have proven to have superior accuracy for the diagnosis of portosystemic vascular anomalies (PSVA) than more commonly used modalities such as sonography and radiographic portography. The use of MR to diagnose portosystemic shunts (PSVA) has undergone significant revision and improvement since being first described by Sequin et al. (1999). Currently, MR portography approaches 100% sensitive and specific for the detection of portosystemic shunts. This level of success of course necessitates appropriate knowledge of the portal vascular system and its variations, as well as familiarity with the appearance of an MR portogram.

The acquisition of a MR portogram utilizes a two-dimensional time-of-flight (2D TOF) sequence. This is a type of gradient recalled echo (GRE). This sequence applies a saturation pulse to a slice volume, which nulls all signals within the volume part acquisition. The blood flowing into the volume can thus be magnetized by an RF pulse and, therefore, the blood is the only detectable signal admitted and detected (Figure 4.11). We have found this sequence to be the most robust, rather than phase contrast venography, for the examination of slower blood velocity associated with PSVA. The improvement in sensitivity and specificity MR portography is related to concurrent application of appropriately sized receiver coils and the administration of gadolinium-based contrast prior to acquisition of the MR portogram to increase the conspicuity of the blood pool. The use of gadolinium, partially or com-pletely, negates the suppression of signal from vessels that are flowing parallel to the slice acquisition. Therefore, the entire vessel even when tortuous is delineated. Like routine abdominal MR imaging, respiratory gating is unnecessary, with the exception of some intrahepatic PSS.

The images produced by TOF sequences are transverse abdominal images that display the major abdominal veins as markedly hyperintense structures on the background of signal suppressed abdominal anatomy (Figure 4.12A–D). The interpretation of these images requires tracing the portal vein along its length and examining its tributaries for anomalous communication with the systemic circulatory system. It is also possible to reconstruct the TOF transverse images into two-dimensional (2D) and three-dimensional (3D) maximum intensity projections, which are also called MIPs (Figure 4.12E, F, respectively).

With the use of MR portography both intra- and extrahepatic PSVAs are easily delineated from their origin to their terminus. When matched to T1- or T2-weighted anatomical images of the abdomen, the precise location of the anomalous vessel can be determined surgically. This information purportedly reduces surgical time, which is critical in these metabolically disturbed patients. With intrahepatic PSVAs (Figure 4.13), the location of the shunt within the hepatic parenchyma is well defined, and the caliber of the anomalous communication can be accurately determined surgically. This information is also important in distinguishing cases, which are surgically amenable from those that are not.

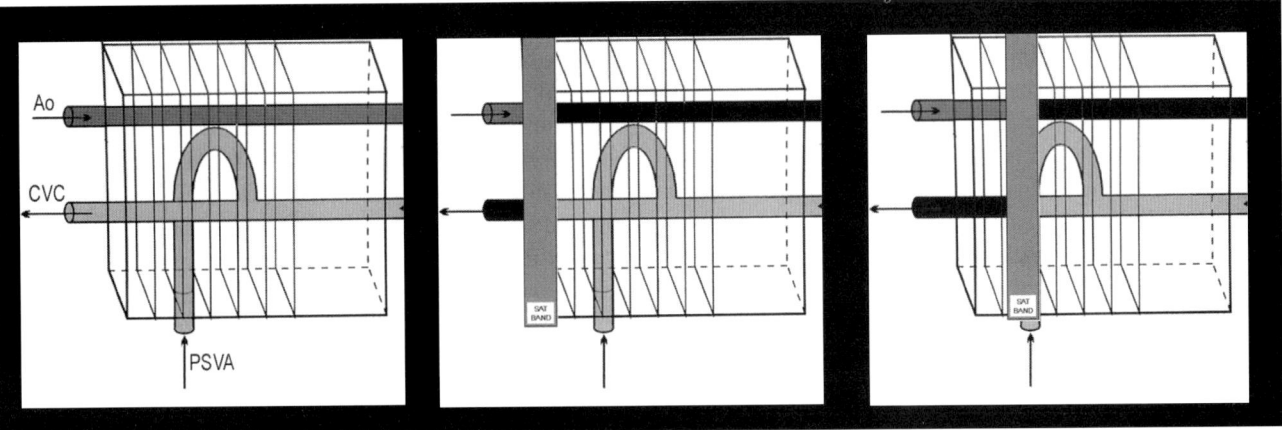

Figure 4.11.   Diagram of the mechanisms of signal suppression used in the production of time-of-flight MR venography to produce MR portograms. (Left) The aorta (dark gray) is represented as the top vessel, with the caudal vena cava (light gray) below with a portosystemic vascular anomaly (PSVA—light gray) communicating with it. (Middle) The saturation band (SAT BAND) is applied sequentially from cranial to caudal for an abdominal venogram, thus is called the marching SAT BAND. It suppresses the signal of the flowing blood (black) downstream. (Right) When vessels lie within the plane of suppression, they are suppressed along their length. This is overcome by administering a gadolinium-based contrast agent.

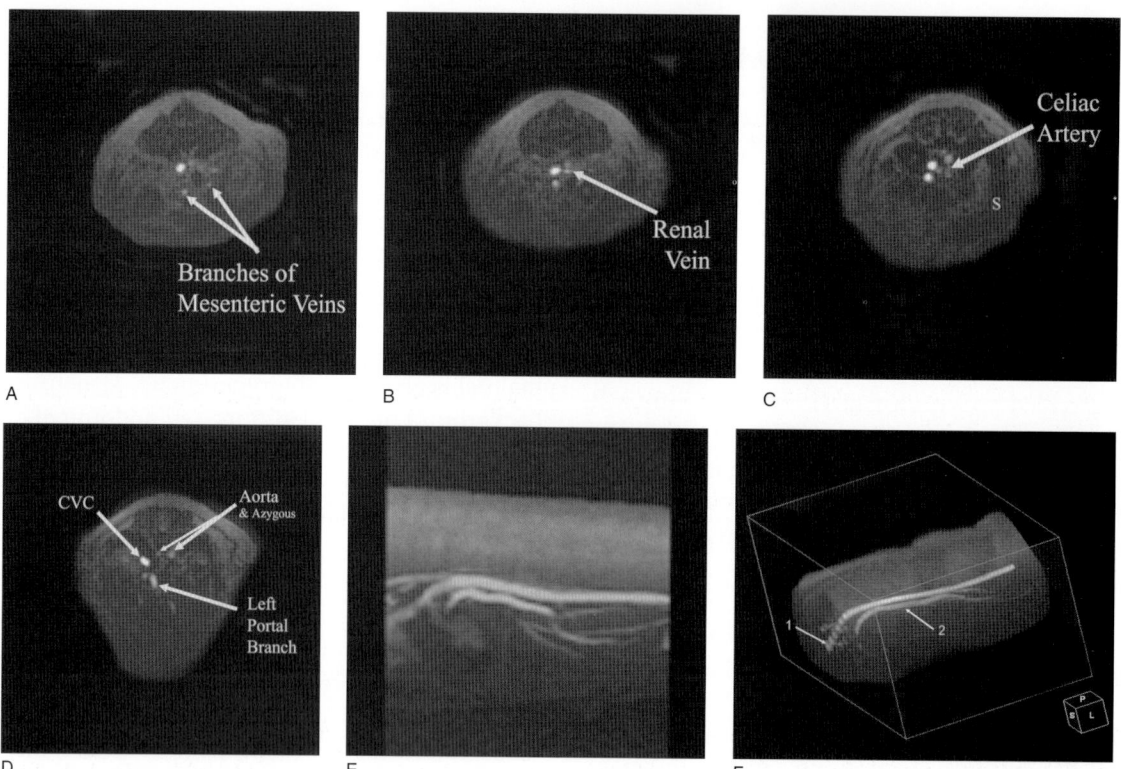

Figure 4.12. Normal MR portograms. (A)–(D) Transverse time-of-flight images showing the normal disposition of portal vein and caudal vena cava from formation of the portal vein by the cranial and caudal mesenteric veins (A) to normal arborization of the portal vein in the liver parenchyma. (E) Two-dimensional maximum intensity projection (MIP). (F) Three-dimensional MIP.

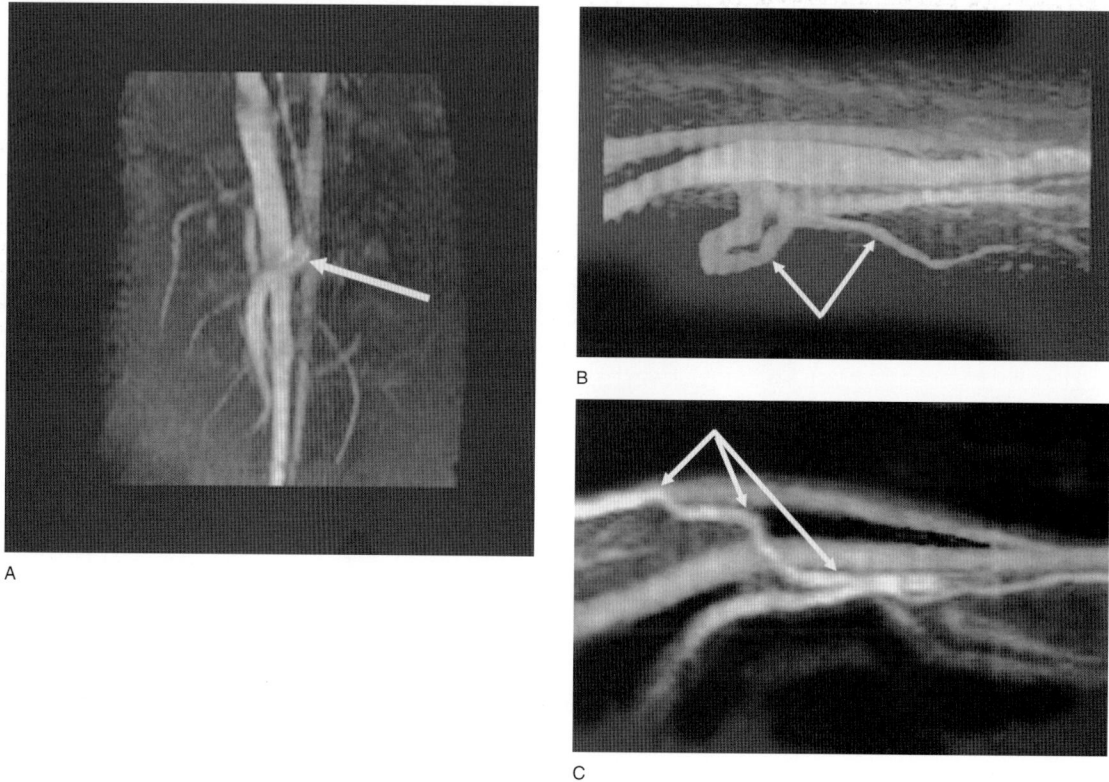

Figure 4.13. Single, extrahepatic portosystemic vascular anomalies (PSVA). (A) Dorsal plane 2D MIP of a portocaval PSVA. (B) Sagittal plane 2D MIP of a right gastric PSVA. Note the markedly dilated pancreaticoduodenal vein (caudally directed arrow). (C) Sagittal plane 2D MIP of a portoazygos PSVA, which measures 3 mm in diameter. This anomalous vessel was not identified on abdominal ultrasound. Because the portal vein is normally sized, the ultrasound diagnosis was negative from a PSVA.

The same benefits are realized with extrahepatic PSVAs (Figure 4.14), with very precise localization available from the MR portogram. Since its inception, MR portography has defined some very abnormal PSVAs (Figure 4.15) that are difficult to delineate well with ultrasound. The ability to distinguish surgically amenable PSVAs is important not only from an emotional but a financial point of view.

In the process of developing MR portography, concurrent studies of the brain of these animals have shown a relatively consistent structural change. A bilateral, common, nearly symmetric hyperintensity is seen in the coronal radiation on T2 and FLAIR sequences

(Figure 4.16). The change is suspected to represent metabolic cerebral disruption associated with hepatic encephalopathy. The MRI abnormality is seen in both animals with clinical signs of hepatic encephalopathy, and those which are assessed to be neurologically normal indicating the presence of subclinical disease. In addition, the severity of this change has been seen to change with medical management alone. In one dog imaged 1 year following placement of an ameroid constrictor on the PSVA, persistence of this hyperintensity on T2 and flair sequences was seen. The histologic correlation of this structural change has not yet been defined and therefore its importance in the clinical management of these patients is unknown.

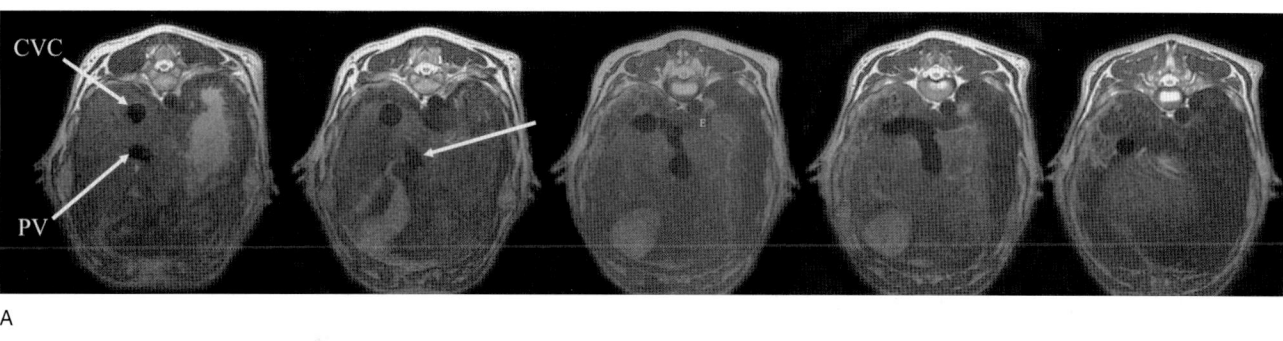

A

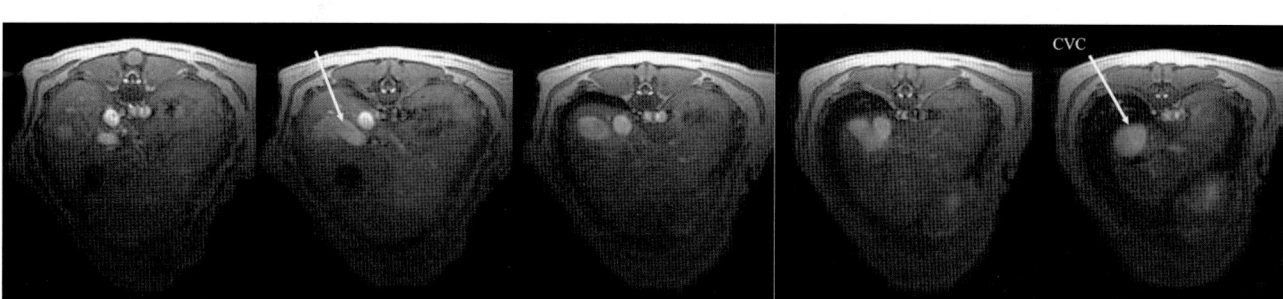

B

Figure 4.14. Single, intrahepatic portosystemic vascular anomalies (PSVA). (A) Transverse T2-weighted images of a left divisional PSVA. Arrows in left image demark the caudal vena cava dorsal to the portal vein at the level of the porta hepatic. The left portal branch is shown in the second image, which communicates with the left hepatic vein at the level of the diaphragm. (B) Transverse gradient recalled echo (GRE) images of a right divisional PSVA. The arrows denoted the anomalous communication between the portal vein and the caudal vena cava, in which the communication is located within the liver parenchyma. This is important pre-operative information.

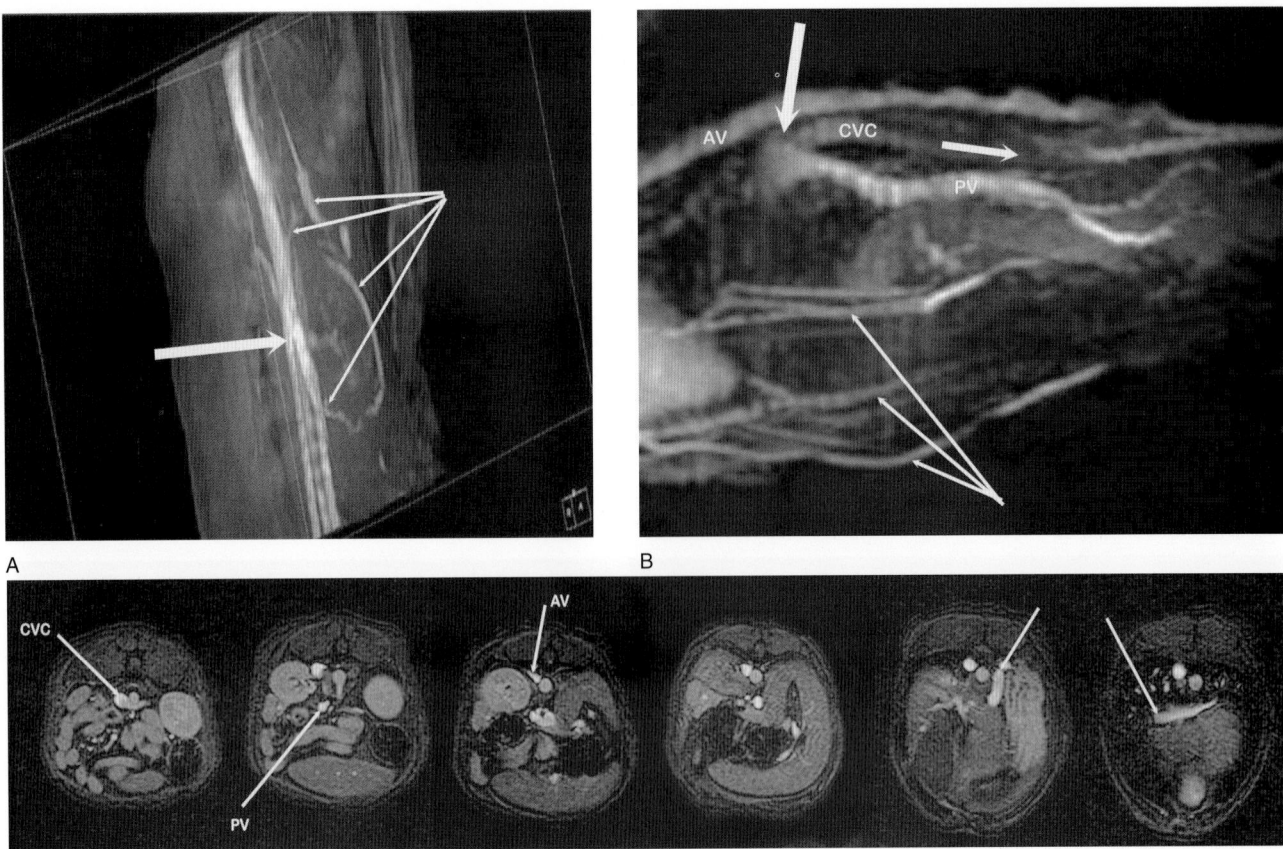

Figure 4.15. Abnormal portosystemic vascular anomalies (PSVA), some which the MR program shows cannot be corrected with surgery. (A) Three-dimensional maximum intensity projection (MIP) of a PSVA located in the retroperitoneum and loops around the left kidney. On the initial abdominal exploration, none of the PSVA could be visualized, but was found with dissection into the retroperitoneal area around the kidney. (B) Sagittal plane 2D MIP of a portal-caval-azygous PSVA. The large arrows denote the intrahepatic communication between the portal vein and the caudal vena cava, which was identified on abdominal ultrasound. However, the blood flow in the caudal vena cava is retrograde and you can see signal detected from this area on the 2D TOF because it is opposite normal. There is also no cranial continuation of the caudal vena cava from the liver to the heart. The communication with the markedly dilated azygos vein is caudal to the pelvic diaphragm, and therefore not seen during the first abdominal exploration. There are numerous enlarged internal thoracic veins (small arrows), forming collateral circulation for the abdomen. (C) Transverse time-of-flight (TOF) images, displayed caudal to cranial, of a caudal vena cava (CVC)—azygos vein (AV) communication and left gastric portosystemic vascular anomaly (PSVA). The left image is at the level of the renal vein entering the CVC. In the next image, the portal vein (PV) has formed and the CVC is now positioned dorsal to the aorta. The fusion of the CVC and the AV is seen in the third image; as well, the PV is crossing midline demarking the beginning of the PSVA. In the fourth image, the PV travels cranially and the right AV is severely dilated accommodating the blood flow of the CVC. The left gastric PSVA is seen medial to the rugae of the stomach and has mild tortuosity. In the far right image, the left gastric PSVA joins the left hepatic branch just caudal to the diaphragm.

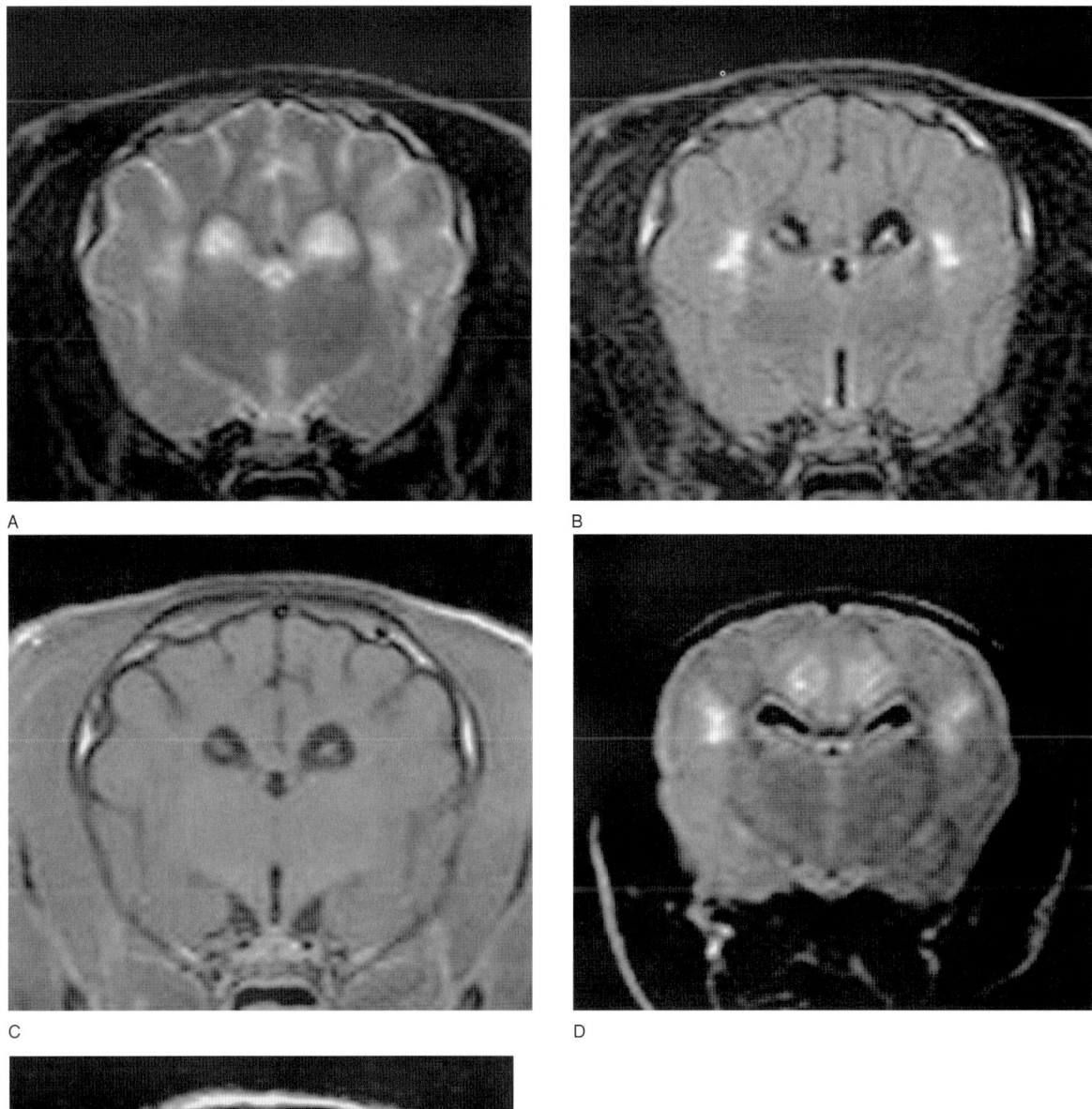

Figure 4.16. Presumed hepatic encephalopathy (HE). (A)–(C) T2-weighted, FLAIR, and post-gadolinium-enhanced T1-weighted images showing bilaterally symmetric hyperintense lesions in the coronal radiation and adjacent gray matter, which do not undergo contrast enhancement. (D)–(E) HE lesions in patients with single extra- and intra hepatic portosystemic vascular anomalies.

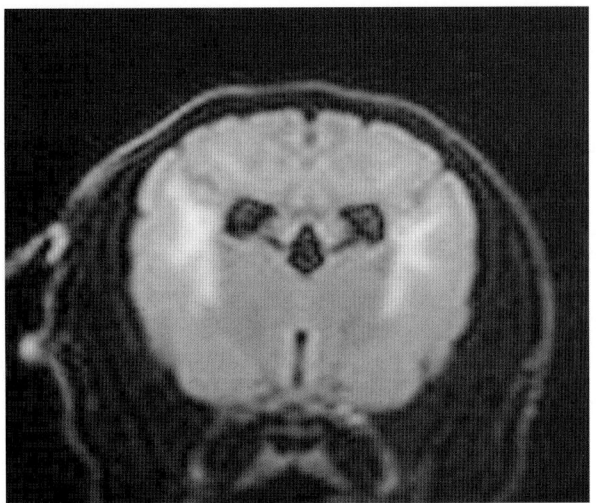

F

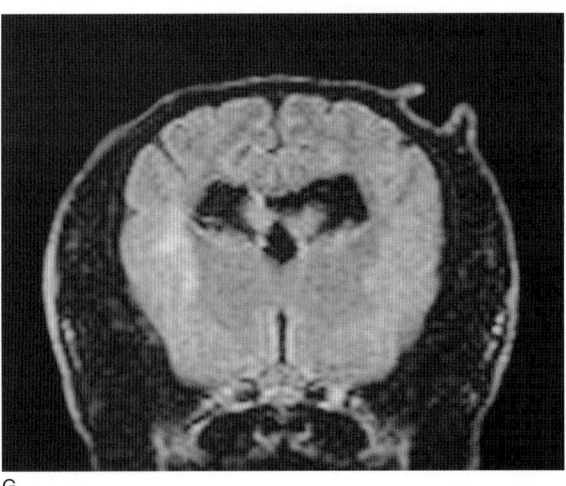

G

Figure 4.16. (*Continued*) (F–H) HE lesions in a patient imaged at presentation (F), 10 weeks following medical management (G) and 1 year following the placement of an ameroid constrictor (H).

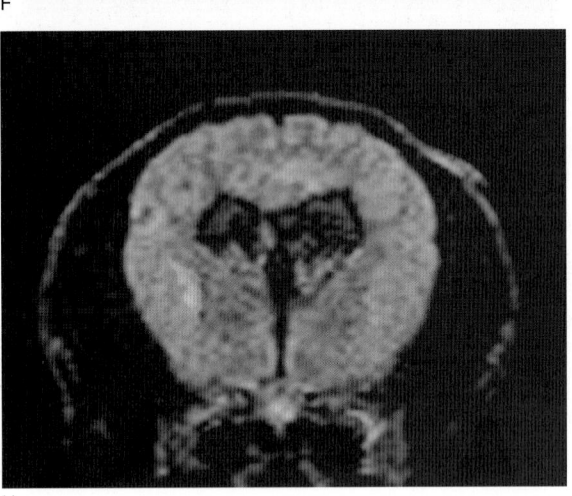

H

OTHER VASCULAR ABNORMALITIES

Aortic and vena cava thromboses can be detected on MR examination of the abdomen or most often when imaging the thoracolumbar spine. Patients with poor vascular flow to the hind limbs may be interpreted as a neurologic disease. The turbulent flow in the aorta often gives a heterogenous appearance on T2-weighted studies (Figure 4.17). Transverse images and 2D TOF studies provide proof of thrombosis (Figure 4.18).

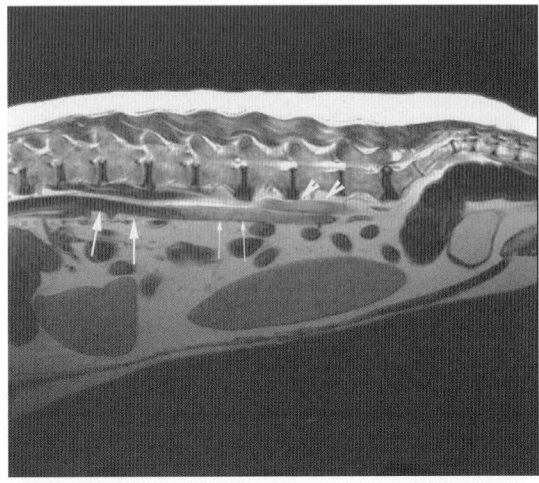

A

Figure 4.17. Normal abdominal aorta. Turbulent flow creates some artifact. (A) T2-weighted sagittal image. Large arrows point to normal lack of signal in fast flowing aortic blood. Small arrows point to increased signal in normal aortal due to turbulent flow and phase shifts. Arrow-heads point to a small area of the vena cava in the slice. (B) Two-dimensional TOF angiogram of the abdominal aorta. Large arrows indicate uniform flow in the aorta. Small arrows point to a small area of vena cava in the slice.

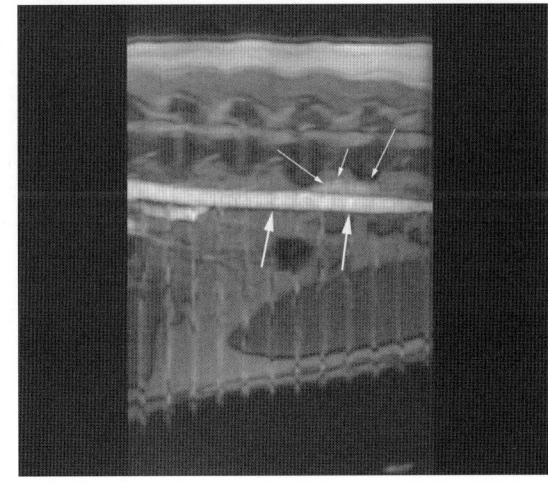

B

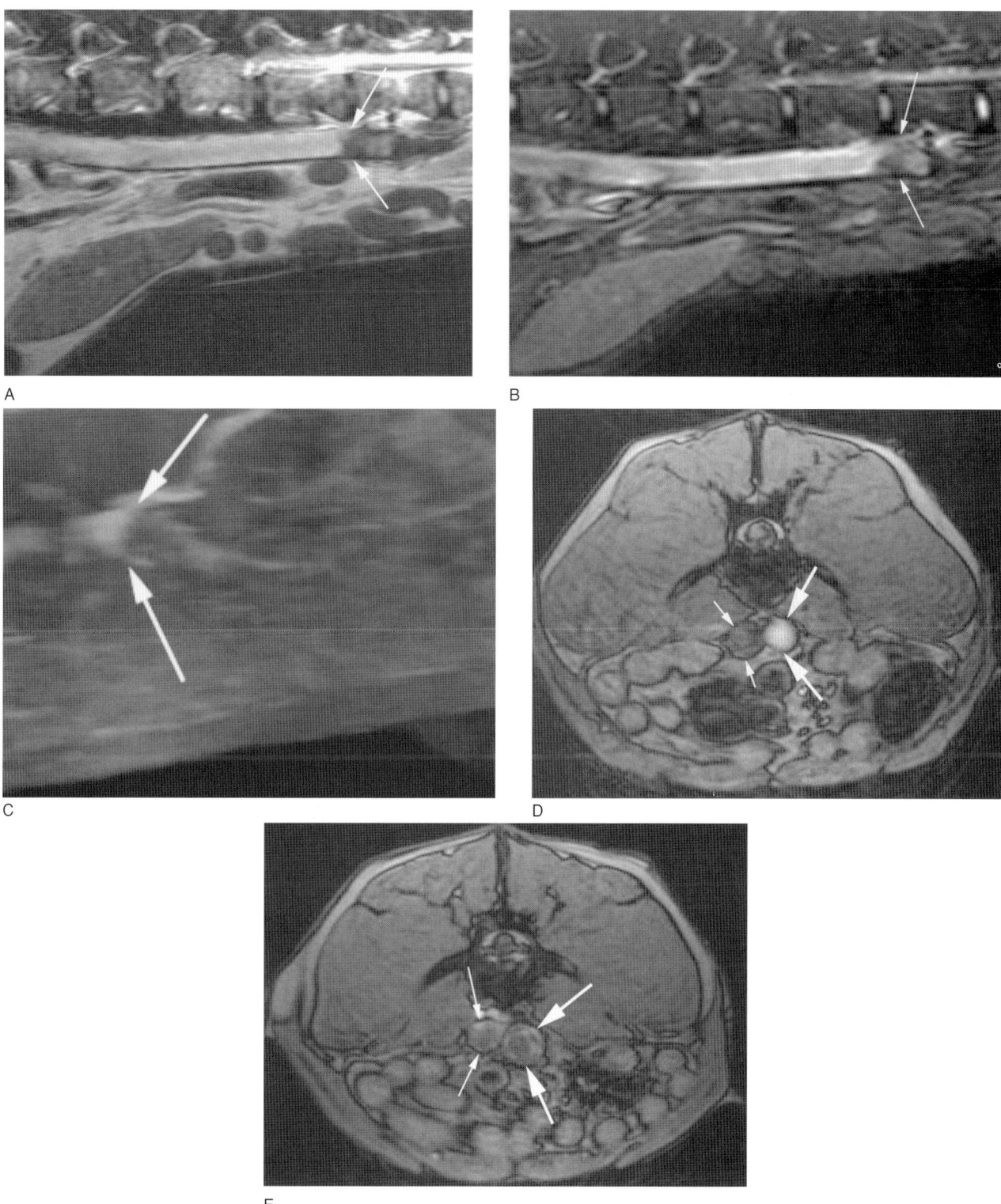

Figure 4.18. Aortic thrombus. (A) T2-weighted sagittal image. Arrows point to the thrombus in the aorta. (B) STIR sagittal image. Arrows point to the thrombus in the aorta. (C) MIP or the 2D TOF angiogram of the abdominal aorta. The arrows point to the start of the thrombus. (D) Source image from 2D TOF angiogram upstream of the thrombus. Small arrows point to the vena cava that is nulled as flow is going the wrong way for this angiogram. Large arrows point to the flow in the aorta. (E) Source image from 2D TOF angiogram just below the start of the thrombus. Small arrows point to vena cava, large arrows to the lack of flow in the aorta.

BIBLIOGRAPHY

Behrend EN and Kemppainen RJ. 2001. Diagnosis of canine hyperadrenocorticism. Vet Clin North Am Small Anim Pract 31(5):985–1003, viii.

Bottcher P, Maierl J, Schicmann T, Glaser C, Weller R, Hoehne KH, et al. 1999. The visible animal project: a three-dimensional, digital database for high quality three-dimensional reconstructions. Vet Radiol Ultrasound 40(6):611–616.

Bourrinet P, Bengele HH, Bonnemain B, Dencausse A, Idee JM, Jacobs PM, et al. 2006. Preclinical safety and pharmacokinetic profile of ferumoxtran-10, an ultrasmall superparamagnetic iron oxide magnetic resonance contrast agent. Invest Radiol 41(3):313–324.

Brofman PJ and Thrall DE. 2006. Magnetic resonance imaging findings in a dog with caudal aortic thromboembolism and ischemic myopathy. Vet Radiol Ultrasound 47(4):334–338.

Chang D, Kim B, Yun Y, Hur Y, Lee Y, Choi M, et al. 2002. Superparamagnetic iron oxide-enhanced magnetic resonance imaging of the liver in beagle dogs. Vet Radiol Ultrasound 43(1):37–42.

Chang SC, Liao JW, Lin YC, Liu Cl, and Wong ML. 2007. Pancreatic acinar cell carcinoma with intracranial metastasis in a dog. J Vet Med Sci 69(1):91–93.

Chowning SL, Susil RC, Krieger A, Fichtinger G, Whitcomb LL, and Atalar E. 2006. A preliminary analysis and model of prostate injection distributions. Prostate 66(4):344–357.

Clifford CA, Pretorius ES, Weisse C, Sorenmo KU, Drobatz KJ, Siegelman ES, et al. 2004. Magnetic resonance imaging of focal splenic and hepatic lesions in the dog. J Vet Intern Med 18(3):330–338.

Dennis R. 2005. Assessment of location of the celiac and cranial mesenteric arteries relative to the thoracolumbar spine using magnetic resonance imaging. Vet Radiol Ultrasound 46(5):388–390.

Diez-Prieto I, Garcia-Rodriguez MB, Rios-Granja MA, Cano-Rabano MJ, Gonzalo-Orden JM, and Perez-Garcia CC. 2001. Diagnosis of renal agenesis in a beagle. J Small Anim Pract 42(12):599–602.

Drost WT, Bahr RJ, Henry GA, and Campbell GA. 1999. Aortoiliac thrombus secondary to a mineralized arteriosclerotic lesion. Vet Radiol Ultrasound 40(3):262–266.

Garamvolgyi R, Petrasi Z, Hevesi A, Jakab C, Vajda Z, Bogner P, et al. 2006. Magnetic resonance imaging technique for the examination of canine mammary tumours. Acta Vet Hung 54(2):143–159.

Garosi LS, Penderis J, McConnell JF, and Jakobs C. 2005. L-2-hydroxyglutaric aciduria in a West Highland white terrier. Vet Rec 156(5):145–147.

Gavin PR. 1997. Future of veterinary radiation oncology. Vet Clin North Am Small Anim Pract 27(1):157–165.

Hahn KA, McGavin MD, and Adams WH. 1997. Bilateral renal metastases of nasal chondrosarcoma in a dog. Vet Pathol 34(4):352–355.

Harder MA, Fowler D, Pharr JW, Tryon KA, and Shmon C. 2002. Segmental aplasia of the caudal vena cava in a dog. Can Vet J 43(5):365–368.

Johnson VS and Seiler G. 2006. Magnetic resonance imaging appearance of the cisterna chyli. Vet Radiol Ultrasound 47(5):461–464.

Khangure MS and Hua J. 1996. Comparative assessment of gadoxetate disodium, manganese dipyridoxal diphosphate, and superparamagnetic iron oxide for enhancement of the liver in dogs. Acad Radiol 3(Suppl. 2):S458–S460.

Llabres-Diaz FJ and Dennis R. 2003. Magnetic resonance imaging of the presumed normal canine adrenal glands [PMID]. Vet Radiol Ultrasound 44(1):5–19.

Muleya JS, Taura Y, Nakaichi M, Nakama S, and Takeuchi A. 1997. Appearance of canine abdominal tumors with magnetic resonance imaging using a low field permanent magnet. Vet Radiol Ultrasound 38(6):444–447.

Munday HS. 1994. Assessment of body composition in cats and dogs. Int J Obes Relat Metab Disord 18(Suppl. 1):S14–S21.

Myers NC, III. 1997. Adrenal incidentalomas. Diagnostic workup of the incidentally discovered adrenal mass. Vet Clin North Am Small Anim Pract 27(2):381–399.

Partington BP and Biller DS. 1995. Hepatic imaging with radiology and ultrasound. Vet Clin North Am Small Anim Pract 25(2):305–335.

Rivera B, Ahrar K, Kangasniemi MM, Hazle JD, and Price RE. 2005. Canine transmissible venereal tumor: a large-animal transplantable tumor model. Comp Med 55(4):335–343.

Sari A, Ozyavuz R, Demirci A, Ercin C, Arslan A, Yuzuncu AK, et al. 1999. MR imaging of renal vein occlusion in dogs. Invest Radiol 34(8):523–529.

Sato T, Aoki K, Shibuya H, Machida T, and Watari T. 2003. Leiomyosarcoma of the kidney in a dog. J Vet Med A Physiol Pathol Clin Med 50(7):366–369.

Stolzenburg JU, Neuhaus J, Liatsikos EN, Schwalenberg T, Ludewig E, and Ganzer R. 2006. Histomorphology of canine urethral sphincter systems, including three-dimensional reconstruction and magnetic resonance imaging. Urology 67(3):624–630.

Suga K, Ogasawara N, Okazaki H, Sasai K, and Matsunaga N. 2001. Functional assessment of canine kidneys after acute vascular occlusion on Gd-DTPA-enhanced dynamic echo-planar MR imaging. Invest Radiol 36(11):659–676.

Tidwell AS, Penninck DG, and Besso JG. 1997. Imaging of adrenal gland disorders. Vet Clin North Am Small Anim Pract 27(2):237–254.

Vitellas KM, Kangarlu A, Bova JG, Bennett WF, Vaswani K, Chakeres DW, et al. 2001. Canine abdominal MRI at 8 Tesla:

initial experience with conventional gradient-recalled echo and rapid acquisition with relaxation enhancement (RARE) techniques. J Comput Assist Tomogr 25(6): 856–863.

Wyse CA, McLellan J, Dickie AM, Sutton DG, Preston T, and Yam PS. 2003. A review of methods for assessment of the rate of gastric emptying in the dog and cat: 1898–2002. J Vet Intern Med 17(5):609–621.

Yasuda D, Fujita M, Yasuda S, Taniguchi A, Miura H, Hasegawa D, et al. 2004. Usefulness of MRI compared with CT for diagnosis of mesenteric lymphoma in a dog. J Vet Med Sci 66(11):1447–1451.

CHAPTER FIVE

THORAX

Patrick R. Gavin and Shannon P. Holmes

ANATOMY

Initial studies of the thorax were not useful due to the motion that occurs with respiratory and the cardiac cycles. Subsequent studies utilizing breathhold techniques and respiratory and cardiac gating have allowed for clear visualization of the thoracic structures.

Normal Anatomy

The appearance of normal anatomy is best seen on T1- and T2-weighted sequences (Figures 5.1–5.4). As noted in the previous chapters, STIR or fat-suppressed sequences are the most robust for detecting pathologic changes and lymph nodes. The heart is best visualized in dorsal and sagittal planes. The dorsal plane is also superior for examining the lungs and mediastinal structures. However, the use of all three planes is preferable for complete evaluation of the thorax, including the thymus, lymph nodes, esophagus, trachea, lungs, heart (and the internal structure of myocardium, valves and chambers), and thoracic wall.

The lungs, due to the presence of air-filled alveoli, are void of signal and appear black. Therefore, it is easy to see soft tissue abnormalities in lung parenchyma using sequences that optimize soft tissue contrast. Atelectasis from general anesthesia is commonly identified in patients imaged in dorsal recumbency. This should not be mistaken for pleural effusion or parenchymal disease; circular and linear signal voids are seen in atelectatic lungs representative of air-filled tertiary bronchi and bronchioles. Similar to the lungs the respiratory tree (trachea and bronchi) is void of signal, but the walls of the airways are hyperintense. The muscle of the heart has low signal intensity on T2-weighted sequences and intermediate signal intensity on T1-weighted sequences. It is best seen on T1- and T2-sequences where the hyperintense mediastinal and pericardial fat delineates its margins. The appearance of the blood within the heart chambers and blood vessels can be hyper- or hypointense, depending on the imaging sequence and the velocity and direction of the blood flow. In addition, it is possible to produce "black-blood" and "white-blood" images of the circulatory system using various imaging sequences. The mediastinal structures will have appearance in accordance with its tissue structure. For example, the esophagus being a muscular tube has intermediate to low signal intensity. Because of general anesthesia, the esophagus can have variable degrees of gas distention. The tracheobronchial and sternal lymph nodes are not routinely identified in normal patients, as they will be nearly isointense to mediastinal fat on T2-weighted sequences.

IMAGING PROCEDURE

Pathologic conditions such as hydrothorax can severely compromise the ability of an imaging modality, such as radiography and computed tomography, to distinguish the fluid within the thoracic cavity from pathology of similar density. While ultrasonography can help, it is difficult to visualize all areas of the thoracic cavity with total confidence. Magnetic resonance imaging allows clear visualization of the difference between fluid within the thoracic cavity and pathologic change (Figure 5.5). Often, sequences to detect pathology utilize T2-weighted sequences and T2-weighted sequences with some type of fat suppression such as the STIR sequence or T2-weighted sequence with fat saturation. The STIR sequence will provide uniform nulling of the fat signal, but is a noisy image. T2 fat-saturation images are more detailed, but the fat-saturation may not be uniform, especially distant to the receiving coil or the isocenter of the magnet.

When the lung is being examined, T1-weighting provides excellent visualization of intrapulmonary abnormalities, as the lack of signal from the lung provides the needed contrast to any abnormality present within the pulmonary parenchyma. T1-weighted images are rapidly obtained and cardiac motion can be negated via cardiac gating or more easily with the acquisition of two sequences in the same plane with the only parameter change being the phase encoding direction to

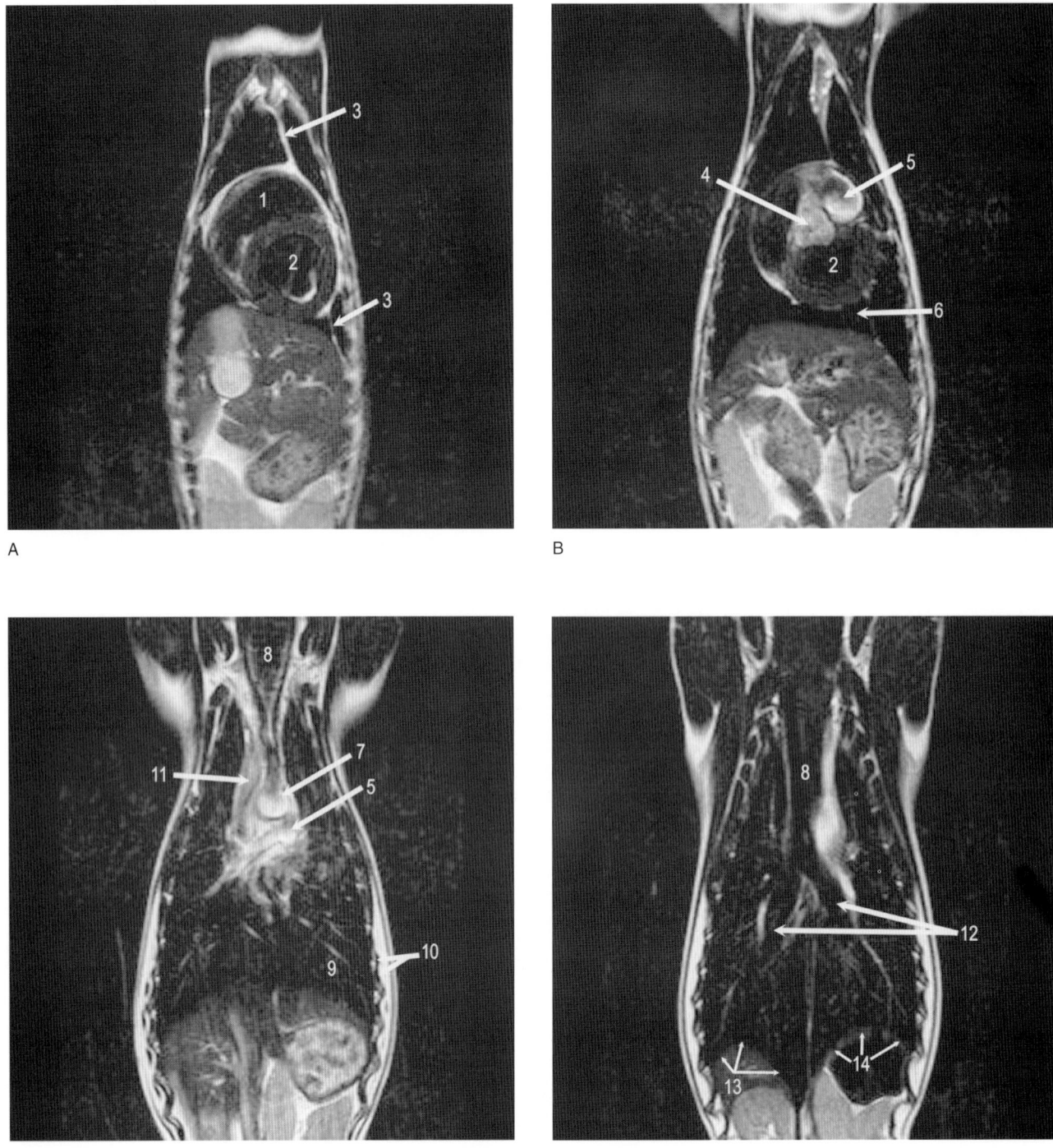

Figure 5.1. (A)–(D) T2-weighted dorsal images. (1) Right ventricle, (2) left ventricle, (3) mediastinum with hyperintense fat, (4) aortic valve, (5) main pulmonary artery, (6) accessory lung lobe, (7) aorta, (8) trachea, (9) left caudal lung with hyperintense blood vessels, (10) ribs and intercostal muscles, (11) esophagus, (12) mainstem bronchi, (13) right diaphragmatic crus, (14) stomach wall and left diaphragmatic crus.

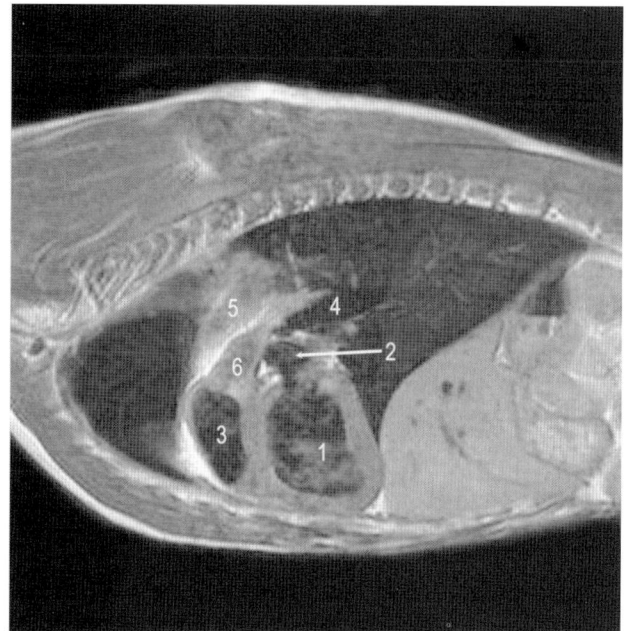

A

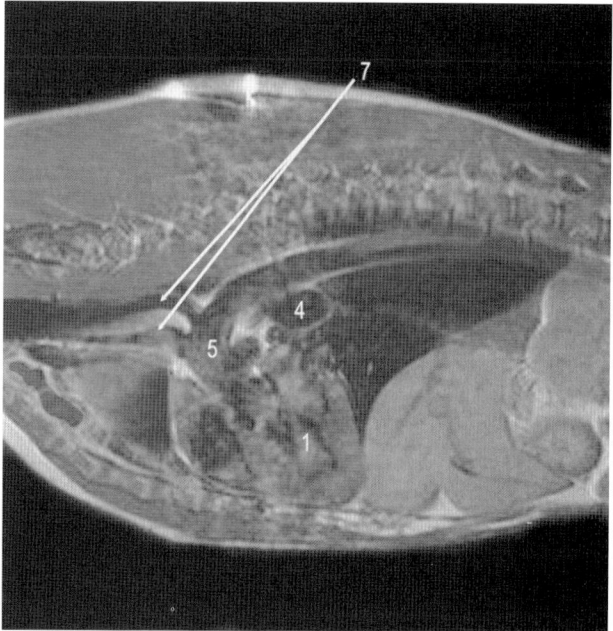

B

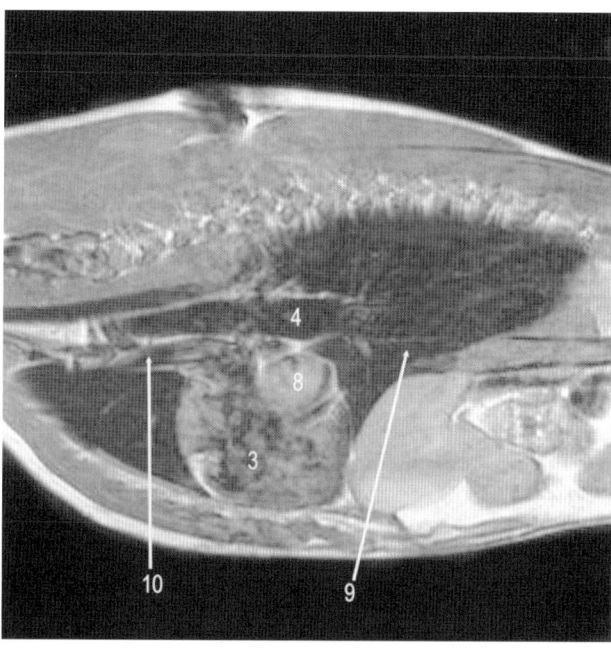

C

Figure 5.2. (A)–(C) T1-weighted sagittal images. (1) Left ventricle, (2) left atrium, (3) right ventricle, (4) trachea and mainstem bronchi, (5) aorta, (6) main pulmonary artery, (7) brachiocephalic trunk and right subclavian artery, (8) right atrium, (9) caudal vena cava, (10) cranial vena cava.

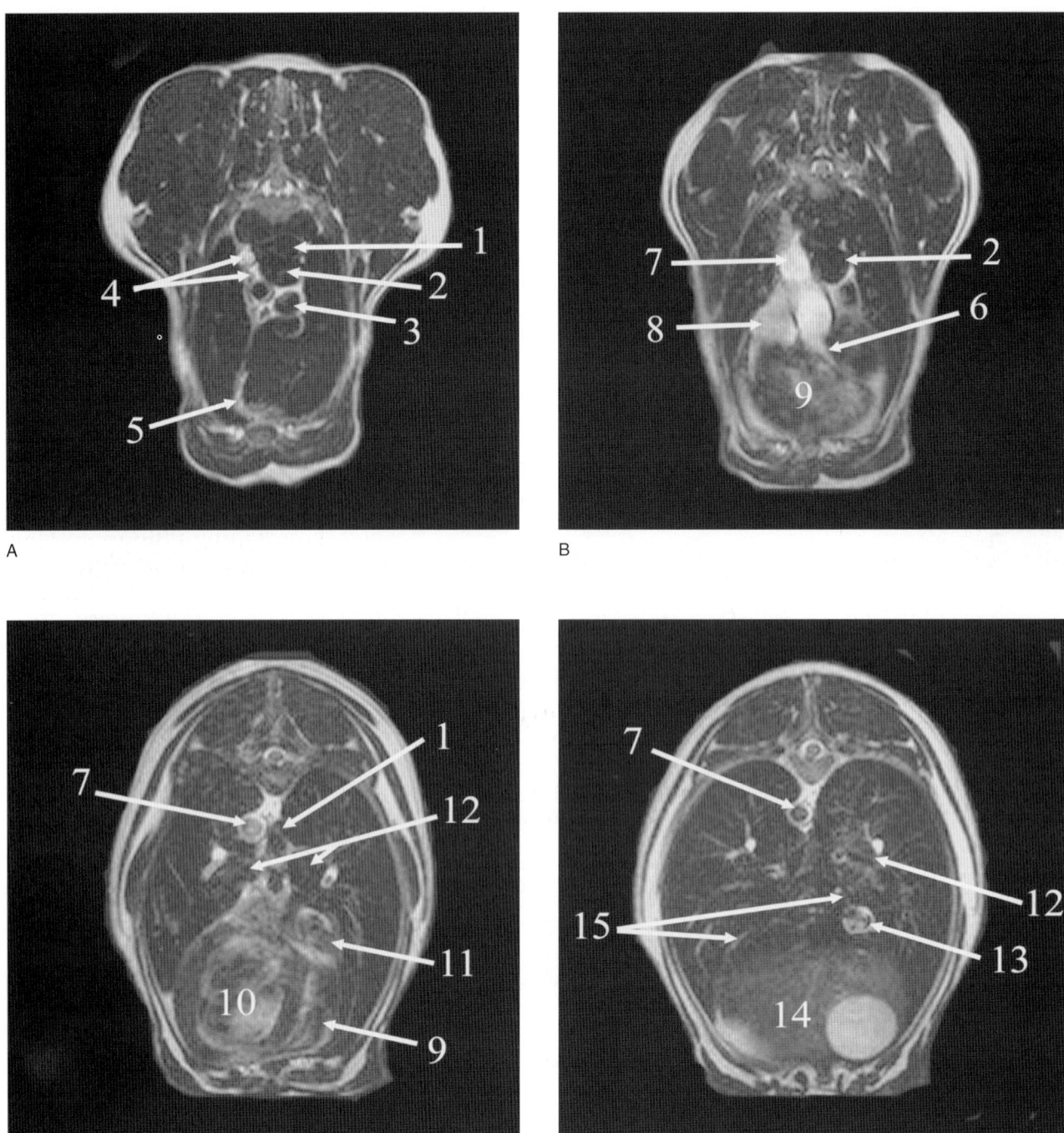

Figure 5.3. 3(A)–(D) T2-weighted transverse images of the thorax acquired with respiratory and cardiac gating. (1) esophagus, (2) trachea left atrium, (3) cranial vena cava with ghosting artifact below in Figure 5.3(A) (4) brachiocephalic trunk and right subclavian artery, (5) fat in cranial mediastinum and location of sternal lymph nodes, (6) coronary artert, (7) aorta, (8) main pulmonary artery, (9) right ventricle, (10) left ventricle, (11) right atrium, (12) mainstem bronchi with paired pulmonary arteries and veins that are white and black respectively, (13) caudal vena cava, (14) liver and gall bladder, (15) caudal mediastium around the accessory lung lobe.

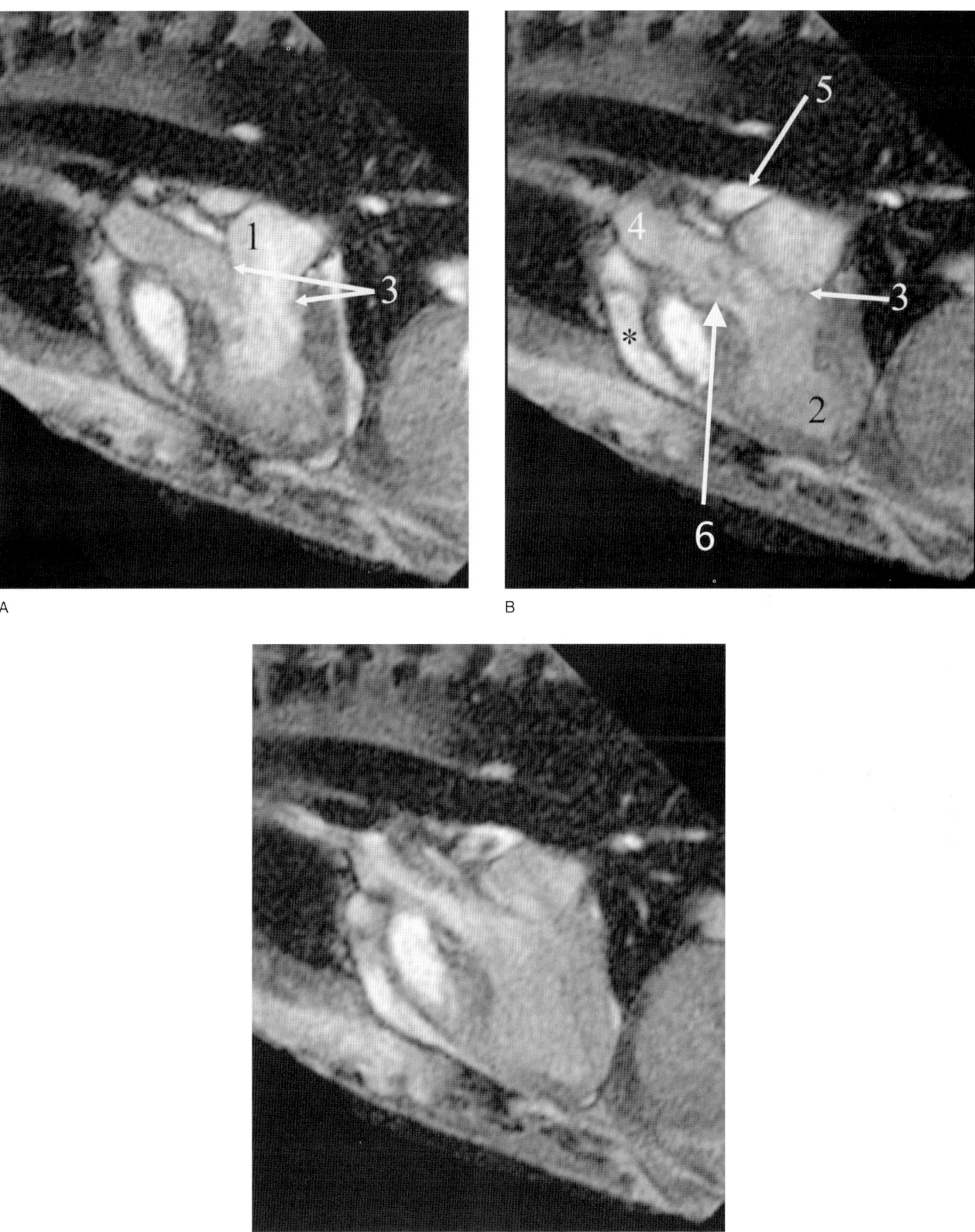

A

B

C

Figure 5.4. Single T2* sagittal image of the cardiac cycle, acquired as CINE loop. A small volume of pericardial fluid (*) star was noted in this patient. (A) Diastolic phase—white blood emptying from left atrium (1) into left ventricle (2) via the open atrioventricular valves (3). (B) Isovolumetric systolic phase—both the AV valve (3) and the aortic valve (6) are closed. The craniocaudal diameter of the left ventricle is reduced and the ventricular wall has increased thickness. The blood in the aorta is of intermediate signal intensity. White blood can be seen in the pulmonary artery (5). (C) Systolic phase—the aortic valve is open and white blood is flowing out.

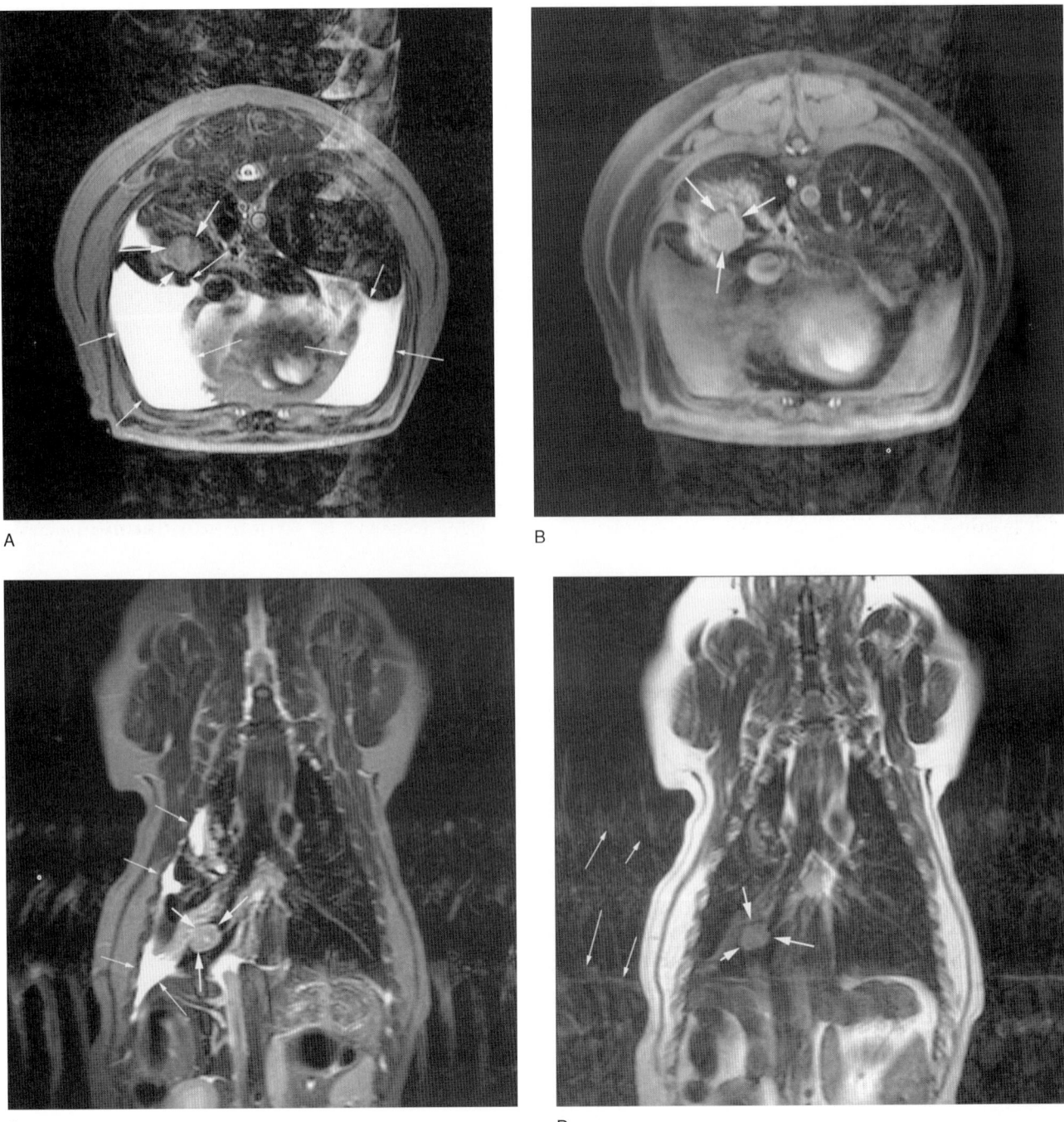

Figure 5.5. (A) T2-weighted fat-suppressed transverse image. Large arrows point to a mass within the pulmonary parenchyma. Small arrows point to the bilateral hydrothorax. The fluid appears homogenous and is dependent, as this patient was scanned in sternal recumbency. Notice the motion artifact from the heart in the background, both above and below the patient. (B) T1-weighted post-contrast image. Some enhancement of the mass can be seen (arrows). Note the enhancement in the heart and in the azygous vein dorsal and to the right of the aorta. The aorta has less enhancement due to high rates of flow. (C) T2-weighted fat-suppressed image in the dorsal plane. Again, fluid can be seen in the thorax with the small arrows, while the large arrows point to the mass. (D) T1-weighted transverse image prior to contrast. The majority of the mass is still readily seen on T1-weighted images without contrast due to the contrast differences between the aerated lung and the nodule. Small arrows point to the flow artifact and the breathing artifact. Obviously, in this case, the phase direction is left to right while in (A) and (B) the phase direction was ventrodorsal.

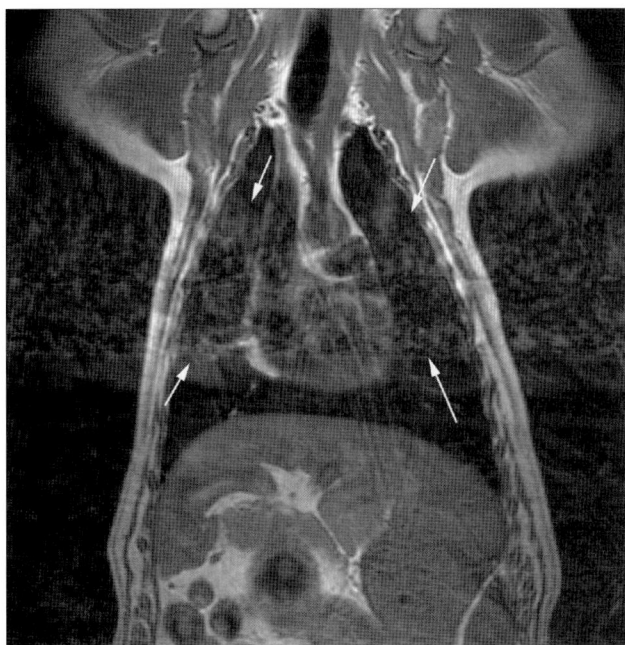

A

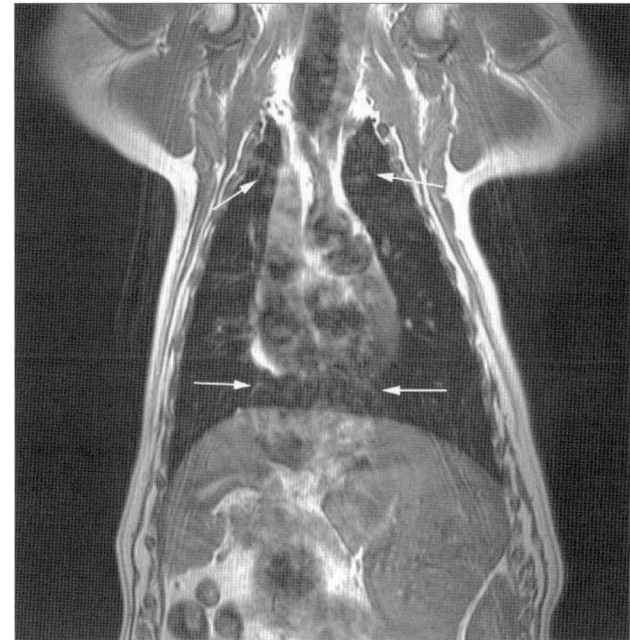

B

Figure 5.6.   Depiction of changing of phase direction to allow visualization of various parts of the lungs and other tissues of the thorax. (A) Phase is left to right. The flow artifact from the heart is shown with the arrows. Note how this can be seen outside of the patient. (B) The phase direction has been changed to head-to-tail. The flow artifact is now basically a midline artifact allowing visualization of the lung lateral to the heart. By swapping phase and frequency directions the entire thoracic cavity can be readily seen, even without sophisticated gaiting. Respiratory and cardiac gaiting and triggering can be done, but can greatly add to the imaging time.

place the cardiac motion artifact in different regions of the thorax (Figure 5.6).

CARDIAC

There are exciting clinical applications and research studies utilizing magnetic resonance for detection of human cardiac abnormalities. While cardiovascular disease, such as arteriosclerosis, is not common in veterinary patients, we have numerous cardiac anomalies and other conditions of the heart including neoplastic conditions which can be examined with MR. The use of gradient echo techniques to allow for rapid visualization can help limit motion artifact. Clear visualization can be obtained of the abnormalities, even without cardiac gaiting (Figures 5.7 and 5.8). The clear visualization of the abnormality, in reference to the anatomical structures, can provide the information needed to properly stage diseases. In our experience, the presence of pericardial effusion can severely hamper the detection of small lesions. The heart moves erratically in the fluid negating any benefit that may be achieved with cardiac gating.

MEDIASTINAL

Thymomas can often be surgically excised if they do not envelope the vasculature of the cranial mediastinum. Many times, the vasculature is merely displaced in a lateral direction from the thymic mass (Figure 5.9). In other types, the mass engulfs the vasculature precluding surgical excision (Figure 5.10).

PULMONARY

MR provides sufficient resolution of pulmonary masses to assess the potential for surgical or other treatments (Figure 5.11). Metastatic lesions can be readily detected when larger than a few millimeters in diameter. Lesions should always be confirmed in more than one plane and more than one type of sequence to avoid overinterpretation of various artifacts. Computed tomography remains the fastest and easiest way to visualize thoracic metastasis. MR can be utilized for this purpose, especially if the patient is already under general anesthesia and being scanned for another malignancy. Studies have shown good ability to detect lesions in the 5 mm

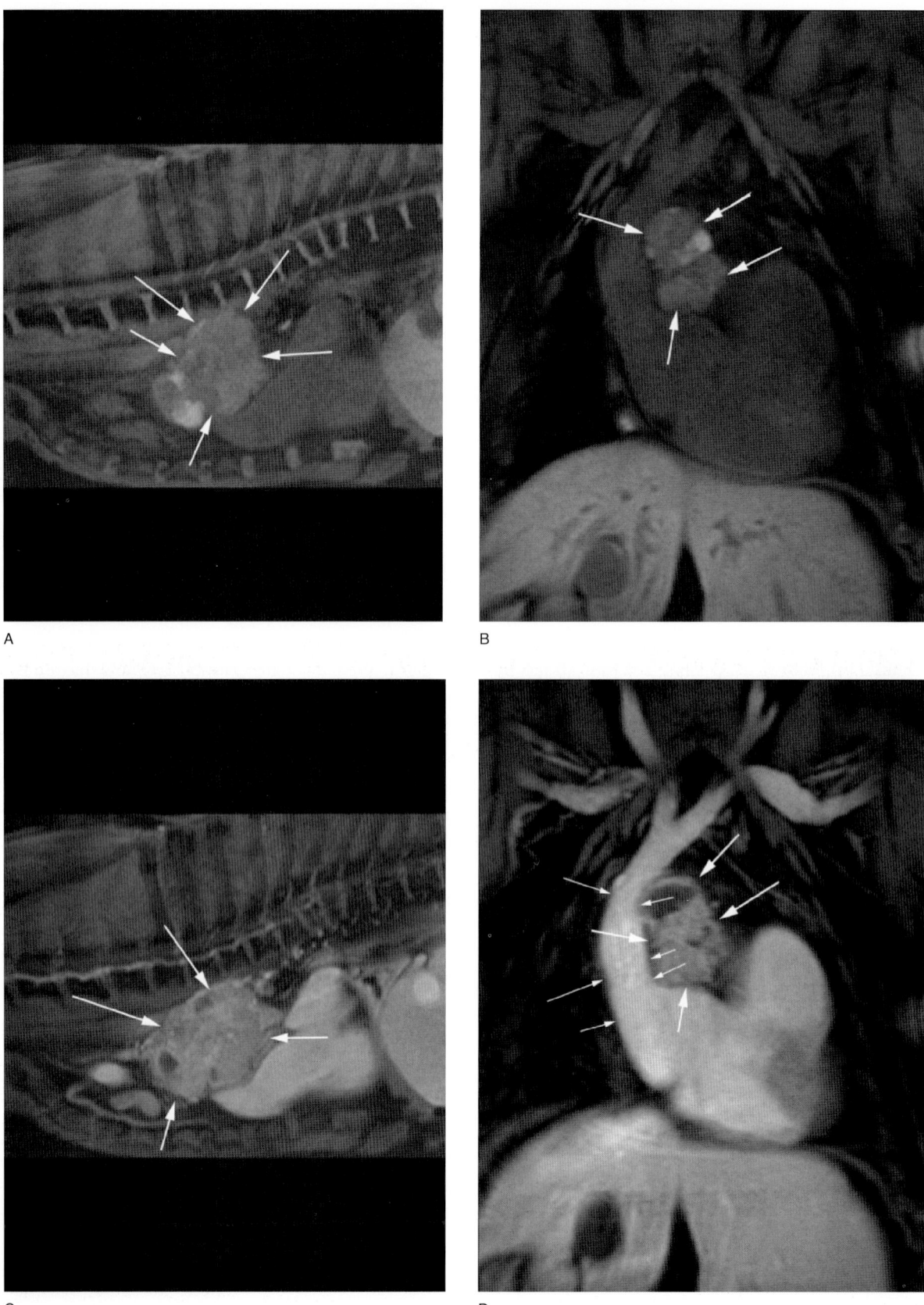

Figure 5.7. Aortic body tumor. (A) T1-weighted pre-contrast fat-suppressed gradient echo image. The mass is highlighted with arrows. (B) Dorsal plane, T1-weighted gradient echo image. The mass can be seen to the left of the aortic arch. (C), (D) T1-weighted gradient echo images post-contrast in the sagittal and dorsal planes, respectively. Mass is readily seen to contrast enhance in a heterogenous manner. Displacement of the aorta (small arrows) by the mass. Mass is readily seen in (D) with large arrows. Gradient echo imaging has less contrast than spin echo sequences, but can be very beneficial due to the high speed imaging for cardiac studies to reduce motion artifact.

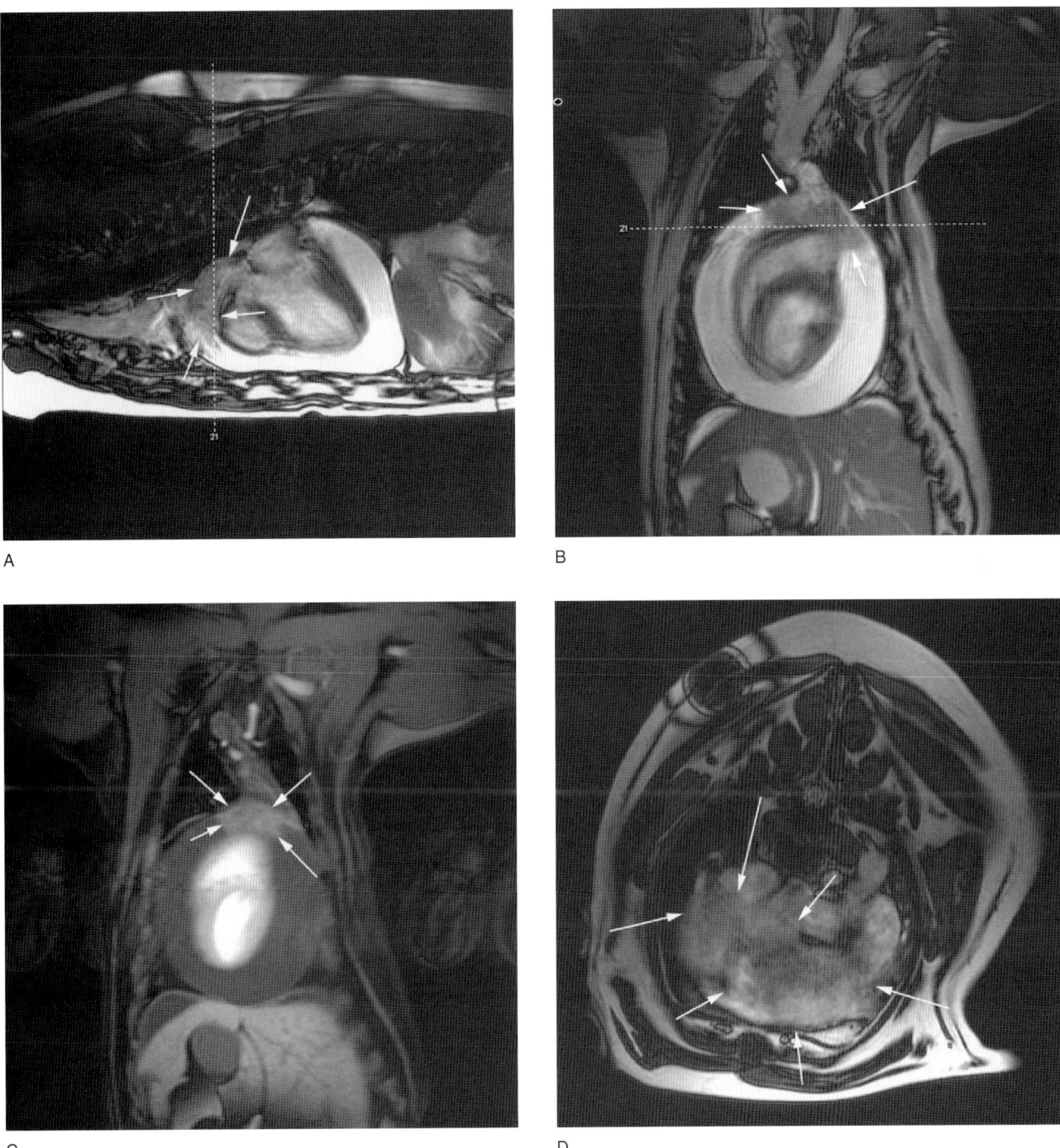

A

B

C

D

Figure 5.8. (A) T2-weighted gradient echo sequence in the sagittal plane. Large amount of fluid in the pericardial sac is readily seen. A mass can be seen, as indicated by the arrows, in the cranial aspect of the pericardial sac. The dotted line shows the slice orientation of (D). (B) T2-weighted gradient echo sequence in the dorsal plane. Again, the fluid in the pericardial sac is easily seen, as well as the mass in the cranial aspect of the sac. Dotted plane shows the slice orientation of (D). (C) T1-weighted post-contrast gradient echo sequence similar in location to (B). The pericardial fluid is now dark in this T1-weighted image, but the enhancement can be seen in the chambers of the heart, as well as enhancement of the mass in the cranial pericardial sac. On transverse imaging, this multilobulated mass in the cranial pericardial sac is seen on the transverse T2-weighted gradient echo sequence. This mass appeared to arise from the right auricle and was diagnosed as a hemangiosarcoma. While the pericardial fluid was readily seen with echocardiography, the mass was poorly visualized. Magnetic resonance imaging showed clear definition of the mass. The magnetic susceptibility artifact seen in the dorsal portion of the patient, parts (A) and (D), is from an identification chip. (D) T2-weighted gradient echo sequence in the transverse plane, located by the dotted line in (B). Arrows indicate the mass from the right auricle.

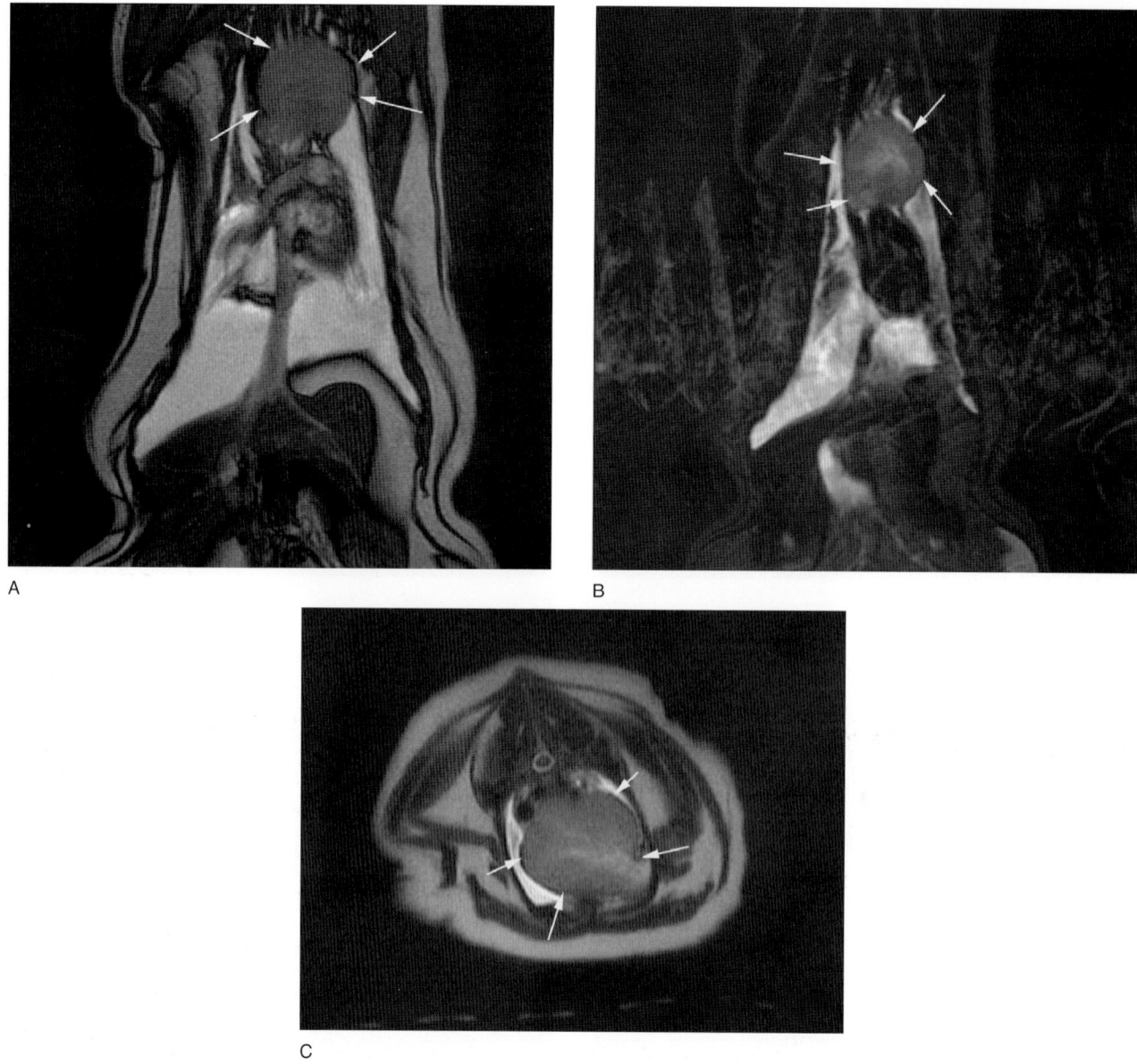

A

B

C

Figure 5.9. Benign thymoma. (A) T2-weighted gradient echo sequence. Arrows show the smooth margination and spherical appearance of the mass in the cranial mediastinum. Fluid can be seen within the thoracic cavity bilaterally. (B) STIR sequence of the thoracic cavity. The mass is readily seen, as is the fluid. Note the increased motion artifact in the STIR sequence. (C) T2-weighted transverse gradient echo sequence showing the smooth margination of the mass. The vascular structures are displaced dorsally by the mass, but they are not surrounded by the mass. This mass was surgically removed in a curative fashion.

diameter range. If the thorax is being visualized, certainly attempts to visualize metastatic nodules, if clinically indicated, will prove worthwhile (Figure 5.12).

Future Thoracic Imaging

Modern high field magnets can provide excellent images of thoracic diseases and should be considered with other imaging options. The superior soft tissue visualization can be of similar benefit in these organ systems. Advanced gating techniques allow for quantitative determination of flow velocities, volumes, and pressure gradients. Cine loops can be obtained in multiple planes. The larger field of view can allow for easier interpretation. With additional experience, this exciting area of investigation will expand to more veterinary imaging centers.

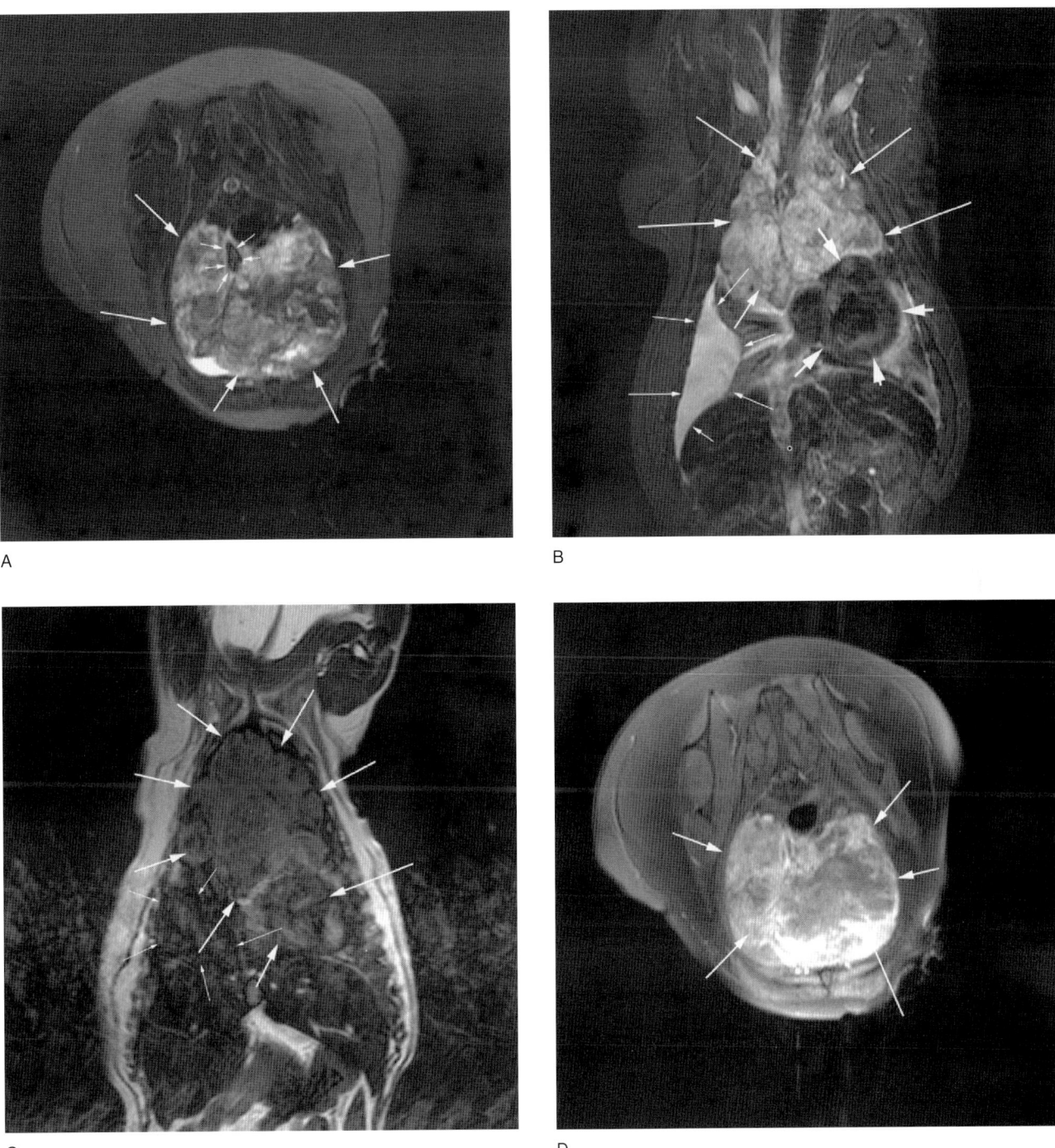

Figure 5.10. (A) T2-weighted gradient echo sequence of a large mass in the cranial mediastinum. The small arrows show the presence of the cranial vena cava within the mass. (B) T2-weighted gradient echo sequence in the dorsal plane. The large arrows show the large mass in the cranial mediastinal region. The small arrows show the presence of fluid within the thoracic cavity on the patient's right-hand side. The arrowheads show the heart being displaced caudally and to the left. (C) T1-weighted pre-contrast image in the same location as (B). Note how in T1-weighted image, while the large mass can be seen, the heart and fluid cannot be seen on T1-weighted. (D) Following the administration of contrast, it shows the heterogenous enhancement of the mass. The mass was proven a thymic carcinoma. The visualization of the vena cava being surrounded by the mass precluded surgical resection.

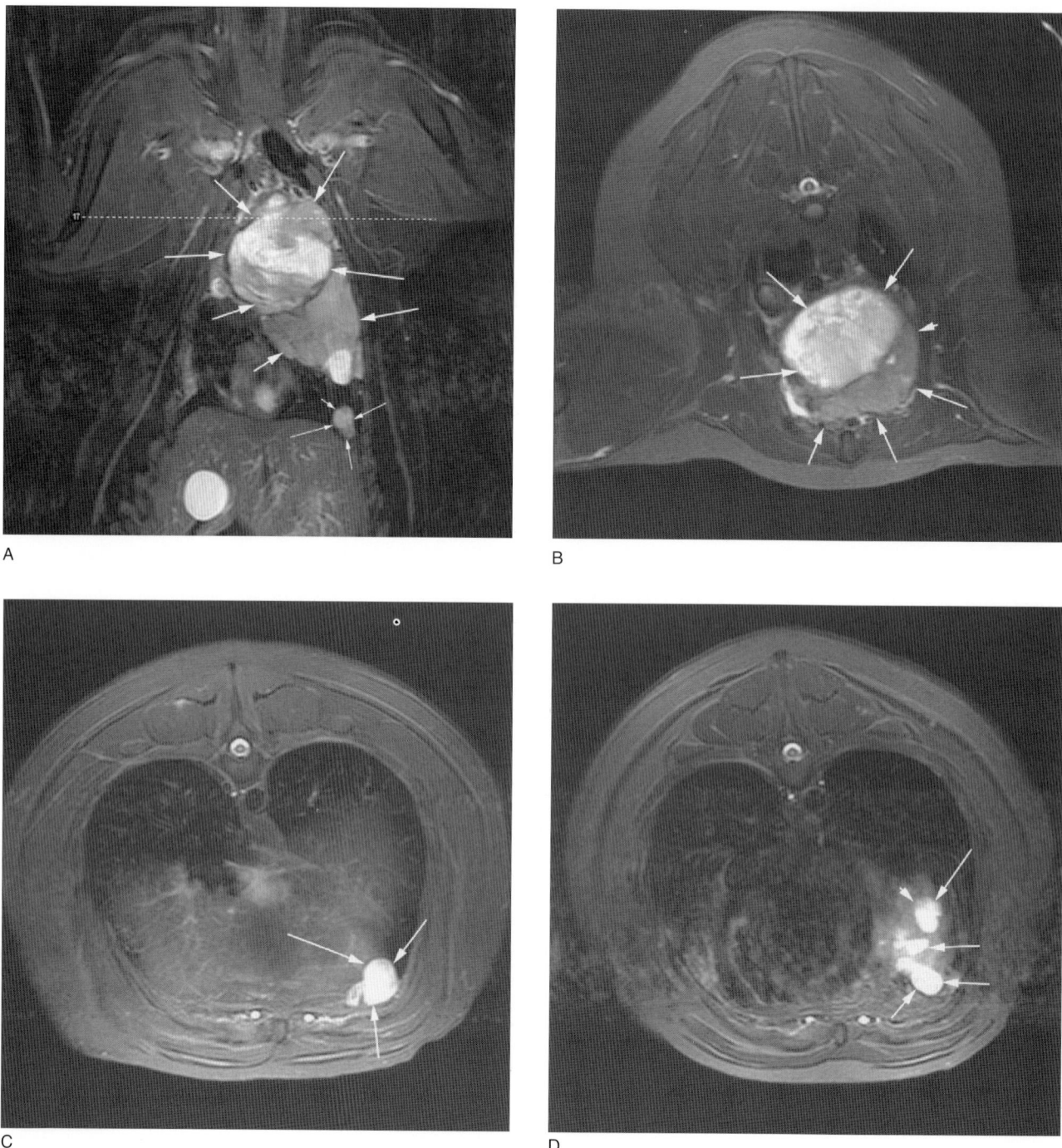

Figure 5.11. Study of a patient with a known large pulmonary mass on radiographs. MR was done to obtain clear visualization of margins for surgical resection. (A) A large heterogenous mass can be seen on the T2-weighted gradient echo sequence in the dorsal plane. Small arrows show the presence of an additional separate lesion within the pulmonary parenchyma. (B) T2-weighted transverse gradient echo image through the large mass. (C) T2-weighted gradient echo sequence through one of the additional masses close to the diaphragm, which was the same mass pointed to by the small arrows in (A). (D) Sequence more cranial, adjacent to the heart. Multiple masses can be seen in the patient's left lung. The discovery of a presumed metastatic mass precludes surgery for a curative procedure.

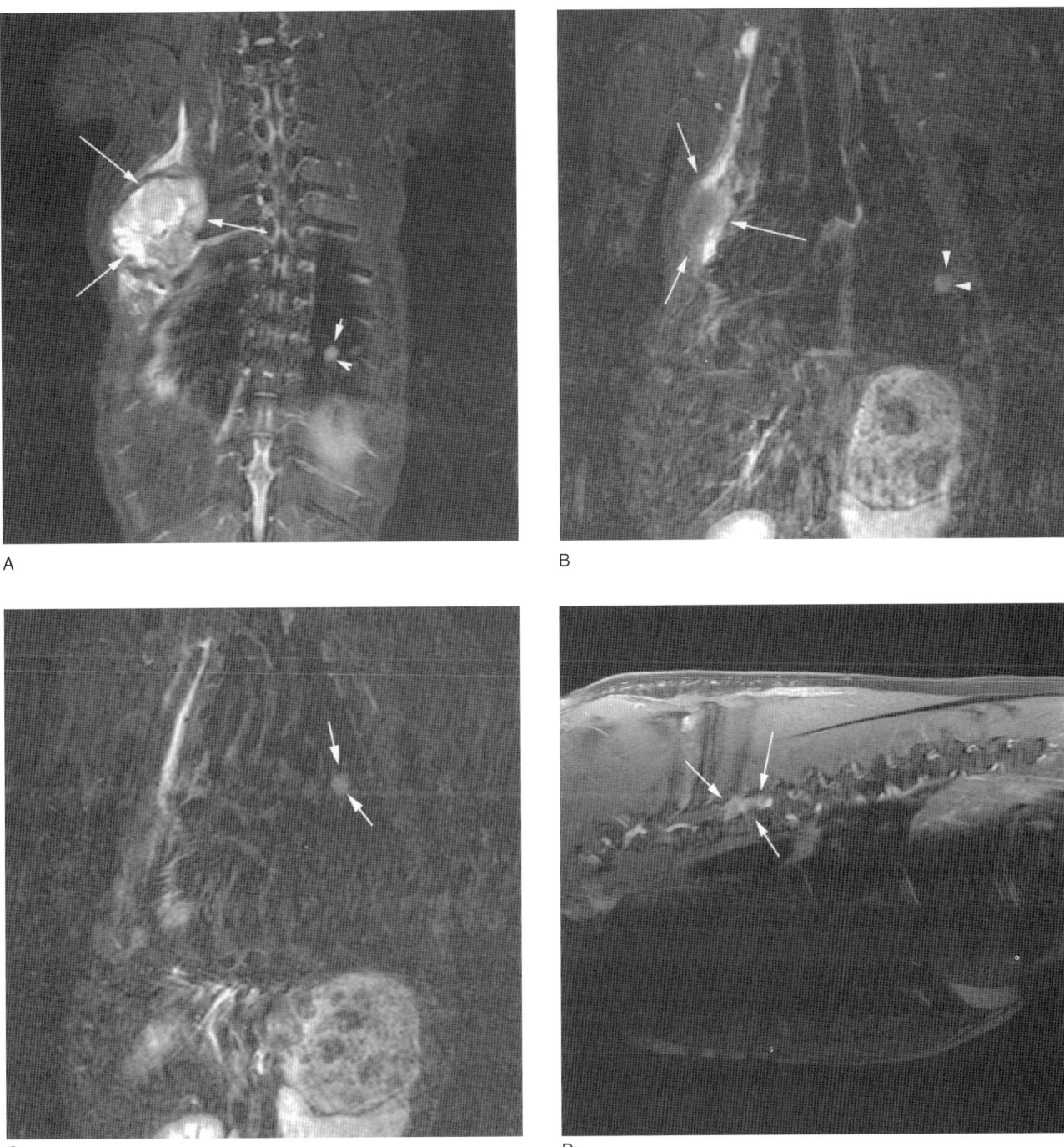

Figure 5.12.   Known mass of the right thoracic wall. Study was done to assess for surgical margins. (A) A large mass can be seen in this T2-weighted fat-suppressed spin-echo sequence. Small arrowheads show the presence of a suspected mass within the pulmonary parenchyma. Some flow artifacts would make this diagnosis suspect. (B), (C) On subsequent examination at different planes, additional pulmonary masses were readily identified. (D) Presence of a mass within the spinal canal in the cranial thoracic spinal column. Presence of pulmonary metastasis, as well as a spinal metastasis, again precluded unnecessary surgery in a curative fashion.

BIBLIOGRAPHY

Aletras AH, Tilak GS, Natanzon A, Hsu LY, Gonzalez FM, Hoyt RF, Jr, et al. 2006. Retrospective determination of the area at risk for reperfused acute myocardial infarction with T2-weighted cardiac magnetic resonance imaging: histopathological and displacement encoding with stimulated echoes (DENSE) functional validations. Circulation 113(15):1865–1870.

Amundsen BH, Helle-Valle T, Edvardsen T, Torp H, Crosby J, Lyseggen E, et al. 2006. Noninvasive myocardial strain measurement by speckle tracking echocardiography: validation against sonomicrometry and tagged magnetic resonance imaging. J Am Coll Cardiol 47(4):789–793.

Chetboul V, Tessier D, Borenstein N, Delisle F, Zilberstein L, Payen G, et al. 2003. Familial aortic aneurysm in Leonberg dogs. J Am Vet Med Assoc 223(8):1159–1162, 1129.

Choi BW. 2006. Differentiation of acute myocardial infarction from chronic myocardial scar with MRI. Korean J Radiol 7(1):1–3.

Dickfeld T, Kato R, Zviman M, Lai S, Meininger G, Lardo AC, et al. 2006. Characterization of radiofrequency ablation lesions with gadolinium-enhanced cardiovascular magnetic resonance imaging. J Am Coll Cardiol 47(2):370–378.

Ferreira AJ, Peleteiro MC, Correia JH, Jesus SO, and Goulao A. 2005. Small-cell carcinoma of the lung resembling a brachial plexus tumour. J Small Anim Pract 46(6):286–290.

Flacke S, Fischer S, Scott MJ, Fuhrhop RJ, Allen JS, McLean M, et al. 2001. Novel MRI contrast agent for molecular imaging of fibrin: implications for detecting vulnerable plaques. Circulation 104(11):1280–1285.

Hsu LY, Natanzon A, Kellman P, Hirsch GA, Aletras AH, and Arai AE. 2006. Quantitative myocardial infarction on delayed enhancement MRI. Part I: animal validation of an automated feature analysis and combined thresholding infarct sizing algorithm. J Magn Reson Imaging 23(3):298–308.

Huynh TV, Bergin CJ, Hauschildt J, Konopka RG, Bloor C, and Buxton R. 1996. Magnetic resonance detection of acute pulmonary emboli in a canine model with pathologic correlation. Acad Radiol 3(12):1019–1024.

Koie H, Kurotobi EN, and Sakai T. 2000. Double-chambered right ventricle in a dog. J Vet Med Sci 62(6):651–653.

Lee DC and Klocke FJ. 2006. Magnetic resonance approaches and recent advances in myocardial perfusion imaging. Curr Cardiol Rep 8(1):59–64.

Liu Y, Sun L, Huan Y, Zhao H, and Deng J. 2006. Effects of basic fibroblast growth factor microspheres on angiogenesis in ischemic myocardium and cardiac function: analysis with dobutamine cardiovascular magnetic resonance tagging. Eur J Cardiothorac Surg 30(1):103–107.

Morino S, Toba T, Araki M, Azuma T, Tsutsumi S, Tao H, et al. 2006. Noninvasive assessment of pulmonary emphysema using dynamic contrast-enhanced magnetic resonance imaging. Exp Lung Res 32(1–2):55–67.

Shea SM, Fieno DS, Schirf BE, Bi X, Huang J, Omary RA, et al. 2005. T2-prepared steady-state free precession blood oxygen level-dependent MR imaging of myocardial perfusion in a dog stenosis model. Radiology 236(2):503–509.

Simor T, Gaszner B, Oshinski JN, Waldrop SM, Pettigrew RI, Horvath IG, et al. 2005. Gd(ABE-DTTA)-enhanced cardiac MRI for the diagnosis of ischemic events in the heart. J Magn Reson Imaging 21(5):536–545.

Storey P, Chen Q, Li W, Seoane PR, Harnish PP, Fogelson L, et al. 2006. Magnetic resonance imaging of myocardial infarction using a manganese-based contrast agent (EVP 1001–1): preliminary results in a dog model. J Magn Reson Imaging 23(2):228–234.

Su MY, Head E, Brooks WM, Wang Z, Muggenburg BA, Adam GE, et al. 1998. Magnetic resonance imaging of anatomic and vascular characteristics in a canine model of human aging. Neurobiol Aging 19(5):479–485.

Tsekos NV, Woodard PK, Foster GJ, Moustakidis P, Sharp TL, Herrero P, et al. 2002. Dynamic coronary MR angiography and first-pass perfusion with intracoronary administration of contrast agent. J Magn Reson Imaging 16(3):311–319.

Vignaud A, Rodriguez I, Ennis DB, DeSilva R, Kellman P, Taylor J, et al. 2006. Detection of myocardial capillary orientation with intravascular iron-oxide nanoparticles in spin-echo MRI. Magn Reson Med 55(4):725–730.

Vilar JM, Arencibia A, Ramirez JA, Gil F, Latorre R, Morales I, et al. 2003. Magnetic resonance imaging of the thorax of three dogs. Vet Rec 153(18):566–568.

Vite CH, Insko EK, Schotland HM, Panckeri K, and Hendricks JC. 1997. Quantification of cerebral ventricular volume in English bulldogs. Vet Radiol Ultrasound 38(6):437–443.

Wagner A, Mahrholdt H, Thomson L, Hager S, Meinhardt G, Rehwald W, et al. 2006. Effects of time, dose, and inversion time for acute myocardial infarct size measurements based on magnetic resonance imaging-delayed contrast enhancement. J Am Coll Cardiol 47(10):2027–2033.

Wray JD and Blunden AS. 2006. Progressive dysphagia in a dog caused by a scirrhous, poorly differentiated perioesophageal carcinoma. J Small Anim Pract 47(1):27–30.

Yang J, Wan MX, and Guo YM. 2004. Pulmonary functional MRI: an animal model study of oxygen-enhanced ventilation combined with Gd-DTPA-enhanced perfusion. Chin Med J (Engl) 117(10):1489–1496.

CHAPTER SIX

HEAD—NON-CNS

Patrick R. Gavin and Shannon P. Holmes

ANATOMY

The entire head can be visualized with magnetic resonance. The common modality to study diseases, such as the nasal cavity, oral cavity, and the middle ear, has been computed tomography. The authors of this text are obviously MR zealots; however, we have found that the use of magnetic resonance generally provided superior imaging of all of these locations. Certainly, when it comes to diseases of the retrobulbar region, magnetic resonance far excels due to superior soft tissue visualization.

IMAGING PROCEDURE

The examination should utilize the strengths of magnetic resonance, that is, the ability to scan in all planes. Therefore, all diseases involving structures such as the nasal cavity should scan from the tip of the nose back through at least the mid portion of the brain (caudal aspect of the skull), at least on the dorsal and sagittal planes. The transverse planes can be localized to the disease process as seen on the previous two planes.

Sequences utilized generally entail STIR sequences for their high sensitivity to the detection of pathologic abnormalities and T1-weighted images before and after contrast. Other than STIR sequences, T2-weighted fat-suppressed images can offer much of the same information. Fat suppression is more difficult to uniformly obtain and that is why most studies utilize the STIR sequence in the nasal cavity. Generally, only one plane prior to contrast is required. These sequences will allow clear visualization of the nasal cavity, retroocular spaces, and the middle ear. In addition, the draining lymph nodes of these regions are also well seen. All structures are clearly visualized (Figure 6.1).

At times, special sequences are utilized. In the case of the ocular studies, it is generally best to perform the T1 post-contrast with fat saturation. One post-contrast without fat saturation should always be acquired. In the case of the middle and inner ear examinations, it is often preferable to perform a very highly T2-weighted sequence to better visualize the cochlear apparatus and the semicircular canals.

NASAL CAVITY

In the nasal cavity, clinicians are often looking for the etiology for a nasal discharge, including epistaxis. The basic rule outs for epistaxis are idiopathic hemorrhage (including that from high blood pressure), nasal infections, nasal fungal infections, and nasal neoplasia. The sequences offered allow clear visualization between obstructive fluid within the sinuses and any obstructing mass. Fungal disease is characterized by loss of turbinates and thickened mucosa, often with the presence of a fungal granuloma within the sinuses. Other diseases can cause loss of turbinates, including chronic bacterial rhinitis; however, it is not accompanied by the thickened mucosa seen with fungal rhinitis (Figure 6.2). Non fungal rhinitis is often characterized by ventral dependence within the nasal cavity that is often bilateral (Figure 6.3).

On rare occasion, a foreign body can be seen associated with the rhinitis. Most foreign bodies are too small to be readily detected. Foreign bodies larger than the size of a grain of rice would be readily detected. Most foreign bodies do not have mobile protons and, therefore, have a low signal intensity on all sequences. Most foreign bodies would be surrounded by an inflammatory fluid and therefore, in T2-weighted images (including STIR), there is a dark mass surrounded by a bright fluid. If contrast is used, then the dark foreign body would be surrounded by a dark fluid and a ring of contrast-enhancing inflammatory tissues.

Nasal neoplasia is generally characterized by turbinate destruction, osseous lysis, and extension into surrounding tissues. The extension can be seen into the frontal sinus, maxillary sinus, and/or sphenoid sinus. In addition, the extension can be seen into the nasal

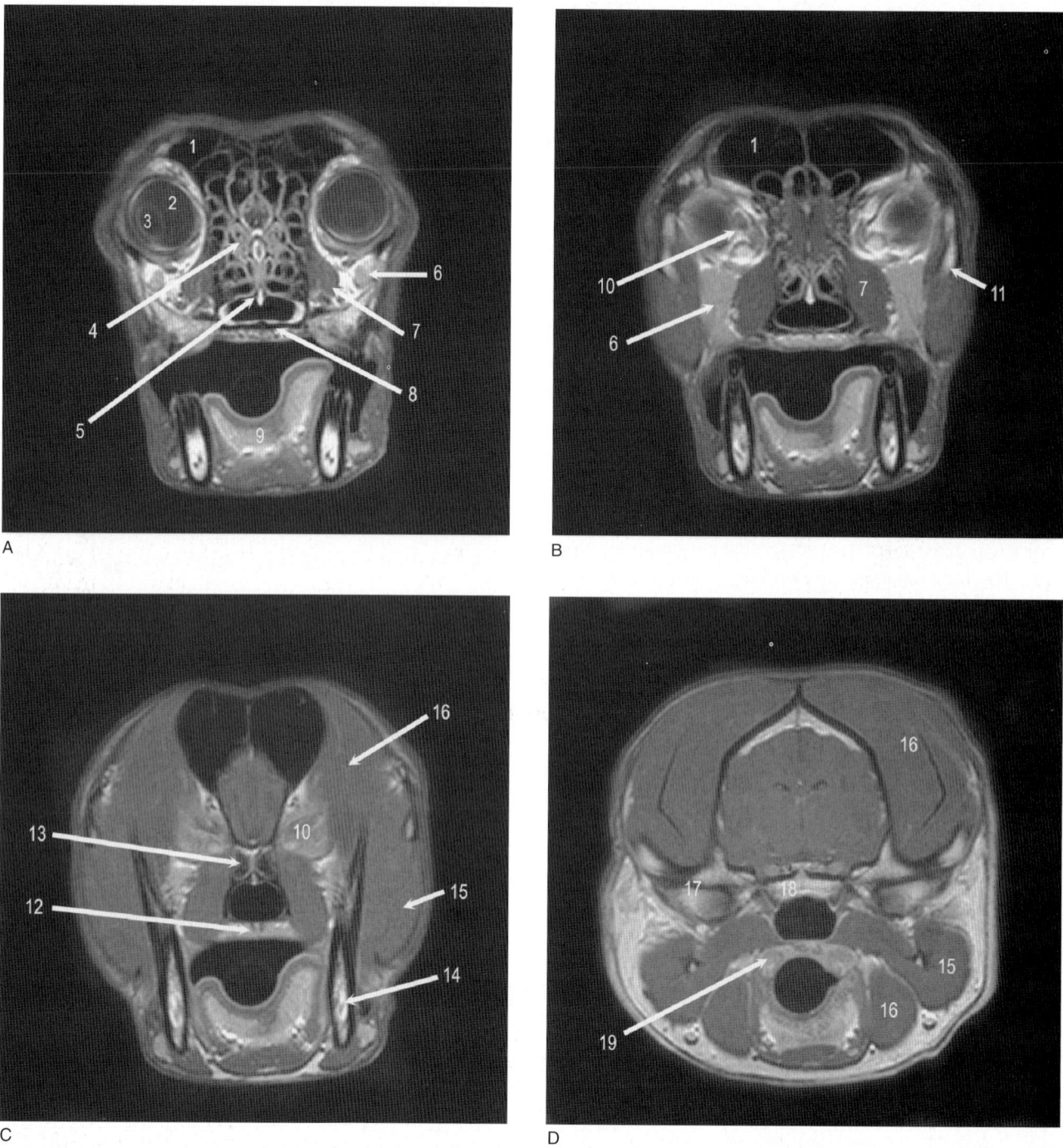

Figure 6.1.   Normal anatomy. (A–F) T1-weighted transverse images of the skull of a dog. (G), (H) T2-weighted sagittal images of the skull of a cat. (I)–(K) T1-weighted images in the dorsal plane of a dog skull. (1) Frontal sinus, (2) vitreous of eye, (3) lens of eye, (4) ethmoid turbinates, (5) vomer at ventral aspect of nasal septum, (6) zygomatic salivary gland, (7) medial pterygoid muscle, (8) hard palate, (9) tongue—being deformed by endotracheal tube, (10) optic nerve and its associated venous plexus within extraocular musculature, (11) zygomatic arch, (12) soft palate, (13) sphenopalatine sinus, (14) mandible, (15) masseter muscle, (16) temporal muscle, (17) temporomandibular joint, (18) basisphenoid bone, (19) tonsilar lymph tissue, (20) tympanic bulla, (21) external auditory meatus, (22) parotid salivary gland, (23) mandibular salivary gland, (24) mandibular lymph nodes, (25) basihyoid of hyoid apparatus, (26) longus capitus muscle, (27) tooth roots, (28) medial retropharyngeal lymph node.

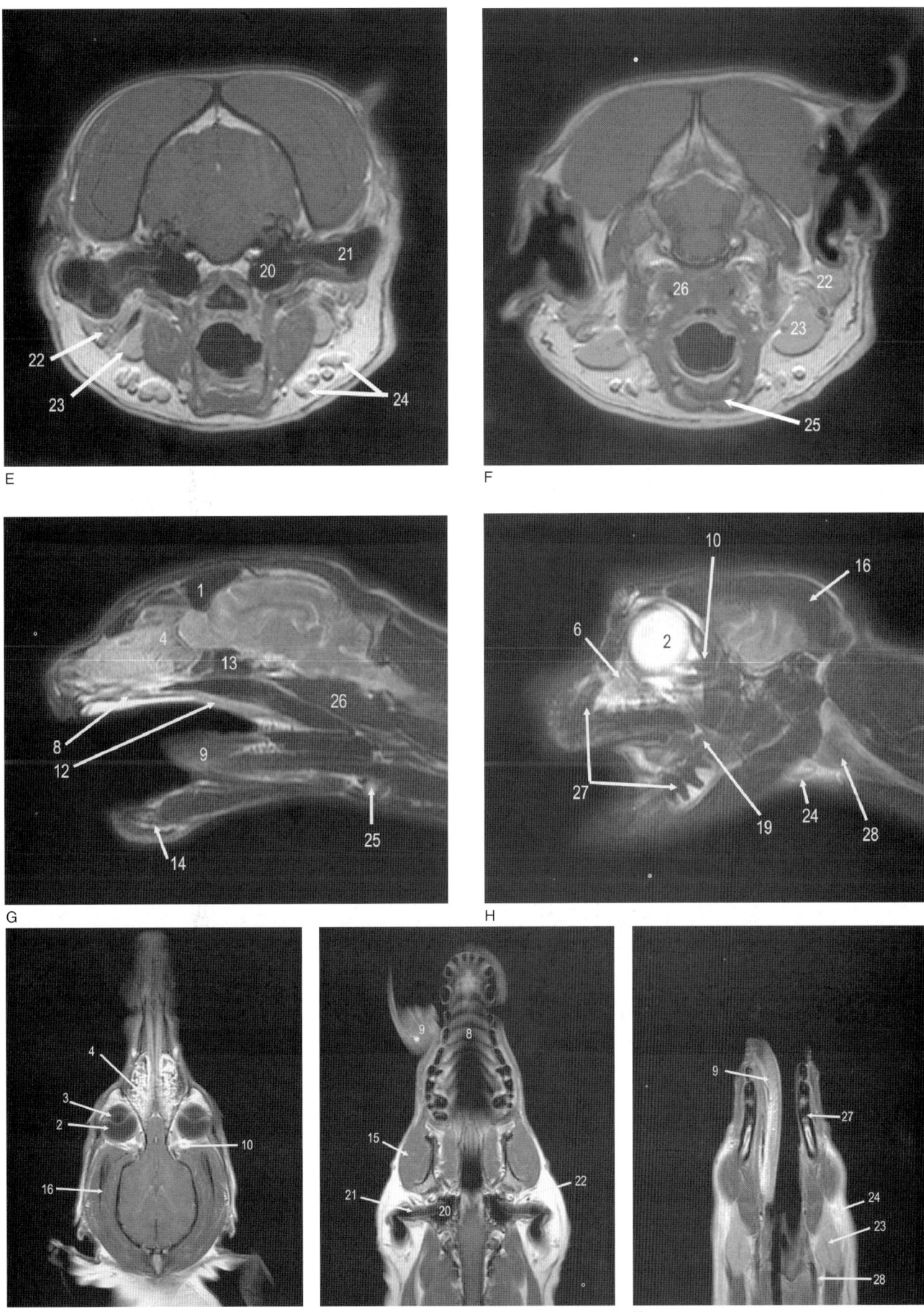

Figure 6.1. (*Continued*)

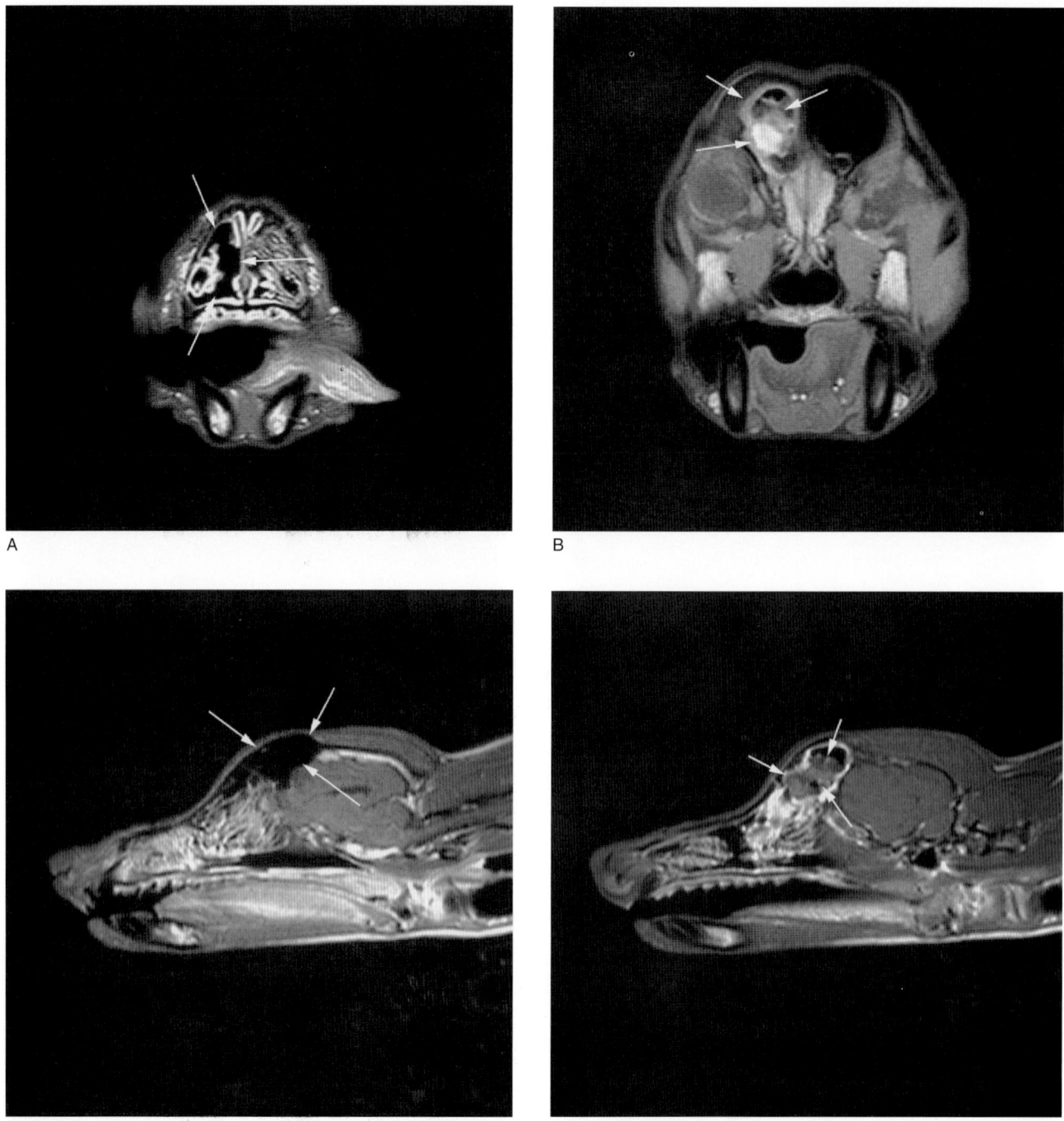

A

B

C

D

Figure 6.2. Fungal rhinitis. (A) T2-weighted transverse imaging showing turbinate lysis and mucosal thickening. (B) Presence of a fungal granuloma in the right frontal sinus and mucosal thickening in a T1-weighted pre-contrast image. (C) Contralateral aerated frontal sinus on the left side in a T2-weighted sagittal image. (D) T1-weighted post-contrast fat-suppressed image showing the frontal granuloma and the contrast enhancement of the mucosa in the right frontal sinus.

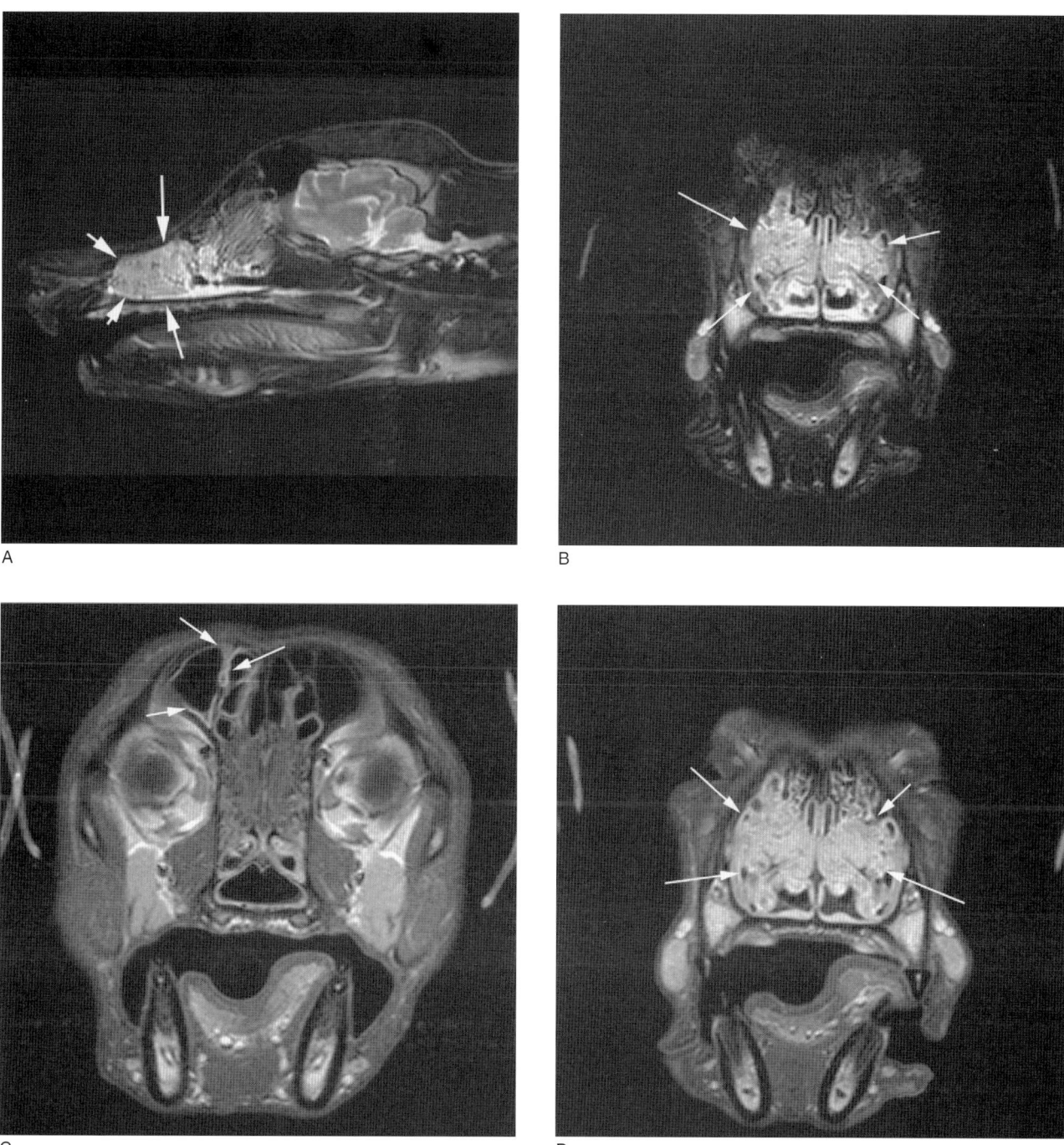

Figure 6.3. Inflammatory rhinitis. (A) T2-weighted sagittal sequence showing increased signal intensity of the nasal cavity. (B) T2-weighted transverse imaging showing the dependence of the increased signal intensity. Patient was scanned in sternal recumbency. (C) The mucosal thickening of the right front sinus. (D) T1-weighted post-contrast study showing the enhancement of the mucosa. The normal nasal mucosa enhances avidly, as does the area associated with the hyperintensity. Such bilateral dependent conditions are due to an inflammatory condition. Biopsies and/or cultures are needed to ascertain if they are infectious.

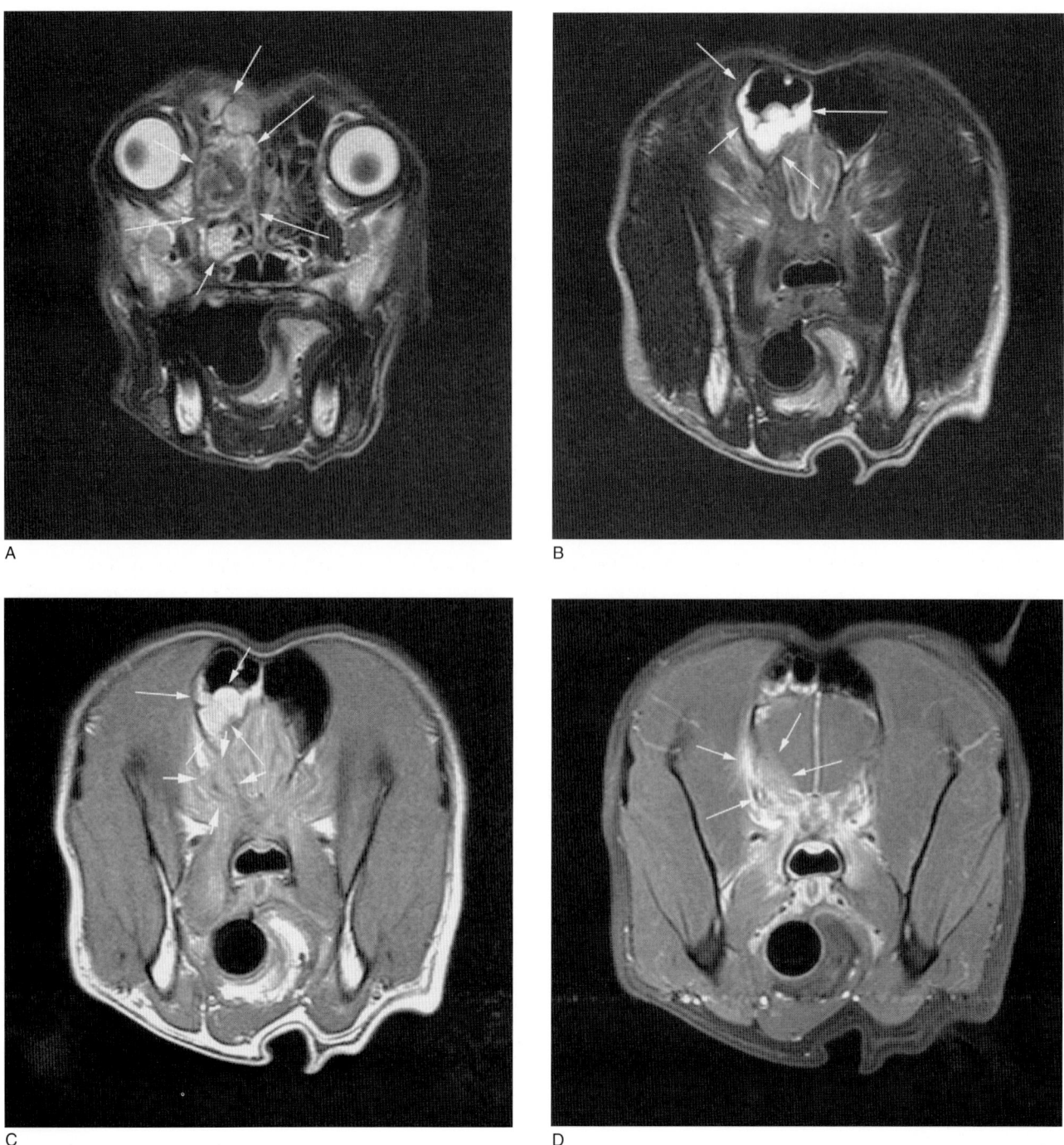

Figure 6.4.   Nasal neoplasm. (A) T2-weighted transverse imaging showing the heterogenous mass in the right nasal cavity and intensities in the right frontal sinus. (B) Slice caudal—showing the increased signal intensity in the right frontal sinus. This lobulated appearance is one of tissue, since there is no air/fluid level. (C) T1-weighted post-contrast enhancement of the area seen in (B). There is avid enhancement of the mass within the nasal cavity. (D) Showing the presence of contrast enhancement involving the meningeal surface of the rostral right brain. This contrast enhancement shows the presence of breaching of the cribriform plate and calvarium.

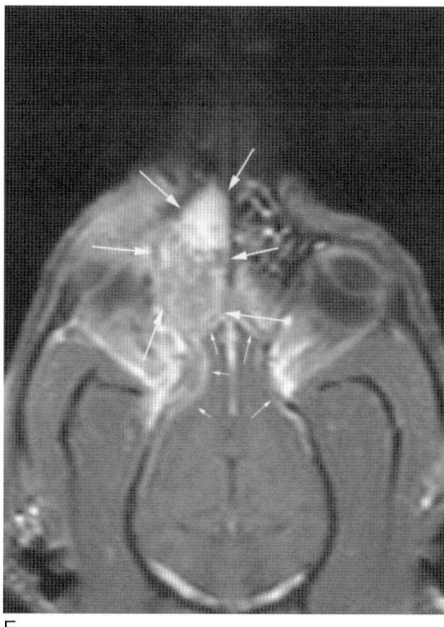 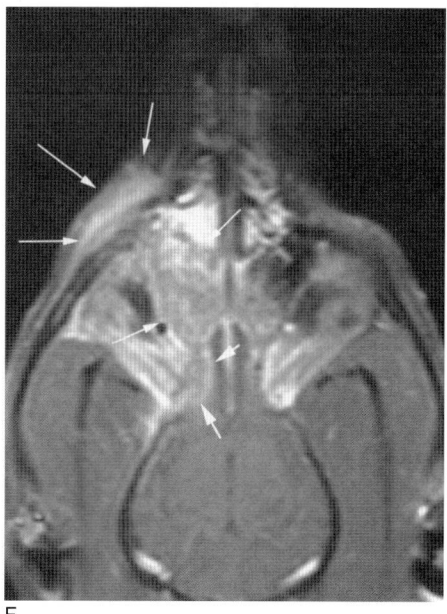

E   F

Figure 6.4. (*Continued*) (E), (F) T1-weighted post-contrast dorsal plane images. The mass in the right nasal cavity is readily seen in both images, and the breaching of the cribriform plate and calvarium with the enhancement encroaching onto the meningeal surface of the rostral right brain is readily seen.

cavity and/or the brain. The cribriform plate is not a linear flat structure as the name would imply. The cribriform plate is a complex curved structure. Therefore, the only clear visualization of the cribriform plate comes with MR examination in the sagittal and dorsal planes. The use of contrast enhancement is often of benefit in detecting cribriform plate extension, as an inflammatory meningitis is the first stage seen with cribriform plate penetration (Figure 6.4).

There can be a homogenous mass in nasal cavity and nasal pharynx extending via the auditory tube into the middle ear. These are termed nasal-pharyngeal polyps (Figure 6.5).

ORAL CAVITY

When studying diseases of the oral cavity, the soft tissue extent of disease is much better delineated with the use of magnetic resonance. When comparing studies with paired CT and magnetic resonance, the lesion is virtually always larger based on the changes in the soft tissues, as visualized with MR. Computed tomography has a difficult time detecting contrast enhancement compared to the normally very vascular oral mucosal tissues, while MR visualizes the chemical structure of the tissues. The electronic density of a soft tissue mass, compared to the surrounding local soft tissues,

would be virtually identical. Therefore, when there is no reason to expect significant contrast enhancement, computed tomography is limited to merely viewing the osseous involvement. With MR, contrast is utilized to visualize the extent of vascularity and the degree of viable tissue compared to nonviable or necrotic tissue (Figures 6.6 and 6.7).

The knowledge of anatomy is often challenged with MR due to the visualization of all tissues and the uncommon loss of symmetry can be a challenge. There can be considerable variation with the appearance of the salivary glands (Figure 6.8).

Not all masses are neoplastic, and with MR the appearance of the tissues and their association with the surrounding soft tissue can help determine if lesions are non-neoplastic and inflammatory (Figure 6.9). Sialocoele can occur in many locations and when the zygomatic salivary gland is involved the appearance on MR helps secure the diagnosis (Figure 6.10). It should be stressed that MR does not replace biopsy and histopathology; if there is any doubt from imaging, those procedures are often necessary.

Dental structures are hypointense on all sequences due to the lack of multiple protons. However, the tooth, including the roots, can be clearly seen due to the intensity differences between the teeth and the surrounding alveolar bone. Therefore, dental disease can be detected. Dental tumors can be readily detected, and the gross extent of the lesion clearly identified. The

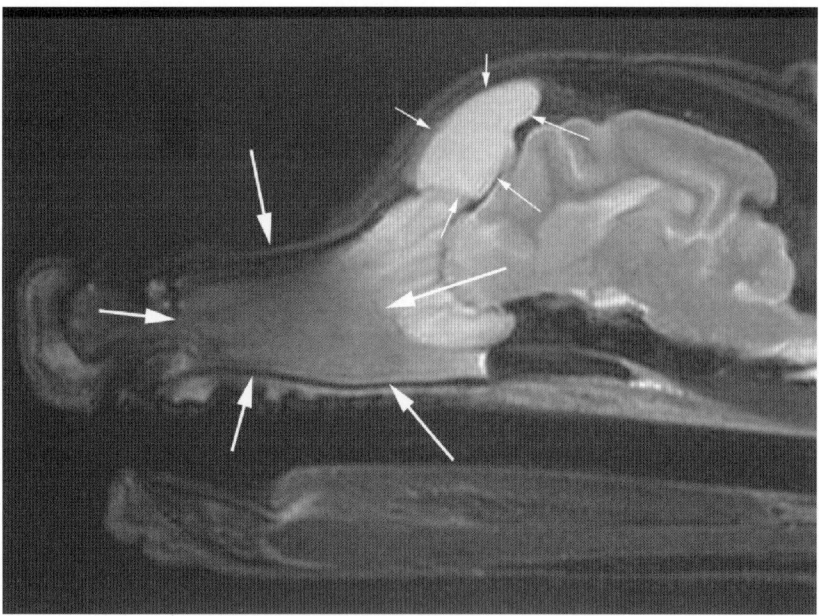

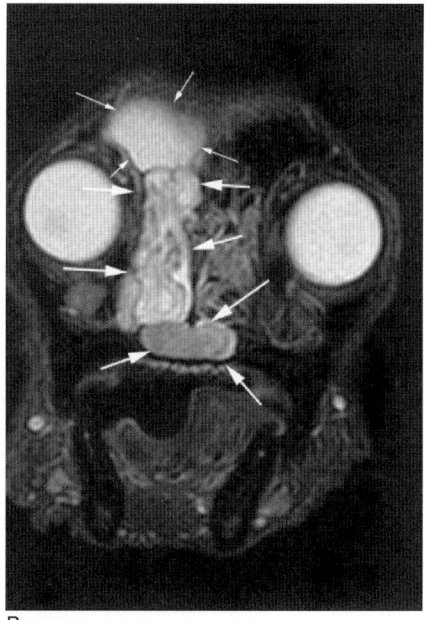

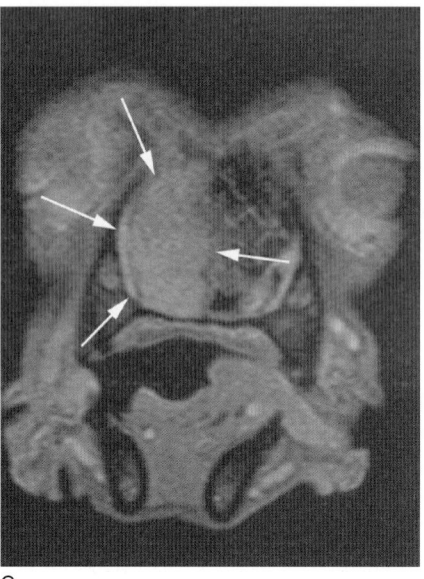

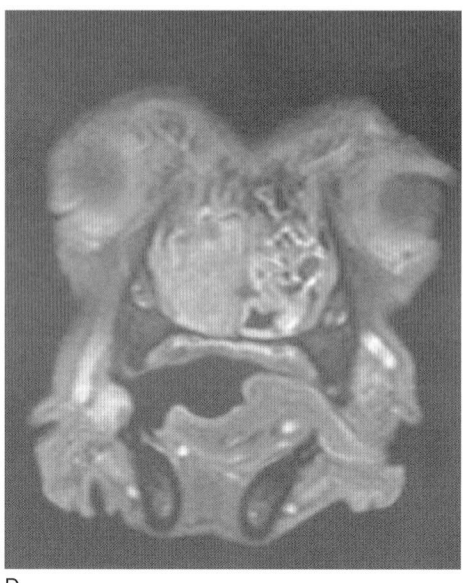

Figure 6.5. Nasal pharyngeal polyp. There is a hyperintensity in T2-weighted sagittal image. (A) There is some heterogeneity to the signal. (B) Showing the increased hyperintensity in the right nasal cavity, the right frontal sinus, and also within the nasal pharynx (larger long arrows). T1-weighted images prior to contrast (C) and post-contrast (D), showing minimal to no enhancement of the tissue within the nasal cavity, as compared to the enhancement of the normal tissues. This homogeneity of the signal in the nasal cavity, without turbinate destruction and without enhancement, is typical of a nasal pharyngeal polyp.

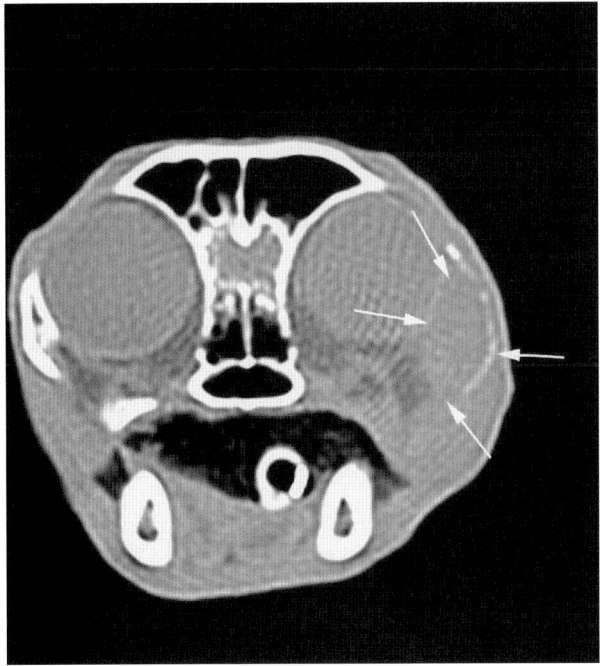
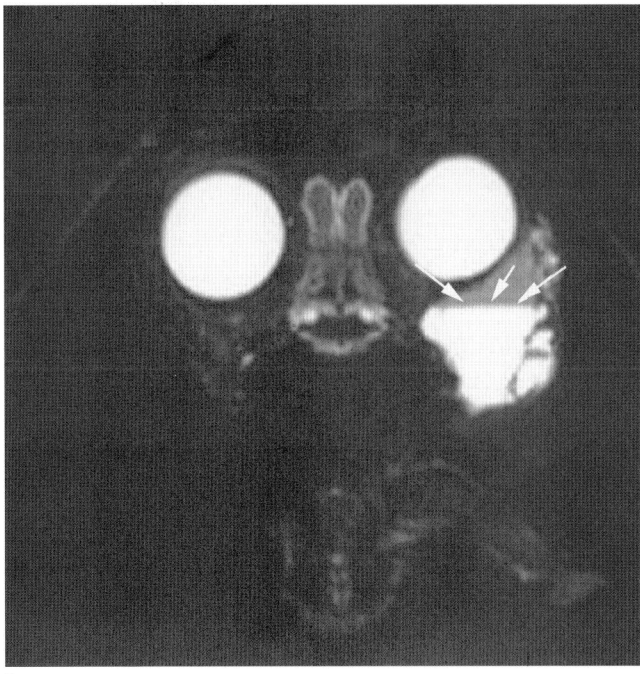

A   B

Figure 6.6.   (A) CT Examination of a cat with "mass" involving the left zygomatic arch region. Lysis and destruction of the zygomatic arch is highlighted with the arrows. This was presumed neoplastic on CT examination. This area did not enhance differently than the surrounding normal tissue. (B) MR STIR transverse sequenced through this similar area. The fluid sediment level could be readily seen, as highlighted by the arrows. Such a homogenous fluid with sediment would be highly indicative of a hematoma or abscess. An abscess with osteomyelitis was confirmed in this case.

study of the head and oral cavity should always include the regional lymph nodes, which would include the mandibular, parotid, and retropharyngeal lymph node structures. Any involvement of the lymph nodes helps lead one to a narrower differential diagnosis (Figure 6.11).

Small, difficult to detect lesions such as tonsillar carcinomas, can often be appreciated both from direct visualization as well as from the metastatic involvement of the regional lymph nodes. In addition to the tonsil, all oral structures including the various structures of the tongue, gingiva, and mucosal surfaces are readily evaluated.

Soft tissue extension beyond midline, in the absence of osseous changes, is better seen with magnetic resonance. At times, the use of contrast enhancement is of little benefit, as the normal mucosa of the nasal and oral cavities is richly vascular and at times, the neoplastic conditions actually enhance less than the corresponding normal tissue. However, contrast is still utilized to determine if the lesion is viable and vascularized.

EXTERNAL, MIDDLE, AND INNER EAR

Magnetic resonance is equally adaptive to viewing all structures of the auditory system, including the external, middle, and inner ear. Sequences utilized are similar to those listed; however, additional sequences that involve highly T2-weighted images are useful to view the cochlear and semicircular canal structures of the inner ear. There are numerous cases of fluid within the middle ear, unilaterally or bilaterally, that are probably not associated with an active infectious condition. In these cases, the fluid is seen on STIR or T2-weighted sequences without any evidence of contrast enhancement to suggest an inflammatory component. This is often called otitis media effusion by our physician colleagues. Such a condition is commonly seen in animals with trigeminal nerve tumors with marked muscle atrophy due to denervation. These animals presumably lose normal function of the auditory tube (eustachian

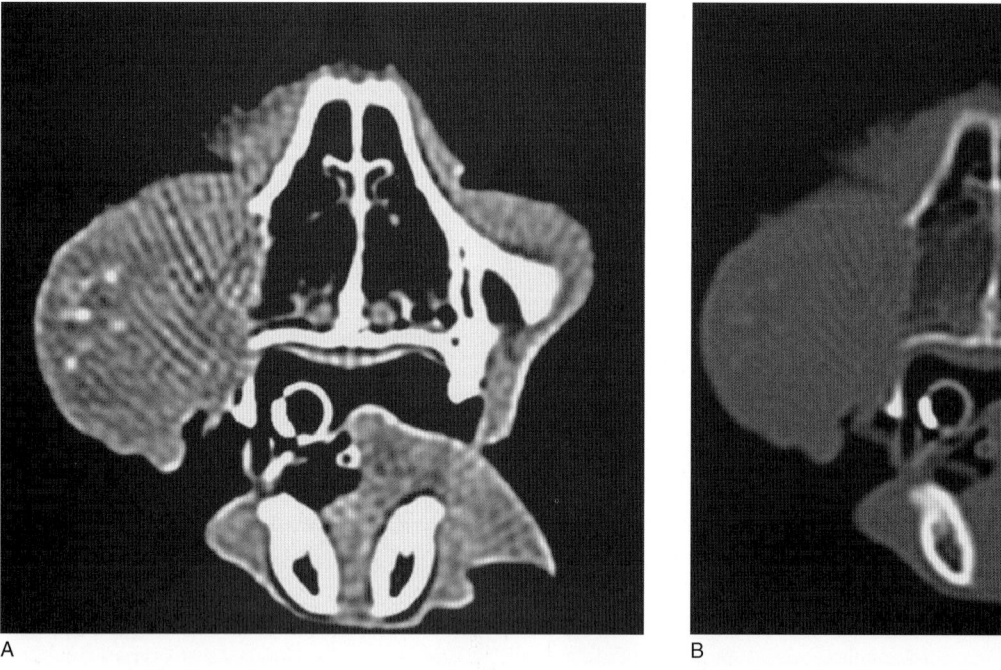

A

B

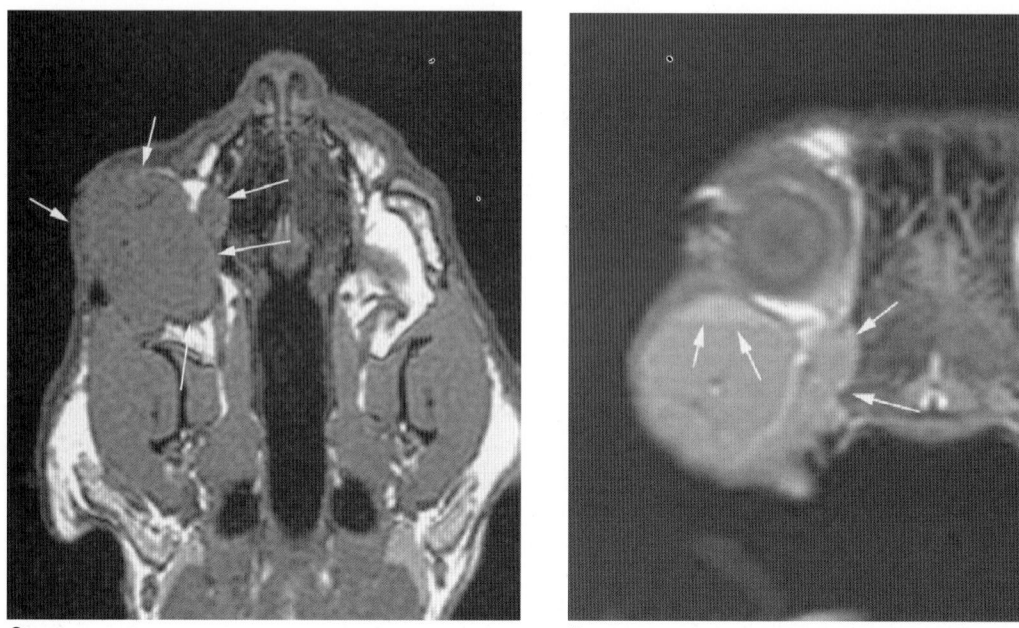

C

D

Figure 6.7. (A), (B) Transverse computed tomographic images through the maxilla. (A) is a soft tissue window and (B) is a bone winder. Lysis of the maxilla is readily seen in both images. The presence of small dense areas within the mass is suggestive of mineralization. Presumptive diagnosis of a carcinoma or adenocarcinoma is made. (C) MR examination of the same patient is a T1-weighted dorsal plane image. The mass is highlighted with the arrows. The lysis of the maxilla is readily seen as the normal maxilla has a high signal intensity on T1-weighted sequences due to the amount of fat within the bone marrow. The difference between the two sides is readily seen. (D) Following the administration of contrast, a T1-weighted transverse image shows no enhancement of the mass and a fluid/sediment level. This was another case of osteomyelitis with abscess formation that was accurately diagnosed on MR. MR has the ability to see osseous lysis as well as CT, but the increased information obtained from signal intensities of the various sequences can be highly useful in a differential diagnosis.

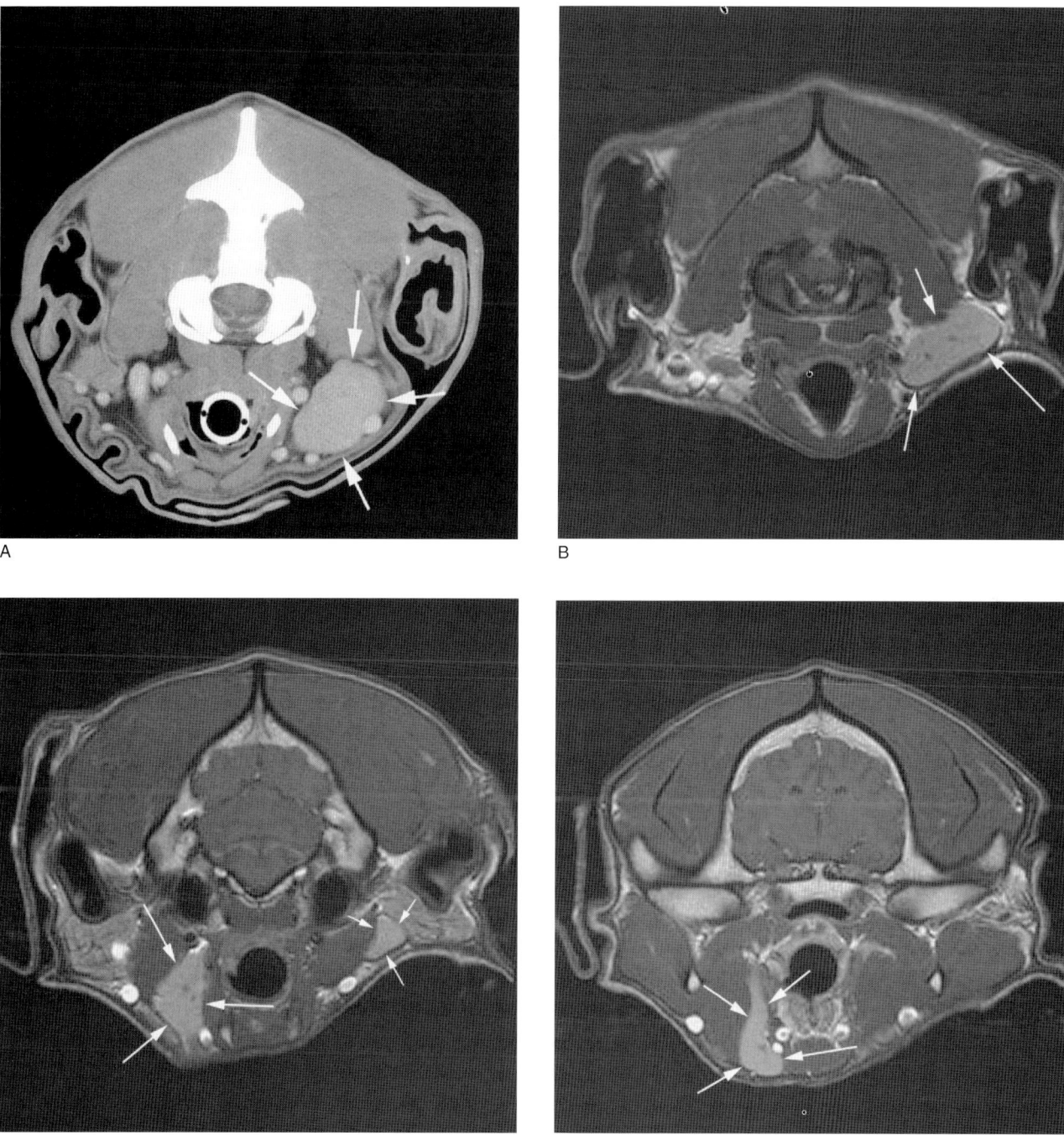

Figure 6.8. (A) CT examination through the atlantooccipital region. A mass was seen on the left side. This mass could also be palpated. Presumptive diagnosis was an enlarged lymph node or a neoplastic condition. (B)–(E) T1-weighted post-contrast MR examinations of this area. (B)–(D) Transverse images at different levels. (B) shows the presence of a normal mandibular salivary gland on the left-hand side. There is no corresponding mandibular salivary gland on the patient's right side. Rostral to (B) and (C) shows the presence of salivary gland. The normal mandibular salivary gland is almost out of view (small arrows). (D) This view is even more rostral through the region of the sella of the mid region of the brain. The sella can be seen in the ventral calvarial region. The arrows show the presence of the elongated mandibular salivary gland that is going into the sublingual region on the patient's right side. The dorsal plane view shows the presence of this aberrant right salivary gland, which is presumed to be a combination of a mandibular salivary gland and a sublingual salivary gland. This type of asymmetry of organs can be seen and obviously has no clinical significance. Computed tomography has the inability to distinguish tissue types compared to the rich information obtained from magnetic resonance imaging.

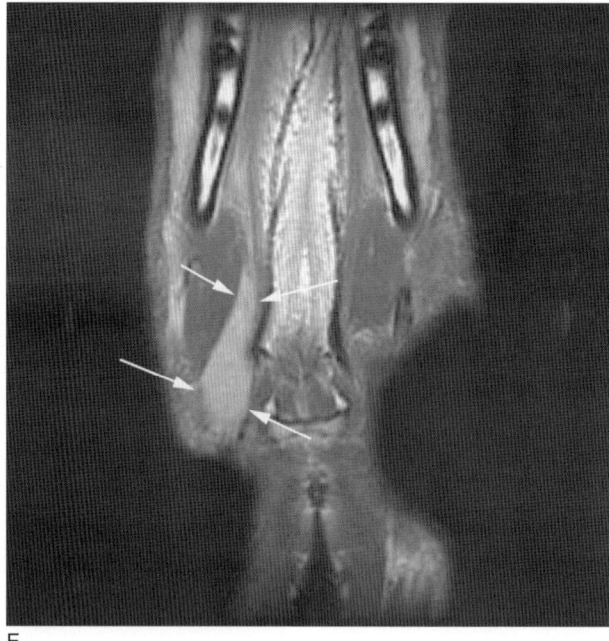

E

Figure 6.8. (*Continued*) (E) Dorsal plane T1 post contrast showing normal enhancement of the aberrant salivary gland.

tube), which most likely leads to fluid buildup within the middle ear.

Areas of otitis media often have higher protein content to the fluid, thickened contrast-enhancing membranes, and often an expansile appearance to the bullae (Figure 6.12). Otitis media that has ruptured through the bullae into the surrounding soft tissues is characterized by a diffuse, poorly marginated cellulitis myositis with regional lymphadenopathy (Figure 6.13). In contrast, neoplastic conditions of these structures are generally well marginated with more central enhancement and a lesser degree of lymphadenopathy (Figure 6.14). Obviously, biopsies with cytopathologic examination are needed to definitively diagnose any condition. However, the magnetic resonance appearance can allow the differential diagnosis to be heavily weighted toward a neoplastic or inflammatory condition. The clear visualization of the abnormalities can help guide the surgeon for either an incisional biopsy or for surgery for either a curative or cytoreductive nature.

ORBIT CONDITIONS

Areas of the orbit can be visualized with ultrasound. However, the ultrasound appearance of retrobulbar structures can be difficult to sort through when they are displaced and modified by pathologic change. The use of magnetic resonance allows clear visualization of all structures, including the palpebral region of the lacrimal gland (normal lacrimal gland not visualized), the zygomatic salivary gland, the interior chamber (posterior chamber), and all structures of the retrobulbar region (Figure 6.1).

Ocular muscles, vessels, and optic nerves are all well visualized. The optic nerve can be difficult to visualize in the normal state. Abnormalities to the optic nerve from either optic nerve neuritis or lesions, including meningioma of the optic nerve, are readily identified (Figure 6.15). Studies of the orbits generally rely heavily on STIR or T2 fat-suppressed images in all three basic planes. T1-weighted images before and after contrast should be performed with fat suppression, if at all possible, due to the large amount of fat present in the retrobulbar region (Figure 6.15). The zygomatic salivary gland is one that is often not considered in our differential diagnoses of orbital disease.

We have taken the liberty of using the zygomatic salivary gland to show the range of diseases that can occur from such an organ. Studies depicted include salivary gland tumors and sialocele (Figures 6.9 and 6.10, respectively). In addition, there can be normal but aberrant or anatomical variations in the placement of the salivary gland (Figure 6.8). These same basic disease processes can occur in any of the anatomical structures of the head. Therefore, with the optic nerve we can

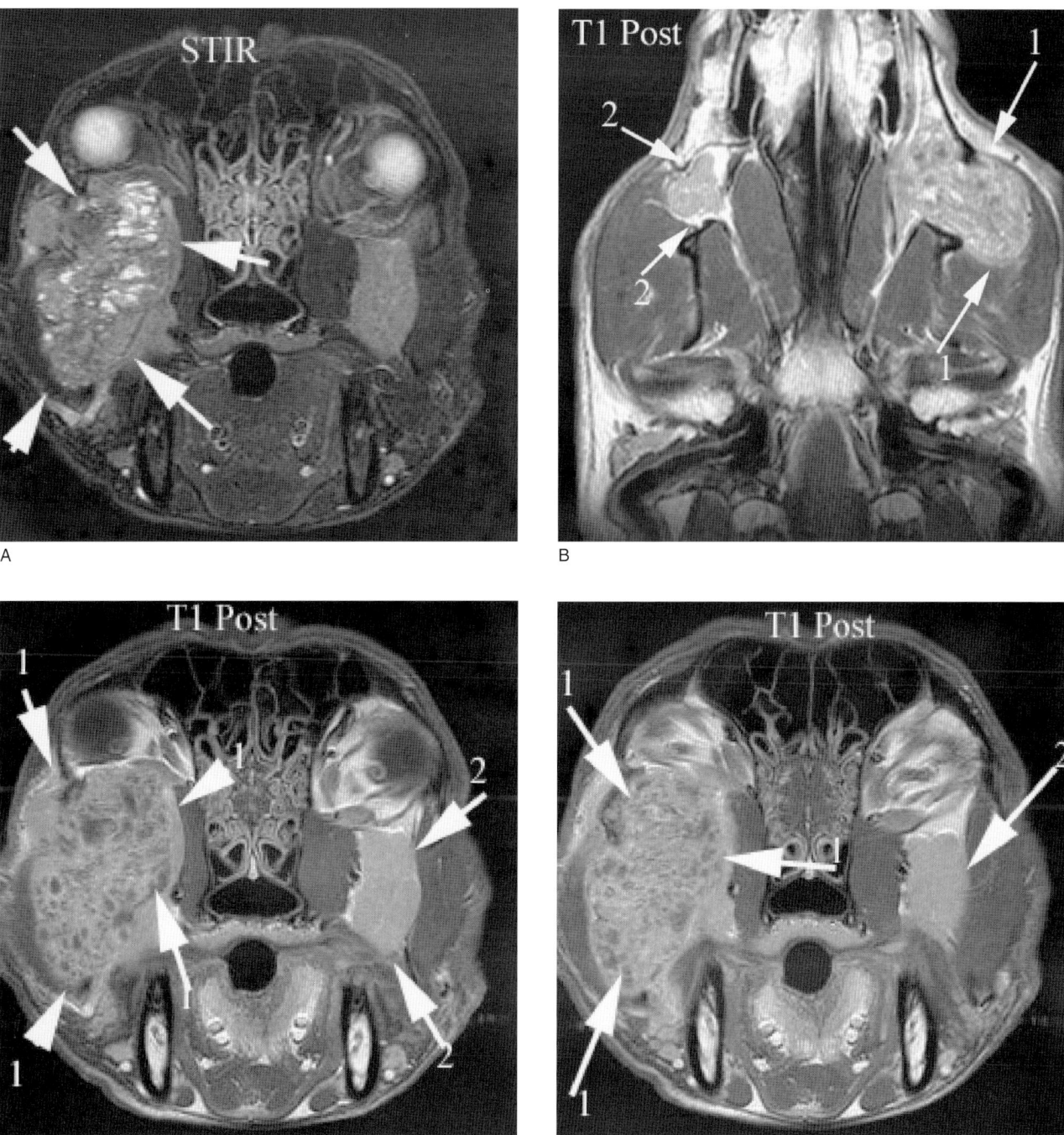

Figure 6.9. Salivary gland adenocarcinoma of the zygomatic salivary gland. (A) STIR sequence. The arrows point to the large mass. The contralateral side shows the normal zygomatic salivary gland. (B) The image is flipped such that the patient's right is to the viewer's right, in this case. Post-contrast image shows the presence of the mass that is indicated by 1, compared to the normal salivary gland, 2. (C) T1 post-contrast image with the normal position of the patient's right to the viewer's left. (D) Adjacent slice from (C), again showing the heterogeneity of the salivary gland mass. This was proven to be salivary carcinoma.

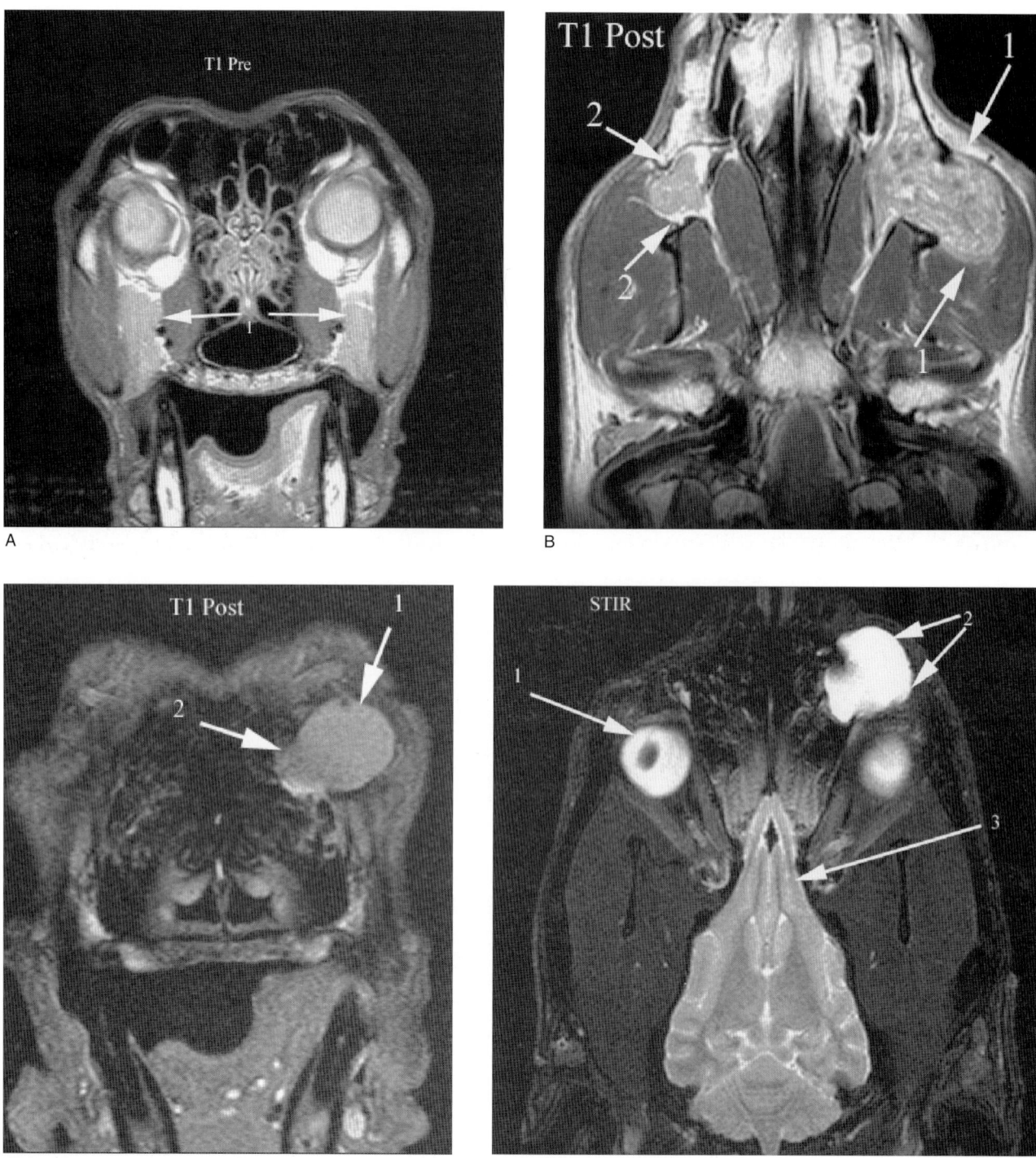

Figure 6.10. (A) T1-weighted pre-contrast image through the level of the zygomatic salivary glands. The arrows show the normal salivary glands. (B) Post-contrast fat-suppressed image showing the normal enhancement pattern of the salivary glands. (C) This view is a few slices rostral to (B). This T1-weighted post-contrast shows the presence of a homogenous spherical "mass." There is no contrast enhancement of this mass. (D) On the dorsal plane, STIR sequence the fluid signal of the mass is readily seen in 2. All fluids are bright on STIR sequences, including the vitreous of the eye (1) and of the cerebral spinal fluid around the brain (3). This fluid mass contained saliva and a diagnosis of a zygomatic sialocele was made.

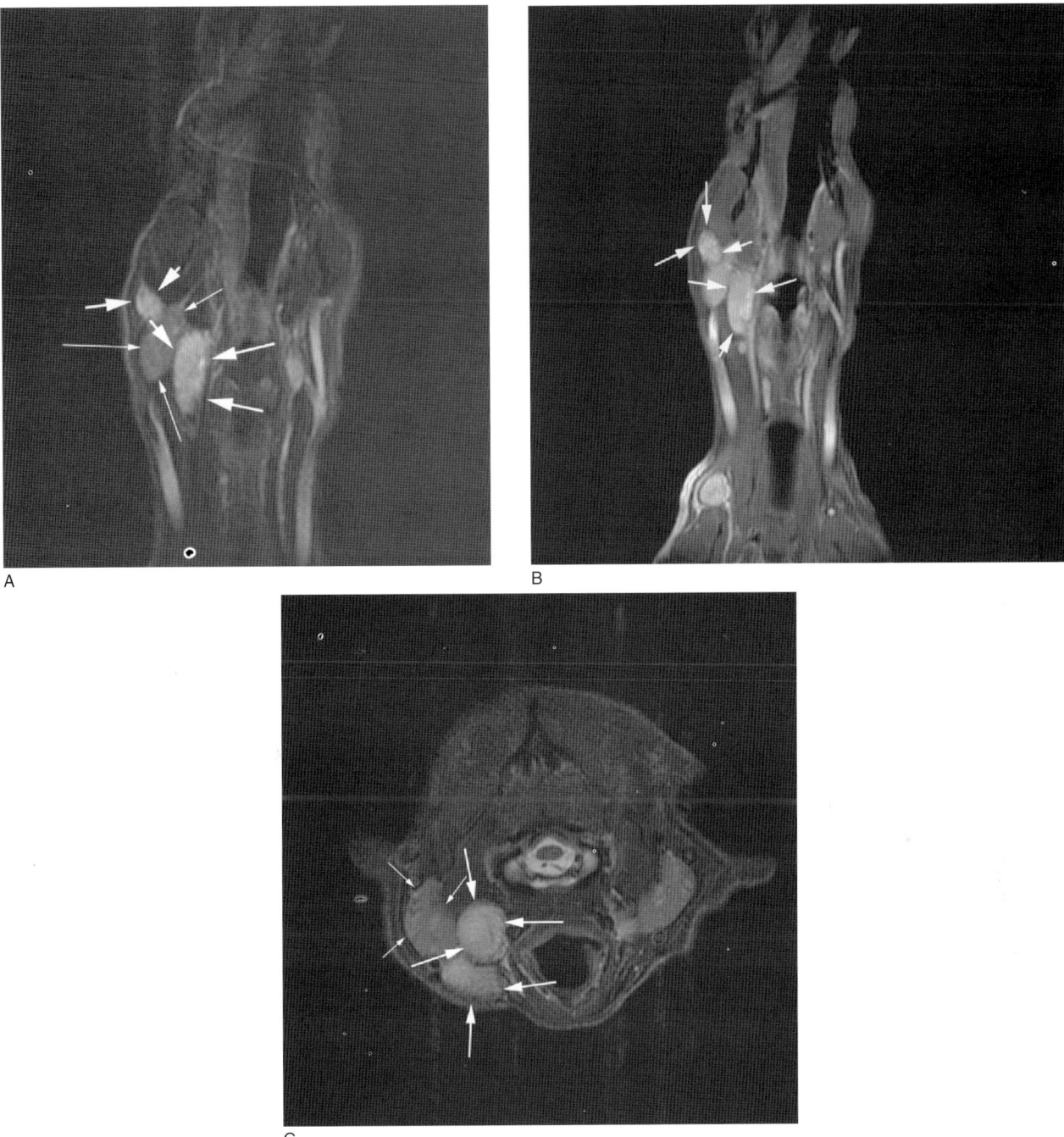

Figure 6.11. Lymphadenopathy. (A) STIR dorsal sequence. The large arrows point to the smaller mandibular lymph node, and the larger retropharyngeal lymph node. Small arrows point to the interposed mandibular salivary gland. (B) T1-weighted post-contrast dorsal plane image. The large arrows point to the same lymph nodes. Note that following contrast enhancement, all the lesions have a similar signal characteristic and one cannot differentiate lymph nodes from the salivary gland. Often, sequences without contrast can be more beneficial in arriving at tissue characterization, as all glandular tissues undergo considerable enhancement. Note that there is an enlarged superficial cervical lymph node (prescapular) lymph node on the ipsilateral side. (C) Transverse STIR sequence, again with the large arrows showing the enlarged mandibular salivary gland in ventral and the retropharyngeal lymph node dorsal to this. Small arrows show the normal mandibular salivary gland. Note the same salivary gland can be seen on the contralateral side. Aspirates indicated only an inflammatory lymphadenitis in this case. There was considerable dental disease in this patient that was presumably the source of the inflammation.

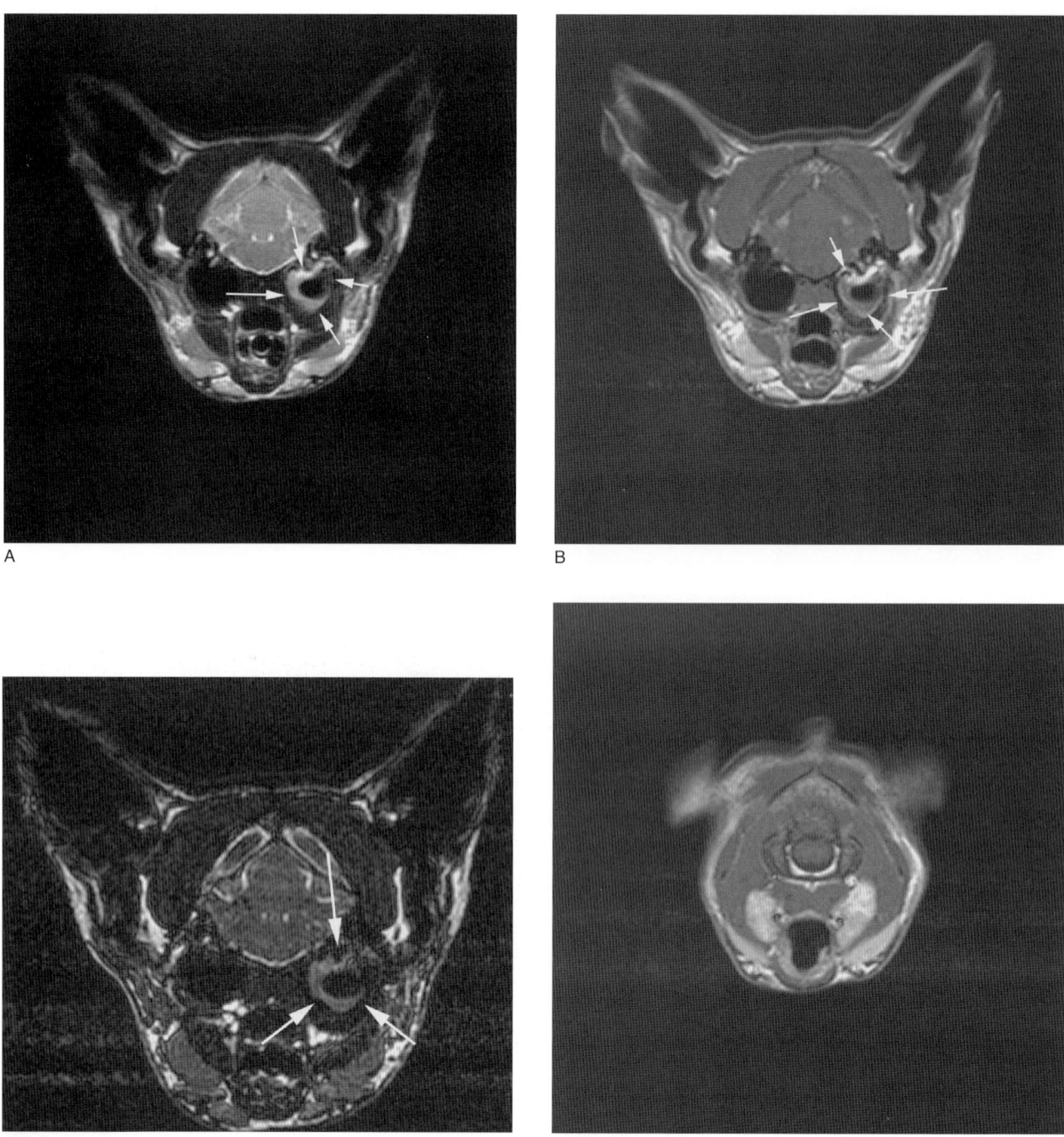

Figure 6.12. Cat with otitis media on the left side. (A) T2-weighted transverse image. Arrows show the presence of fluid with an air/fluid level in the left middle ear. (B) T1-weighted post-contrast showing only minimal enhancement of the lining of the tympanic bulla. There is no enhancement of the majority of the lesion. (C) Heavily T2-weighted image performed for visualization of fluid within the tissue. This "tympanic bullae series" shows the presence of the fluid and no involvement of the area of the inner ear. (D) Enlarged retropharyngeal lymph nodes, bilateral. Lymphadenitis is often bilateral, as the lymphatics in the head can have multiple drainage patterns.

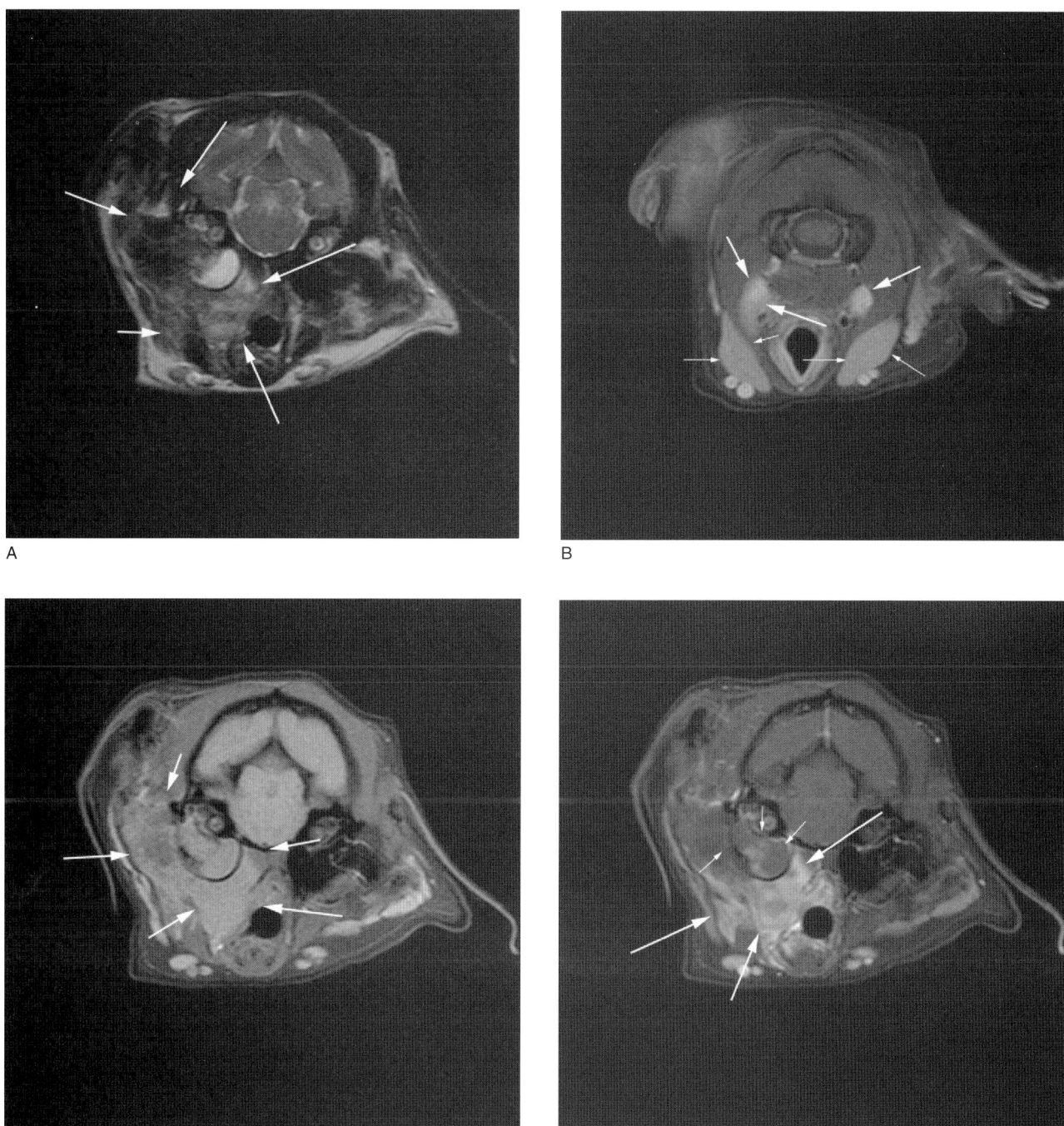

Figure 6.13. (A) T2-weighted transverse image. The arrows show the presence of a large heterogenous lesion in the patient's right side. There is a fluid signal within the right tympanic bulla. (B) Large arrows show the presence of mild lymphadenopathy of the retropharyngeal lymph nodes. The small arrows show the normal mandibular salivary glands. (C) T1-weighted pre-contrast image. (D) Post-contrast T1-weighted image. Note how much of the fluid signal in the middle ear did not enhance as well as some of the tissue immediately external to the middle ear, while there was avid enhancement of the pharyngeal tissue. The enhancement is poorly marginated and tends to follow fascial planes. This was proven to be cellulitis, presumed from extension of the otitis externa and otitis media on that side. Patient was successfully treated with antimicrobial therapy.

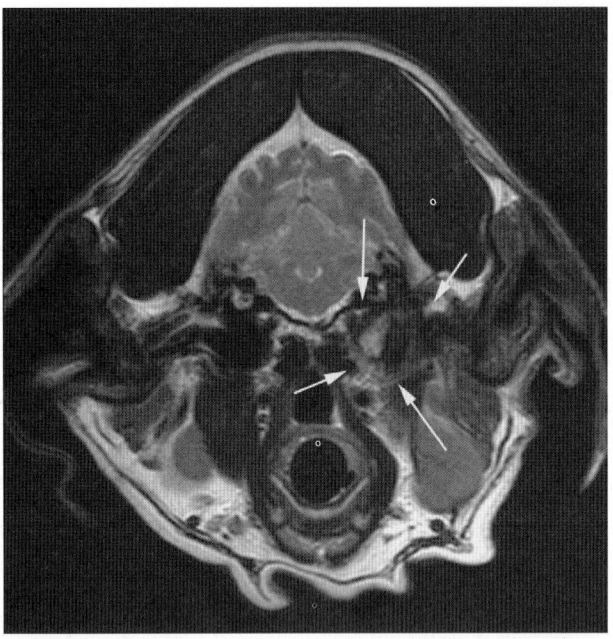

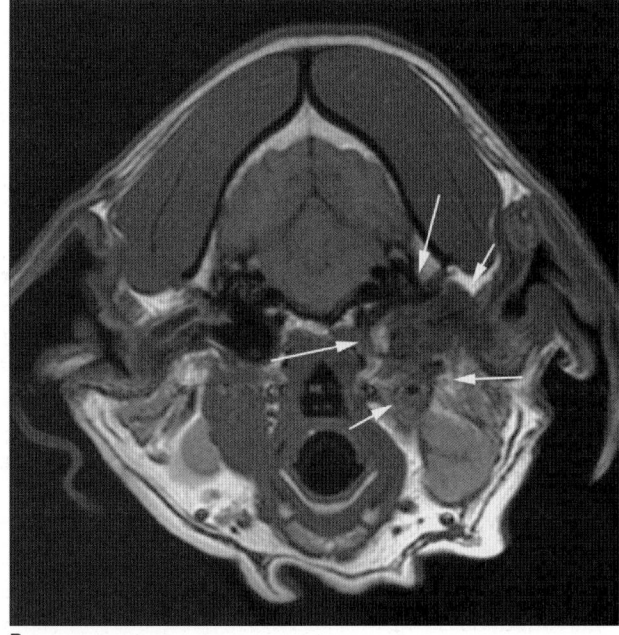

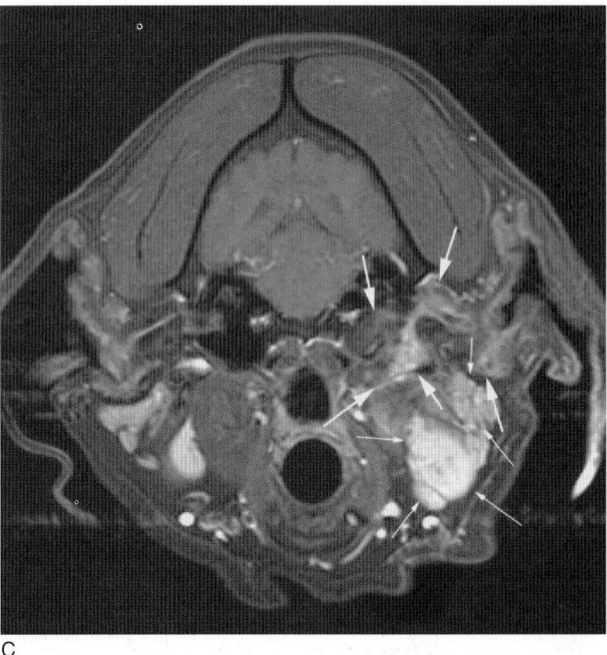

Figure 6.14. (A) T2-weighted transverse image. Lack of normal aeration of the tympanic bulla is seen. There appears to be tissue outside of the tympanic bulla that is abnormal. (B) T1-weighted pre-contrast study. (C) T1-weighted post-contrast fat-suppressed image. Note how much of the tissue within the external ear and middle ear does enhance. This is indicated with the large arrows. The small arrows point to the enhancement of the normal parotid and mandibular salivary glands. Biopsy indicated this was a ceruminous gland carcinoma.

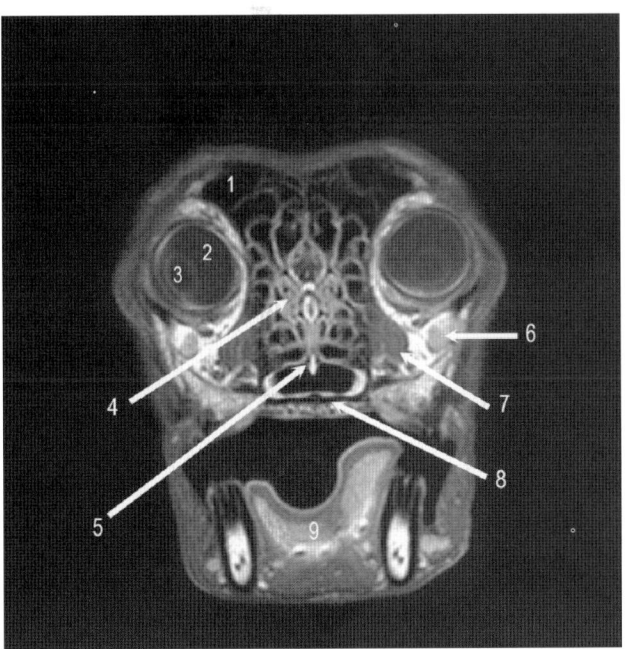

A

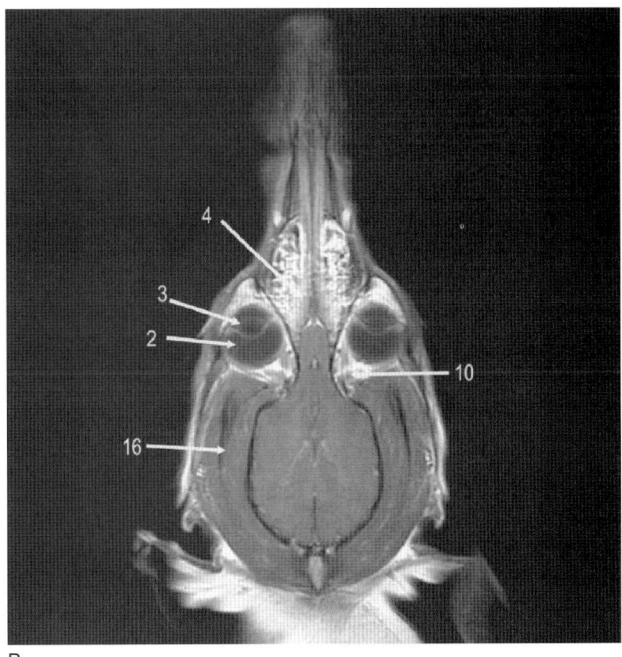

B

Figure 6.15.   Normal eye: (A) T1 transverse; (B) T1 coronal. (1) Frontal sinus, (2) vitreous of eye, (3) lens of eye, (4) ethmoid turbinates, (5) vomer at ventral aspect of nasal septum, (6) zygomatic salivary gland, (7) medial pterygoid muscle, (8) hard palate, (9) tongue—being deformed by endotracheal tube, (10) optic nerve and its associated venous plexus within extraocular musculature.

have inflammatory or neoplastic conditions. Generally, these can be differentiated due to margination, vascular supply, and degree of homogeneity of their chemical structure.

Retrobulbar lesions are clearly seen, and the imaging characteristics help diagnose benign abscesses from more serious lesions (Figures 6.16 and 6.17).

OTHER

In some cases, the animal is presented with an abnormal physical appearance, such as atrophy of the temporal musculature. Universal atrophy of the temporal muscle generally involves an abnormal trigeminal nerve. Trigeminal nerve problems can be from an inflammatory process, a diffuse neoplastic process including lymphoma, or a nerve sheath tumor. While MR is not highly specific at differentiating these diseases, with unilateral lesions the degree of nerve enlargement often helps differentiate between neuritis and a nerve sheath tumor. Since the region is very difficult to biopsy, one of the

main methods for differential diagnosis is through repeat examination within a few months to determine the progress of the disease.

There have been many cases where the animal presents with vague signs such as inability to open its mouth or difficulty eating, and the MR examination reveals large tumors of the skull. Many of these tumors are multilocular osteosarcomas (Figure 6.18). Many of these animals have had a radiographic examination. Standard orthogonal radiographs of the skull can miss numerous lesions. Even with the many special views of the skull, diseases can be missed, as it must be remembered that it takes a large increase or decrease in the bone marrow content to be radiographically visible. The example shown of a large tumor within the skull was a clinical case that had received prior high quality radiographic examination that was deemed normal. Currently, it is this author's recommendation that if cross-sectional imaging is available, it should be used for examination of the skull in virtually all cases. While magnetic resonance imaging is preferable in many cases, computed tomography offers a great advantage over standard radiographic examination.

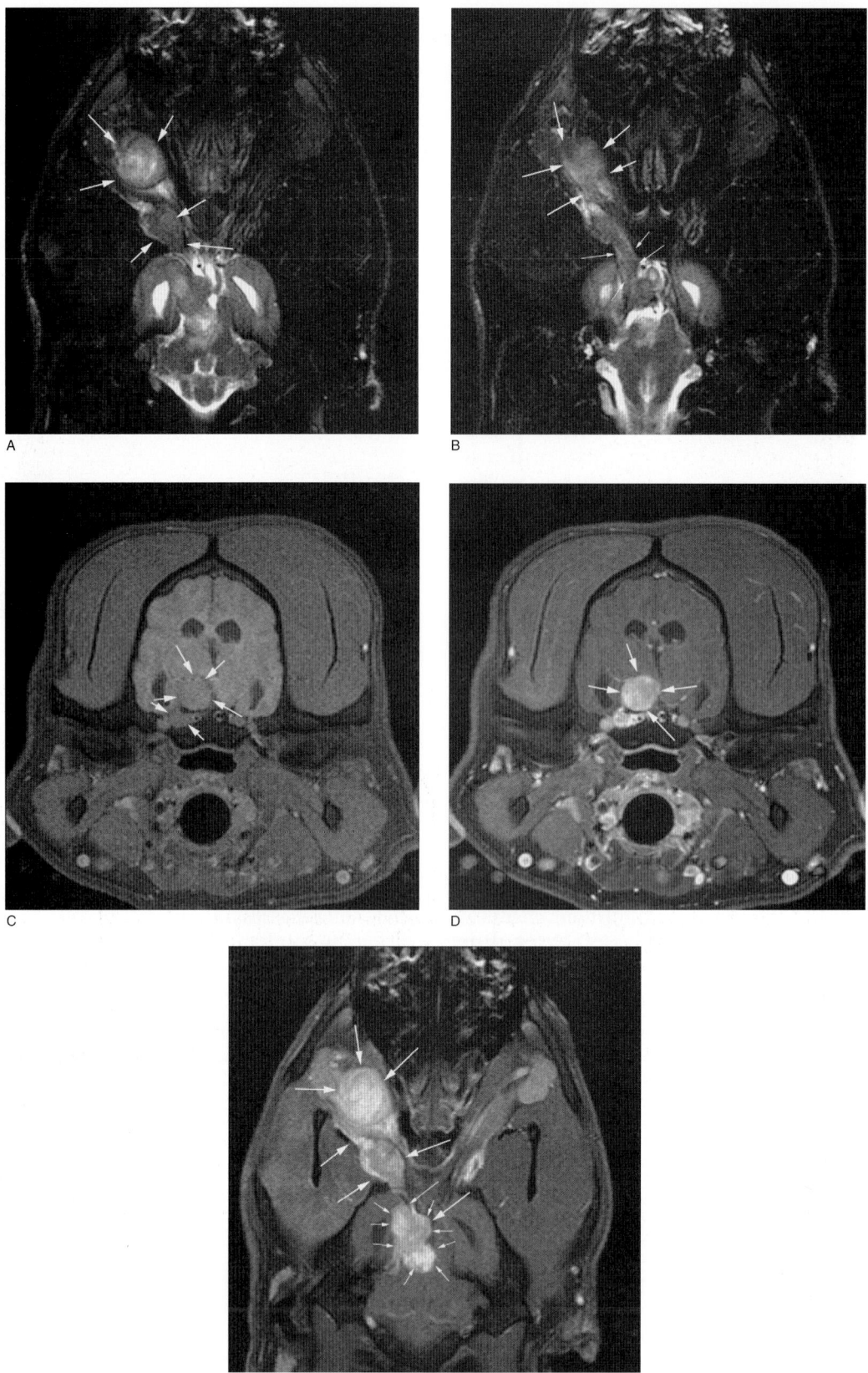

Figure 6.16. Meningioma of the optic nerve. (A), (B) Heterogeneity of the mass in the retrobulbar region on the right-hand side is seen on (A) and (B) STIR sequences in the dorsal plane. (B) This shows the large mass in the retrobulbar area with the large arrows while the intracranial extension of the mass through the optic foramen is highlighted with the small arrows. (C) T1-weighted pre-contrast transverse image. The avid enhancement of the extension of this tumor into the calvarium is seen. (D) Transverse T1 post-contrast. Arrows indicate the contrast-enhancing optic nerve. (E) Dorsal plane image in the similar location to (B). The avid enhancement of the retrobulbar portion of the meningioma is readily seen, as indicated with the large arrows, while the intracranial extension of the mass along the optic nerve is highlighted with the small arrows. This was proven to be an optic nerve meningioma. The intracranial extension proved that surgical excision was not a viable curative option.

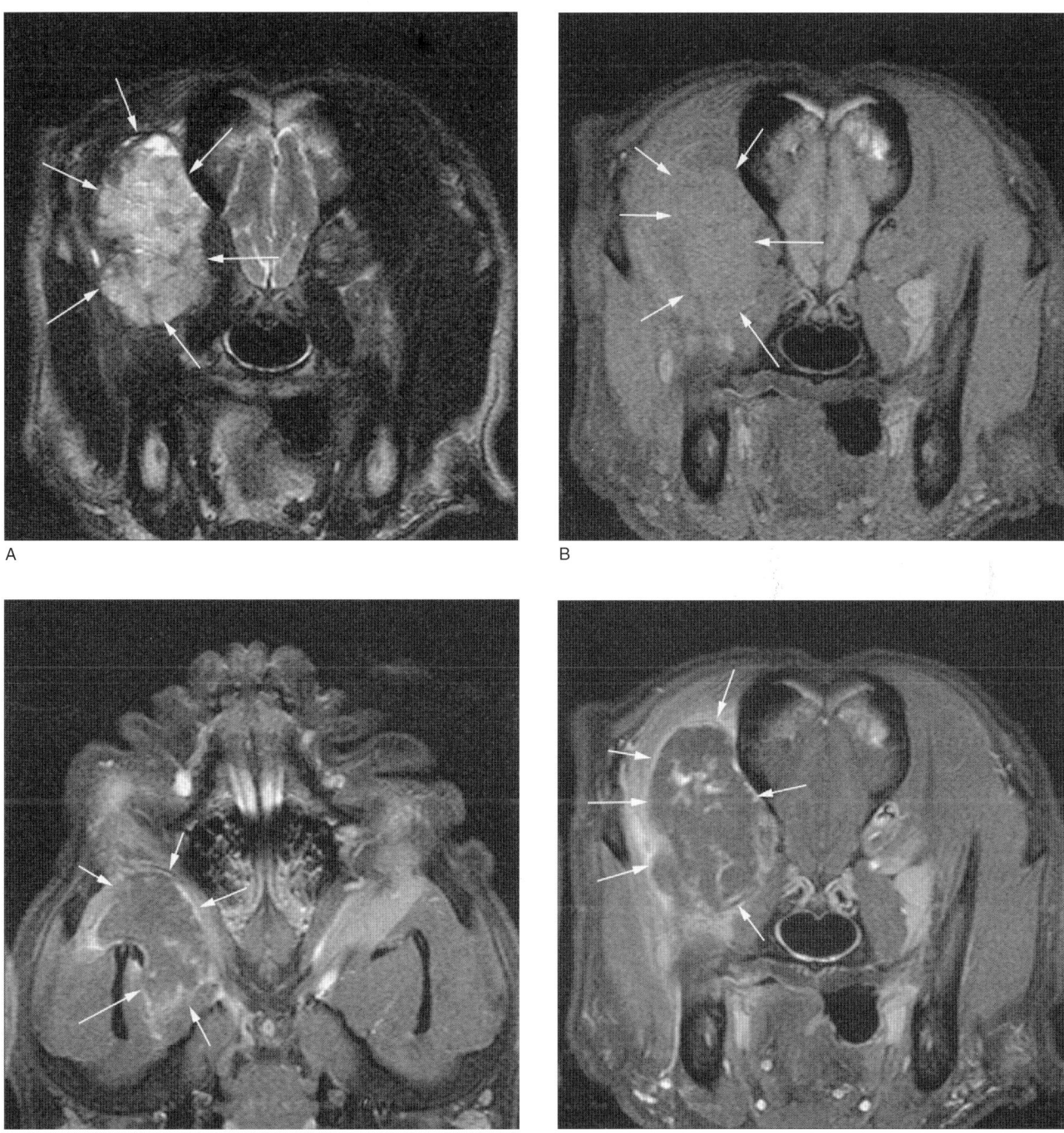

Figure 6.17. (A) Large heterogenous mass on T2-weighted transverse imaging in the right retrobulbar region. (B) T1-weighted pre-contrast image through the same area. Note how the mass is very difficult to see on T1-weighting compared to the T2-weighted image. (C), (D) T1-weighted fat-suppressed images post-contrast. Note how the vast majority of the mass does not enhance and only a peripheral enhancement is seen as well as some wispy enhancement along fascial planes. This large mass was a retrobulbar abscess. Plant material was found within the abscess.

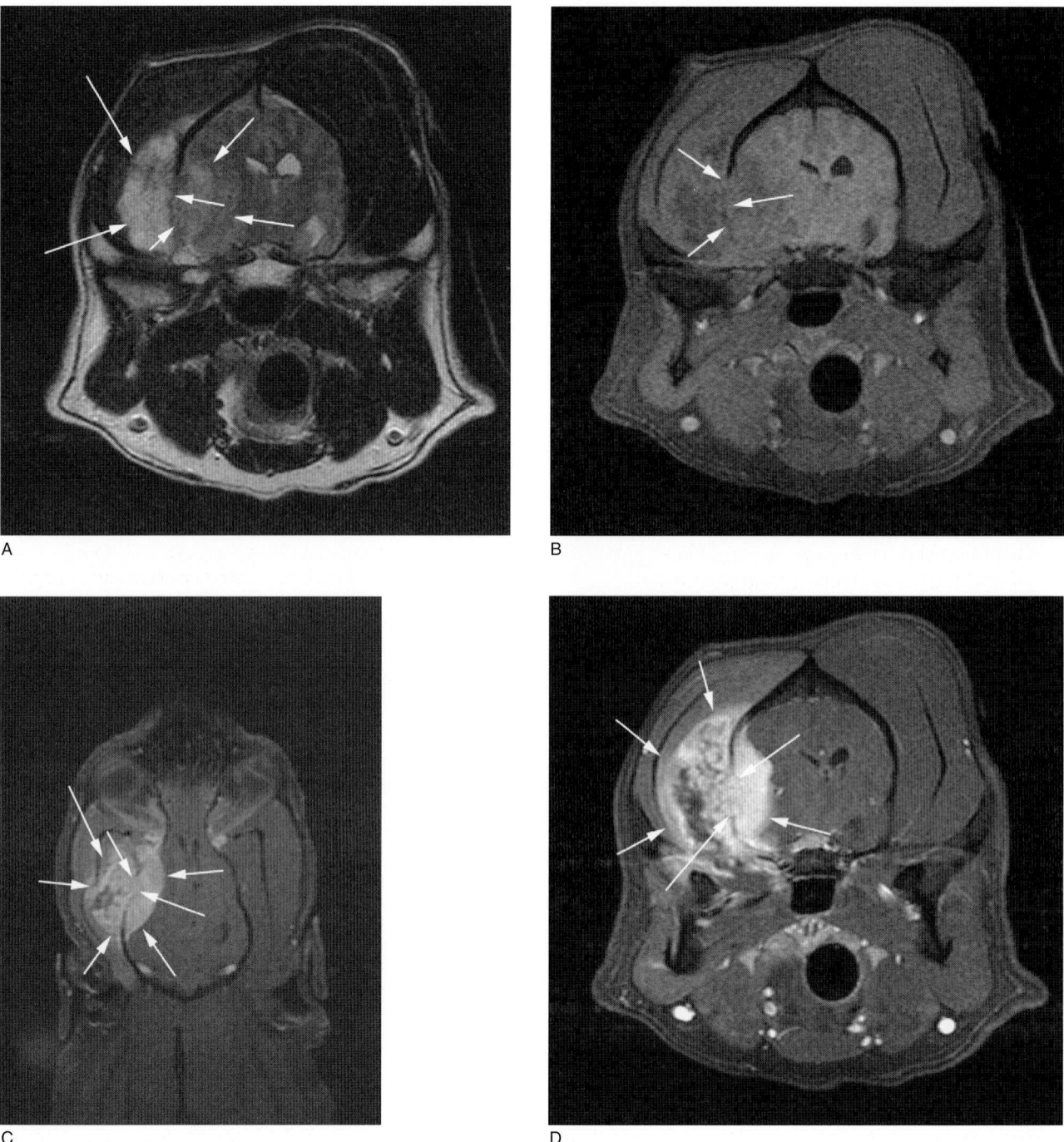

Figure 6.18. (A) T2-weighted transverse imaging showing marked atrophy of the temporalis muscle on the patient's right side. A large mass is seen that is hyperintense. Loss of some of the calvarium can be seen. There appears to be a mass effect with a midline shift of the brain to the patient's left. (B) T1-weighted pre-contrast image. While the mass is poorly seen in T1-weighted images, the lysis of the calvarium is readily seen. The normal dark signal of the calvarium has been lost in the area, as indicated with the arrows. (C) Coronal image—post-contrast, fat suppressed. The avid enhancement of this mass can be seen both inside and outside of the normal calvarium. Midline shift is readily seen. (D) T1-weighted post-contrast transverse fat-suppressed image. The enhancement of the mass is readily seen as well as the lysis of the calvarium. Mass was proven to be a multilocular osteochondrosarcoma. This mass was not seen with standard orthogonal views on skull radiographs.

CONCLUSION

Abnormalities can be visualized in any of the tissues within the head. These include all the structures of the eye, retrobulbar space, all the various tissues of the nasal cavity and oral cavity, middle ear, and accessory structures including the salivary glands and lymph nodes. Cases shown in this chapter represent many of the most common conditions seen to date. However, it should be stressed that magnetic resonance has the ability to see the skeletal structures as well as *any* of the soft tissues of the head.

This chapter has shown the broad use of magnetic resonance to image numerous organ systems. We have long known of the insensitive, nonspecific nature of skull radiography. Computed tomography was a large advancement. Magnetic resonance offers an even further advance in the imaging and clear delineation of abnormalities of the skull and tissues of the head. In many aspects, magnetic resonance imaging helps provide a narrower differential diagnosis and certainly clearer determination of disease borders.

BIBLIOGRAPHY

Barthez PY, Schaafsma IA, and Pollak YW. 2006. Multimodality image fusion to facilitate anatomic localization of 99mTC-pertechnetate uptake in the feline head. Vet Radiol Ultrasound 47(5):503–506.

Bischoff MG and Kneller SK. 2004. Diagnostic imaging of the canine and feline ear. Vet Clin North Am Small Anim Pract 34(2):437–458.

Caruso K, Marrion R, and Silver G. 2002. What is your diagnosis? Retrobulbar mass indenting the inferior aspect of the right globe. J Am Vet Med Assoc 221(11):1553–1554.

Chang Y, Thompson H, Reed N, and Penderis J. 2006. Clinical and magnetic resonance imaging features of nasopharyngeal lymphoma in two cats with concurrent intracranial mass. J Small Anim Pract 47(11):678–681.

Clifford C, Jennings D, Maslin WR, and Weigand C. 2000. What is your neurologic diagnosis? Unilateral otitis externa or media, cerebellar meningioma, and a solitary mammary adenoma. J Am Vet Med Assoc 216(8):1217–1219.

Cullen CL, Grahn BH, and Wolfer J. 2000. Diagnostic ophthalmology. Mesenchymal orbital tumor with adjacent bony invasion. Can Vet J 41(9):723–724.

Dennis R. 2000. Use of magnetic resonance imaging for the investigation of orbital disease in small animals. J Small Anim Pract 41(4):145–155.

De Rycke LM, Saunders JH, Gielen IM, van Bree HJ, and Simoens PJ. 2003. Magnetic resonance imaging, computed tomography, and cross-sectional views of the anatomy of normal nasal cavities and paranasal sinuses in mesaticephalic dogs. Am J Vet Res 64(9):1093–1098.

Dvir E, Kirberger RM, and Terblanche AG. 2000. Magnetic resonance imaging of otitis media in a dog. Vet Radiol Ultrasound 41(1):46–49.

Ellison GW, Donnell RL, and Daniel GB. 1995. Nasopharyngeal epidermal cyst in a dog. J Am Vet Med Assoc 207(12):1590–1592.

Endo H, Taru H, Nakamura K, Koie H, Yamaya Y, and Kimura J. 1999. MRI examination of the masticatory muscles in the gray wolf (Canis lupus), with special reference to the M. temporalis. J Vet Med Sci 61(6):581–586.

Garosi LS, Dennis R, and Schwarz T. 2003. Review of diagnostic imaging of ear diseases in the dog and cat. Vet Radiol Ultrasound 44(2):137–146.

Garosi LS, Lamb CR, and Targett MP. 2000. MRI findings in a dog with otitis media and suspected otitis interna. Vet Rec 146(17):501–502.

Guilliard MJ, Banks AR, Baxter CJ, and Mayo AK. 1999. What is your diagnosis? Mouth neoplasms. J Small Anim Pract 40(1):1, 35.

Jeffery N. 2005. Ethmoidal encephalocoele associated with seizures in a puppy. J Small Anim Pract 46(2):89–92.

Johnson VA and Seiler G. 2006. Magnetic resonance imaging appearance of the Cisterna chyli. Vet Radiol Ultrasound 47(5):461–464.

Kafka UC, Carstens A, Steenkamp G, and Symington H. 2004. Diagnostic value of magnetic resonance imaging and computed tomography for oral masses in dogs. J S Afr Vet Assoc 75(4):163–168.

Kato K, Nishimura R, Sasaki N, Matsunaga S, Mochizuki M, Nakayama H, et al. Magnetic resonance imaging of a canine eye with melanoma. J Vet Med Sci 67(2):179–182.

Kneissl S and Probst A. 2006. Magnetic resonance imaging features of presumed normal head and neck lymph nodes in dogs. Vet Radial Ultrasound 47(6):538–541.

Kneissl S, Probst A, and Konar M. 2004. Low-field magnetic resonance imaging of the canine middle and inner ear. Vet Radiol Ultrasound 45(6):520–522.

Larocca RD. 2000. Unilateral external and internal ophthalmoplegia caused by intracranial meningioma in a dog. Vet Ophthalmol 3(1):3–9.

Lipsitz D, Levitski RE, and Berry WL. 2001. Magnetic resonance imaging features of multilobular osteochondrosarcoma in 3 dogs. Vet Radiol Ultrasound 42(1):14–19.

McConnell JF, Hayes A, Platt SR, and Smith KC. 2006. Calvarial hyperostosis syndrome in two bullmastiffs. Vet Radiol Ultrasound 47(1):72–77.

Miwa Y, Matsunaga S, Kato K, Ogawa H, Nakayama H, Tsujimoto S, et al. 2005. Choroidal melanoma in a dog. J Vet Med Sci 67(8):821–823.

Owen MC, Lamb CR, Lu D, and Targett MP. 2004. Material in the middle ear of dogs having magnetic resonance imaging for investigation of neurologic signs. Vet Radiol Ultrasound 45(2):149–155.

Petite AF and Dennis R. 2006. Comparison of radiography and magnetic resonance imaging for evaluating the extent of nasal neoplasia in dogs. J Small Anim Pract 47(9):529–536.

Pownder S, Fidel JL, Saveraid TC, Gailbreath KL, and Gavin PR. 2006. What is your diagnosis? Incidental melanosis of a salivary gland lesion. J Am Vet Med Assoc 229(2):209–210.

Saunders JH, Clercx C, Snaps FR, Sullivan M, Duchateau L, van Bree HJ, et al. 2004. Radiographic, magnetic resonance imaging, computed tomographic, and rhinoscopic features of nasal aspergillosis in dogs. J Am Vet Med Assoc 225(11):1703–1712.

Sturges BK, Dickinson PJ, Kortz GD, Berry WL, Vernau KM, Wisner ER, et al. 2006. Clinical signs, magnetic resonance imaging features, and outcome after surgical and medical treatment of otogenic intracranial infection in 11 cats and 4 dogs. J Vet Intern Med 20(3):648–656.

Tolwani R, Hagan C, Runstadler J, Lyons H, Green S, Bouley D, et al. 2004. Magnetic resonance imaging and surgical repair of cleft palate in a four-week-old canine (Canis familiaris): an animal model for cleft palate repair. Contemp Top Lab Anim Sci 43(6):17–21; quiz 58.

Varejao AS, Munoz A, and Lorenzo V. 2006. Magnetic resonance imaging of the intratemporal facial nerve in idiopathic facial paralysis in the dog. Vet Radiol Ultrasound 47(4):328–333.

Vazquez JM, Arencibia A, Gil F, Ramirez JA, Gonzalez N, Sosa CD, et al. 1998. Magnetic resonance imaging of the normal canine larynx. Anat Histol Embryol 27(4):263–270.

Willis CK, Quinn RP, McDonell WM, Gati J, Parent J, and Nicolle D. 2001. Functional MRI as a tool to assess vision in dogs: the optimal anesthetic. Vet Ophthalmol 4(4):243–253.

Xia Y, Moody JB, and Alhadlaq H. 2002. Orientational dependence of T2 relaxation in articular cartilage: a microscopic MRI (microMRI) study. Magn Reson Med 48(3):460–469.

CHAPTER SEVEN

CANCER IMAGING

Susan L. Kraft

INTRODUCTION

MR has been used for cancer imaging for many years to diagnose brain and spinal cord tumors, in the context of its long-standing and well-developed neuroradiology application. Its utility for non-neurological cancers has evolved more slowly, especially in veterinary medicine in which economics and availability mandate the recommended imaging strategy. The potential advantages of MR for cancer diagnosis and staging are irrefutable, and its use for this purpose is increasing along with greater access and affordability.

The basic concepts regarding MR physics have been reviewed in Chapter 1. MR's greatest strength is soft tissue imaging, and its portrayal of pathology results in a "virtual autopsy." MR's aptitude for multiplanar imaging is especially useful to identify tumor margins relative to involved or susceptible surrounding anatomy (Figure 7.1). Furthermore, the ability to characterize a lesion with MR can improve specificity and diagnostic accuracy by evaluating the combined pattern of a tumor's altered signal intensity from a series of pulse sequences. This provides a wealth of information about tumor morphology, composition, margins, and presence of secondary complications. MR depicts tumor heterogeneity and disorganization since the grayscale images reflect not just a tumor's water and fat content, but also evolving hemorrhage, necrosis, edema, proteinaceous fluid, even melanin. Even so, many tumor types and some noncancerous pathology can have similar abnormal signal intensity patterns, so biopsy or cytology may still be necessary to verify diagnosis.

Cortical bone structures are depicted as areas of black signal void and bone landmarks are not as obvious as on CT images. Tissue mineralization and periosteal bone production can be more difficult to detect with MR until fairly well developed. However, tumor osteolysis and invasion through cortical bone is readily visible on MR (Figure 7.1).

TECHNICAL CONSIDERATIONS FOR CANCER MR

For proper detection, mapping, and staging of a cancer, an MR examination of the affected area should include multiple imaging planes in conjunction with at least two types of pulse sequences, using an appropriate coil. Either a STIR or T2-weighted pulse sequence are suggested due to their sensitivity to pathology, combined with pre- and postcontrast T1-weighted scans for anatomic detail (Figure 7.2). This type of examination can entail imaging times of 0.5–1.5 h with the animal under general anesthesia. Besides a working knowledge of MR interpretation, the evaluator should know the typical routes of cancer extension and metastasis, and have a detailed knowledge of anatomy.

The STIR pulse sequence is excellent for cancer imaging. The details of performing a STIR sequence have been described in the chapter on MR physics (Chapter 1). STIR imaging suppresses the signal from fat and renders it dark gray or hypointense. As a result, the hyperintense signal from cancer pathology stands out noticeably against the darkened tissue background (Figure 7.2). It is important that STIR imaging be done prior to, and not after, contrast enhancement with paramagnetic contrast media. The tumor's contrast enhancement could potentially be masked due to suppression by the STIR's inversion recovery pulse.

Fat-saturated T2-weighted imaging is an alternative to the STIR pulse sequence, and with smaller FOV can have excellent image quality (Figure 7.2). Fat saturation is an MR technique that uses a selective pulse tuned to the frequency of fat to suppress its signal during imaging. Like the STIR sequence, fat saturation will render fatty tissues dark, thereby highlighting pathology which has a hyperintense signal. The disadvantage is that with some MR instruments, fat saturation over a large FOV can be incomplete and uneven, plus

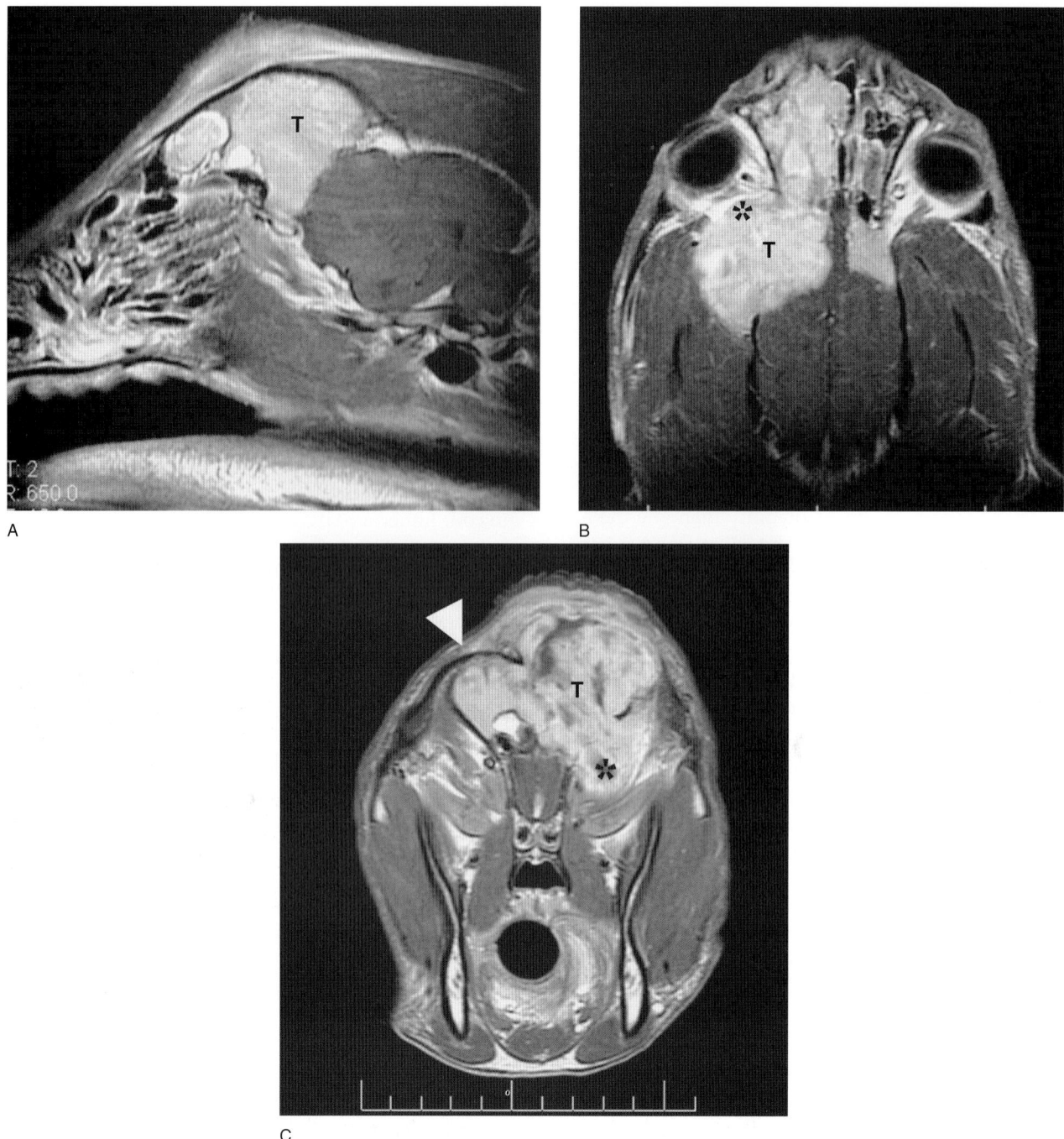

Figure 7.1. Multiplanar postcontrast T1-weighted MR images of a dog with a multilobular osteosarcoma (T) showing extensive invasion within the frontal sinuses. The tumor extent is best illustrated by assessing the combination of sagittal (A), dorsal (B), and transverse (C) images. Retrobulbar invasion is also apparent (* in parts (B) and (C)). In part (C), cortical osteolysis is evident by absence of the hypointense line representing the frontal cortex ipsilaterally (compare to the contralateral frontal cortex marked by the white arrowhead).

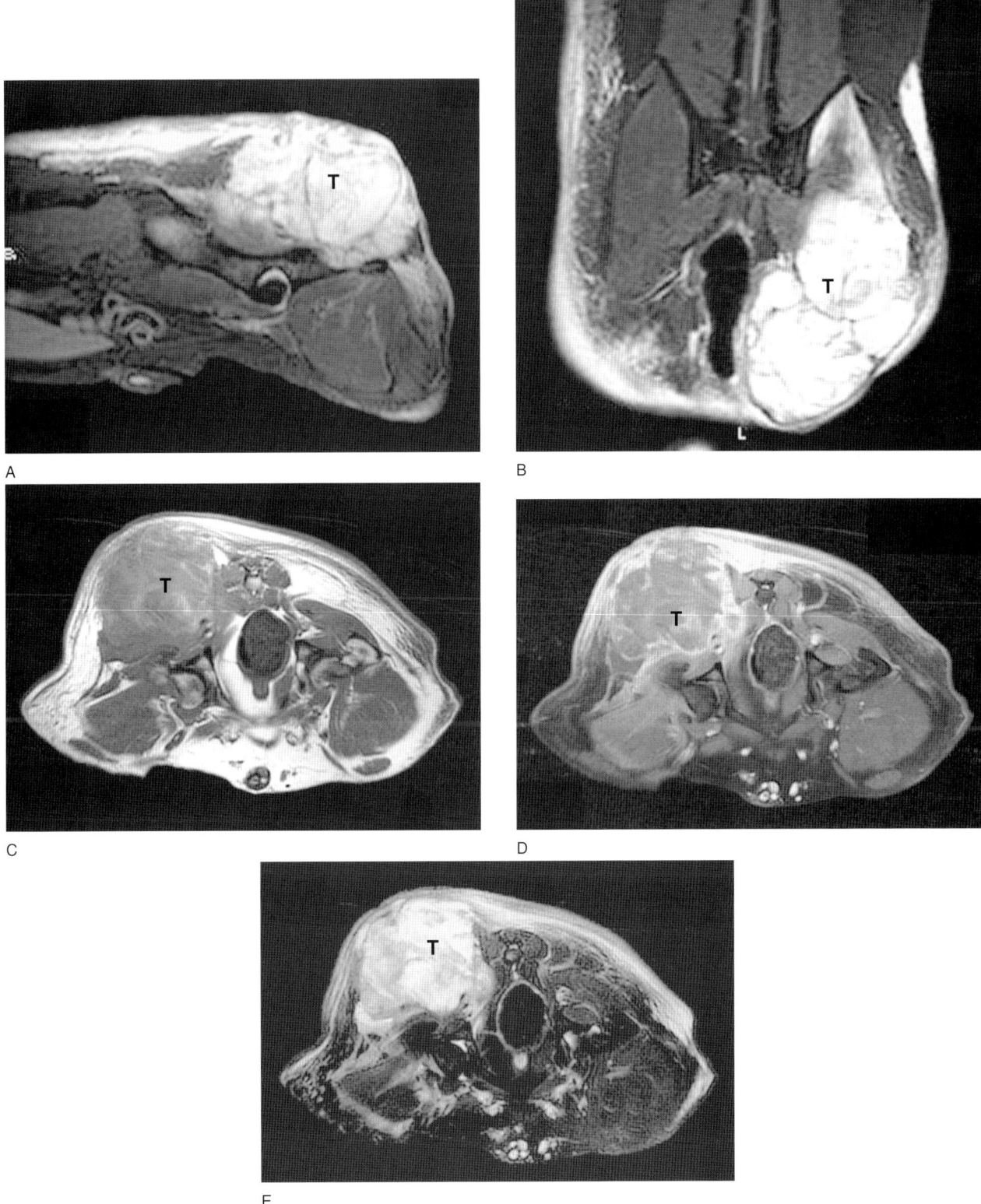

Figure 7.2. Multiplanar, multi-pulse sequence MR images of a dog with a soft tissue sarcoma dorsal to the hip, including sagittal and dorsal STIR (A) and (B), transverse pre- and fat-saturated postcontrast T1-weighted (C) and (D), and fat-saturated transverse T2-weighted image (E). The diffuse subcutaneous T1 contrast enhancement and hyperintense T2 signal is related to peritumor reactive inflammation.

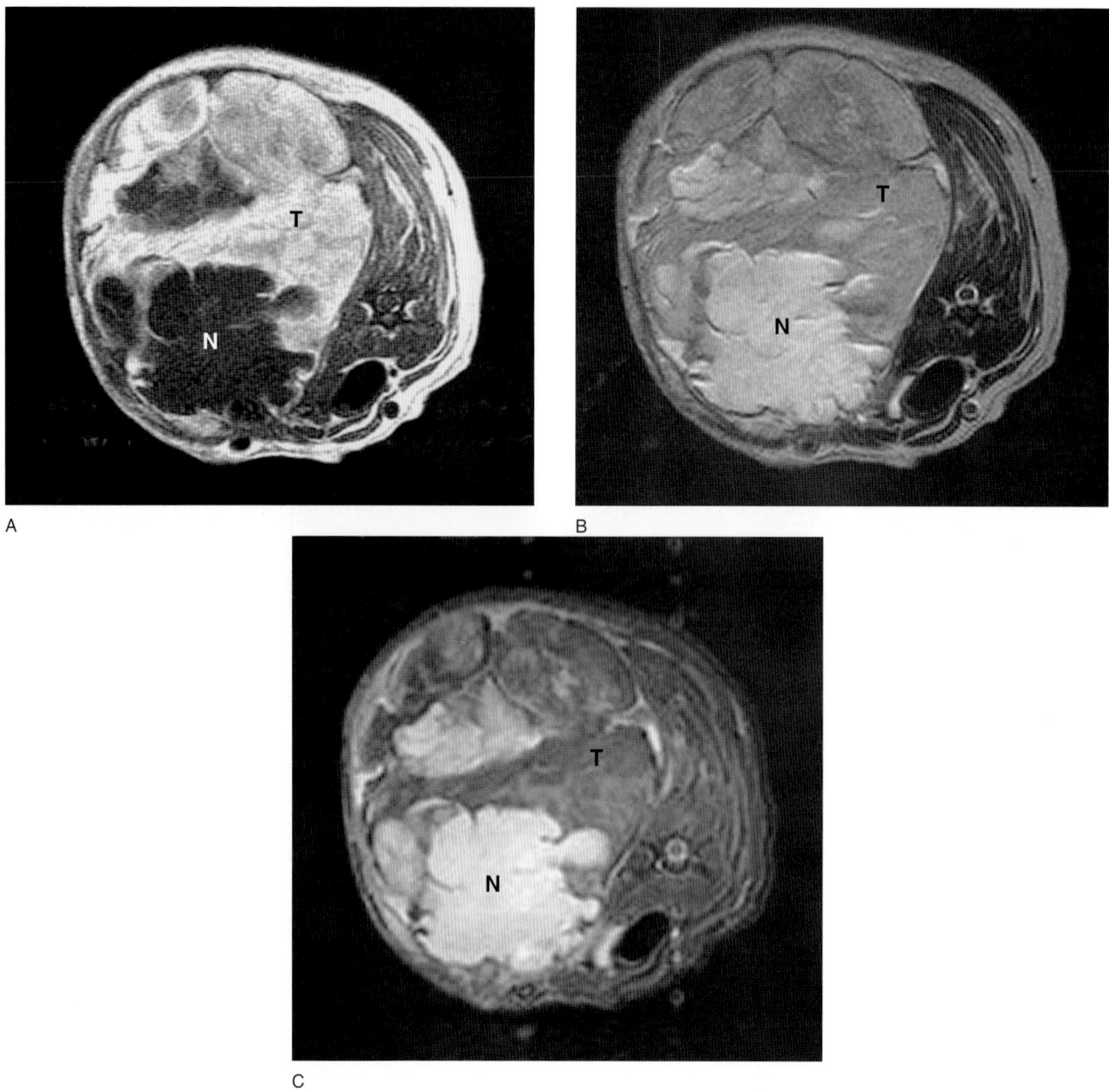

Figure 7.3. Transverse T1-weighted (A), fat-saturated T2-weighted (B), and STIR (C) MR images from a dog with a large cervical necrotic lipoma (T). Note that the signal intensity of the tumor parenchyma is similar to that of subcutaneous fat on each image. The ventral tumor region has signal characteristics consistent with fluid and/or necrosis (N).

the technique increases scan time. In comparison, fat suppression using a STIR sequence is uniform over even large FOV giving it more consistent quality. Use of fat-suppression imaging can also be used diagnostically to confirm the presence of adipose content in a tumor (Figure 7.3).

Despite MR's excellent contrast resolution, injection of paramagnetic contrast media is useful for detecting some benign and lower grade malignant tumors, which can be relatively isointense to surrounding tissues. The visibility of gadolinium contrast agents with MR is much greater than iodine contrast agents with CT. Contrast enhancement also aids in delineating tumor margins from surrounding secondary pathology such as edema and hemorrhage. Use of fat saturation during postcontrast T1-weighted scans helps further to distinguish contrast-enhanced tumor margins from subcutaneous, epidural, or bone marrow fat when imaging spinal, skeletal tumors, and subcutaneous tumors (Figure 7.2). Another technique used is to subtract the precontrast or "mask" images from the postcontrast images leaving only the enhancement.

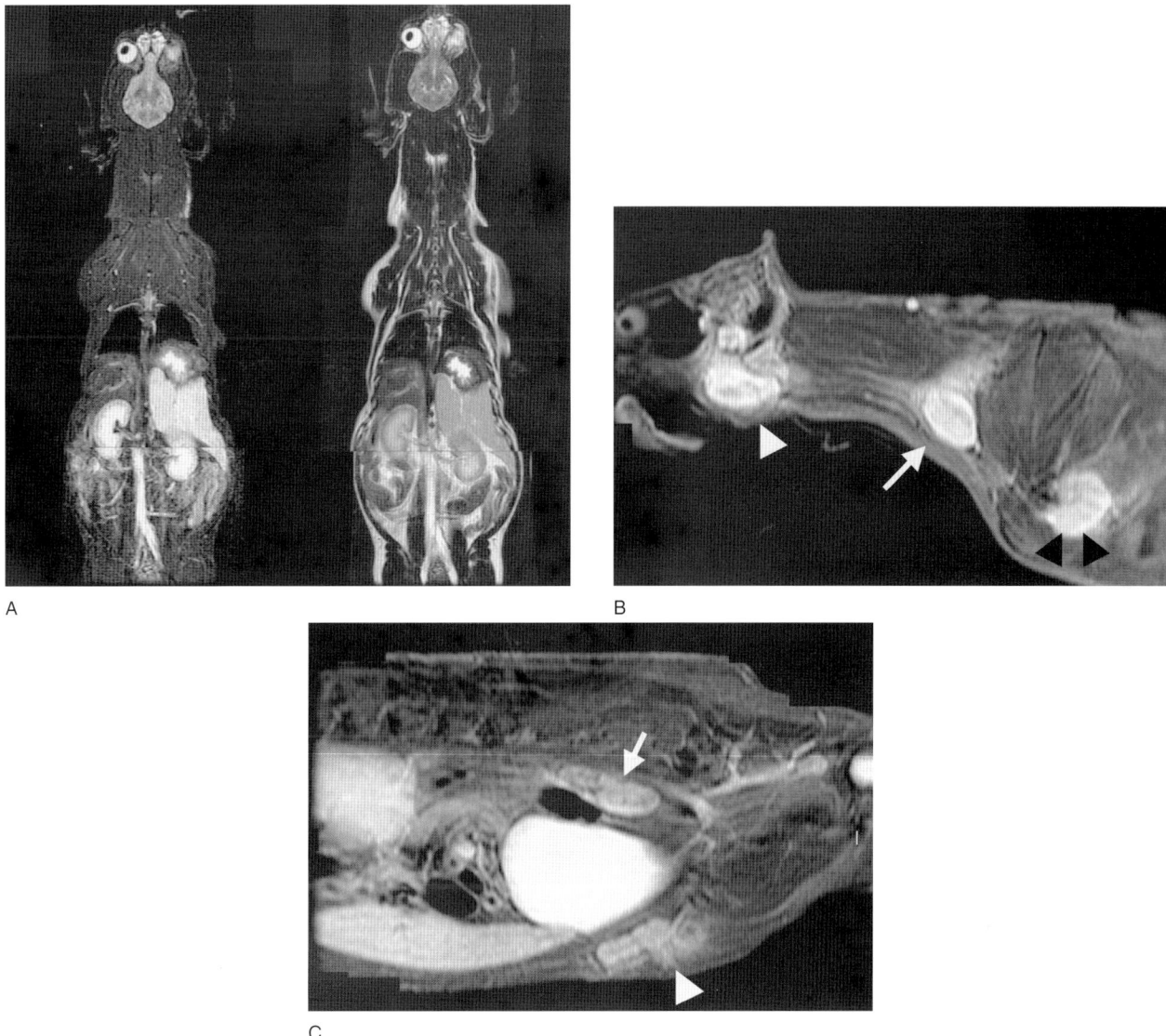

Figure 7.4.   Dorsal plane whole body STIR ((A), left) and T2-weighted ((A), right) MR images of a normal dog. Parts (B) and (C) are sagittal STIR MR images showing multiple enlarged lymph nodes in a dog with lymphoma, including the mandibular (white arrowhead in (B)), superficial cervical (white arrow (B)), axillary (black arrowheads in (B)), medial iliac (white arrow in (C)), and inguinal lymph nodes (white arrowhead in (C)).

WHOLE BODY MR FOR CANCER STAGING

Whole body MR is potentially a single imaging method that could replace traditional imaging to stage cancer. In the past, whole body MR had the disadvantages of prolonged scan times and image degradation due to motion artifact. Technical improvements and new imaging strategies are evolving to achieve practical scan times along with acceptable image quality. Techniques for whole body MR are being developed for veterinary patients (Figure 7.4). In comparison to PET (which is also a highly sensitive cancer staging modality), MR is more available, less expensive, and does not lead to patient radiation exposure. Whole body MR is more sensitive than CT or 99m-Tc-MDP bone scintigraphy to skeletal metastases from various malignancies and also to bone marrow infiltration from lymphoma. Occult canine and human bone marrow lymphoma has been detected with whole body MR since it provides a global view of the marrow, even when biopsy results are negative.

MR Imaging Techniques for Radiation Therapy Planning

Radiation therapy planning systems have traditionally used CT scan data, but some systems can also utilize MR images. Despite its poorer contrast resolution, CT images are the source of tissue electron density values that are used for dosimetric heterogeneity corrections. Those density data cannot be obtained directly during MR imaging. A recent veterinary study by Lyons et al. (2007), however, compared treatment plans created with and without consideration of electron density data. The study showed only a 1.0 ± 0.86% difference in mean dose delivered to 95% of the tumor volume. MR images can suffer from geometric inaccuracy and artifact due to local magnetic field distortions, particularly at the periphery of images away from the central axis, which could be important if delivering spatially focused therapy such as radiosurgery. Finally, it is easier to simulate a radiation treatment setup (patient positioning and landmarks to an anatomic isocenter) during CT scanning than with MR due to the use of receiver coils and lack of triangulating laser light systems in most MR suites. Recent publications, however, have shown excellent repositioning accuracy using MR and positioning aids.

Still, due to the known advantages of MR for depicting tumors and their margins, it is important to incorporate MR into target definition whenever possible. A multimodality approach for radiation treatment planning is the trend in human medicine, through use of fused CT-MR, CT-MR-single photon emission computed tomography (SPECT), or PET results so that treatment incorporates the complementary information from each modality. Also, open MR scanners specially designed for radiation therapy planning are being built that have geometric distortion corrections and landmarking systems.

In select situations, MR has already proven to be superior to CT for radiation and surgical treatment planning. An example is human vestibular schwannoma, in which CT has limitations due to artifacts at the skull base. Three-dimensional postcontrast MR is the choice method for radiosurgery planning of these tumors with measurably lower post-treatment morbidity. The same principles would apply for small caudal fossa brain tumors in animal patients.

Imaging Residual Tumor and Tumor Recurrence

An increasing number of veterinary cancer patients are undergoing surgery, radiation and/or chemotherapy, and enjoying longer life spans. Imaging is being requested with increasing frequency to detect residual tumor when surgical margins are found to be inadequate, or later to detect tumor recurrence and distinguish that from radiation fibrosis or necrosis. The distinction between residual tumor and postradiation or postsurgical reactive tissue or inflammation is difficult to make in the early post-treatment phase (Figure 7.5). Postsurgical studies should be done in the first 2 days or have a delay of at least 3–4 weeks after surgery in order to allow postsurgical inflammation to subside so that images can be interpreted accurately regarding the presence of residual tumor. Immediate postsurgical scanning can be done as it takes about 3 days to get surgical inflammation. A delay of at least several months post-treatment is recommended for a baseline scan to monitor for subsequent tumor recurrence. Granulation tissue and developing fibrosis after an aggressive surgery or after radiation therapy can have similar characteristics to neoplasia. After 3–6 months, mature scar tissue is hypocellular and low in signal in T2 images, thereby allowing it to be distinguished from active tumor recurrence.

Physiological and Molecular Imaging With MR

MR techniques that assess tumor physiology are becoming an inherent part of clinical cancer imaging. Diffusion MR imaging shows an improvement in tumor water mobility if there is a positive response to therapy (Figure 7.6). BOLD imaging is now attracting interest as a method of mapping tumor hypoxia. Dynamic contrast-enhanced MR provides information about tumor perfusion and angiogenesis, and can indicate response to treatment. MR angiography can identify the major vessels supplying a tumor and its degree of vascularity (Figure 7.7). Cancer can also be assessed metabolically using MR spectroscopy to improve diagnostic specificity and evaluate response to therapy (Figure 7.8).

The newest frontier in MR is molecular imaging involving the use of targeted contrast agents linked to

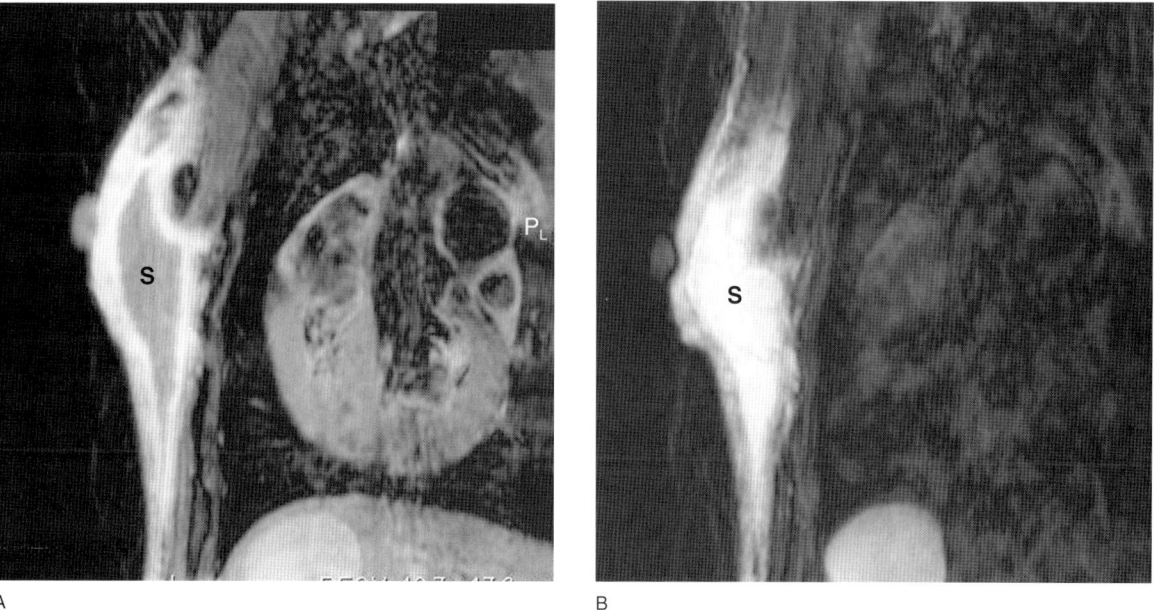

Figure 7.5. Dorsal plane postcontrast fat-saturated T1-weighted (A) and STIR (B) MR images made a week after incomplete surgical resection of a liposarcoma. It is not possible to distinguish residual tumor from the contrast-enhancing margins (T1) and diffuse signal hyperintensity (STIR) of this postsurgical seroma (S).

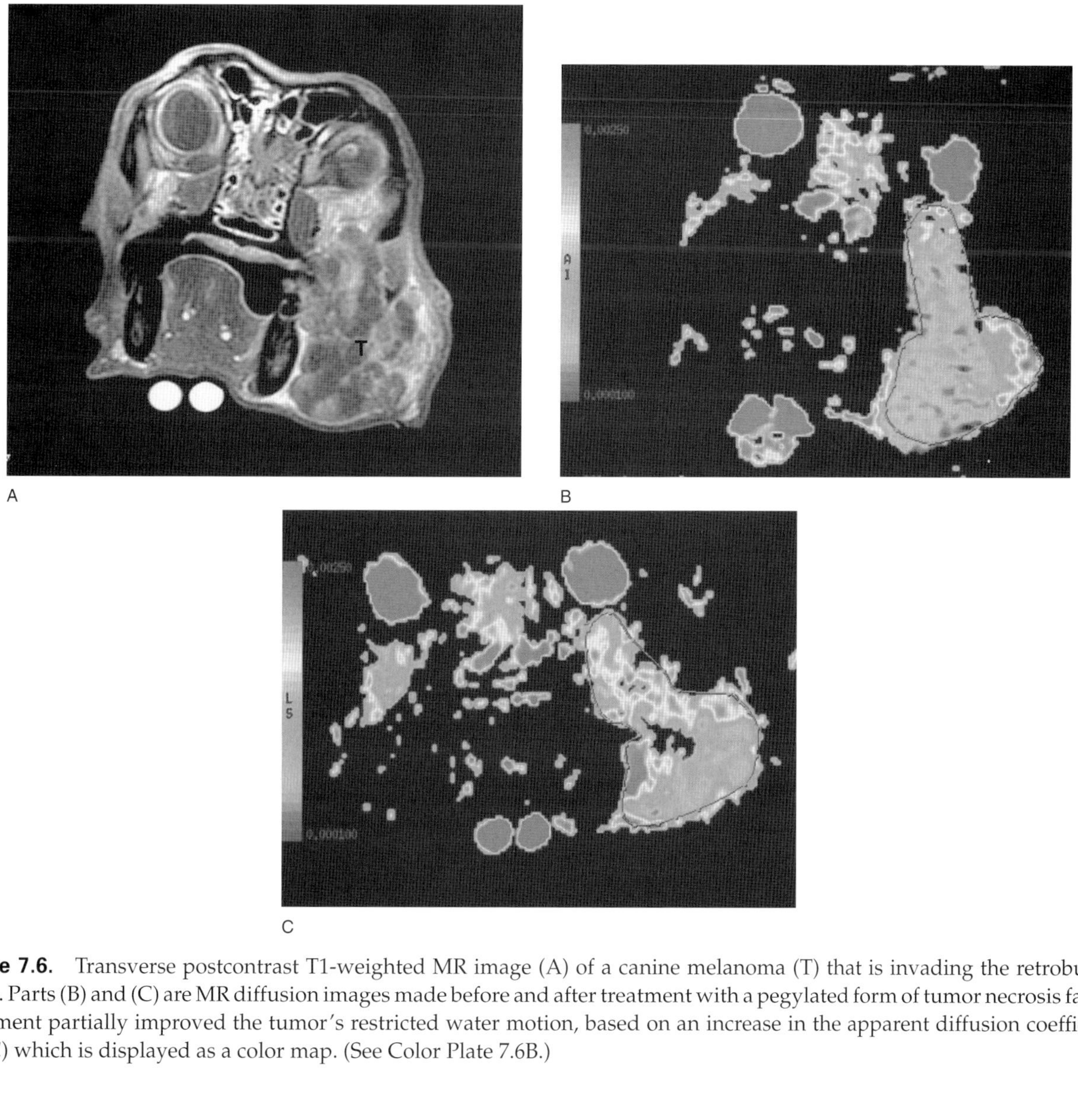

Figure 7.6. Transverse postcontrast T1-weighted MR image (A) of a canine melanoma (T) that is invading the retrobulbar space. Parts (B) and (C) are MR diffusion images made before and after treatment with a pegylated form of tumor necrosis factor. Treatment partially improved the tumor's restricted water motion, based on an increase in the apparent diffusion coefficient (ADC) which is displayed as a color map. (See Color Plate 7.6B.)

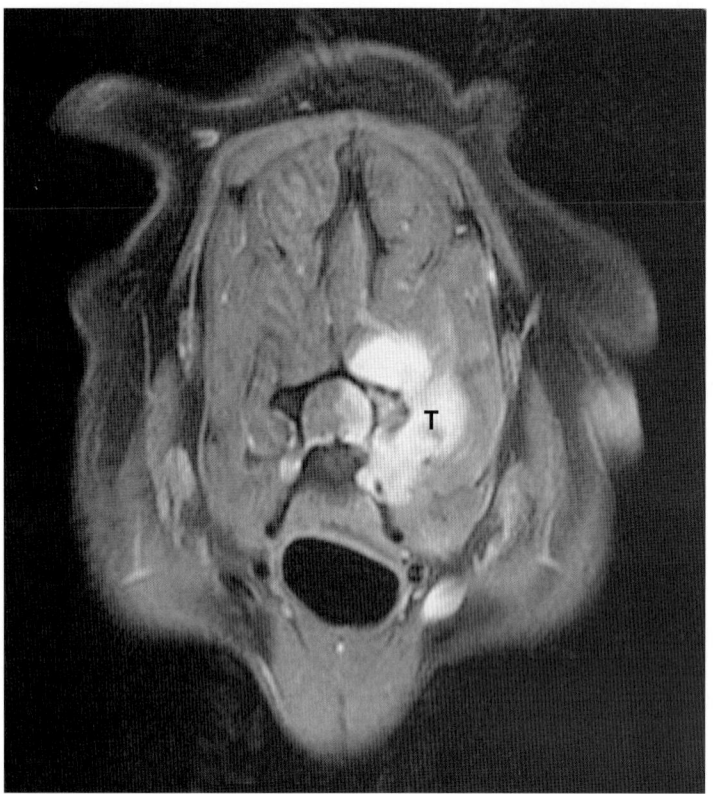
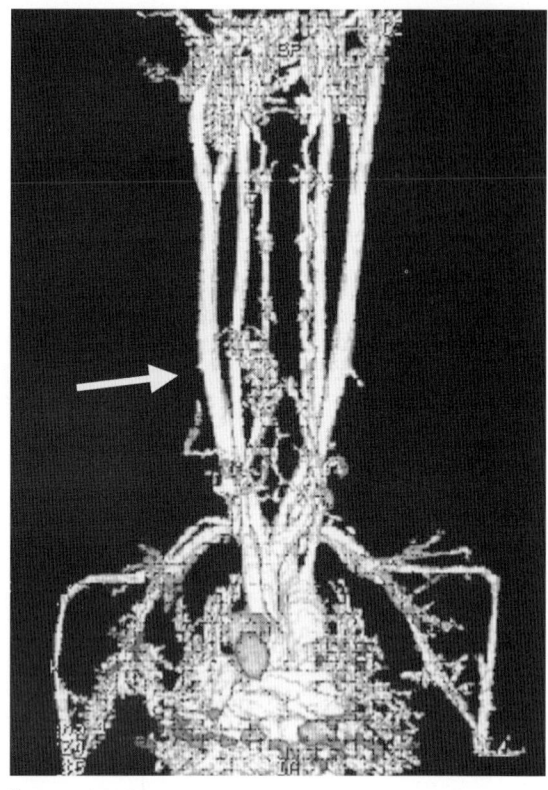

A   B

Figure 7.7. Transverse postcontrast T1-weighted MR image (A) of a vertebral osteosarcoma (T), and an MR angiogram (B) showing the tumor vasculature (arrow) branching off the carotid artery.

cellular biomarkers, receptor, gene, or substrate probes. These methods have the promise of combining the functional sensitivity of PET scanning with high-resolution anatomic images from MR.

The assessment of tumor physiology with MR generally requires contemporary state-of-the-art MR scanners with advanced software, higher field strength, stronger and faster gradient systems. Veterinary oncology will benefit from physiological and molecular MR imaging as high-caliber MR equipment becomes more available to veterinarians. Ultimately, these methods will further improve diagnostic sensitivity and specificity, accuracy of tumor staging, allow us to identify positive responders to therapy and eventually to tailor a patient's treatment based on the response documented with MRI/MRS.

SPECIFIC AREAS

Nervous System Tumors

MR is unquestionably the method of choice for detection and diagnosis of nervous system tumors, and this is its best-understood use in veterinary medicine

(Figures 7.9 and 7.10). Numerous publications are now available on brain, spinal cord, cranial, and peripheral nerve tumor diagnosis in the dog and cat. An entire chapter (Chapter 2, Section 1) has been dedicated to this subject in this reference. Neoplasia of the nervous system usually results in hyperintense signal in T2 and FLAIR images and hypointensity in T1-weighted images. The occasional nervous system tumor that remains isointense in T2 and T1 images is usually detectable on MR after contrast enhancement with gadolinium DTPA (Figure 7.9). Rarely, a low-grade glioma will have relatively normal vasculature (and intact blood brain barrier) and therefore be poor or non-contrast enhancing and/or too small to cause noticeable mass effect or edema. MR provides the best chance of detecting these lesions via abnormal signal intensity caused by the infiltrate. Central nervous system (CNS) lesions that are small, poorly enhancing, or located in the brainstem region, are best seen with MR and can be missed on CT scans.

Accurate tumor margins are especially important in treatment planning for CNS lesions to spare normal surrounding tissue while treating the entire tumor volume. MR with gadolinium-based contrast enhancement of

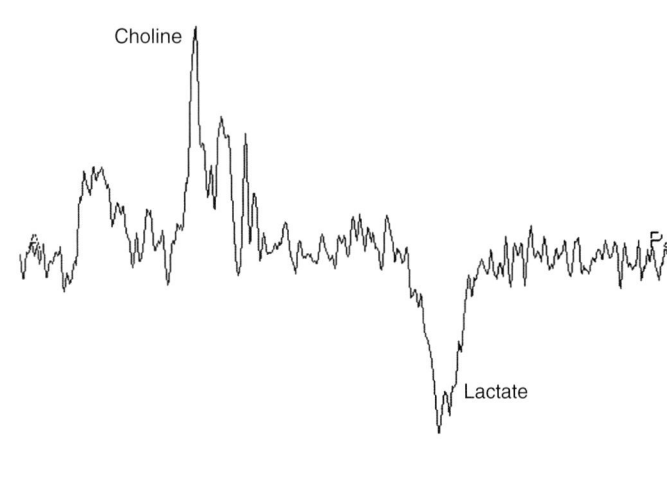

A   B

Figure 7.8. Transverse plane T2-weighted image of a dog with a nasal carcinoma invading the brain (T) (A). Part (B) shows the biochemical spectra from the tumor within the white voxel shown on the image. The spectra indicates the presence of abnormal lactate (signifying necrosis) and elevated choline (associated with increased cell membrane turnover).

human brain tumors has been reported to equal or exceed the area of enhancement of the same lesions with iodine-based contrast media from CT images, and may correspond better to tumor margins. Even so, contrast-enhanced tumor margins still underestimate the edge of more infiltrative tumor types such as human malignant gliomas. This has been demonstrated through human studies using comparative stereotactic biopsies and also by evidence from multivoxel MR spectroscopy in which cancer-like metabolic spectra have been found outside the contrast-enhancing tumor margins.

Despite MR having the best sensitivity to nervous system lesions and excellent lesion characterization, its specificity is not absolute. Non-neoplastic lesions such as abscesses and infarcts can have features similar to cancer (Figure 7.11). Biopsy of CNS lesions in veterinary patients is frequently impractical or undesirable. MR spectroscopy is improving diagnostic specificity for human brain tumors and initial investigations are underway in veterinary medicine.

Tumors of the Head

MR's multiplanar imaging is particularly advantageous when imaging the complex anatomy of the head. MR should be considered when imaging head tumors that have an extensive soft tissue component, and especially when there is concern regarding possible CNS invasion (Figure 7.12). Dural, pial, or brain parenchymal invasion can be detected using fat-suppressed postcontrast T1-weighted imaging.

MR is excellent for tumor characterization and can show the location and size of ocular lesions better than ophthalmoscopy or ultrasonography (Figure 7.13). Its advantage over CT for examining the orbit and retrobulbar space is the ability to image in an oblique plane parallel to the optic cone (Figure 7.13). In a study by Dennis (2000), MR provided more accurate diagnoses of orbital disease in 25 dogs and cats compared to radiography and ultrasound.

MR provides excellent images of the nasal passages, turbinates, and sinuses. Besides its sensitivity to cribriform plate destruction, MR allows tumor tissue to be distinguished from exudate based on differing signal intensity and exudate's lack of contrast enhancement (Figure 7.14). The combined T1 and T2 signal intensity pattern varies depending upon an exudate's degree of inspissation and protein content. T1-weighted signal intensity increases with protein content until it exceeds 28%, at which point exudate decreases in intensity. Tumors of the sinonasal region tend to be intermediate in signal in T2-weighted images with a more diffuse or solid form of enhancement, whereas sinusitis and rhinitis have higher T2 signal intensity and rim enhancement of inflamed mucosa.

MR of neoplasia involving the ear has been described in veterinary patients. Thin slice volume scans with MR are best to see the full extent of invasion of malignant cancer into the middle and inner ear, intralabyrinthine structures, cranial nerves VII and VIII, cerebellopontine angle, and brainstem nuclei due to lack of artifact in the brainstem region (Figure 7.15).

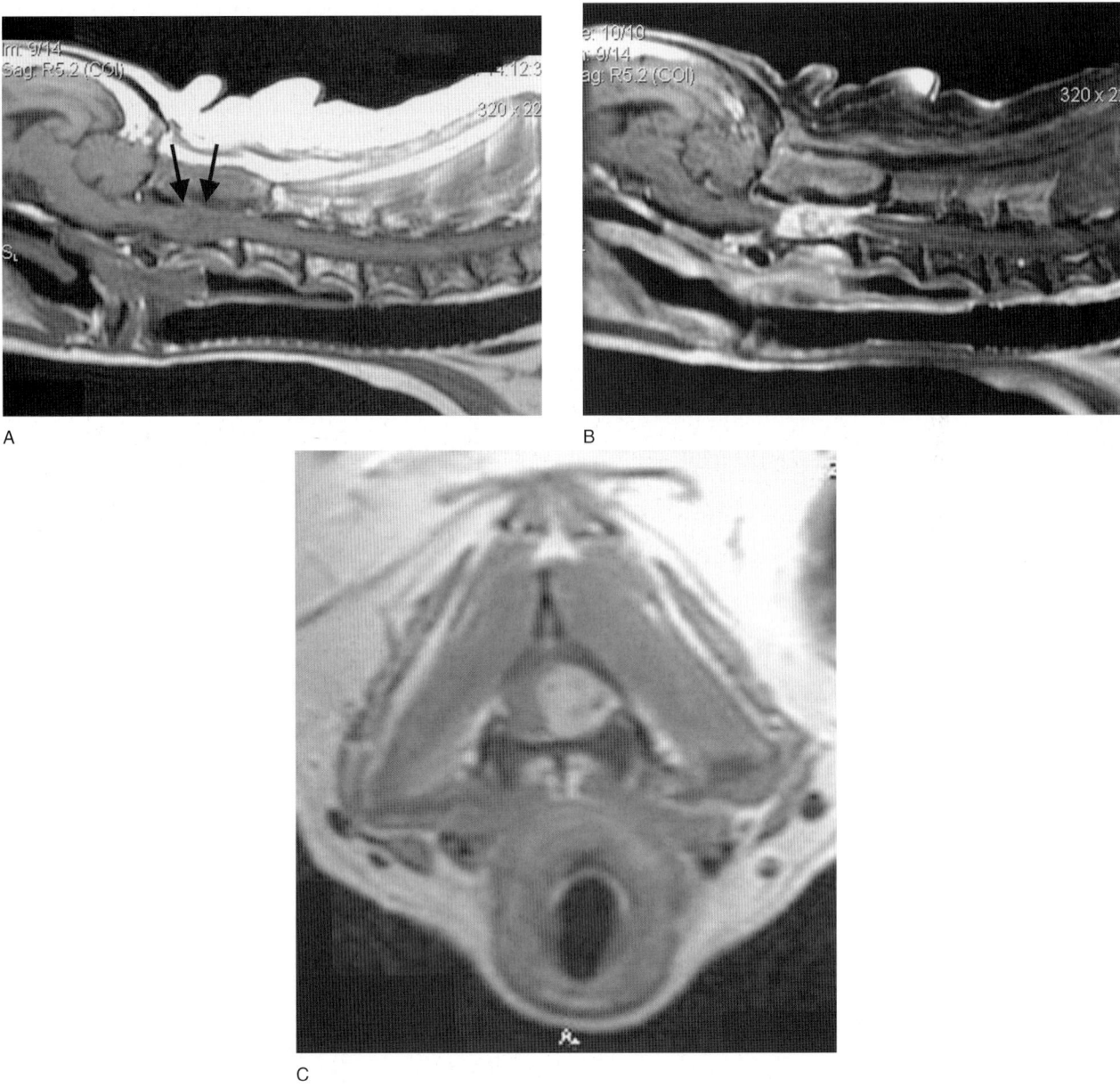

Figure 7.9. Sagittal pre- and postcontrast (parts (A) and (B), respectively) and transverse (C) postcontrast T1-weighted MR images of a dog with cervical spinal meningioma. The tumor is slightly hypointense relative to the spinal cord before contrast enhancement (black arrows in (A)) but is quite visible after contrast enhancement.

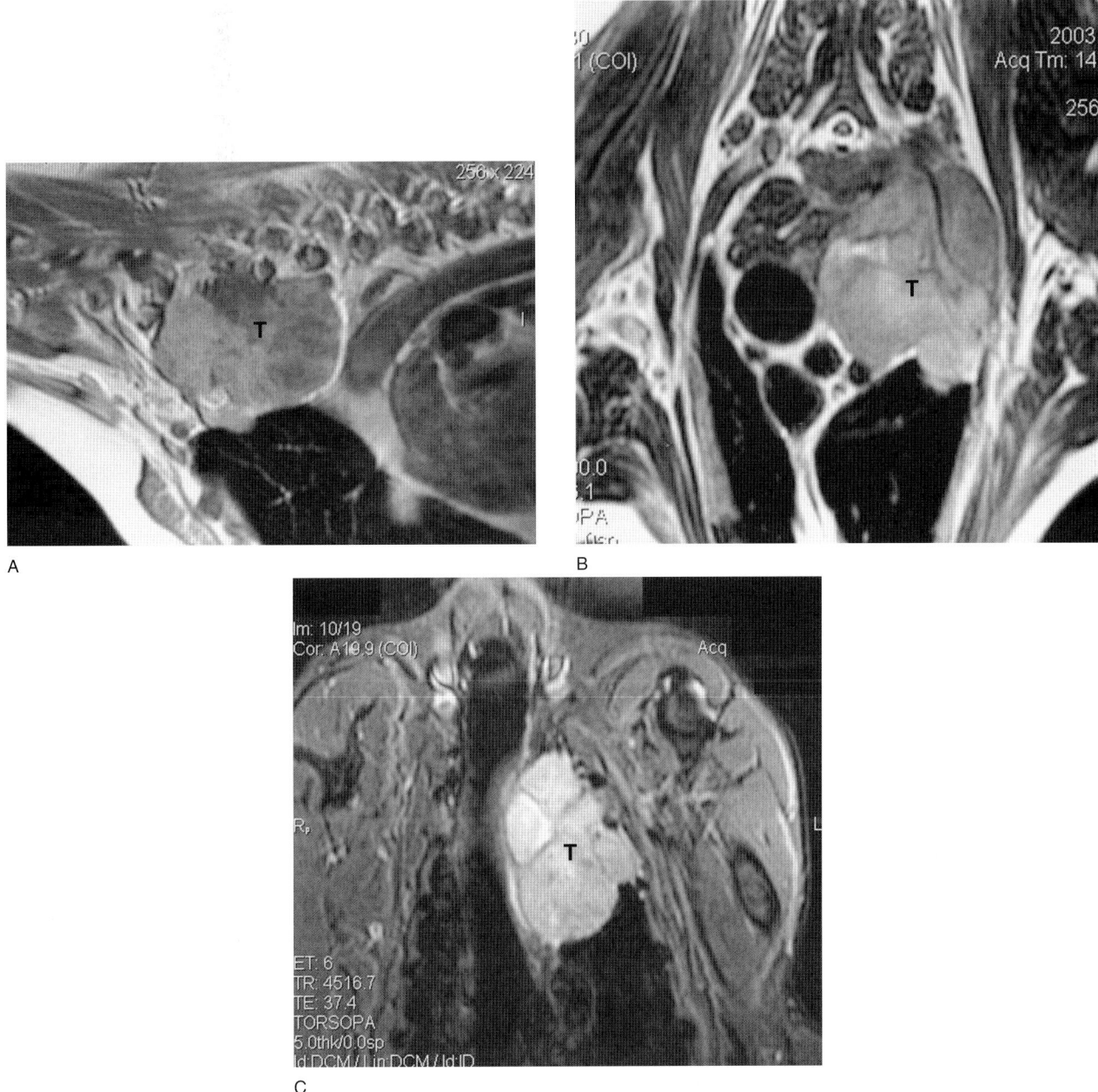

Figure 7.10.   Sagittal fat-saturated postcontrast T1-weighted (A), transverse T2-weighted (B), and dorsal STIR (C) MR images of a neurofibroma (T) extending parasagittally and ventrally from a cranial thoracic spinal nerve root. The multiplanar capabilities of MRI make it excellent for assessing full anatomic extent of peripheral nerve sheath tumors.

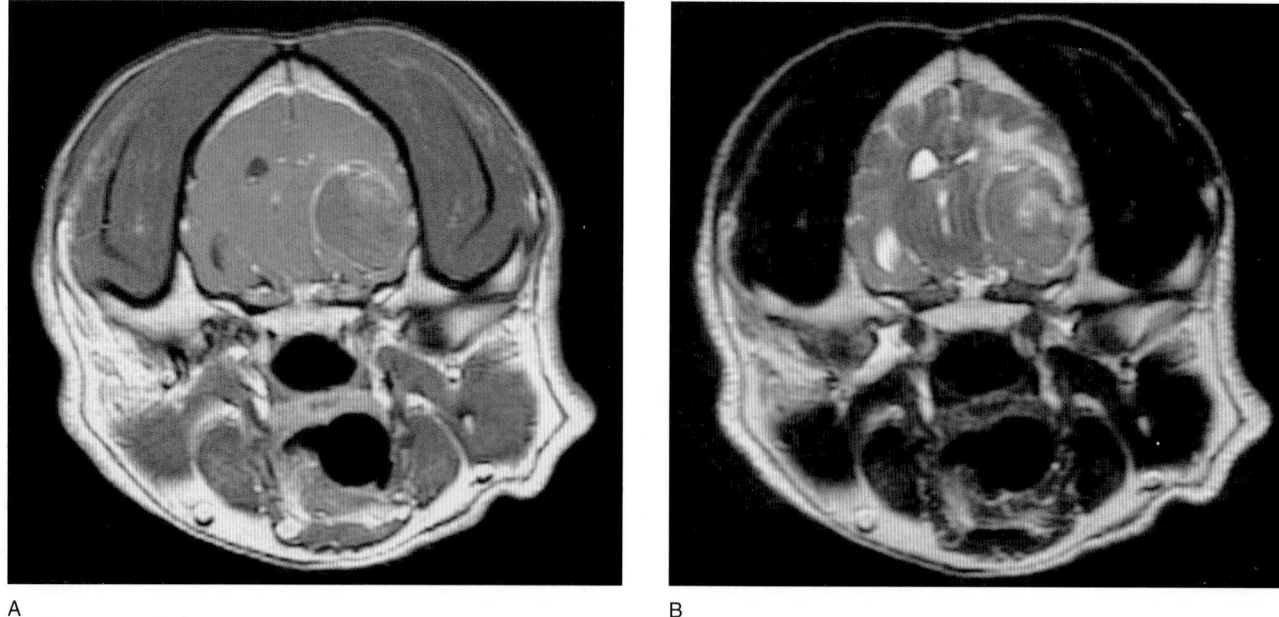

A   B

Figure 7.11.   Transverse postcontrast T1 (A) and T2 (B) MR images of a dog's ring-enhancing cerebral lesion with a mild mass effect and perilesional edema. These features are common with intra-axial brain tumors such as oligodendroglioma, however this was due to malacia and a blood clot secondary to an inflammatory vasculitis of unknown etiology.

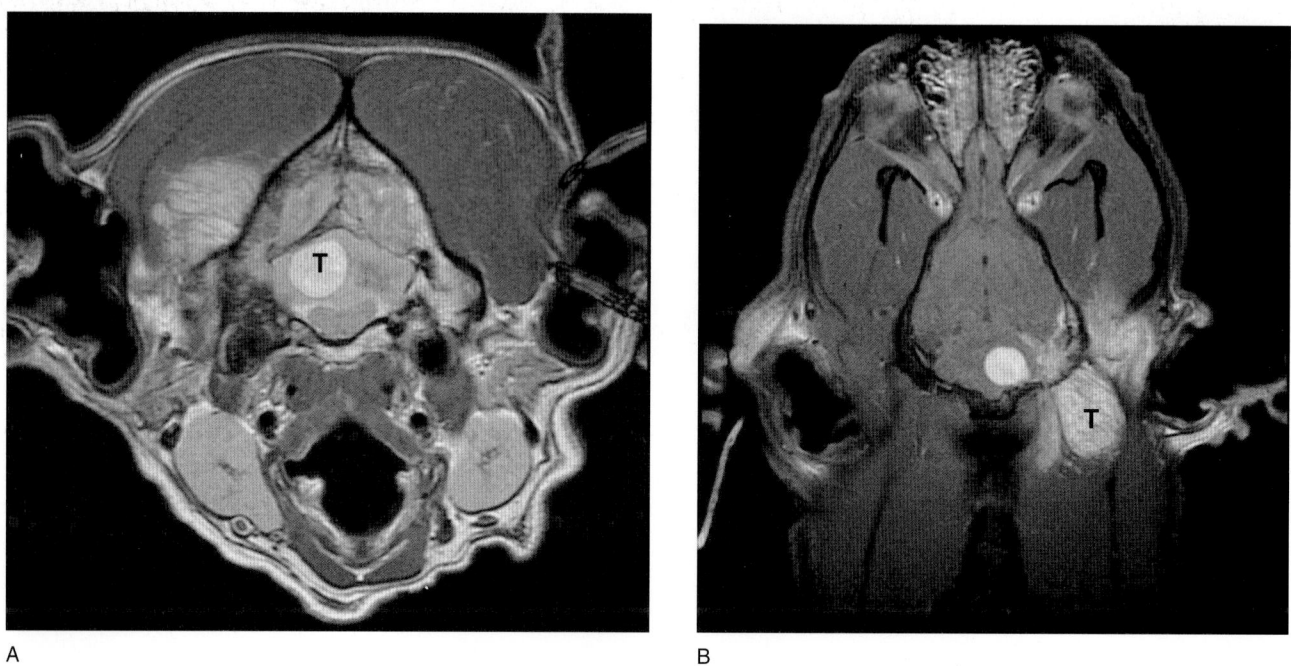

A   B

Figure 7.12.   Transverse (A) and dorsal plane (B) postcontrast T1-weighted MR images from a dog with a chondroblastic osteosarcoma that has invaded the calvaria (T). Note the hyperintensity and unsharp cortical bone margin due to osteolysis at the invasive area.

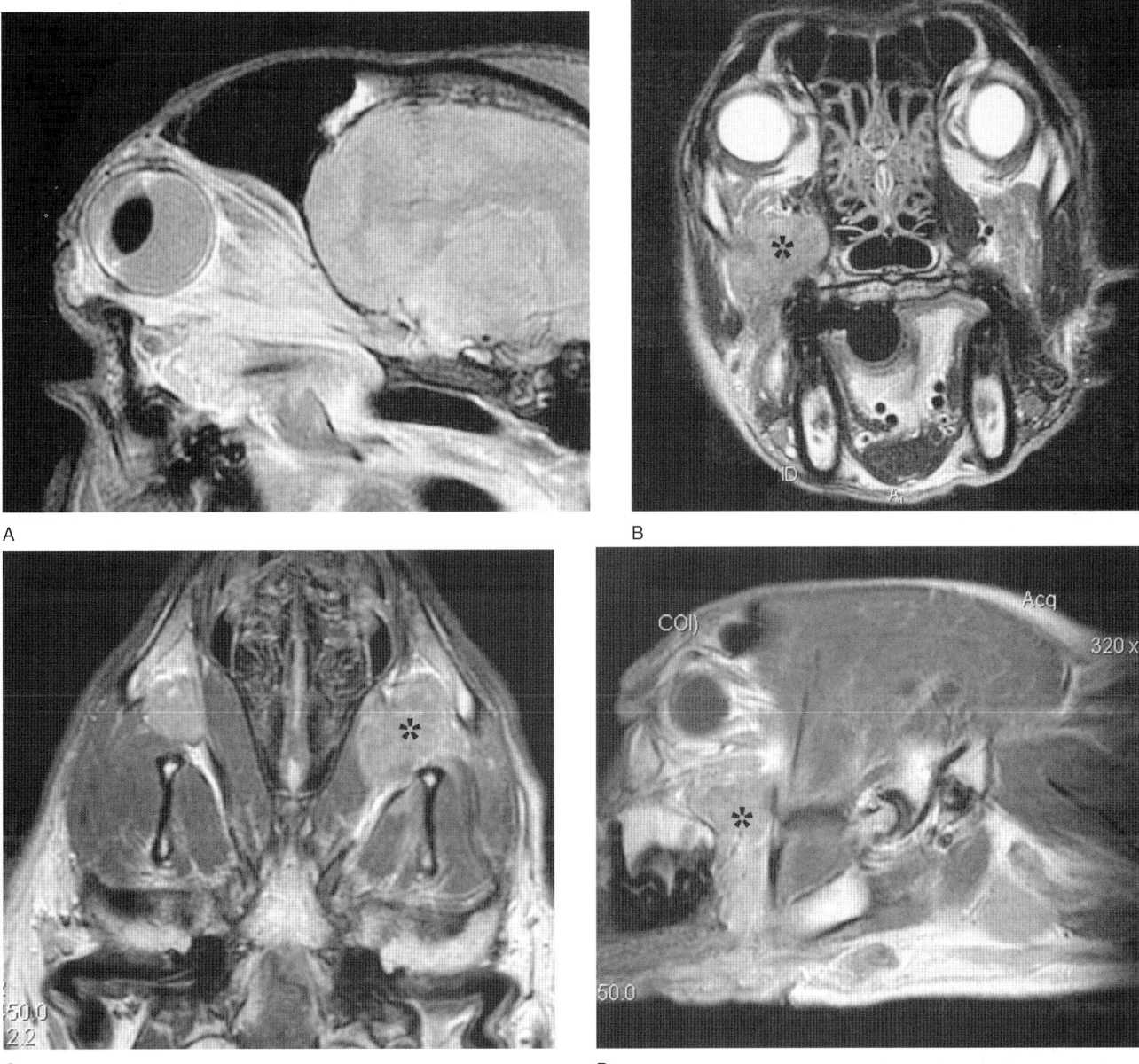

Figure 7.13. The ability to image obliquely with MRI is especially useful for ophthalmologic imaging. Part (A) is a proton density oblique plane MR image of a normal dog's optic cone. Transverse T2-weighted (B), dorsal (C), and sagittal (D) postcontrast T1-weighted images are shown of a small canine retrobulbar melanoma (*). Careful comparison with the opposite side allows its detection.

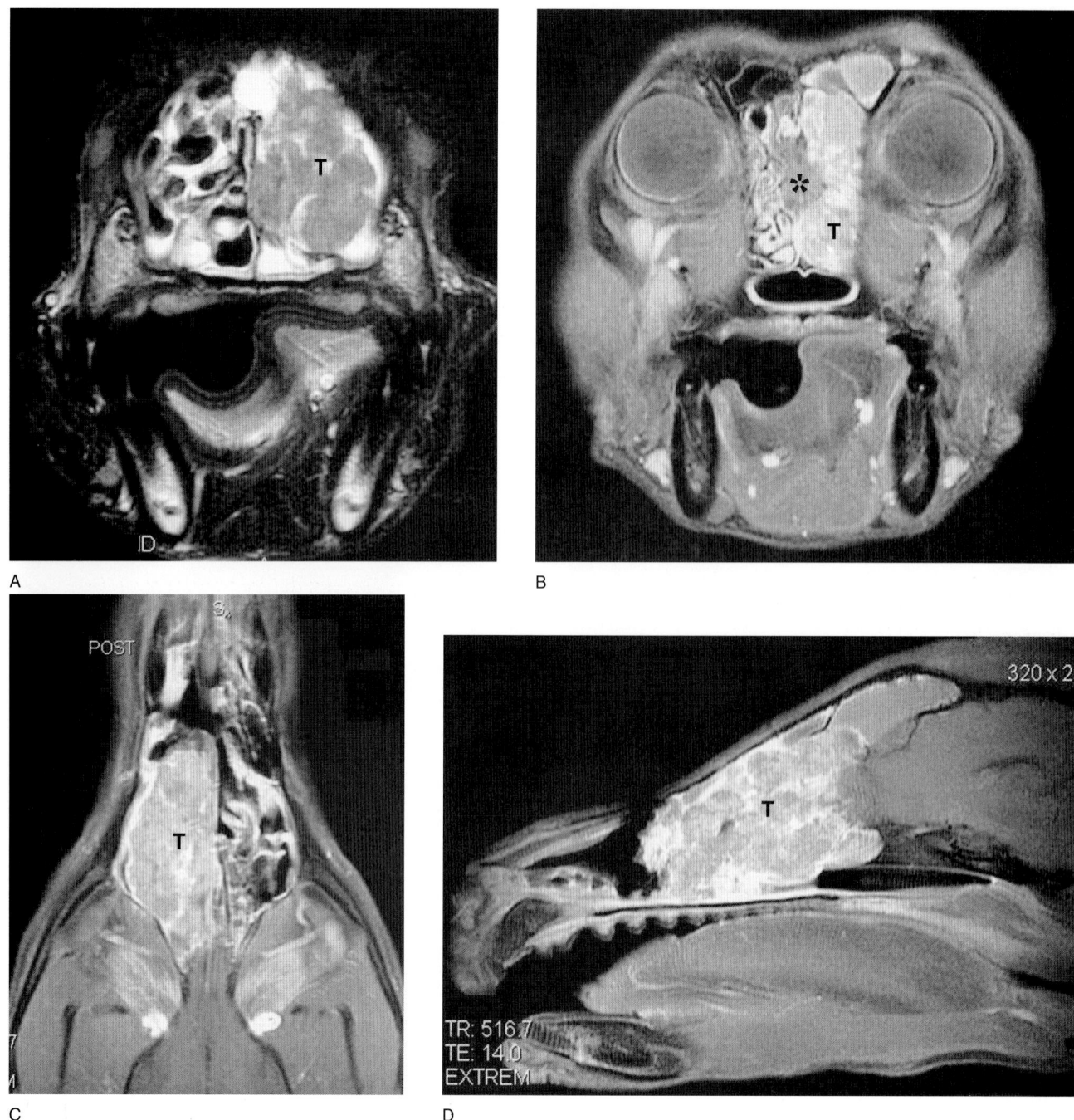

Figure 7.14. Transverse T2-weighted (A), fat-saturated transverse (B), dorsal (C), and sagittal (D) postcontrast T1-weighted MR images of a nasal adenocarcinoma (T). Note in the T2-weighted image the hyperintense exudate interspersed around the tumor. In the T1-weighted images, frontal sinus fluid is homogeneous and less intense than the enhancing tumor tissue. The * marks the olfactory lobe of the brain in (B). Early calvarial erosion is seen on these views.

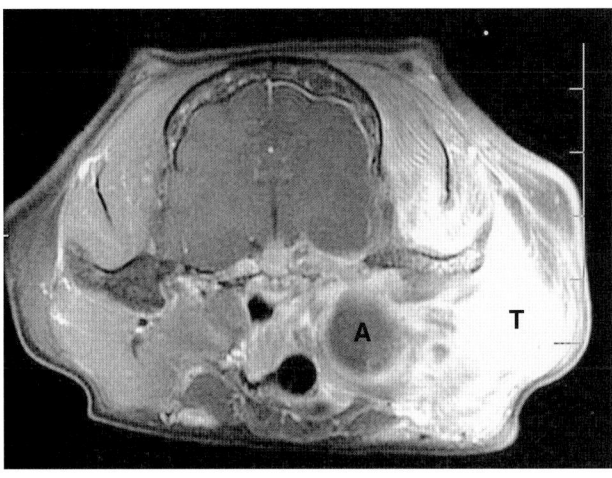
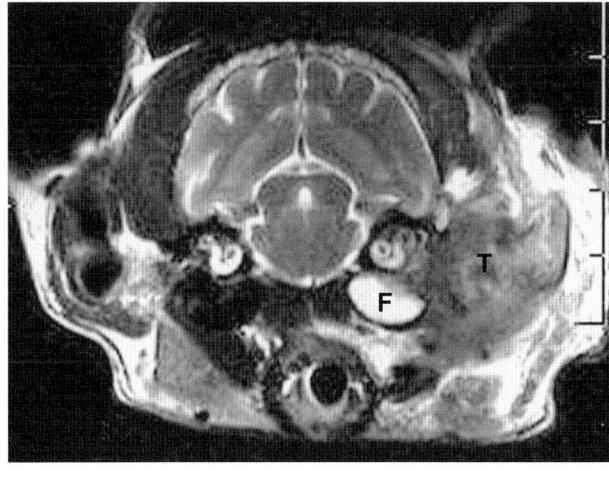

A   B

Figure 7.15. Transverse postcontrast T1-weighted (A) and T2-weighted (B) MR images of a cat with invasive squamous cell carcinoma of the ear canal that had also formed a necrotic abscess (A). Also note the contrast enhancement of the inner margin of the skull base and meninges from local invasion and inflammation. In the T2-weighted image, the middle ear contains hyperintense fluid (F).

MR of Musculoskeletal and Bone Marrow Cancers

MR is the modality of choice in human medicine for musculoskeletal cancer, because it excels at delineating tumor margins from neurovascular and skeletal structures. MR is more sensitive than CT to soft tissue tumor infiltrate within fat, muscle, tendon, bone, and allows better identification of blood vessels (Figure 7.16). For primary bone tumors, MR has been found to be better than CT and radiography for determining extraosseous and intramedullary tumor margins, joint and neurovascular involvement, and skip lesions, all of which are critical factors for limb spare surgery or curative-intent radiation therapy (Figure 7.17). Recurring tumors can be visualized in the presence of nonferrous metal orthopedic implants. Dynamic-contrast-enhanced MR of both human and canine osteosarcomas has shown promise in predicting percent tumor necrosis, an important prognostic indicator that can also be used to evaluate response to neoadjuvant chemotherapy.

As previously stated, MR's sensitivity to skeletal metastases and bone marrow infiltrate exceeds that of CT and 99m-Tc-MDP bone scintigraphy. The MR appearance of canine bone marrow changes with age and varies geographically due to the relative distribution of yellow (fatty) versus red (cellular) bone marrow. An adult dog's yellow fatty bone marrow is hyperintense relative to musculature in T1- and T2-weighted images, and hypointense in STIR or fat-suppressed T1- and T2-weighted images. Primary or metastatic lesions lead to a reversal of those signal intensities, resulting in mottled to uniformly hypointense regions in T1 images and hyperintensity in STIR images (Figure 7.17). Although the STIR pulse sequence is quite sensitive to bone marrow cancer, false positives can occur due to other pathology such as edema, inflammation, and conversion of yellow to red bone marrow during certain diseases.

Tumors of the Thorax

There is great untapped potential for MR of thoracic neoplasia in veterinary medicine. Historically, the respiratory and cardiac motion artifact and slower scan times associated with earlier MR equipment resulted in an inability to match the lung image quality that can be obtained using CT. Advances have been made in MR to reduce motion artifact and it is now considered suitable for thoracic imaging. Those advances include faster breath-hold gradient echo imaging, respiratory compensation, and respiratory and cardiac gating. Suitable spatial and contrast resolutions can now be achieved with MR to detect lung metastases. MR has been shown to detect lung nodules as small as 5 mm with similar sensitivity as CT, and lung nodules and masses are now being imaged in veterinary patients (Figures 7.18 and 7.19).

The multiplanar feature of MR allows lesions involving curved structures such as the rib cage or diaphragm to be accurately depicted, and MR is being used with increasing frequency for human tumors of the mediastinum, thoracic wall, cardiovascular structures, and diaphragm (Figures 7.20 and 7.21).

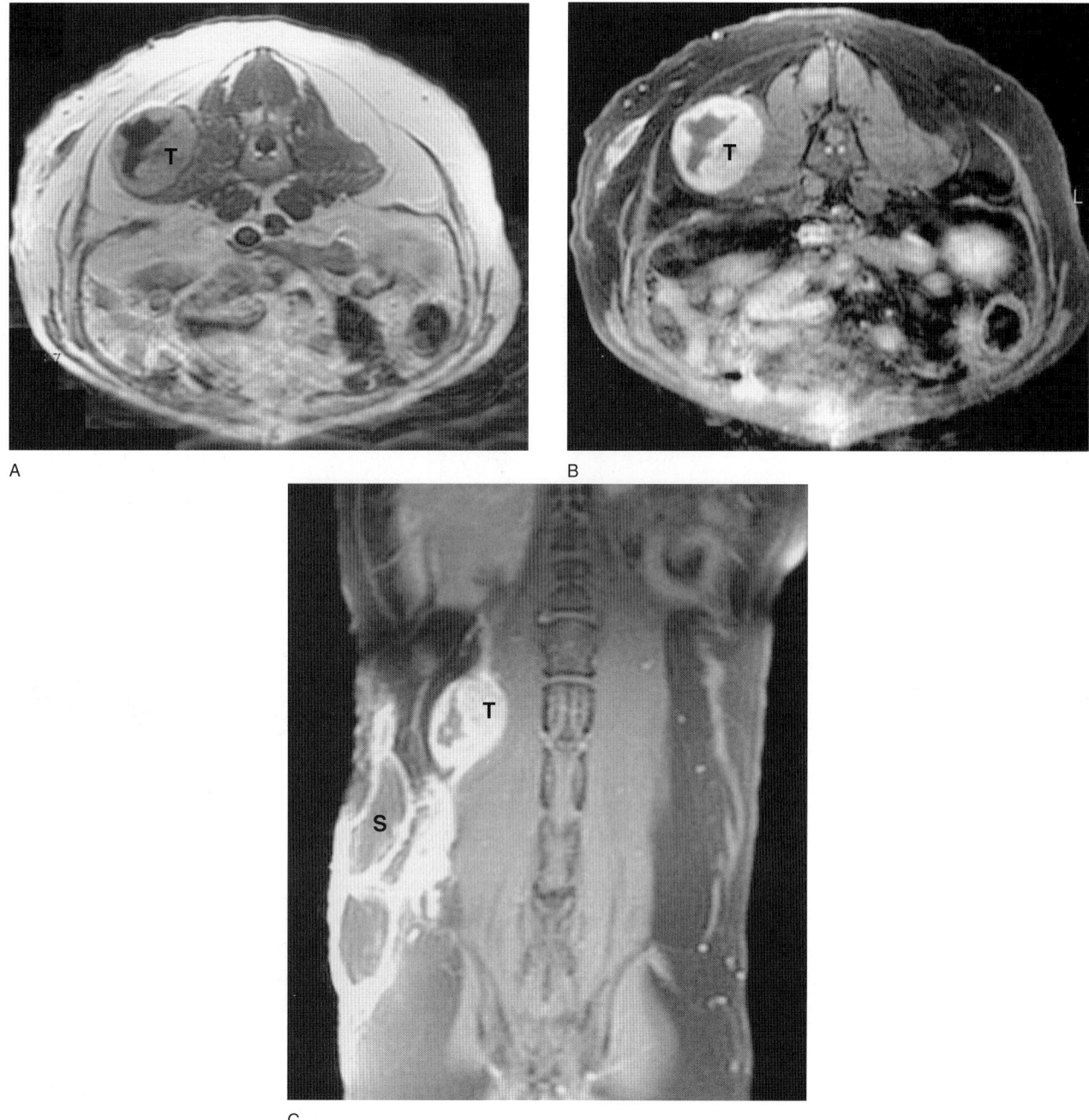

Figure 7.16. Transverse T1-weighted precontrast (A), fat-saturated postcontrast (B), and dorsal plane postcontrast (C) MR images from a dog with rapid recurrence of a hemangiosarcoma metastasis (T) in the muscle along the flank. The muscular tumor was incompletely excised 1 week ago, along with a splenectomy for the primary hemangiosarcoma. The metastasis has a nonenhancing necrotic center, and there is a seroma (S) along the flank whose margins blend with the contrast-enhancing tumor.

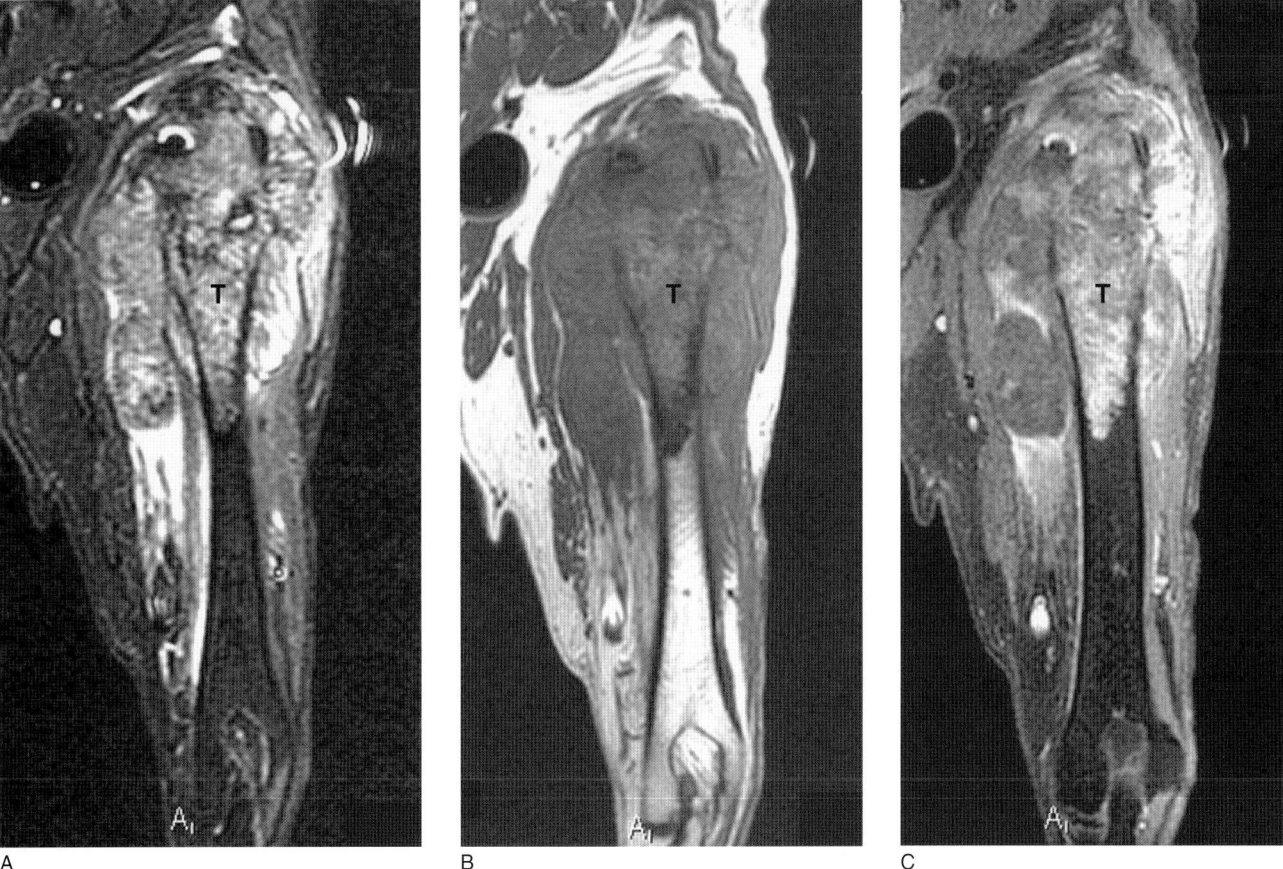

Figure 7.17.   Coronal STIR (A), T1-weighted precontrast (B), and postcontrast fat-saturated (C) MR images of a proximal humeral osteosarcoma (T) in a dog. The intramedullary margin is well defined, but there is an extensive extramedullary component with tissue reaction extending to the vasculature medial to the distal humerus.

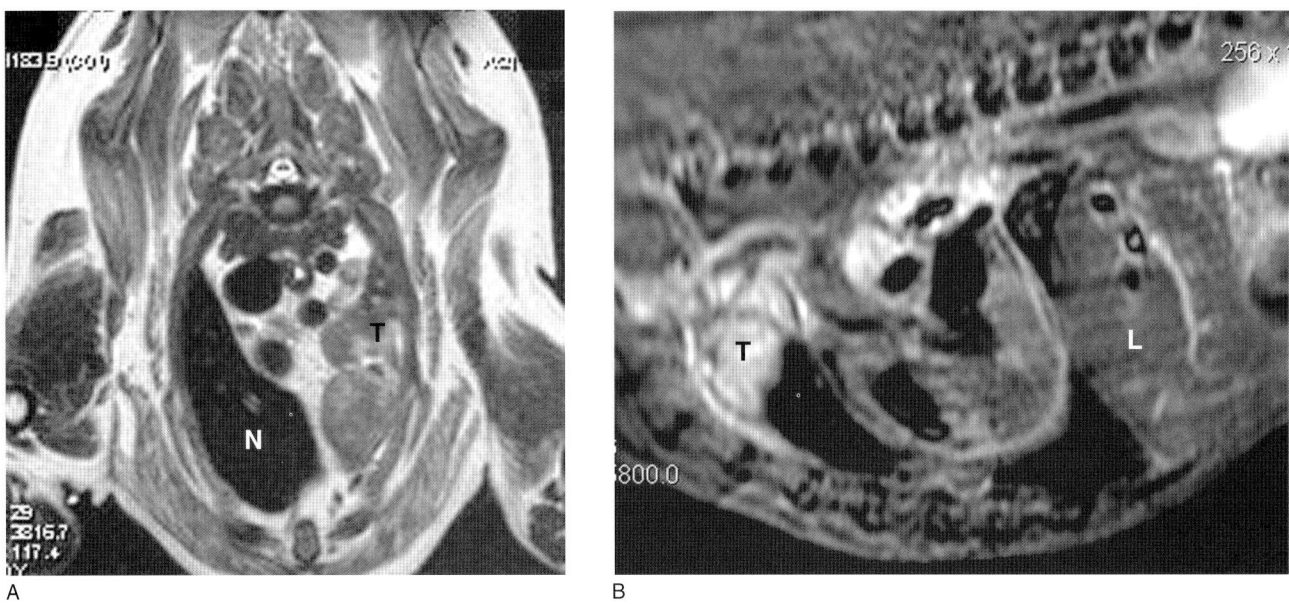

Figure 7.18.   Transverse T2-weighted (A) and sagittal STIR (B) MR images of a dog with a primary lung tumor (presumably, based on signalment, history, and radiographic appearance) in the cranial lung lobe (T). The normal contralateral lung lobe is hypointense (N). Normal liver (L) is seen caudal to the heart and diaphragm on sagittal view.

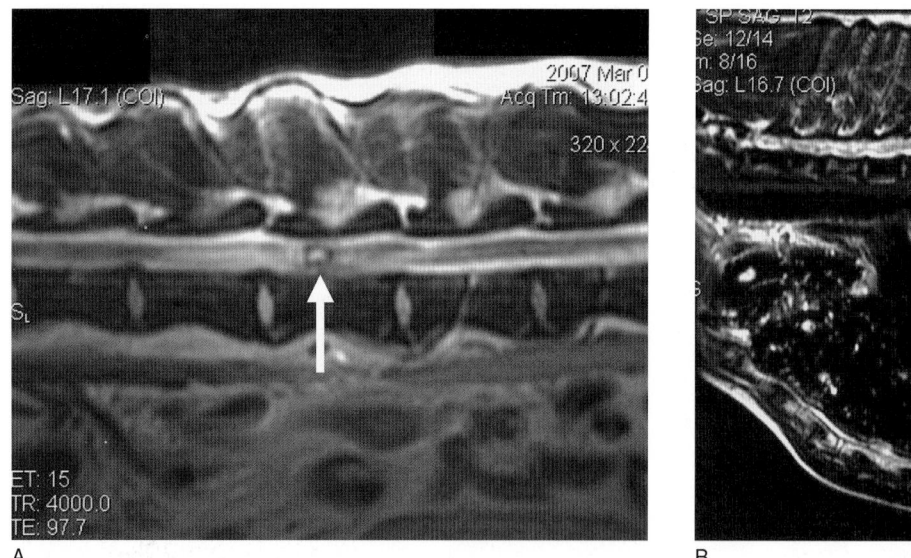
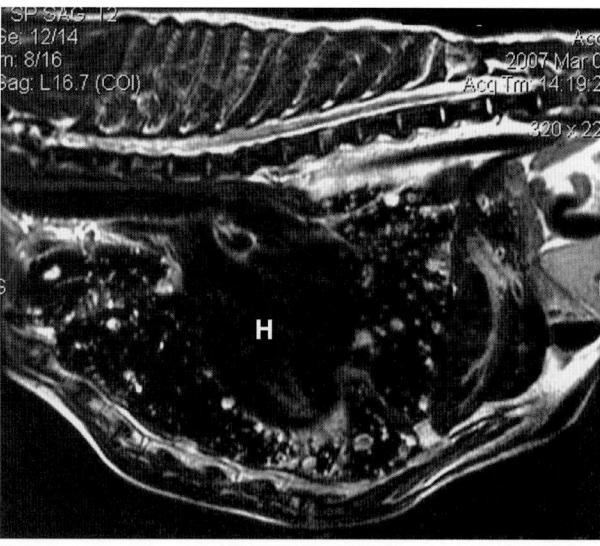

A   B

Figure 7.19.   Transverse T2-weighted MR image of a metastatic hemangiosarcoma (white arrow) in a dog that presented for upper motor neuron signs to the hind limbs (A). Numerous hyperintense variably sized metastases are apparent in the lungs on the sagittal STIR MR image of this dog's thorax surrounding the heart (H) (B).

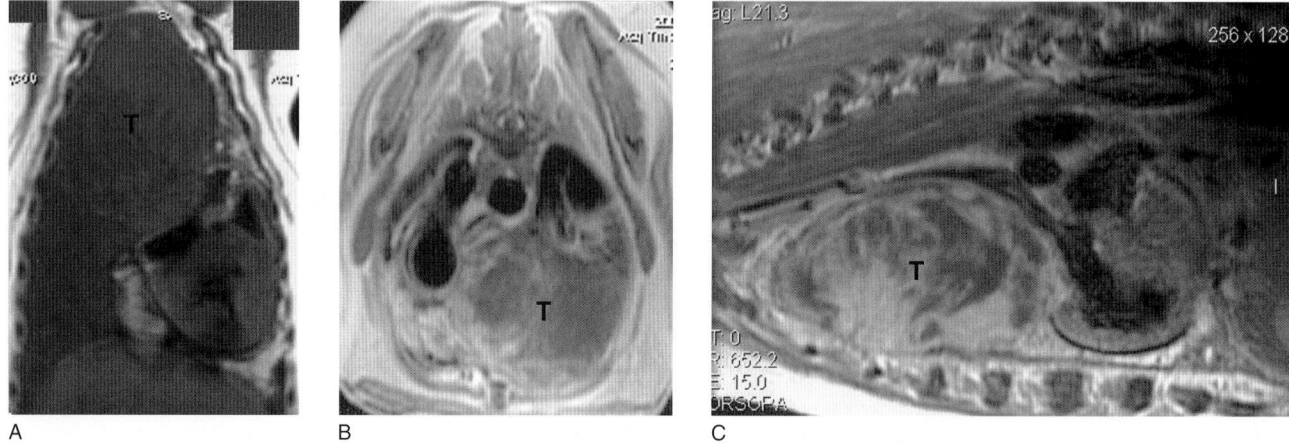

A   B   C

Figure 7.20.   Dorsal plane precontrast T1-weighted (A), transverse (B), and sagittal (C) postcontrast T1-weighted MR images of a large mediastinal liposarcoma (T) in a dog's thorax. Note the marked cardiac displacement.

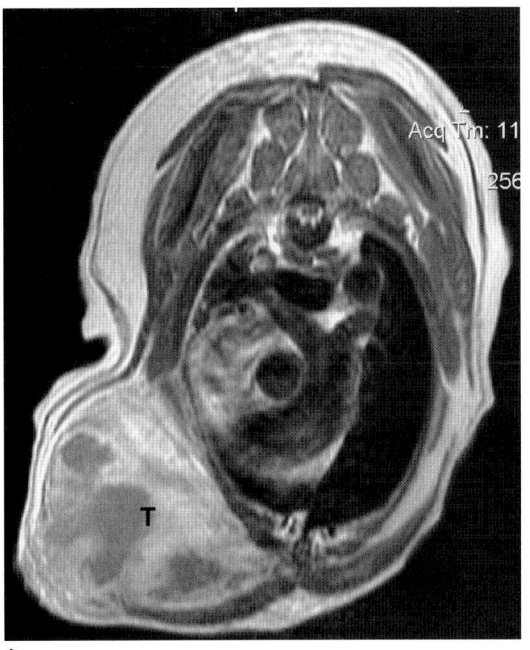
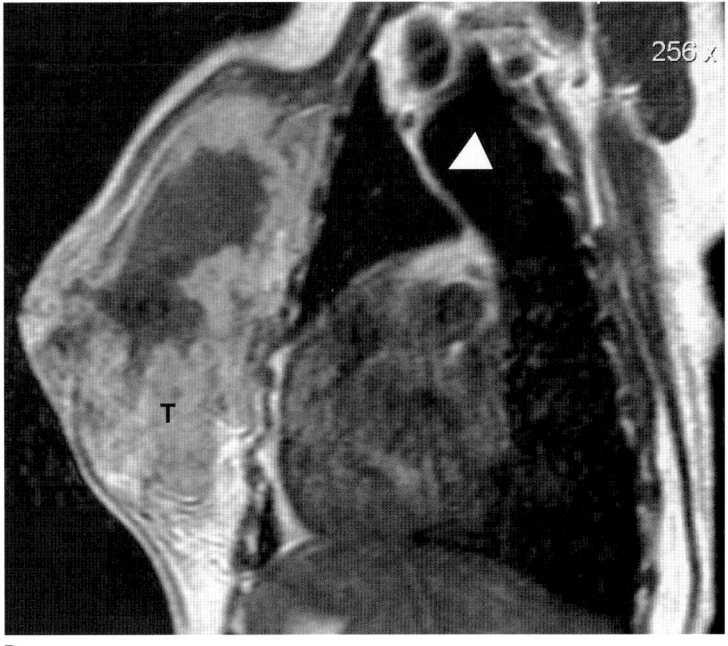

A   B

Figure 7.21. Transverse (A) and dorsal plane (B) postcontrast T1-weighted MR images from a dog with a myxosarcoma of the chest wall (T). The hypointense lungs are separated by the cranioventral mediastinal reflection (white arrowhead in (B)).

Tumors of the Abdomen and Pelvis

Very few reports are available on abdominal MR in veterinary patients, largely due to the widespread availability and relative low cost of radiographs and diagnostic ultrasound but there are many promising applications (Figures 7.22–7.25). Faster MR scan techniques minimize artifacts from bowel motion, and multiple applications are being evaluated for human abdominal cancer imaging. Those will guide future developments in veterinary medicine; one advantage is that the needed general anesthesia in animals reduces bowel motion.

MR is considered the best and first choice for human hepatic imaging, but more commonly a screening CT precedes a more focused MR exam of the abdomen. Multiphase contrast-enhanced MR is highly sensitive and specific for detecting human hepatocellular carcinoma (and also for abdominal metastatic disease) compared to contrast-enhanced CT. Human liver nodules seen on ultrasound imaging that cannot be found on MR are classified as pseudolesions and not even biopsied. Similarly, a prospective MR study by Clifford et al. (2004) of 23 dogs resulted in a 90% specificity in differentiating 35 benign hyperplastic nodules from malignant nodules of the liver or spleen, indicating a potential for noninvasive diagnostic specificity compared to ultrasound imaging (Figures 7.23 and 7.24). Detection of early or small malignant nodules of the spleen can be more challenging due to similarities in signal intensity between normal spleen and tumors.

MR's gastrointestinal applications have been slower to develop due to lack of an effective intraluminal contrast media and efficacy of existing techniques. Its use for human GI cancers is increasing, however, in conjunction with gadolinium IV contrast and faster scan techniques. MR is now a recognized methodology for human preoperative distant staging of gastrointestinal cancers and detecting intestinal wall infiltrate. In a veterinary case report by Yasuda et al. (2004), MRI's usefulness in distinguishing mesenteric lymphoma from adjacent adhesions and bowel has been demonstrated.

CONCLUSION

MR's advantages are well accepted in veterinary medicine for examining neoplasia of the brain, spinal cord and spine, cranial and peripheral nerves, and for other structures of the head. The veterinary use of MR for cancer of the musculoskeletal system, thorax, and abdomen is undergoing active evolution. Exciting new promising applications of MR for cancer are in transition from a research to a clinical veterinary setting, including whole body MR, physiological, and metabolic imaging.

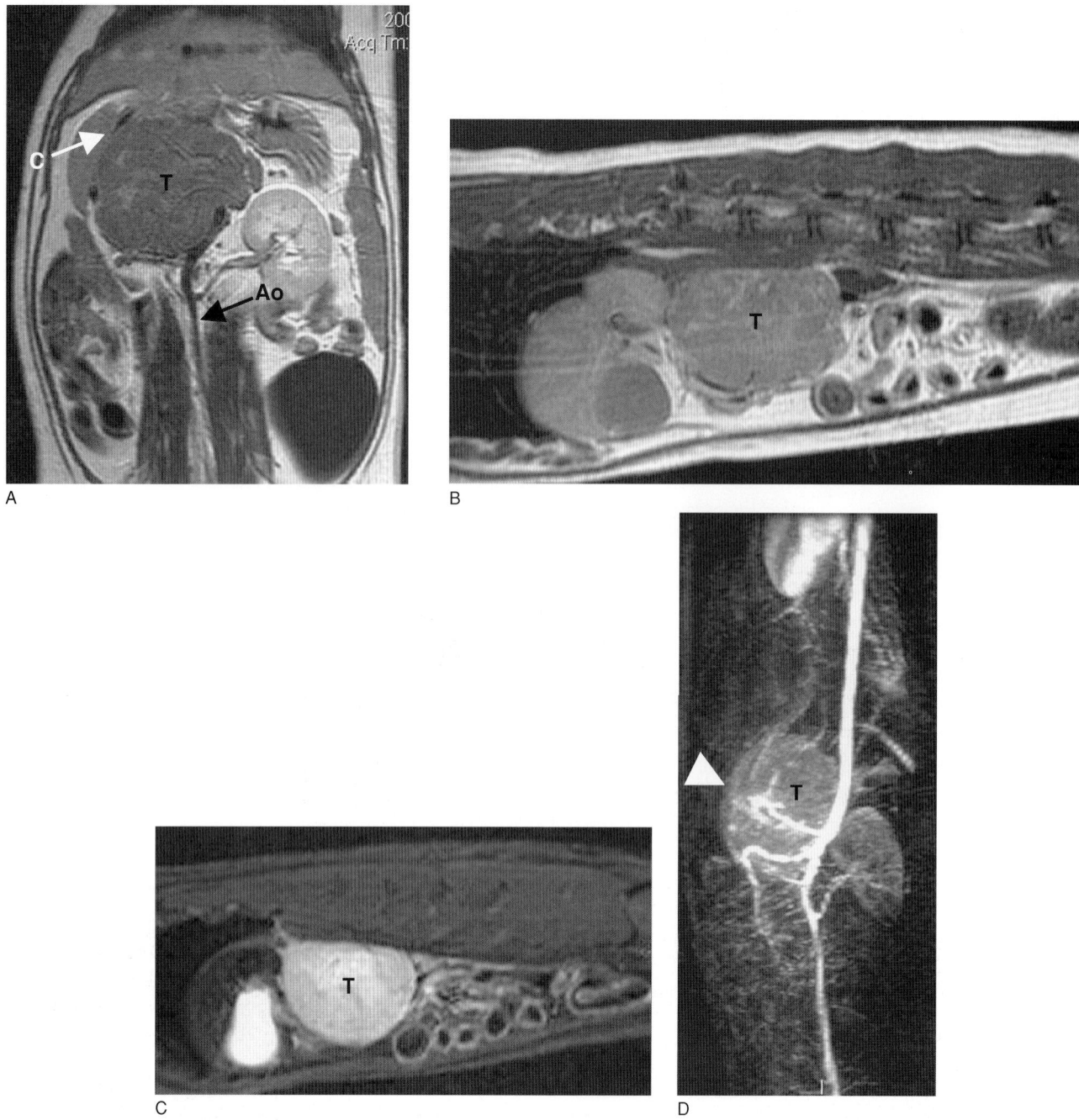

Figure 7.22. MRI is well suited for imaging invasive abdominal masses and the adjacent vasculature. Dorsal plane (A) and sagittal (B) precontrast T1-weighted MR images and sagittal STIR (C) MR images are shown of a large feline adrenal adenoma. The mass was compressing and displacing the caudal vena cava rightward (indicated by the "C" and white arrow in (A)) and the aorta leftward ("Ao" and black arrow in (A)). An MR angiogram shows the tumor vasculature branching from the aorta cranial to the right renal artery (white arrowhead in (D)).

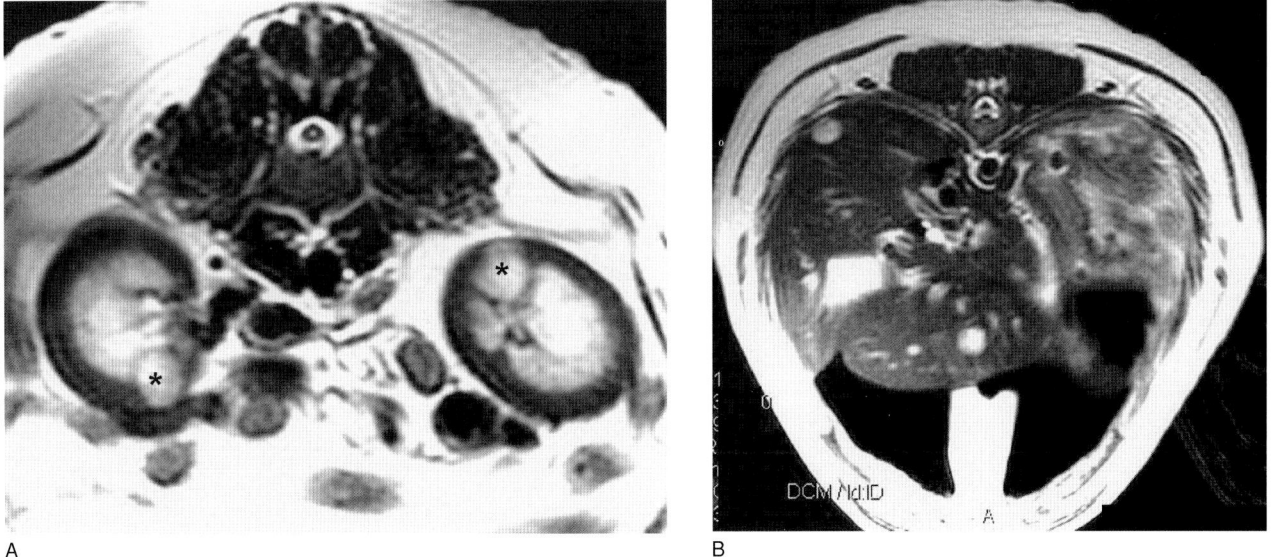

Figure 7.23. Transverse T2-weighted MR images of hemangiosarcoma metastases in both kidney cortices (* in (A)) and in the liver (hyperintense nodules in (B)) in the same dog shown in Figure 7.19.

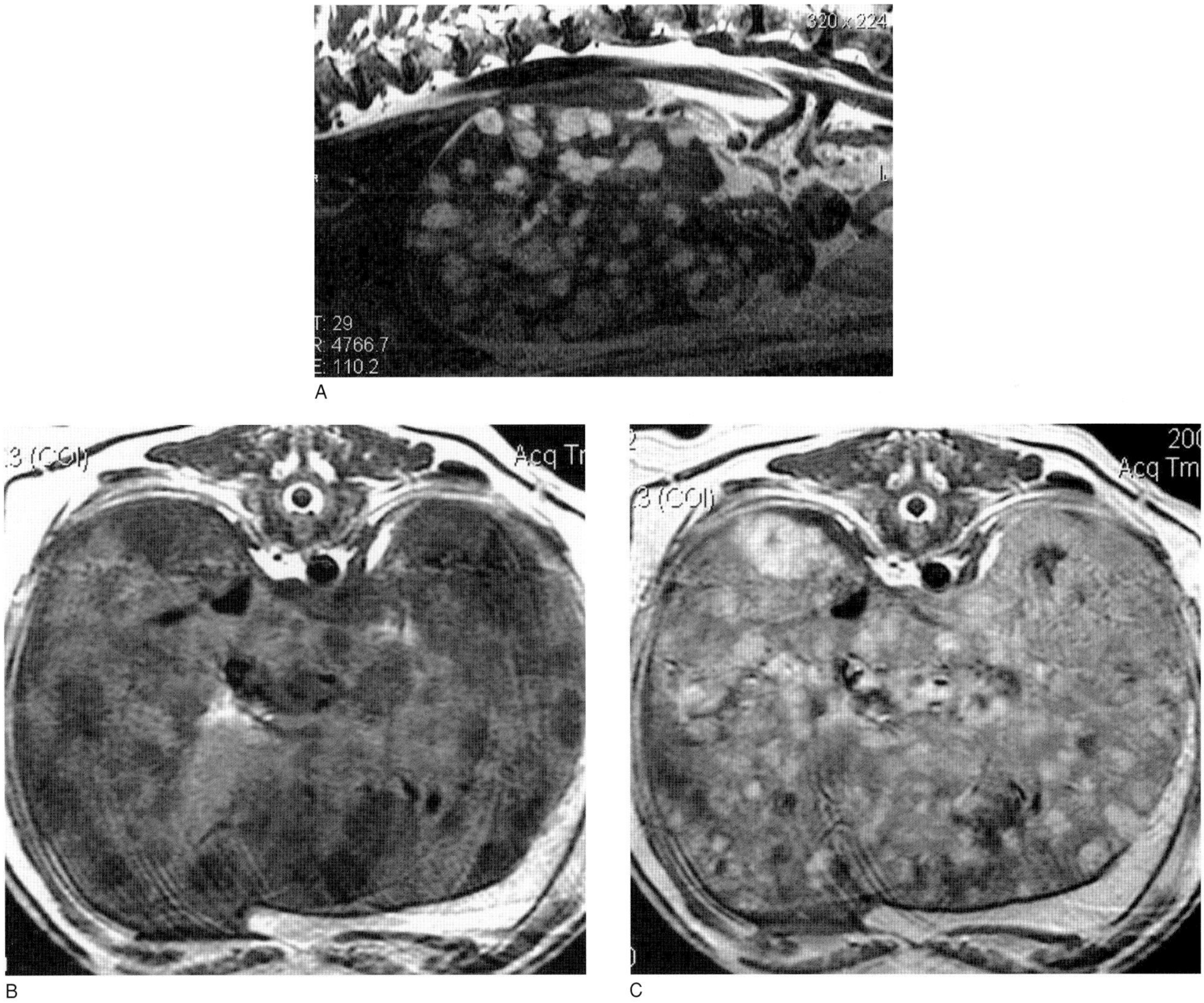

A

B

C

Figure 7.24. Sagittal T2-weighted (A), transverse pre- (B), and postcontrast T1-weighted MR images (C) of the liver from a dog that presented for an MRI of the lumbar spine. Although the cause of the neurological deficits were not identified on the MRI, numerous liver nodules were found and liver enzymes and clotting times were elevated. Neoplasia was the presumed diagnosis but histological verification could not be obtained.

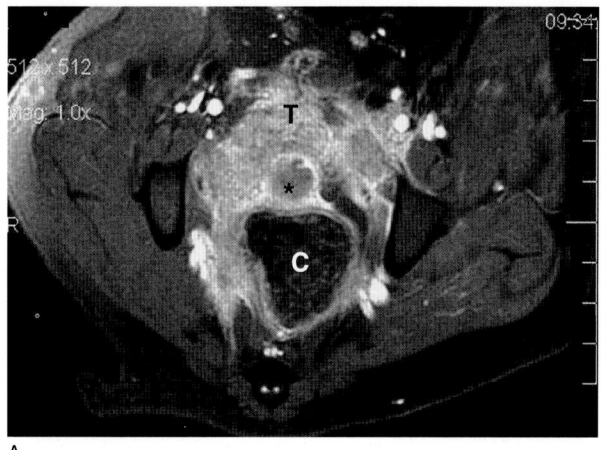
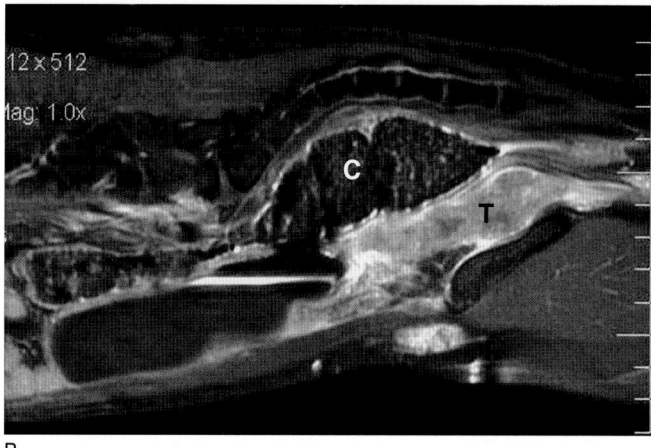

A   B

Figure 7.25. Transverse (A) and sagittal (B) fat-saturated postcontrast T1-weighted MR images from a dog with a transitional cell carcinoma (T) of the urethra. The urethra is marked with a * in (A) and the colon with a white "C" on both views.

ACKNOWLEDGMENTS

Special thanks to Ms. Betsy Sestina, Billie Arceneaux, and Melinda Wilhelm for their excellent technical assistance, and to my neurology, oncology and pathology colleagues of Colorado State University's Veterinary Medical Center for their many contributions.

BIBLIOGRAPHY

Armbrust LJ, Hoskinson JJ, Biller DS, and Wilkerson M. 2004. Low-field magnetic resonance imaging of bone marrow in the lumbar spine, pelvis, and femur in the adult dog. Vet Radiol Ultrasound 45:393–401.

Bagley RS, Wheeler SJ, Klopp L, Sorjonen DC, Thomas WB, Wilkens BE, et al. 1998. Clinical features of trigeminal nerve-sheath tumor in 10 dogs. J Am Anim Hosp Assoc 34:19–25.

Balaban RS and Hampshire VA. 2001. Challenges in small animal noninvasive imaging. Ilar J 42:248–262.

Barentsz J, Takahashi S, Oyen W, Mus R, De Mulder P, Reznek R, et al. 2006. Commonly used imaging techniques for diagnosis and staging. J Clin Oncol 24:3234–3244.

Calvo BF and Semelka RC. 1999. Beyond anatomy: MR imaging as a molecular diagnostic tool. Surg Oncol Clin N Am 8:171–183.

Chenevert TL, Meyer CR, Moffat BA, Rehemtulla A, Mukherji SK, Gebarski SS, et al. 2002. Diffusion MR: a new strategy for assessment of cancer therapeutic efficacy. Mol Imaging 1:336–343.

Chin T, Chang S, and Dillion W. 2002. Brain and spinal cord tumors. In: David PR, Bragg G, and Hricak H (eds), Oncologic Imaging, WB Saunders, Philadelphia, pp. 133–159.

Chong V, Fan Y, Mukerji SK. 2002. Malignancies of the nasopharynx and skull base. In: David PR, Bragg G, and Hricak H (eds), Oncologic Imaging, WB Saunders, Philadelphia, pp. 182–201.

Choyke PL, Dwyer AJ, and Knopp MV. 2003. Functional tumor imaging with dynamic contrast-enhanced magnetic resonance imaging. J Magn Reson Imaging 17:509–520.

Clifford CA, Pretorius ES, Weisse C, Sorenmo KU, Drobatz KJ, Siegelman ES, et al. 2004. Magnetic resonance imaging of focal splenic and hepatic lesions in the dog. J Vet Intern Med 18:330–338.

Daniel GB and Mitchell S. 1999. The eye and orbit. Clin Tech Small Anim Pract 14:160–169.

Davis GJ, Kapatkin AS, Craig LE, Heins GS, and Wortman JA. 2002. Comparison of radiography, computed tomography, and magnetic resonance imaging for evaluation of appendicular osteosarcoma in dogs. J Am Vet Med Assoc 220:1171–1176.

Dennis R. 2000. Use of magnetic resonance imaging for the investigation of orbital disease in small animals. J Small Anim Pract 41:145–155.

Duesberg CA, Feldman EC, Nelson RW, Bertoy EH, Dublin AB, and Reid MH. 1995. Magnetic resonance imaging for diagnosis of pituitary macrotumors in dogs. J Am Vet Med Assoc 206:657–662.

Dyke J, Panicek D, Healey J, Meyers P, Huvos A, Schwartz L, et al. 2003. Osteogenic and ewing sarcomas: estimation of necrotic fraction during induction chemotherapy with dynamic contrast-enhanced MR imaging. Radiology 228:271–278.

Eustace SJ, Walker R, Blake M, and Yucel EK. 1999. Whole-body MR imaging. Practical issues, clinical applications, and future directions. Magn Reson Imaging Clin N Am 7:209–236.

Follen M, Levenback CF, Iyer RB, Grigsby PW, Boss EA, Delpassand ES, et al. 2003. Imaging in cervical cancer. Cancer 98:2028–2038.

Forrest L. 1999. The head: excluding the brain and orbit. Clin Tech Small Anim Pract 14:170–176.

Friedman WA and Foote KD. 2003. Linear accelerator-based radiosurgery for vestibular schwannoma. Neurosurg Focus 14 (5):1–8.

Garosi LS, Dennis R, Penderis J, Lamb CR, Targett MP, Cappello R, et al. 2001. Results of magnetic resonance imaging in dogs with vestibular disorders: 85 cases (1996–1999). J Am Vet Med Assoc 218:385–391.

Garosi LS, Dennis R, and Schwarz T. 2003. Review of diagnostic imaging of ear diseases in the dog and cat. Vet Radiol Ultrasound 44:137–146.

Ghanem N, Uhl M, Brink I, Schafer O, Kelly T, Moser E, et al. 2005. Diagnostic value of MR in comparison to scintigraphy, PET, MS-CT and PET/CT for the detection of metastases of bone. Eur J Radiol 55:41–55.

Gore R and Yaghmai V. 2002. Esophageal cancer. In: David PR, Bragg G, and Hricak H (eds), Oncologic Imaging, WB Saunders, Philadelphia, pp. 359–390.

Hathcock JT. 1995. Low field magnetic resonance imaging characteristics of cranial vault meningiomas in 13 dogs. Vet Radiol Ultrasound 37:257–263.

Hosten N, Wust P, Beier J, Lemke AJ, and Felix R. 1998. MR-assisted specification/localization of target volumes. Aspects of quality control. Strahlenther Onkol 174(Suppl 2):13–18.

Kafka UC, Carstens A, Steenkamp G, and Symington H. 2004. Diagnostic value of magnetic resonance imaging and computed tomography for oral masses in dogs. J S Afr Vet Assoc 75:163–168.

Kalmar JA, Eick JJ, Merritt CR, Shuler SE, Miller KD, McFarland GB, et al. 1988. A review of applications of MR in soft tissue and bone tumors. Orthopedics 11:417–425.

Kato K, Nishimura R, Sasaki N, Matsunaga S, Mochizuki M, Nakayama H, et al. 2005. Magnetic resonance imaging of a canine eye with melanoma. J Vet Med Sci 67:179–182.

Kippenes H, Gavin PR, Bagley RS, Silver GM, Tucker RL, and Sande RD. 1999. Magnetic resonance imaging features of tumors of the spine and spinal cord in dogs. Vet Radiol Ultrasound 40:627–633.

Kippenes H, Gavin PR, Sande RD, Rogers D, and Sweet V. 2003. Accuracy of positioning the cervical spine for radiation therapy and the relationship to GTV, CTV and PTV. Vet Radiol Ultrasound 44:714–719.

Kneissl S, Probst A, and Konar M. 2004. Low-field magnetic resonance imaging of the canine middle and inner ear. Vet Radiol Ultrasound 45:520–522.

Kraft SL. 2007. Magnetic resonance imaging characteristics of peripheral nerve sheath tumors of the canine brachial plexus in 18 dogs. Vet Radiol Ultrasound 48:1–7.

Kraft S, Ashton E, Ehrhart E, Sestina L, Arceneaux B, Thamm D, et al. 2007. Estimation of % tumor necrosis by 3D compartmental analysis of dynamic contrast-enhanced MR in spontaneous canine osteosarcomas, in Proceedings of the International Society of Magnetic Resonance in Medicine, Berlin Germany, p. 564

Kraft SL and Gavin PR. 1999. Intracranial neoplasia. Clin Tech Small Anim Pract 14:112–123.

Kraft SL, Gavin PR, DeHaan C, Moore M, Wendling LR, and Leathers CW. 1997. Retrospective review of 50 canine intracranial tumors evaluated by magnetic resonance imaging. J Vet Intern Med 11:218–225.

Kraft SL, Trncic N, and LaRue S. 2006. MR and CT of dynamic contrast enhancement decreased after single dose irradiation of canine tumors. In Proceedings of the American College of Veterinary Radiology. Vet Radiol Ultrasound 47:118.

Lappas J and Maglinte D. 2002. Gastrointestinal malignancies. In: David PR, Bragg G, and Hricak H (eds), Oncologic Imaging, WB Saunders, Philadelphia, pp. 419–433.

Lipsitz D, Higgins RJ, Kortz GD, Dickinson PJ, Bollen AW, Naydan DK, et al. 2003. Glioblastoma multiforme: clinical findings, magnetic resonance imaging, and pathology in five dogs. Vet Pathol 40:659–669.

Loevner LA. 2002. Paranasal sinus neoplasms. In: David PR, Bragg G, and Hricak H (eds), Oncologic Imaging, WB Saunders, Philadelphia, pp. 160–181.

Lyons J, Thrall DE, and Pruitt AF. 2007. Comparison of isodose distributions in canine brain in the heterogeneity corrected versus uncorrected treatment plans usig 6 Mv photons. Vet Radiol Ultrasound 48:292–296.

Mah D, Steckner M, Palacio E, Mitra R, Richardson T, and Hanks GE. 2002. Characteristics and quality assurance of a dedicated open 0.23 T MR for radiation therapy simulation. Med Phys 29:2541–2547.

McConnell JF, Platt SR, Penderis J, Abramson C, and Dennis R. 2006. Use of MR spectroscopy in the investigation of canine brain disease. In Proceedings of European Association of Veterinary Diagnostic Imaging. Vet Radiol Ultrasound 47:421.

Mellanby RJ, Jeffery ND, Baines EA, Woodger N, and Herrtage ME. 2003. Magnetic resonance imaging in the diagnosis of lymphoma involving the brachial plexus in a cat. Vet Radiol Ultrasound 44:522–525.

Mentzel HJ, Kentouche K, Sauner D, Fleischmann C, Vogt S, Gottschild D, et al. 2004. Comparison of whole-body STIR-MR and 99mTc-methylene-diphosphonate scintigraphy in children with suspected multifocal bone lesions. Eur Radiol 14:2297–2302.

Miwa Y, Matsunaga S, Kato K, Ogawa H, Nakayama H, Tsujimoto S, et al. 2005. Choroidal melanoma in a dog. J Vet Med Sci 67:821–823.

Muleya JS, Taura Y, Nakaichi M, Nakama S, and Takeuchi A. 1997. Appearance of canine abdominal tumors with magnetic resonance imaging using a low field permanent magnet. Vet Radiol Ultrasound 38:444–447.

Munden R and Bragg D. 2002. Primary malignancies of the thorax. In: David PR, Bragg G, and Hricak H (eds), Oncologic Imaging, WB Saunders, Philadelphia, pp. 313–341.

Platt SR, Graham J, Chrisman CL, Collins K, Chandra S, Sirninger J, et al. 1999. Magnetic resonance imaging and ultrasonography in the diagnosis of a malignant peripheral nerve sheath tumor in a dog. Vet Radiol Ultrasound 40:367–371.

Randall EK, Lana S, Avery A, Olver C, and Kraft S. 2005. Whole-body MR: a prospective comparison to routine diagnostic evaluation in staging lymphoma in dogs. In

Proceedings of the American College of Veterinary Radiology. Vet Radiol Ultrasound 47:115.

Ross BD, Moffat BA, Lawrence TS, Mukherji SK, Gebarski SS, Quint DJ, et al. 2003. Evaluation of cancer therapy using diffusion magnetic resonance imaging. Mol Cancer Ther 2:581–587.

Rubin P, Brasacchio R, and Katz A. 2006. Solitary metastases: illusion versus reality. Semin Radiat Oncol 16:120–130.

Schmidt T, Reinshagen M, Brambs HJ, Adler G, Rieber A, Tirplitz CV, et al. 2003. Comparison of conventional enteroclysis, intestinal ultrasound and MR-enteroclysis for determining changes in the small intestine and complications in patients with Crohn's disease. Z Gastroenterol 41:641–648.

Sherar M. 2005. Imaging in oncology. In: Tannock IF, Hill RP, Bristow RG, and Harrington L (eds), The Basic Science of Oncology, McGraw Hill, New York, pp. 249–260.

Sheu M, Chang C, Wang J, and Yen M. 2001. MR staging of clinical stage I and IIa cervical carcinoma: a reappraisal of efficacy and pitfalls. Eur J Radiol 38:225–231.

Sostman HD, Prescott DM, Dewhirst MW, Dodge RK, Thrall DE, Page RL, et al. 1994. MR imaging and spectroscopy for prognostic evaluation in soft-tissue sarcomas. Radiology 190:260–275.

Stockberger S and Maglinte D. 2002. Colorectal cancer. In: David PR, Bragg G, and Hricak H (eds), Oncologic Imaging, WB Saunders, Philadelphia, pp. 434–477.

Takagi S, Tsunoda S, and Tanaka O. 1998. Bone marrow involvement in lymphoma: the importance of marrow magnetic resonance imaging. Leuk Lymphoma 29:515–522.

Tanimoto A, Yuasa Y, Imai Y, Izutsu M, Hiramatsu K, Tachibana M, et al. 1992. Bladder tumor staging: comparison of conventional and gadolinium-enhanced dynamic MR imaging and CT. Radiology 185:741–747.

Thomas WB. 1996. Magnetic resonance imaging features of primary brain tumors in dogs. Vet Radiol Ultrasound 37:20–27.

Troxel MT, Vite CH, Massicotte C, McLear RC, Van Winkle TJ, Glass EN, et al. 2004. Magnetic resonance imaging features of feline intracranial neoplasia: retrospective analysis of 46 cats. J Vet Intern Med 18:176–189.

Tsunoda S, Takagi S, Tanaka O, and Miura Y. 1997. Clinical and prognostic significance of femoral marrow magnetic resonance imaging in patients with malignant lymphoma. Blood 89:286–290.

Tucker DW, Olsen D, Kraft SL, Andrews GA, and Gray AP. 2000. Primary hemangiosarcoma of the iliopsoas muscle eliciting a peripheral neuropathy. J Am Anim Hosp Assoc 36:163–167.

Turrel JM, Fike J, and LeCouteur RA. 1986. Computed tomographic characteristics of primary brain tumors in 50 dogs. J Am Vet Assoc 188:851–856.

Wallack ST, Wisner ER, Werner JA, Walsh PJ, Kent MS, Fairley RA, et al. 2002. Accuracy of magnetic resonance imaging for estimating intramedullary osteosarcoma extent in preoperative planning of canine limb-salvage procedures. Vet Radiol Ultrasound 43:432–441.

Wisner E and Pollard R. 2004. Trends in veterinary cancer imaging. Vet Comp Oncol 2:49–74.

Yamaguchi H, Minami A, Kaneda K, Isu K, and Yamawaki S. 1992. Comparison of magnetic resonance imaging and computed tomography in the local assessment of osteosarcoma. Int Orthop 16:285–290.

Yasuda D, Fujita M, Yasuda S, Taniguchi A, Miura H, Hasegawa D, et al. 2004. Usefulness of MR compared with CT for diagnosis of mesenteric lymphoma in a dog. J Vet Med Sci 66:1447–1451.

Yin FF, Das S, Kirkpatrick J, Oldham M, Wang Z, and Zhou SM. 2006. Physics and imaging for targeting of oligometastases. Semin Radiat Oncol 16:85–101.

INDEX